The Handbook of Mental Health Communication

Handbooks in Communication and Media

This series aims to provide theoretically ambitious yet accessible volumes devoted to the major fields and subfields within communication and media studies. Each volume sets out to ground and orientate the student through a broad range of specially commissioned chapters, while also providing the more experienced scholar and teacher with a convenient and comprehensive overview of the latest trends and critical directions.

The Handbook of Rhetoric and Public Address, *edited by Shawn J. Parry-Giles and J. Michael Hogan*
The Handbook of Global Communication and Media Ethics, *edited by Robert S. Fortner and P. Mark Fackler*
The Handbook of Communication and Corporate Social Responsibility, *edited by Øyvind Ihlen, Jennifer Bartlett, and Steve May*
The Handbook of Gender, Sex, and Media, *edited by Karen Ross*
The Handbook of Global Health Communication, *edited by Rafael Obregon and Silvio Waisbord*
The Handbook of Global Media Research, *edited by Ingrid Volkmer*
The Handbook of Global Online Journalism, *edited by Eugenia Siapera and Andreas Veglis*
The Handbook of Communication and Corporate Reputation, *edited by Craig E. Carroll*
The Handbook of Media and Mass Communication Theory, *edited by Robert S. Fortner and P. Mark Fackler*
The Handbook of International Advertising Research, *edited by Hong Cheng*
The Handbook of Psychology of Communication Technology, *edited by S. Shyam Sundar*
The Handbook of Magazine Studies, *edited by Miglena Sternadori and Tim Holmes*
The Handbook of European Communication History, *edited by Klaus Arnold, Paschal Preston, and Susanne Kinnebrock*
The Handbook of Public Sector Communication, *edited by Vilma Luoma-aho and María José Canel*
The Handbook of Applied Communication Research, 2 Volume Set, *edited by H. Dan O'Hair and Mary John O'Hair*
The Handbook of Listening, *edited by Debra L. Worthington and Graham D. Bodie*
The Handbook of Communication Rights, Law, and Ethics, *edited by Loreto Corredoira, Ignacio Bel Mallen, and Rodrigo Cetina Preusel*
The Handbook of Strategic Communication, *edited by Carl H. Botan*
The Handbook of Peer Production, *edited by Mathieu O'Neil, Christian Pentzold, and Sophie Toupin*
The Handbook of Crisis Communication, second edition, *edited by W. Timothy Coombs and Sherry J. Holladay*
The Handbook of Critical Intercultural Communication, second edition, *edited by Thomas K. Nakayama and Rona Tamiko Halualani*
The Handbook of Social and Political Conflict, *edited by Sergei A. Samoilenko and Solon Simmons*

The Handbook of Mental Health Communication

Edited by

Marco C. Yzer and Jason T. Siegel

WILEY Blackwell

Published by John Wiley & Sons, Inc., Hoboken, New Jersey.
Published simultaneously in Canada.

Library of Congress Cataloging-in-Publication Data Applied for:

Hardback ISBN: 9781394179862; epdf: 9781394179886; epub: 9781394179893

Cover Design: Wiley
Cover Image: © wildpixel/Getty Images

Set in 9.5/12pt ITC Galliard Std by Straive, Pondicherry, India

Contents

List of Contributors

Elayne Ahern
University of Limerick
Ireland

Dolores Albarracín
University of Pennsylvania
United States

Jennifer Alvidrez
National Institutes of Health
United States

John Anagnost
University of California Los Angeles
United States

Seth Asafo
University of Ghana Medical School
Ghana

Dzifa Attah
University of Ghana Medical School
Ghana

Rachel Banawa
University of California Los Angeles
United States

Crystal L. Barksdale
National Institutes of Health
United States

Dror Ben-Zeev
University of Washington
United States

Tibor Bosse
Radboud University
The Netherlands

Rachel E. Brenner
Twilio
United States

Gert-Jan de Bruijn
University of Antwerp
Belgium

Sarah Caban
University of Illinois Urbana-Champaign
United States

Minhey Chung
University of Illinois Urbana-Champaign
United States

Patrick Corrigan
Illinois Institute of Technology
United States

William D. Crano
Claremont Graduate University
United States

Wenhao Dai
Lawrence University
United States

Jolynn Childers Dellinger
Duke University
United States

David J. A. Dozois
Western University
United States

Valerie A. Earnshaw
University of Delaware
United States

Daniel Eisenberg
University of California Los Angeles
United States

Jonas Everaert
Tilburg University
The Netherlands

Christopher M. Falco
Claremont Graduate University
United States

Annie B. Fox
MGH Institute of Health Professions
United States

Maria Ftanou
University of Melbourne
Australia

Frances J. Griffith
Yale University
United States

Gregory Guldner
HCA Healthcare
United States

Patrick J. Heath
Gustavus Adolphus College
United States

Fakhra Jabeen
Radboud University
The Netherlands

Ashley Johnston
University of California Los Angeles
United States

Anthony F. Jorm
University of Melbourne
Australia

Ava Kikut-Stein
Harvard University
Dana-Farber Cancer Institute
United States

Rudy Sunrin Kim
University of Maryland
United States

Stefanie Kirchner
Medical University of Vienna
Austria

Lola Kola
King's College London
United Kingdom

BRiTE Center
University of Washington
United States

Daniel G. Lannin
Illinois State University
United States

Nancy Lau
University of Washington School of Medicine
United States

Seattle Children's Research Institute
United States

Collene Lawhorn
National Institutes of Health
United States

Monica Luciana
University of Minnesota
United States

Haijing Ma
University of Houston-Victoria
United States

Laura Marciano
Harvard University
Dana-Farber Cancer Institute
United States

Sabrina Menezes
Claremont Graduate University
United States

Supriya Misra
San Francisco State University
United States

Mohammad Mousavi
University of Delaware
United States

Gabriela C. M. Murphy
Western University
United States

Tara Muschetto
Claremont Graduate University
United States

Xiaoli Nan
University of Maryland
United States

Angela Nicholas
University of Melbourne
Australia

Thomas Niederkrotenthaler
Medical University of Vienna
Austria

Seth M. Noar
University of North Carolina at Chapel Hill
United States

Ruth A. Osoro
Pennsylvania State University
United States

Caroline Ostrand
University of Minnesota
United States

Jane Pirkis
University of Melbourne
Australia

Brian Quick
University of Illinois Urbana-Champaign
United States

Xueli Qiu
University of Delaware
United States

Jenna Reno
RTI International
United States

Jacob A. Rohde
RTI International
United States

Benjamin D. Rosenberg
Dominican University of California
United States

Romy RW
Loyola Marymount University
United States

Kat Schwartz
National Institutes of Health
United States

Jason T. Siegel
Claremont Graduate University
United States

Sydney C. Simmons
Yale University
United States

Tom Smeets
Tilburg University
The Netherlands

Rachel A. Smith
Pennsylvania State University
United States

Brian Southwell
RTI International
United States

Tasha Straszewski
Claremont Graduate University
United States

Cara N. Tan
Claremont Graduate University
United States

Teresa L. Thompson
University of Dayton and University of Kansas-Edwards
United States

Benedikt Till
Medical University of Vienna
Austria

Nataliya Turchmanovych-Hienkel
Illinois Institute of Technology
United States

Miranda Twiss
Illinois Institute of Technology
United States

K. Viswanath
Harvard University
Dana-Farber Cancer Institute
United States

David L. Vogel
Iowa State University
United States

Lisa M. W. Vos
Tilburg University
The Netherlands

René Weber
University of California Santa Barbara
United States

Kevin Wombacher
University of Illinois
United States

Kylie Woodman
University of California Santa Barbara
United States

Xingman Wu
University of Maryland
United States

Jia Yan
University of Illinois Urbana-Champaign
United States

Fei Ying
Western University
United States

Marco C. Yzer
University of Minnesota
United States

Nan Zhao
Iowa State University
United States

Xin Zhao
University of Washington School of Medicine
United States

Seattle Children's Research Institute
United States

Xuan Zhu
Mayo Clinic
United States

Xun Zhu
University of Kentucky
United States

Preface

In a 2023 opinion piece in *Time* magazine, Gabriel Boric (who at the time of writing is the President of the Republic of Chile) and Dr. Tedros Adhanom Ghebreyesus (who at the time of writing is Director-General of the World Health Organization) argued that mental health is a fundamental human right. Boric and Adhanom Ghebreyesus stressed that the extensive detrimental effects of mental illness and poor mental well-being on individual, public, and societal health call for a large-scale, multisectoral response from a wide array of stakeholders. There are essentially two parts to such a response. One focuses on the structural environment of mental health and mental illness and includes efforts by various stakeholders, who separately or in collaboration, improve structural conditions of people's lives, invest in mental health care capacity, and strengthen access to mental health care. The other focuses on how people think, feel, and act regarding mental health and mental illness and includes the promotion of mental health in whole populations as well as in specific priority groups such as people who currently have severe mental illness.

Purposefully planned mass communication messages are a potentially useful tool to promote mental health. Indeed, there is a long history of the use of mass media messages to promote mental health. This does not mean, however, that message-based mass communication interventions have proven to be generally effective. There are many reasons why mental health mass communication interventions may not work; for example, such interventions compete with many other media messages for an audience's attention in an increasingly cluttered media environment, there may not be sufficient funding available to ensure prolonged exposure, and social norms around mental health may not be conducive to favorable responses in some cases. Perhaps even more important, however, is the lack of an established knowledge base; the scientific domain of mental health mass communication remains in its infancy.

To enhance knowledge of how mental health mass communication can effectively be used as a tool for mental health promotion, scientific knowledge of how to create effective mental health messaging must be shared across domains. There already exists excellent work from researchers across the communication discipline who have investigated means of improving the lives of people experiencing mental health challenges. However, a lack of intellectual research space shared by mental health communication scholars among themselves and with scholars from other disciplines has minimized the potential impact of this work. Even worse, siloed research can lead to the use of messages that can harm the very people they were meant to help—people with mental illness. This contention was the impetus for this handbook.

The *Handbook of Mental Health Communication* was designed based on the notion that optimizing mass communication messaging approaches to mental health requires the integration of insights from various disciplines relevant to communicating mental health. There exists a wealth of knowledge of the psychopathological, social, epidemiological, political, and etiological aspects of mental health and mental illness, and much is known about communication principles that can inform the development of messages on a variety of health issues. An amalgamation of this literature is a necessary and exciting next step in evolving the burgeoning mental health mass communication field.

The *Handbook of Mental Health Communication* brings together a wealth of diverse conceptual frameworks and empirical lines of research that collectively offer complementary insights for optimizing mental health mass communication. The 33 chapters in this handbook are written by 85 outstanding experts worldwide. Integrating diverse insights from various disciplines makes the handbook of interest to a broad audience. We hope that the handbook will be a resource for those who want to use messaging to improve the lives of people with mental illness.

There are seven parts to this handbook. The chapters in each part address different aspects of primary questions that need to be understood before designing mental health mass communication messages. In part I, Lisa Vos and colleagues, Elayne Ahern, Caroline Ostrand and Monica Luciana, and Fei Ying and colleagues review the causes, manifestations, and consequences of biased information processing in mental illness. In part II, Romy RW and colleagues, Brian Quick and colleagues, Seth Noar and colleagues, David Vogel and colleagues, Annie Fox and colleagues, and Anthony Jorm discuss definitional and measurement issues related to a wide array of mental health communication concepts, such as information seeking, message effectiveness perceptions, self-stigma, and mental health literacy. We next move to issues related to the global dominance of digital information platforms. In part III, Kylie Woodman and Rene Weber, Fakhra Jabeen and colleagues, Nancy Lau and colleagues, and Jolynn Dellinger unpack the dangers of digital media for mental health and how their potential can be leveraged for improving mental health. In part IV, Crystal Barksdale and colleagues, Frances Griffith and Sydney Simmons, Sabrina Menezes and Gregory Guldner, and Laura Marciano and colleagues speak to the complex question of what needs to be done to ensure that mental health messaging improves mental health outcomes in special populations, given the strong causal effects of structural factors on mental illness and well-documented evidence that health message campaigns can exacerbate mental health disparities and communication inequalities.

In part V, Xun Zhu and colleagues, Ashley Johnson and colleagues, Tara Muschetto and Jason Siegel, and Miranda Twiss and colleagues discuss various ways messages can inadvertently increase stigma of mental illness and alternative message approaches that can reduce stigma. In part VI, Christopher Falco and Benjamin Rosenberg, Thomas Niederkrotenthaler and colleagues, Tasha Straszewski and Jason Siegel, Marco Yzer and Xuan Zhu, and Jason Siegel and Cara Tan review research on message strategies that offer exciting potential for improving mental health outcomes. Part VII includes essays by Teresa Thompson, Wenhao Dai and Dolores Albarracín, Jenna Reno and colleagues, and Bill Crano in which they reflect on their prolific and essential work in domains other than mental health and advance ideas lessons learned from their work that can be applied to mental health communication. For the final chapter, we accepted the challenge of highlighting how all the chapters in the book can come together to offer a helpful path ahead for mental health communication efforts. We proudly cite every chapter in the book and provide one of many recommendations that can come from the culmination of the Handbook's chapters.

This brief overview of the chapters in this *Handbook of Mental Health Communication* illustrates the wide range of questions that must be addressed when one considers developing mental health messages. Some questions directly ask about message aspects, whereas others ask about contextual, psychopathological, and other noncommunication issues. A comprehensive picture of the mental health communication landscape emerges when all these chapters are put together. To maximize the integration of ideas, we also asked all authors to include their thoughts on what their review meant as advice for those who want to use messaging for mental health promotion. This handbook's wealth of insights is not the final word about what we can do to optimize and safeguard mental health communication. It is a beginning. We hope this handbook will lead to a conversation among scholars, practitioners, and others for whom mental health and mental illness are essential, sparking interest in new research. This will ultimately converge in a significantly strengthened knowledge base on mental health communication.

Acknowledgments

Mental health is close to our hearts. We believe this handbook can make a real contribution to efforts that improve the lives of people with mental illness. For that reason alone, working on this project has been gratifying, humbling, and energizing. We have been similarly thrilled by the opportunity to work with and be supported by such an amazing group of people. Our collaborative work has underscored how significant an interaction effect can be.

Considerable credit goes to Nicole Allen at Wiley and Dr. Teri Thompson, founding editor of the journal *Health Communication*. Our collective paths crossed thanks to them. We are thankful to them for their reliably strong support throughout this entire project.

We are filled with gratitude for the expert contributions from all authors, who generously contributed their time and wisdom because they believed in the importance of this book's mission.

We wish to acknowledge the assistance of Zach Buttram, Yuming Fang, and Noel Perez. Their careful attention to detail and positive demeanor greatly helped the preparation of the book materials during the final stages of the project.

We owe a debt of gratitude to our departments for their support. We also are hugely thankful for the support we received from so many of our colleagues, whose helpful thoughts and patience when we made them listen to our long updates had a significant effect on the success of this project. We particularly recognize Dr. Rebekah Nagler and Dr. Jen Lueck. We also acknowledge the deep respect we have for the guidance we have received over the years from our mentors, Dr. Marty Fishbein and Dr. Bill Crano.

Dr. Siegel would also like to thank the past and present members of the Depression and Persuasion Research Lab. They believed in the importance of this scholarship and that it would make a useful contribution to the field and the plight of those with mental illness.

Dr. Yzer expresses his deep appreciation for the unwavering support and mentorship from Aaltjo and Ge Yzer.

Our families have been and are hugely important for our work. We are grateful for their inspiration, encouragement, and support as well as for their astute feedback and many other contributions. Thank you, Amanda and Satoko. Thank you, Erin, Anet, and Sven. Thank you, Maya and Shaw.

Last, we sincerely thank every person who has participated in our research studies. All of the chapters in this book are in the service of advancing understanding of how we can best develop mass communication messages that can help reduce the plight of people with mental illness.

All of the chapters ultimately also are the result of the willingness of our participants to share their personal experiences with us. An anonymous participant wrote to us after completion of one of our studies:

"Hey. I wanted to write and say I appreciate studies that cover stuff like this. As someone who as attempted suicide in the past, it's not an easy thing to talk about but I do when given the chance to help someone."

This leaves us with pride in the collective work represented in this book and a keen sense of responsibility for doing the right work and doing that work right.

Marco C. Yzer
Jason T. Siegel

Reference

Boric, G., & Adhanom Ghebreyesus, T. (2023, October 13). Mental health is a universal right. *Time*. https://time.com/collection/time100-voices/6323214/mental-health-care-delivery-who-chile/

Introduction

1

Mental Health Mass Communication: Using Messages to Relieve the Plight of People With Mental Illness

Marco C. Yzer[1] and Jason T. Siegel[2]

[1] University of Minnesota

[2] Claremont Graduate University

Introduction

Mental health challenges have become one of the leading public health issues of our time, negatively affecting the well-being of millions of people globally (World Health Organization, 2022). In response, there have been significant mass communication efforts to promote mental health. Mass communication interventions "expose high proportions of large populations to messages through routine uses of existing media" (Wakefield et al., 2010, p. 1261). Mass communication interventions have been used, for example, to reduce the stigma of mental illness in the general population or to encourage seeking professional help among people with mental illness (e.g. Foulkes & Andrews, 2023; Tam et al., 2024).

The broader mental health communication field includes any scholarship and professional application of communication content, processes, and outcomes related to mental health (Aldrich & Quintero-Johnson, 2021). Subfields of mental health communication include, among others, *interpersonal communication,* such as conversations with a professional care provider to talk about one's mental illness, *media portrayals* of mental illness in entertainment media and news media, *technological features* of social media that facilitate sharing mental health information, and, the focus of this chapter, mass-communicated *messaging* that promotes mental health.

Mental health mass communication shares a focus on how communication content, processes, and outcomes affect mental health with other subfields of mental health communication but is uniquely different in the approach to those communication factors. We define mental health mass communication as *the academic study and practice of purposefully planned mass communication messages designed to improve the plight of people with mental illness by, for example, promoting mental health awareness, reducing stigma, or encouraging help-seeking behaviors.*

In this chapter we discuss various aspects of mental health mass communication. We put forth a set of principles that offer actionable guidance for optimizing and safeguarding mental health messaging. We begin with a discussion of the significance of mental illness as a global public health issue to contextualize the need for effective mental health mass communication.

The Handbook of Mental Health Communication, First Edition.
Edited by Marco C. Yzer and Jason T. Siegel.

The Need for Mental Health Mass Communication: The Global Burden of Mental Illness

Prevalence data make clear that mental illness is a massive global public health issue. Several sources of global mental illness prevalence data support this contention. For example, the World Health Organization's world mental health surveys (Harvard Medical School, 2023; Kessler et al., 2006) collect prevalence data on anxiety disorders, mood disorders, impulse control disorders, and substance disorders from over 30 countries. In one analysis of world mental health survey data collected between 2001 and 2021, the lifetime prevalence of any mental disorder was about 29%; the morbid risk of any mental disorder by age 75 was 46% for males and 53% for females; and major depression (both males and females), alcohol use disorder (males), and phobia disorders (females) were the most prevalent mental disorders (McGrath et al., 2023).

The Global Burden of Diseases, Injuries, and Risk Factors study (GBD) collects data on over 350 causes of adverse health outcomes (Murray, 2020). In an analysis of 2019 data on 369 diseases and injuries across 294 countries, depression and anxiety were the 13th and 24th leading causes of loss of life years (Vos et al., 2020). The GBD database suggests that in 2019, the global prevalence of mental illness was as high as 970 million people or one in eight people. Anxiety (301 million) and depression disorders (280 million) were most prevalent. Among other mental disorders, the prevalence of alcohol use disorder was estimated to be 108 million; attention deficit or hyperactivity disorder 85 million; drug use disorder 58 million; conduct disorder 40 million; bipolar disorder 40 million; schizophrenia 24 million; and eating disorders 13 million (Institute of Health Metrics and Evaluation, 2024). These prevalence estimates may differ between regions in the world. For example, an analysis of world health surveys between 2001 and 2012 suggested that the prevalence of posttraumatic stress disorder (PTSD) was 3.9% across 24 mostly upper- to high-income countries (Koenen et al., 2017). In contrast, the prevalence of PTSD in 2019 was as high as 27% in 12 countries affected by war (Hoppen et al., 2021).

Whether global prevalence rates of mental illness are rising is a debated question, partly because of methodological issues in studies that may have led to an interpretation of demographic changes in the past decades as increasing prevalence trends (Baxter et al., 2013; Richter et al., 2019). What is less debated is that the COVID-19 pandemic has contributed to an increase in mental illness. For example, a recent initiative has examined the impact of the COVID-19 pandemic on depression and anxiety disorders (COVID-19 Mental Disorders Collaborators, 2021). Estimates from a meta-analysis of 48 data sources that represented 204 countries suggested that global prevalence rates of depression increased from 193 million to 246 million people during the COVID-19 pandemic, and prevalence rates of anxiety increased from 298 million to 374 million. For both depression and anxiety disorders, both prevalence and increase in prevalence were higher for females than for males and higher for younger age groups than older age groups (COVID-19 Mental Disorders Collaborators, 2021).

Most epidemiological research reports the prevalence of mental illnesses either as prevalence estimates based on survey participants' self-reported disorder severity or self-reported diagnoses (Kessler et al., 2006) or as counts of medical health data, such as treatment data or insurance claims (Global Burden of Disease Collaborative Network, 2020). However, people can have poor mental health even if they do not meet the criteria for a formal mental illness diagnosis. In addition, many people who may meet the diagnosis criteria for mental illness are not able to see a health professional for their symptoms and are therefore not formally diagnosed. This means that most published prevalence data underestimate the number of people who suffer from mental illness symptoms. In addition, mental illness prevalence data are not available for many countries or suffer from methodological problems, which makes an accurate estimate of the global burden of mental illness difficult (Baxter et al., 2013). This underscores that mental illness is common, which makes it even more tragic that mental illness continues to be stigmatized and that people with mental illness often feel alone in their predicament.

The Role of Mass Communication in Reducing the Burden of Mental Illness

Mass communication messaging interventions have a demonstrated potential for producing positive health outcomes, ranging from health knowledge and beliefs to health behaviors (Noar, 2006; Wakefield et al., 2010). Whereas competing factors such as cluttered media environments and firmly rooted social norms, among many others, certainly challenge the success of mass communication interventions, the likelihood of producing positive changes demonstrably improves when principles of mass communication intervention effectiveness are adhered to. These include the use of mechanisms of effects theories as a basis for message design, careful pretesting of messages, and the use of intervention design and dissemination tools that maximize exposure, among others (Noar, 2006; Wakefield et al., 2010; Willoughby & Noar, 2022).

With great power comes great responsibility. Mental health mass communication exists in a complex system of multilevel factors that interact and reciprocally influence mental health (Allen et al., 2014). These factors are outlined in social determinants of mental health frameworks, which explain the causal role of a range of structural and malleable factors such as economic opportunities, racism, educational attainment, access to media, and many others (Alegría et al., 2018; Marciano et al., 2025). Social determinants of mental health frameworks imply that the use of mental health mass communication to improve mental health is not a decision that should be made without considering other factors that influence mental health. For example, messages that promote self-care activities to cope with mental illness will not be optimally effective or even ethically suspect if structural factors that cause mental illness are not addressed in other interventions. As another example, when designing a message intervention to encourage people to seek help for mental illness, one must ensure that there are sufficient professional care options and that people have access to these. An important implication is that communication must be matched to what is feasible. For example, a campaign that encourages help-seeking may not be appropriate if there are insufficient treatment resources. However, if that is the case, messages that increase social support for people with mental illness would be helpful. Particular communication campaigns might be inappropriate for some goals, but there are always ways to use alternative communication for the betterment of people with mental illness.

Mental Health Mass Communication: Objectives, Messages, and Audiences

When it is clear that mass communication is an appropriate tool to consider in a particular setting for improving the plight of people with mental illness, decisions need to be made to develop mass communication messages. Central to these decisions are three interrelated factors: the objectives of mental health mass communication, the messages that are used to reach those objectives, and the audiences for whom the messages are intended.

Objectives

Whereas intuitively, mental health mass communication may be expected to primarily focus on reducing mental illness symptomatology and reducing stigma toward people with mental illness, prevention efforts that focus on maintaining mental health, interventions that seek to strengthen well-being, and efforts to convince policymakers to implement mental health-related system changes also are the province of mental health mass communication. Thus, the ultimate objective of mental health mass communication to relieve the plight of people with mental illness can be achieved by a wide array of interventions. This means that those who want to use messaging to strengthen mental health and reduce mental illness must think imaginatively about all the different ways that mental health can be improved.

Messages

Mental health mass communication messages can be thought of as content about mental health or mental illness that is presented in various formats, disseminated through many channel types, and conveyed using a wide range of strategies. For a discussion of theory-based, systematic ways to determine mental health message content, see Yzer and Zhu (2025).

Message Format and Channel Types

Mass communication messages come in various formats that relate to embodiment (e.g. a printed brochure, a 30-second video advertisement, billboards, and bumper stickers) and dissemination channels (e.g. print, broadcast, and digital media). Mental health mass communication uses the full spectrum of message formats. Large-scale campaigns typically use different formats and channels to reach multiple audiences over an extended period (for an illustrative review, see Foster, 2018).

Message Strategies

Message strategies pertain to the types of appeal and message features used to express the content of the message. An essential focus of mental health mass communication scholarship is on testing these strategies for mental health promotion purposes. For example, Lueck (2017) tested the effects of framing information about help-seeking for depression in terms of positive outcomes of help-seeking and adverse outcomes of not seeking help. Straszewski and Siegel (2018) tested the effects of message-induced savoring (i.e. focusing attention on positive feelings and experiences) on help-seeking for depression. Quintero Johnson et al. (2021) tested the effects of narrative perspective (i.e. that of a bystander, first person, or third person) on recall of mental illness information and attitudinal beliefs about mental illness. For an overview of mental health message components and strategies, see RW et al. (2025) and Siegel and Yzer (2025).

Given the multitude of message formats and strategies, the number of possible message configurations is infinitely large (Cappella, 2006). This requires systematic, theory-based research to identify those message configurations that maximize the match between the message and audience characteristics relevant to message attention and processing. For example, which dissemination channel should be selected is a function of how much members of an intended audience rely on various channels as part of their media diet, and which format and strategy should be selected is a function of how cognitive characteristics of intended audience members challenge or facilitate message engagement and processing. We return to this contention in greater detail when we present principles of effective mental health mass communication.

Audiences

There are two primary questions when considering audiences of mental health mass communication efforts. The first question pertains to audience segmentation: Who needs to be addressed? A second question asks: What needs to be known about these audiences, that is, which audience characteristics have meaningful implications for messaging?

Concerning the question of who needs to be reached, it is helpful to consider that messages can improve conditions for people with mental illness through direct and indirect pathways (Hornik & Yanovitzky, 2003). A direct pathway means that people with mental illness are the target audience of a message intervention. In direct pathway interventions, messages aim to educate or persuade people with mental illness by directly speaking to them. The mechanism of effects is that when people with mental illness engage with a message themselves, learning processes are induced that can lead to awareness, knowledge, belief change, and action. In contrast, an indirect pathway means that people with mental illness are *not* the target audience of a message intervention, even if the ultimate objective is to relieve the plight of people with mental illness.

Two types of audiences exist in indirect pathway interventions. First, messages can aim to persuade institutions such as news media and policymakers of the importance of mental health and, in doing so, rely on institutional change processes. Second, messages can aim to encourage the public or social network members to support others who have mental illness and, in doing so, rely on interpersonal influence processes. In indirect pathway interventions, the mechanism of effects is that, for example, more frequent and more accurate reporting on mental illness in news media, implementation of policies that improve mental health care, and strengthened motivation and skills to support social network members with mental illness create a supportive environment that improves conditions for people with mental illness (Herrman, 2001; Woodman & Weber, 2025).

Principles of Effective Mental Health Mass Communication

Considerations of objectives, messages, and audiences are essential for developing mass communication interventions across all health domains. Communicating mental health additionally faces several challenges that are unique to the mental health domain. Those who want to use mass communication for mental health must be cognizant of these challenges in order to optimize and safeguard mental health messaging. This section presents several principles of effective mental health mass communication that can guide the research and development of mental health messages. Four principles pertain to message development research, and three to message testing research.

Message Development Principles

Principle 1: Develop Systematic Research Programs

We highlighted that mental health mass communication involves a complex set of interacting factors, analogous to a 5,000-piece jigsaw puzzle where each piece is essential but must be considered in the context of the entire picture. This requires a systematic, programmatic approach to mental health mass communication research. A wealth of research insights are available for developing those research programs. First, one can lean upon the existing communication literature, which offers much guidance (Quick et al., 2025; RW et al., 2025). In addition, consider contributions from other disciplines, given that many questions that mental health message scientists must address originate outside the realm of communication (e.g. what are the pathological characteristics of particular mental disorders? Which structural factors that cause mental illness are malleable?). Research across all subdomains of psychology, communication, sociology, medicine, public health, anthropology, and likely others we failed to mention have insights that must be applied.

We rely on basic science as the foundation of our work. There is a need for basic researchers to be the masters of their domain, but given the goal of improving the lives of people with mental illness, those accepting this mission do not have the luxury of being field-specific. All contributions must be considered and utilized regardless of the field in which they are published. Note that this has implications for research funding. Whereas many basic science grant opportunities exist in the mental health domain, grant mechanisms for communication-centered projects on mental health are sparse. Researchers must use their grantsmanship to explain the significance of mass communication research on particular mental disorders to grant reviewers who may not be very familiar with mental health mass communication science. An integrative, interdisciplinary approach is central to successful mental health communication grant applications.

Further Recommendation: Continue the Trend of Research Transparency. The integrity of research programs is imperative for safeguarding mental health communication messaging (see John et al. 2012 for a foundational piece on this topic). Research practices that must be adhered to include reporting all the dependent measures collected as part of a study, reporting studies that do not support hypotheses, and acknowledging that unexpected findings go against a priori hypotheses.

In this spirit, we caution against perhaps understandable practices given the publication pressure many academic researchers feel, but that are never acceptable from a research integrity perspective. These include slicing single data collections into multiple studies and presenting new terms for existing concepts. These practices lead to a disjointed literature and the loss of relevant findings, which hinders scientific progress. Overstating the success of a messaging approach by failing to report nonsignificant dependent measures or reporting only studies that support hypotheses can lead to the selection of messaging approaches that, in actuality, are not very successful. These behaviors are problematic in all research, but such behaviors in mental health communication research can risk lives.

Principle 2: Consider Cognitive Characteristics of Message Recipients

When designing messages for people with mental illness, the cognitive characteristics of the particular mental disorder must be thoroughly understood, as these can significantly bias how people process information. Biased information processing in mental illness has been widely documented across a wide variety of mental disorders (MacLeod, 2012). The implication of biased information processing for mental health communication is that a mental health promotional message will be perceived through the lens of the particular mental disorder, which may not be the same as the message designer intended.

The implications of biased information processing in mental disorders must be considered when designing messages for people with a particular mental disorder (Yzer & Siegel, in press). For example, schizophrenia is associated with an impaired ability to focus on salient information and an increased sensitivity to distraction. This means that people with schizophrenia may be more easily overwhelmed by messages and focus on peripheral rather than focal message elements (Braff, 1993). Borderline personality disorder (BPD) is associated with a reduced ability to recognize other people's emotions accurately. This implies that people with BPD may incorrectly interpret messages that use images and language that portray emotional expressions (Niedtfeld et al., 2016). PTSD is associated with a heightened interpretation of ambiguous situations as threatening to oneself. This means that people with PTSD may feel at increased risk for harm if they see a message that uses ambiguous imagery or language (Bomyea et al., 2017). As a last example, negative self-knowledge schemas in depression lead to an expectation of negative experiences and outcomes as well as a reappraisal of positive, disconfirming information (Kube et al., 2020). This implies that messages that emphasize positive information, such as the notion that depression is not one's fault, may inadvertently reinforce existing negative self-information among people with depression (Lienemann et al., 2013).

Whereas the idea that in order to effectively communicate mental health, one must understand mental health science seems self-evidently true, integrating psychopathology and communication principles is not yet the norm in mental health mass communication scholarship, although promising exceptions certainly exist (for review, see Siegel et al., 2017; Yzer & Siegel, in press). We implore researchers and practitioners to begin their intervention projects with a thorough analysis of the nature and extent of biased information processing in their audience. Next, translate these to implications for message design. Partnerships with psychopathology experts are recommended for ensuring that cognitive aspects of mental illness are respected in message design.

This can be an exciting part of the research process, as message developers must find synergy between the clinical psychology literature on processing and the persuasion literature. For example, the idea that people with depression process self-relevant information in a particularly negatively biased fashion (Bargh & Tota, 1988) led Siegel and colleagues to use Walster and Festinger's (1962) overheard communication technique to reduce self-focus and maximize message success (Siegel et al., 2015). This also led Hollar and Siegel (2020) to explore the utility of self-distancing. Beck's theorizing on how the depressogenic schema can be temporarily thwarted (Beck, 2002) led Siegel and Thomson (2017) to test the positive emotion infusion technique.

Further Recommendation: Expand the Knowledge Base to All Mental Illnesses. Extant research in the mental health mass communication literature primarily focuses on depression disorders, anxiety disorders, or nonspecified mental health or mental illness. Collectively, these studies have importantly advanced knowledge of help-seeking beliefs, intentions, and behavior as a function of particular message configurations (e.g. Quintero Johnson et al., 2021; Siegel et al., 2017) and of positive and negative effects of messaging on the stigma of mental illnesses (e.g. Corrigan, 2016; Foster, 2018). At the same time, the primary attention to depression and anxiety disorders and on nonspecified mental illness makes clear that mental health communication principles regarding other mental disorders largely remain uncharted territory. Exceptions exist; Woodman and Weber (2025), for example, connect the cognitive basis of gaming disorder with the effectiveness of immersive messaging strategies for people with gaming disorder. Nevertheless, it is safe to say that many other mental disorders have received little or no research attention in the mental health mass communication literature. It is exciting that the knowledge base of mental health mass communication is growing, yet it is concerning that this is primarily true for depression and anxiety disorders only.

The paucity of mental health mass communication research on mental disorders other than depression and anxiety would not be a concern if it can be assumed that findings about message effects on depression and anxiety or nonspecified mental health and mental illness outcomes can be generalized to all mental disorders. This, however, is unlikely to be accurate, as biased information processing manifests itself in uniquely different ways in different mental disorders. Each mental disorder has unique cognitive characteristics that must be understood to decide whether messaging is a viable option and, if so, what the implications of these specific cognitive features of the particular illness are for how particular message configurations are processed. Further complicating matters is the high prevalence of comorbidity in mental illness (McGrath et al., 2020). For example, the implications of depression symptoms for information processing for someone who is afflicted with major depression may well be different than the implications for information processing for someone whose depression symptoms co-occur with BPD.

Thus, we call for mental health mass communication research on all mental disorders, including their comorbidities. This may require significant effort. For example, the nature of some disorders may make it very difficult to find research volunteers who are severely affected.

Principle 3: Anticipate Unintended Message Effects

It is imperative to realize that a message can backfire, that is, have unintended adverse effects. For example, it is not uncommon for those creating mental health promotion messages to underestimate how individual differences in message receivers (e.g. the presence of mental illness symptomatology) affect message processing. This can be a costly mistake. For example, research findings suggest that directly addressing depressed individuals in help-seeking messaging may lead those individuals to be even less inclined to seek help for their depression than they would have been without seeing those messages (Lienemann et al., 2013).

Relatedly, one must consider that unintended effects are possible when a message is seen by people not in the intended audience. A mass communication message that is created for people with mental illness will also be seen by people without mental illness. Similarly, if a mass communication message is created to change perceptions of the public, people with mental illness will see these messages as well. There is good evidence that well-intended large-scale campaigns that aim to reduce mental illness stigma in the general population can inadvertently lead to ***increased*** self-stigma among people with mental illness (Corrigan, 2016), for example, because antistigma messages can make the negative self-perceptions that people with certain mental disorders have more accessible (Siegel et al., 2017).

The possibility of unintended adverse message effects implies that in contrast to the saying that something is better than nothing, in mental health mass communication, something is ***not always*** better than nothing. However, when researchers are mindful that their interventions can have unintended effects, steps can be taken to prevent adverse effects. For example, many unintended negative research participation effects on people with mental illness can be prevented by matching a message to the cognitive characteristics of mental illness so that biased processing of the message will be less likely. In addition, studies can be designed to ensure that participants leave the study in a better place than when they came in. For example, Siegel adds a positive emotion infusion task to the end of his studies. In a positive emotion infusion task, participants reflect on a positive experience and how they felt during that experience, which has been shown to elevate positive feelings and even help-seeking intentions (e.g. Straszewski & Siegel, 2018).

Principle 4: Match Messages to Cultural Meanings of Mental Health and Illness

Our discussion of the interrelatedness of objectives, messages, and audiences spoke to the contention that the effectiveness of a mental health message is a function of the match between the message and audience characteristics that are relevant for message attention and processing. In addition to cognitive characteristics of mental illness (see Principle 2), cultural factors deserve particular attention as an audience characteristic that must be considered in message design. The language that is used to talk about mental illness reflects cultural values that should be respected in messaging. For example, because of a history of gendered racism and oppression, many African American women have developed what has been named a superwoman schema that dictates the need to always be strong. In addition to existing disparities in access to mental health care, the superwoman schema negatively affects professional help-seeking as that violates the normative expectation to be strong, suppress emotions, and prioritize caring for others over self-care (Woods-Giscombe et al., 2016). This means that messaging for African American women may need to avoid language about formal treatment and, more generally, should avoid any language or imagery that may inadvertently reinforce stigma. Barksdale et al. (2025) argue that mental health communication messages that focus on culturally diverse populations should focus on health equity through fairness, inclusivity, and justice by using messages that include accessibility, representation, and community engagement and that use culturally and linguistically appropriate information.

Message Testing Principles

Principle 5: Test Messages Meant for People with Mental Illness Among Participants With Mental Illness

The discussion thus far has made clear that researchers should anticipate the likelihood that people with mental illness will attend to, interpret, and remember messages that are directed to them in a biased manner. This means that research conducted to assess messages that are meant to be beneficial for people with mental illness should include participants with mental illness.

As the extent of biased information processing increases as a function of mental illness severity, samples that include a relatively even distribution of participants along a mental illness' symptom severity continuum will be best able to demonstrate at which level of severity particular message strategies will produce diverging effects. Alternatively, when researchers are interested only in the question of whether a particular message configuration works for people with heightened mental illness (and not in the question of whether people with varying mental illness severity respond differently to the same message), they should recruit only participants with heightened levels of mental illness. Both of these situations require purposive sampling strategies. See Bell et al. (2010) and Lienemann and Siegel (2019) for excellent examples.

Purposive sampling of people with mental illness is essential for research that aims to speak to the question of which message configurations and strategies are beneficial for people with mental illness. Of course, having the right sampling strategy does not guarantee an optimal actual sample. For example, participants with heightened mental illness may not be representative of the population of people who have the particular illness, as the very same psychiatric symptoms that are the impetus for the research may make participation in a study very hard or undesirable (Kanuch et al., 2016; Lally et al., 2018). Conversely, mental health severity may also be a motivator for research participation. For example, Pfeiffer et al. (2010) found in a sample of patients at a mental health care organization that patients with relatively more severe mental illness and more extended treatment history were more likely to volunteer for mental health outpatient research. These examples underscore that researchers must give painstaking attention to their participant recruitment to be confident that their sample allows them to draw conclusions about which messages are most promising for those people for whom these messages are supposed to be beneficial. Online participant-sourcing platforms, available in many but unfortunately not yet in all regions of the world, offer avenues for finding research participants that were near impossible prior to online data collection. For example, Yzer and Zhu (2025) recruited participants from the Prolific platform. They used background data that Prolific had collected from their panel members about depression diagnoses for purposively sampling people with depression.

Principle 6: Recognize Your Implicit Assumptions About Mental Health

The proposition to develop systematic mental health communication research programs by integrating contributions from multiple disciplines implies the need for careful conceptualization of primary variables. By definition, a conceptualization of a variable implies a set of assumptions about that variable, and often these assumptions are unrecognized. This may be particularly consequential for mental health. Consider, for example, the core concepts of mental health and mental illness. Mental health and mental illness have been conceptualized as semantic opposites on a single bipolar continuum (Zhao & Tay, 2023), which means that mental health is the absence of mental illness, and alternatively as two distinct concepts that can correlate but do not necessarily always do (the dual continua model; Iasiello et al., 2024; Keyes, 2005; Manderscheid et al., 2010), which implies that a person may not have a mental illness yet may not have positive mental health. A bipolar interpretation of mental health as the absence of mental illness implies that assessment of symptoms can be sufficient to measure mental health, whereas the dual continua model implies that mental health and mental illness can be and should be measured separately (Keyes, 2005; Westerhof & Keyes, 2010). Beyond measurement implications, a conceptualization of mental health and mental illness as distinct broadens the scope of mental health mass communication from reducing symptoms of mental illness to strengthening mental health among people who may or may not have mental illness (Marciano et al., 2025).

In addition, in the psychopathology literature, mental illness has been conceptualized as categorical or dimensional (Ostrand & Luciana, 2025). A categorical approach conceptualizes mental illness as a syndrome of symptoms, which produces descriptive categories of distinct mental disorders. This is the basis of the widely used *Diagnostic and Statistical Manual of Mental Disorders*, currently in its fifth edition (DSM-5; American Psychiatric Association [APA], 2022). DSM-5 describes each specific mental disorder in terms of symptoms. The presence and duration of these symptoms are the diagnostic criteria for mental disorders. For example, a person is diagnosed with major depression when they report that they experienced at least five of nine symptoms (e.g. trouble concentrating, feeling worthless) in a 2-week period, and when one of those symptoms is depressed mood or loss of interest in activities (APA, 2022). Alternatively, a dimensional conceptualization of mental illness proposes various aspects or dimensions of mental illness. It describes those as continuums, moving away from a threshold-based interpretation of mental illness and allowing for individualized descriptions that cut across categorical disorders (Cuthbert, 2022; Krueger & Bezdjian, 2009).

Different conceptualizations of mental illness have measurement implications. Categorical measures tend to ask about the presence and duration of symptoms specific to a disorder, whereas dimensional measures assess task performance, physiological responses, and digital phenotyping, among others (Cuthbert, 2022). Measurement variability also exists within the same conceptualizations. For example, Newson et al. (2020) reviewed 126 categorical assessment instruments for 10 mental disorders. They found that the consistency of symptom assessments within disorders was as low as 29% (for bipolar disorder and schizophrenia) and no higher than 58% (for obsessive-compulsive disorder).

Principle 7: First, Do No Harm

Research on mental health mass communication has several ethical implications. To begin, before inviting people with mental illness to a research study on mental illness, one must ask whether it is possible that participating in the study worsens symptoms. For example, Boothroyd (2000) reported results from exit interviews with 668 adults with severe mental illness who had been part of a 12-month study on the effects of two mental health managed care plans. He found that whereas most participants did not report adverse outcomes, some did; 9% reported that participating in the study made them anxious, 17% feared that their responses could be disclosed, and 17% thought the questions were invasive. A comparative analysis showed that these proportions were much higher than those obtained in community samples of participants who did not have mental illness. Jorm et al. (2007) reported more encouraging findings. They reviewed 46 studies that assessed the association between mental disorder symptoms and emotional responses to research participation. They found that less than 10% of participants reported distress across settings. In studies that focused on traumatic or otherwise adverse experiences, distress rates were higher. Findings from studies that included markers of longer-term effects showed no indications of persistent effects. Notwithstanding these encouraging findings, Jorm et al. (2007) cautioned that care must be given to ensure that research protocols are maximally protective against untoward effects of research participation on people with mental illness. We fully support this contention.

A second set of ethical questions concerns the outcomes of mental health mass communication interventions. Consider, for example, that a common goal of many mental health mass communication interventions is to encourage people to seek help if they have mental illness. What if such interventions are successful? Counterintuitively, there may be reasons for concern if an intervention successfully encourages people to seek help. Typically, help-seeking interventions do not include a second arm that supports people when the intervention helps them take the step to seek help. At the very least, researchers need to determine whether there, in fact, are treatment or care options available for their participants. These can be included at the end of research instruments, for example, as a list of resources.

As a last example, implementing new media technologies before the implications of those technologies are fully understood can produce unexpected outcomes. Artificial intelligence (AI) technologies present a particularly relevant case at the time of writing. AI is increasingly used for easily accessible online mental health support. However, it may offer less appropriate feedback than human counselors (Morris et al., 2018) and result in unethical sharing of personal information because data privacy regulation has not been fully established (Dellinger, 2025).

Conclusions

Mental health mass communication has compelling potential for relieving the plight of people who have mental illness. It is one of many tools that will be maximally effective when used together with other intervention tools, particularly those that ensure concurrent availability of treatment options (Wakefield et al., 2010). Indeed, whereas mental health mass communication has significant potential, it is not a tool that is advisable under all circumstances. For example, if environmental factors do not facilitate or even obstruct mental health care, mental health mass communication that encourages seeking treatment is not effective or even appropriate.

Once it has been determined that mental health mass communication is appropriate in a particular setting, several issues must be considered to optimize and safeguard mental health messaging. In this chapter, we discussed those issues and proposed several principles of effective mental health mass communication messaging. We hope these principles will catalyze interest among scholars, lead to conversations that refine the principles, and spur exciting new research on mental health communication. This will ultimately converge in a significantly strengthened mental health mass communication messaging that can improve the lives of people with mental illness.

References

Aldrich, R. S., & Quintero-Johnson, J. M. (2021). Mental health, mental illness, and suicide. In T. L. Thompson & N. G. Harrington (Eds.), *The Routledge handbook of health communication* (3rd ed., pp. 63–76). Routledge.

Alegría, M., NeMoyer, A., Bagué, I. F., Wang, Y., & Alvarez, K. (2018). Social determinants of mental health: Where we are and where we need to go. *Current Psychiatry Reports*, *20*(11), 95. https://doi.org/10.1007/s11920-018-0969-9

Allen, J., Balfour, R., Bell, R., & Marmot, M. (2014). Social determinants of mental health. *International Review of Psychiatry*, *26*(4), 392–407. https://doi.org/10.3109/09540261.2014.928270

American Psychiatric Association. (2022). *Diagnostic and statistical manual of mental disorders* (3rd ed., text rev.). https://doi.org/10.1176/appi.books.9780890425787

Bargh, J. A., & Tota, M. E. (1988). Context-dependent automatic processing in depression: Accessibility of negative constructs with regard to self but not others. *Journal of Personality and Social Psychology*, *54*(6), 925–939. https://doi.org/10.1037//0022-3514.54.6.925

Barksdale, C. L., Lawhorn, C., Alvidrez, J., & Schwartz, K. (2025). Considerations for optimizing mental health communication to advance mental health equity. In M. C. Yzer & J. T. Siegel (Eds.), *Handbook of mental health communication*. Wiley.

Baxter, A. J., Patton, G., Scott, K. M., Degenhardt, L., & Whiteford, H. A. (2013). Global epidemiology of mental disorders: What are we missing? *PLoS One*, *8*(6), e65514. https://doi.org/10.1371/journal.pone.0065514

Beck, A. T. (2002). Cognitive models of depression. In L. Robert & E. T. Dowd (Eds.), *Clinical advances in cognitive psychotherapy: Theory and application* (pp. 29–61). Springer.

Bell, R. A., Paterniti, D. A., Azari, R., Duberstein, P. R., Epstein, R. M., Rochlen, A. B., & Kravitz, R. L. (2010). Encouraging patients with depressive symptoms to seek care: A mixed methods approach to message development. *Patient Education and Counseling*, *78*, 198–205. https://doi.org/10.1016/j.pec2009.07.007

Bomyea, J., Johnson, A., & Lang, A. J. (2017). Information processing in PTSD: Evidence for biased attentional, interpretation, and memory processes. *Psychopathology Review, 4*(3), 218–243. https://doi.org/10.5127/pr.037214

Boothroyd, R. A. (2000). The impact of research participation on adults with severe mental illness. *Mental Health Services Research, 2*, 213–222. https://doi.org/10.1023/A:1010112503631

Braff, D. L. (1993). Information processing and attention dysfunctions in schizophrenia. *Schizophrenia Bulletin, 19*(2), 233–259. https://doi.org/10.1093/schbul/19.2.233

Cappella, J. N. (2006). Integrating message effects and behavior change theories: Organizing comments and unanswered questions. *Journal of Communication, 56*(S1), S265–S279. https://doi.org/10.1111/j.1460-2466.2006.00293.x

Corrigan, P. W. (2016). Lessons learned from unintended consequences about erasing the stigma of mental illness. *World Psychiatry, 15*(1), 67–73. https://doi.org/10.1002/wps.20295

COVID-19 Mental Disorders Collaborators. (2021). Global prevalence and burden of depressive and anxiety disorders in 204 countries and territories in 2020 due to the COVID-19 pandemic. *Lancet, 398*, 1700–1712. https://doi.org/10.1016/S0140-6736(21)02143-7

Cuthbert, B. N. (2022). Research domain criteria (RDoC): Progress and potential. *Current Directions in Psychological Science, 31*(2), 107–114. https://doi.org/10.1177/09637214211051363

Dellinger, J. (2025). Mental health apps and privacy: Misunderstandings and messaging. In M. C. Yzer & J. T. Siegel (Eds.), *Handbook of mental health communication*. Wiley.

Foster, J. (2018). Mental health campaigns and social representations theory: A consideration. *Papers on Social Representation, 26*(2), 4.1–4.21. https://doi.org/10.17863/CAM.28049

Foulkes, L., & Andrews, J. L. (2023). Are mental health awareness efforts contributing to the rise in reported mental health problems? A call to test the prevalence inflation hypothesis. *New Ideas in Psychology, 69*, 101010. https://doi.org/10.1016/j.newideapsych.2023.101010

Global Burden of Disease Collaborative Network. (2020). *Global burden of disease study 2019 (GBD 2019)*. Institute for Health Metrics and Evaluation.

Harvard Medical School. (2023). *The world mental health survey initiative*. https://www.hcp.med.harvard.edu/wmh/index.php

Herrman, H. (2001). The need for mental health promotion. *Australian & New Zealand Journal of Psychiatry, 35*(6), 709–715. https://doi.org/10.1046/j.1440-1614.2001.00947.x

Hollar, S. M., & Siegel, J. T. (2020). Self-distancing as a path to help-seeking for people with depression. *Social Science and Medicine, 245*, 1–9. https://doi.org/10.1016/j.socscimed.2019.112700

Hoppen, T. H., Priebe, S., Vetter, I., & Morina, N. (2021). Global burden of post-traumatic stress disorder and major depression in countries affected by war between 1989 and 2019: A systematic review and meta-analysis. *BMJ Global Health, 6*(7), e006303. https://doi.org/10.1136/bmjgh-2021-006303

Hornik, R., & Yanovitzky, I. (2003). Using theory to design evaluations of communication campaigns: The case of the national youth anti-drug media campaign. *Communication Theory, 13*(2), 204–224. https://doi.org/10.1111/j.1468-2885.2003.tb00289.x

Iasiello, M., van Agteren, J., Ali, K., & Fassnacht, D. B. (2024). Positive psychology is better served by a bivariate rather than bipolar conceptualization of mental health and mental illness: A commentary on Zhao & Tay (2022). *Journal of Positive Psychology, 19*(2), 337–341. https://doi.org/10.1080/17439760.2023.2179935

Institute of Health Metrics and Evaluation. (2024). *Global Health Data Exchange (GHDx)*. Retrieved May 2, 2024, from https://vizhub.healthdata.org/gbd-results.

John, L. K., Loewenstein, G., & Prelec, D. (2012). Measuring the prevalence of questionable research practices with incentives for truth telling. *Psychological Science, 23*(5), 524–532. https://doi.org/10.1177/0956797611430953

Jorm, A. F., Kelly, C. M., & Morgan, A. J. (2007). Participant distress in psychiatric research: A systematic review. *Psychological Medicine, 37*(7), 917–926. https://doi.org/10.1017/S0033291706009779

Kanuch, S. W., Cassidy, K. A., Dawson, N. V., Athey, M., Fuentes-Casiano, E., & Sajatovic, M. (2016). Recruiting and retaining individuals with serious mental illness and diabetes in clinical research: Lessons learned from a randomized, controlled trial. *Journal of Health Disparities Research and Practice, 9*(3), 115–126.

Kessler, R. C., Haro, J. M., Heeringa, S. G., Pennell, B.-E., & Bedirhan Üstün, T. (2006). The World Health Organization world mental health survey initiative. *Epidemiology and Psychiatric Sciences, 15*(3), 161–166. https://doi.org/10.1017/S1121189X00004395

Keyes, C. L. M. (2005). Mental illness and/or mental health? Investigating axioms of the complete state model of health. *Journal of Consulting and Clinical Psychology, 73*(3), 539–548. https://doi.org/10.1037/0022-006X.73.3.539

Koenen, K. C., Ratanatharathorn, A., Ng, L., McLaughlin, K. A., Bromet, E. J., Stein, D. J., Karam, E. G., Meron Ruscio, A., Benjet, C., Scott, K., Atwoli, L., Petukhova, M., Lim, C. C. W., Aguilar-Gaxiola, S., Al-Hamzawi, A., Alonso, J., Bunting, B., Ciutan, M., de Girolamo, G., . . . Kessler, R. C. (2017). Posttraumatic stress disorder in the World Mental Health Surveys. *Psychological Medicine, 47*(13), 2260–2274. https://doi.org/10.1017/S0033291717000708

Krueger, R. F., & Bezdjian, S. (2009). Enhancing research and treatment of mental disorders with dimensional concepts: Toward DSM-V and ICD-11. *World Psychiatry, 8*(1), 3–6. https://doi.org/10.1002/j.2051-5545.2009.tb00197.x

Kube, T., Schwarting, R., Rozenkrantz, L., Glombiewski, J. A., & Rief, W. (2020). Distorted cognitive processes in major depression: A predictive processing perspective. *Biological Psychiatry, 87*(5), 388–398. https://doi.org/10.1016/j.biopsych.2019.07.017

Lally, J., Watkins, R., Nash, S., Shetty, H., Gardner-Sood, P., Smith, S., Murray, R. M., & Gaughran, F. (2018). The representativeness of participants with severe mental illness in a psychosocial clinical trial. *Frontiers in Psychiatry, 9*, 654. https://doi.org/10.3389/fpsyt.2018.00654

Lienemann, B. A., & Siegel, J. T. (2019). A mixed methods approach to creating depression public service announcements by collaborating with people with depressive symptomatology. *Journal of Health Communication, 24*(11), 801–820. https://doi.org/10.1080/10810730.2019.1670762

Lienemann, B. A., Siegel, J. T., & Crano, W. D. (2013). Persuading people with depression to seek help: Respect the boomerang. *Health Communication, 28*(7), 718–728. https://doi.org/10.1080/10410236.2012.712091

Lueck, J. A. (2017). Matching message design and depressed cognition: An exploration of attention patterns for gain- and loss-framed depression help-seeking messages. *Journal of Health Communication, 22*(7), 593–603. https://doi.org/10.1080/10810730.2017.1324538

MacLeod, C. (2012). Cognitive bias modification procedures in the management of mental disorders. *Current Opinion in Psychiatry, 25*(2), 114–120. https://doi.org/10.1097/YCO.0b013e32834fda4a

Manderscheid, R. W., Ryff, C. D., Freeman, E. J., McKnight-Eily, L. R., Dhingra, S., & Strine, T. W. (2010). Evolving definitions of mental illness and wellness. *Preventing Chronic Disease, 7*(1), A19.

Marciano, L., Kikut-Stein, A., & Viswanath, K. (2025). Communication, equity, and mental well-being: The road ahead. In M. C. Yzer & J. T. Siegel (Eds.), *Handbook of mental health communication*. Wiley.

McGrath, J. J., Al-Hamzawi, A., Alonso, J., Altwaijri, Y., Andrade, L. H., Bromet, E. J., Bruffaerts, R., de Almeida, J. M. C., Chardoul, S., Chiu, W. T., Degenhardt, L., Demler, O. V., Ferry, F., Gureje, O., Haro, J. M., Karam, E. G., Karam, G., Khaled, S. M., Kovess-Masfety, V., . . . Zaslavsky, A. M. (2023). Age of onset and cumulative risk of mental disorders: A cross-national analysis of population surveys from 29 countries. *Lancet Psychiatry, 10*(9), 668–681. https://doi.org/10.1016/S2215-0366(23)00193-1

McGrath, J. J., Lim, C., Plana-Ripoll, O., Holtz, Y., Agerbo, E., Momen, N., Mortensen, P., Pedersen, C., Abdulmalik, J., & Aguilar-Gaxiola, S. (2020). Comorbidity within mental disorders: A comprehensive analysis based on 145,990 survey respondents from 27 countries. *Epidemiology and Psychiatric Sciences, 29*, e153. https://doi.org/10.1017/S2045796020000633

Morris, R. R., Kouddous, K., Kshirsagar, R., & Schueller, S. M. (2018). Towards an artificially empathic conversational agent for mental health applications: System design and user perceptions. *Journal of Medical Internet Research, 20*(6), e10148. https://doi.org/10.2196/10148

Murray, C. J. L. (2020). The global burden of disease study at 30 years. *Nature Medicine, 28*, 2019–2026. https://doi.org/10.1038/s41591-022-01990-1

Newson, J. J., Hunter, D., & Thiagarajan, T. C. (2020). The heterogeneity of mental health assessment. *Frontiers in Psychiatry, 11*, 76. https://doi.org/10.3389/fpsyt.2020.00076

Niedtfeld, I., Defiebre, N., Regenbogen, C., Mier, D., Fenske, S., Kirsch, P., Lis, S., & Schmahl, C. (2016). Facing the problem: Impaired emotion recognition during multimodal social information processing in borderline personality disorder. *Journal of Personality Disorders, 31*(2), 273–288. https://doi.org/10.1521/pedi_2016_30_248

Noar, S. M. (2006). A 10-year retrospective of research in health mass media campaigns: Where do we go from here? *Journal of Health Communication, 11*(1), 21–42. https://doi.org/10.1080/10810730500461059

Ostrand, C., & Luciana, M. (2025). Neural correlates of psychopathology: Implications for the processing of persuasive health messages. In M. C. Yzer & J. T. Siegel (Eds.), *Handbook of mental health communication*. Wiley.

Pfeiffer, P. N., Szymanski, B., Dhawan, N., DiFranco, D., Valenstein, M., & Zivin, K. (2010). Is there an "unhealthy volunteer effect" in mental health outpatient research? *Psychiatry Research, 176*(2–3), 224–228. https://doi.org/10.1016/j.psychres.2009.07.016

Quick, B., Caban, S., Chung, M., & Yan, J. (2025). Introducing health communication science to mental health researchers: An examination of information seeking, processing, and dissemination frameworks. In M. C. Yzer & J. T. Siegel (Eds.), *Handbook of mental health communication*. Wiley.

Quintero Johnson, J. M., Sangalang, A., & Park, S. Y. (2021). First-person, third-person, or bystander? Exploring the persuasive influence of perspective in mental health narratives. *Journal of Health Communication, 26*(4), 225–238. https://doi.org/10.1080/10810730.2021.1916658

Richter, D., Wall, A., Bruen, A., & Whittington, R. (2019). Is the global prevalence rate of adult mental illness increasing? Systematic review and meta-analysis. *Acta Psychiatrica Scandinavica, 140*(5), 393–407. https://doi.org/10.1111/acps.13083

RW, R., Xingman, W., Kim, R. S., & Nan, X. (2025). A typology of health communication variables relevant for mental health. In M. C. Yzer & J. T. Siegel (Eds.), *Handbook of mental health communication*. Wiley.

Siegel, J. T., Lienemann, B. A., & Rosenberg, B. D. (2017). Resistance, reactance, and misinterpretation: Highlighting the challenge of persuading people with depression to seek help. *Social and Personality Psychology Compass, 11*(6), e12322. https://doi.org/10.1111/spc3.12322

Siegel, J. T., Lienemann, B. A., & Tan, C. (2015). The overheard communication technique: Influencing people with depression to seek help. *Clinical Psychological Science, 3*(2), 242–255. https://doi.org/10.1177/2167702614542846

Siegel, J. T., & Thomson, A. (2017). Positive emotion infusions of elevation and gratitude: Increasing help-seeking among people with elevated levels of depressive symptomatology. *Journal of Positive Psychology, 12*(6), 509–524. https://doi.org/10.1080/17439760.2016.1221125

Siegel, J. T., & Yzer, M. C. (2025). Maximizing mental health communication: The IIFF model of help-seeking. In M. C. Yzer & J. T. Siegel (Eds.), *Handbook of mental health communication*. Wiley.

Straszewski, T., & Siegel, J. T. (2018). Positive emotion infusions: Can savoring increase help-seeking intentions among people with depression? *Applied Psychology: Health and Well Being, 10*(1), 171–190. https://doi.org/10.1111/aphw.12122

Tam, M. T., Wu, J. M., Zhang, C. C., Pawliuk, C., & Robillard, J. M. (2024). A systematic review of the impacts of media mental health awareness campaigns on young people. *Health Promotion Practice*. Advance online publication. https://doi.org/10.1177/15248399241232646

Vos, T., Lim, S. S., Abbafati, C., Abbas, K. M., Abbasi, M., Abbasifard, M., . . . Bhutta, Z. A. (2020). Global burden of 369 diseases and injuries in 204 countries and territories, 1990–2019: A systematic analysis for the Global Burden of Disease Study 2019. *Lancet, 396*(10258), 1204–1222. https://doi.org/10.1016/S0140-6736(20)30925-9

Wakefield, M. A., Loken, B., & Hornik, R. (2010). Use of mass media campaigns to change health behavior. *Lancet, 376*(9748), 1261–1271. https://doi.org/10.1016/S0140-6736(10)60809-4

Walster, E., & Festinger, L. (1962). The effectiveness of "overheard" persuasive communications. *Journal of Abnormal and Social Psychology, 65*(6), 395–402. https://doi.org/10.1037/h0041172

Westerhof, G. J., & Keyes, C. L. M. (2010). Mental illness and mental health: The two continua model across the lifespan. *Journal of Adult Development, 17*, 110–119. https://doi.org/10.1007/s10804-009-9082-y

Willoughby, J. F., & Noar, S. M. (2022). Fifteen years after a 10-year retrospective: The state of health mass mediated campaigns. *Journal of Health Communication, 27*(6), 362–374. https://doi.org/10.1080/10810730.2022.2110627

Woodman, K., & Weber, R. (2025). Cracking the code of gaming disorder: Effective communication for parents, children, and policy makers. In M. C. Yzer & J. T. Siegel (Eds.), *Handbook of mental health communication*. Wiley.

Woods-Giscombe, C., Robinson, M. N., Carthon, D., Devane-Johnson, S., & Corbie-Smith, G. (2016). Superwoman schema, stigma, spirituality, and culturally sensitive providers: Factors influencing African American women's use of mental health services. *Journal of Best Practices in Health Professions Diversity: Research, Education and Policy, 9*(1), 1124–1144. https://doi.org/10.1177/1049732310361892

World Health Organization. (2022). *World mental health report: Transforming mental health for all*. World Health Organization. https://iris.who.int/handle/10665/356119

Yzer, M., & Siegel, J. T. (in press). Recipient-focused research on depression help-seeking messaging. In G. J. De Bruijn & H. Vandebosch (Eds.), *Handbook of communication science: Vol. 15. Health, media, and communication*. De Gruyter Mouton.

Yzer, M. C., & Zhu, X. (2025). A research protocol for determining depression help-seeking message content. In M. C. Yzer & J. T. Siegel (Eds.), *Handbook of mental health communication*. Wiley.

Zhao, M. Y., & Tay, L. (2023). From ill-being to well-being: Bipolar or bivariate? *Journal of Positive Psychology, 18*(5), 649–659. https://doi.org/10.1080/17439760.2022.2109204

Part I

Mental Illness and Information Processing

2

Emotional Information-Processing Biases in Psychopathology

Lisa M. W. Vos[1], Tom Smeets[1], and Jonas Everaert[1,2]
[1] Tilburg University
[2] KU Leuven

People are bombarded with emotional information as they go about their day-to-day lives. Imagine that you call a friend, and he reacts grumpy and annoyed when he picks up the phone. In appraising his response, you may think, "He is not happy to hear from me," or "Something must have happened that is making him upset." During the ensuing phone conversation your friend says that he is not able to have dinner with you today. As he did not greet you warmly when he picked up the phone, you may think, "He just does not want to see me." Alternatively, because of the higher pitch of his voice, you may think, "He must be so stressed and busy with work." As these potential musings imply, how people process emotional cues in everyday life situations determines how people make sense of social situations. People's interpretations of emotional and ambiguous situations play an important role in shaping their emotions and behaviors as well as their mental health (Hirsch et al., 2016).

Cognitive theories have long implicated information-processing biases in the onset, maintenance, and recurrence of depression and anxiety (Beck & Haigh, 2014; Chen et al., 2020; Everaert et al., 2017b; Hirsch et al., 2016). These theories have inspired a wealth of empirical research examining preferential processing of certain types of emotional information in basic as well as higher-order cognitive processes, that is, the ways people attend to and remember emotional events as well as the ways people interpret emotional events (Beck & Haigh, 2014; De Raedt & Koster, 2010; Ingram, 1984; Joormann et al., 2007; Williams et al., 1997). The extensive work in this area has provided evidence for attention, interpretation, and memory biases in both depression and anxiety (LeMoult & Gotlib, 2019; MacLeod & Mathews, 2012). Accumulating work is also uncovering systemic interactions between these basic and higher-level information-processing biases (Everaert et al., 2020a) as well as how they derail socio-affective processes leading to increased risk for developing depression and anxiety.

Research has hitherto largely focused on elucidating the role of individual factors (e.g., attention bias) in depression and anxiety. While this is instrumental to understanding individual risk mechanisms and their role in depression or anxiety, this approach cannot characterize how cognitive, affective, and social risk mechanisms work together to confer risk for complex multifactorial mental health conditions such as depression and anxiety. This chapter reviews prior work and casts a comprehensive framework for understanding the role of information-processing biases in depression and anxiety by integrating findings from cognitive, affective, and social science approaches to psychopathology. Such attempts to integrate findings from research on information-processing biases and related fields of affective and social sciences are urgently needed to build a more comprehensive understanding of depression and anxiety.

The Handbook of Mental Health Communication, First Edition.
Edited by Marco C. Yzer and Jason T. Siegel.

Grounded in prior research, we argue that biases in basic cognitive processes such as attention and memory are instrumental to understanding biases in higher-level cognitive processes such as interpretation. We further propose that distorted interpretations of (social) situations in turn dysregulate various affective and social processes to erode social relationships and impact networks, as such setting the stage for depression and anxiety. In what follows, we begin by briefly reviewing current research findings on attention, interpretation, and memory processes in depression and anxiety. We then elaborate on how attention–memory interactions shape interpretation processes. Next, we highlight potential pathways from interpretation processes to depression and anxiety. Then, we outline various recommendations for clinically applied settings. We conclude with promising directions for future research.

Current Research on Attention, Memory, and Interpretation Biases

Theories postulate that depression and anxiety are caused in part by biases in basic processes of attention and memory. In line with theoretical predictions, systematic reviews and meta-analyses have provided evidence for two types of attention biases in depression, namely, an attention bias toward negative self-relevant information (Armstrong & Olatunji, 2012; Peckham et al., 2010) and an attenuated attention bias toward positive or rewarding stimuli (Armstrong & Olatunji, 2012; Winer & Salem, 2016). Regarding anxiety, meta-analyses and integrative reviews found evidence for an attentional bias toward threat-related stimuli (Armstrong & Olatunji, 2012; Bar-Haim et al., 2007; Cisler & Koster, 2010; Pergamin-Hight et al., 2015; Van Bockstaele et al., 2014). This attention bias in anxiety is characterized by increased vigilance or attentional orienting toward threat (Armstrong & Olatunji, 2012).

Concerning memory processes, extensive research has linked depression to difficulties in working memory operations such as inhibition (overriding dominant or prepotent responses), shifting (switching between mental sets or tasks), and updating (adding or discarding of working memory contents) that result in a biased representation of more negative and less positive material (Askelund et al., 2019; Joormann, 2010; Koster et al., 2011). With respect to anxiety, previous studies found that both state and trait anxiety are associated with impaired working memory performance such as the inability to inhibit irrelevant information from gaining access to working memory, which in turn impairs the ability to maintain relevant information (Moran, 2016; Shi et al., 2019).

Moreover, studies have examined both explicit long-term memory (i.e., more effortful and controlled storage of consciously accessible knowledge) and implicit long-term memory (i.e., storing nonconsciously accessible knowledge expressed through behavior or performance). There is strong evidence that depression is marked by biases in explicit memory, with depressed individuals recalling significantly more negative memories and fewer positive memories (Barry et al., 2004; Everaert et al., 2022; Matt et al., 1992; Watkins, 2002; Williams et al., 2007). Regarding implicit memory, depression is linked to increased implicit recall of negative information and decreased implicit recall of positive information when there is a congruence between the depth of processing (e.g., perceptual, conceptual) at encoding and retrieval (Gaddy & Ingram, 2014). Regarding anxiety, empirical evidence for a memory bias for threatening information in anxiety is limited to memory processes that rely on control cognitive operations that require participants to engage in self-initiated memory search processes in the absence of external recall cues (Herrera et al., 2017; Mitte, 2008). Extensive research also found that anxious individuals recall less positive information compared with nonanxious individuals (Herrera et al., 2017).

In addition to biases in basic processes, theories have postulated that higher-level cognitive processes such as interpreting ambiguous emotional information are also affected in depression and anxiety. Empirical research suggests that both depression and anxiety are characterized by a tendency to draw more negative and/or fewer positive interpretations in ambiguous situations. A comprehensive meta-analysis suggests that people with both clinical and subclinical forms of depression tend to draw more negative and fewer positive interpretations to resolve ambiguous situations (Everaert et al., 2017b). Regarding anxiety, research found that people with generalized anxiety disorder exhibit a general interpretation bias toward threat (Hirsch et al., 2016). Finally, people with social anxiety are more likely to interpret socially ambiguous situations more negatively (Chen et al., 2020).

Extending the focus on positive and negative biases, recent work is considering context sensitivity of interpretation processes and adopts a more dynamic approach. Indeed, inferring negative or positive interpretations may not always be adaptive or maladaptive (Everaert et al., 2018; Mehu & Scherer, 2015). Whether negative or positive interpretations encourage (mal)adaptive behavior likely depends on the fluctuating demands of a situation in which the interpretations are made. To capture the toxic nature of interpretation processes, recent research has started to examine inflexibility in revising interpretations based on information that disconfirms initial interpretations. This work has found that depression and social anxiety severity is linked with inflexibility in revising negative but not positive interpretations based on disconfirmatory information (Everaert et al., 2018, 2020b). That is, even in the face of positive information about the outcome of a situation, individuals with higher depression and anxiety levels are less inclined to update their initial negative interpretations based on new information. Importantly, this inflexibility is not accounted for by interpretation bias.

In summary, empirical research is generally consistent with the notion that depression and anxiety are marked by aberrant processing of emotional information at the level of attention, memory, and subsequent interpretation. Emerging dynamic approaches may better capture the toxic nature of such cognitive biases. Importantly, these distorted cognitive processes are not mere correlates of depression and anxiety; evidence suggests that such distortions may cause symptoms and predict them across time (Creswell & O'Connor, 2011; Everaert et al., 2021, 2022; Fodor et al., 2020; Hallion & Ruscio, 2011; Herrera et al., 2017; Menne-Lothmann et al., 2014; Songco et al., 2020). Cognitive biases may thus confer a risk to experiencing depression and anxiety, representing transdiagnostic vulnerability factors.

Mechanisms Underlying Distorted Interpretation: Attention and Memory Bias

Interpreting ambiguous situations represents a higher-level cognitive operation that involves integrating and weighing different aspects of a situation to construct new mental representations that resolve the ambiguity (Everaert, 2021; Everaert et al., 2020a). This process of ambiguity resolution is expected to rely on a set of basic attention and memory operations (Blanchette & Richards, 2010; Everaert, 2021; Everaert et al., 2020a). Because depression and anxiety feature mood-congruent biases in attention allocation and memory retrieval (see aforementioned evidence), these information-processing biases plausibly contribute to the skewed generation and selection of interpretations. These attention and memory biases may shape how individuals with depression and anxiety make sense of ambiguous situations.

In interpreting ambiguous situations, it is plausible that the generation of interpretations is guided by prior knowledge and/or experiences in similar situations (i.e., cognitive representations; Wittenborn et al., 2016). This knowledge can be consciously retrieved or rather automatically triggered from long-term memory by allocating attention toward cues in the environment. A negative attention bias and attenuated positive attention bias may make more negative than positive long-term memory accessible (e.g., previous conflicts with close friends), thereby setting the stage for a congruent bias in interpretation generation (e.g., "My friend is mad at me," "My friend does not want to see me"). In considering generated interpretations, the different options must be held online in working memory and the most plausible interpretation must be selected from its competitors. Difficulties in working memory operations and biases in attention are likely to influence this selection process (Everaert et al., 2020a). Difficulties in inhibiting negative representations, shifting between negative and positive representations, and updating working memory by removing irrelevant negative material may result in a disproportionate representation of negative versus positive interpretations in working memory (at the expense of positive interpretations). These biased working memory contents may then guide attention toward matching (external) information (e.g., your friend canceling your dinner plans), which may in turn bias what is subsequently encoded and maintained in working memory (e.g., "Nobody wants to go out with me"). These bidirectional influences between working memory and external attention bias may increase the likelihood that a negative and not a positive interpretation is selected as the most plausible explanation for that particular situation. The selected interpretation may then be encoded into long-term memory and hence influence what is available for later retrieval from long-term memory when ambiguity is encountered. This may instigate a self-maintaining cycle of increasingly negative as well as less positive information-processing, shaping one's views about the self (e.g., "I'm a terrible friend"), others (e.g., "People do not care about me"), and future (e.g., "No one will ever like me").

Emerging research examining interactions between cognitive biases in psychopathology is generally consistent with this combined cognitive bias hypothesis (Everaert & Koster, 2020; Everaert et al., 2020a). Various studies have shown that biased attention toward negative stimuli predicts higher proportions of negative interpretations in individuals with more severe symptoms of depression (Everaert et al., 2013, 2017b; Sanchez et al., 2015). For example, in one study (Everaert et al., 2014), participants with varying self-reported levels of depressive symptom severity were asked to complete a Scrambled Sentences Test (SST; Wenzlaff & Bates, 1998). In this test, participants unscramble emotional sentences in either a positive or negative manner (e.g., "born winner am loser a I" into either "I am a born loser" or "I am a born winner;" Everaert et al., 2014). When participants were unscrambling the sentences, biases in attention toward negative (e.g., "loser") vs. positive (e.g., "winner") words were measured using eye-tracking. Results showed that a bias in fixation frequency favoring negative words was related to a higher proportion of SST sentences that were unscrambled negatively (i.e., negative interpretations). This suggests that, when attention is biased and prioritizes negative stimuli, more negative interpretations are derived. Moreover, a recent study on social anxiety provided further evidence in support of the association between attention and interpretation biases in the processing of emotional facial expressions (Leung et al., 2022). In this study, participants were asked to label various emotional expressions as quickly and accurately as possible (e.g., happy, angry, sad, disgust, fear). Facial stimuli displaying subtle expressions (i.e., low-intensity emotion) were then used to measure interpretation bias. Results showed that, regardless of social anxiety levels, attention bias toward angry (but not disgusted) faces was associated with more negative interpretations of these angry expressions. This interpretation bias in turn predicted better recognition of the faces displaying anger. Importantly, experimental work supports a causal influence of attention bias on interpretation bias for threat-relevant material (White et al., 2011).

In addition to the influence of attention bias on interpretation bias, biased interpretations may, in theory, guide the allocation of attention to matching emotional information. Yet no evidence has been found for the reverse effect of interpretation bias on attention. In a recent study (LeMoult et al., 2017), adolescents suffering from clinical depression completed a cognitive training procedure to induce a positive bias when resolving ambiguous information. Results showed that while the cognitive training procedure successfully induced a positive interpretation bias, there was no transfer of the training on the attention bias task.

With respect to memory processes, current research suggests that working memory difficulties are involved in how people with depressive or anxiety symptoms interpret ambiguous information. In particular, our recent work suggests that both difficulties in shifting between emotionally negative working memory representations and the updating of working memory to discard negative representations are uniquely related to depression-linked interpretation biases (Everaert et al., 2017a). In that study, both shifting and updating difficulties had an indirect effect on depression severity through negative interpretation bias. In addition, some evidence suggests that long-term memory recall is affected by interpretation biases (Everaert et al., 2014). A study in clinically depressed individuals modified interpretation biases through experimental manipulation to examine its impact on long-term memory (Joormann et al., 2015). The results showed that an induced positive interpretation bias resulted in more positive interpretations and improved recall of these interpretations on a memory test. In addition, two studies revealed empirical evidence for the association between biases in interpretation and memory in social anxiety (Hertel et al., 2008). In particular, how situations are interpreted affects what socially anxious individuals remember about the situation. These inaccurate memories may in turn influence future interpretations of other social situations.

Summing up, current evidence suggests that attention biases filter negative information in the environment to modulate the interpretation of ambiguity. Interpretation biases in turn may not guide attention toward congruent information in the environment. Furthermore, working memory difficulties may modulate the information that is considered when interpreting ambiguity, and these biased interpretations may then be stored in long-term memory, setting the stage for recall biases as observed in depression or anxiety. Unfortunately, similar research on cognitive mechanisms in interpretation inflexibility is missing. Yet difficulties in working memory operations seem particularly relevant to understand inflexibility when initial negative interpretations are violated by novel positive information.

Pathways from Aberrant Interpretations of Ambiguity to Depression and Anxiety

While research has made important progress in identifying distorted interpretation processes in psychopathology, the potential pathways driving the interpretation of ambiguity remain understudied. Existing research points to important affective and social–behavioral mechanisms connecting interpretation processes to depression and anxiety.

Affective Pathways

Biased and inflexible interpretations of ambiguity may increase the risk for depression and anxiety by dysregulating emotional responding and emotion regulation (Mehu & Scherer, 2015). Several studies have investigated the causal impact of interpretation biases on emotional responding. This research has used cognitive training methods to manipulate interpretation biases and test how the induced biases are related to responses on a stress induction task. Current findings suggest that induced positive interpretation biases are related to smaller increases in heart rate during the anticipation of a social–evaluative speech task (Joormann et al., 2015) as well as more positive and less negative emotions following a failure task (Cowden Hindash & Rottenberg, 2017). Positive interpretation biases may thus have a benign influence on stress reactivity. In a similar vein, research suggesting reinterpreting stress as helpful has shown that this mindset is related to improved stress appraisals, cardiovascular reactivity, daily cortisol levels, well-being, and anxiety symptoms in adolescents (Yeager et al., 2022). Linking interpretation bias to social emotions, one study examined whether biased interpretations of socially ambiguous situations predict as well as maintain loneliness in youth (Lau et al., 2021). However, they found a concurrent rather than a causal relation, suggesting that the tendency to infer threatening interpretations of social situations maintains feelings of loneliness.

To date, still little is known about how emotional disturbances in ambiguity resolution predict problems in the dynamic unfolding of emotions in daily life (Houben et al., 2015; Kuppens & Verduyn, 2017). Initial research connecting interpretation processes measures in the lab to emotions experienced in real life found that negative interpretation bias was linked to heightened daily negative affect and decreased daily positive affect (Puccetti et al., 2023). A highly interesting avenue for future research is to explore whether inflexible negative interpretations consistently evoke similar negative emotions (e.g., sadness, fear) regardless of the past and current attributes of a situation, thereby setting the stage for higher levels of stability in elevated negative and blunted positive emotions in depression and anxiety.

There is increasing research that aims to uncover how biased and inflexible negative interpretations of ambiguous information are involved in initiating and perpetuating the maladaptive pattern of emotion regulation strategy usage characteristic of depression (Joormann & Stanton, 2016; Joormann & Vanderlind, 2014) and anxiety (Everaert et al., 2020b). Cross-sectional studies have repeatedly shown that interpretation biases are associated with higher levels of rumination and lower levels of positive reappraisal in subclinical and clinical forms of depression (Everaert et al., 2017a; Krahé et al., 2019; Mor et al., 2014; Wisco et al., 2014). Regarding anxiety, previous research found that social anxiety may inhibit positive interpretations of socially ambiguous situations, which in turn, might predict diminished cognitive reappraisal (Romano et al., 2020). Going beyond cross-sectional data, a recent study tested the predictive role of cognitive biases and emotion regulation strategies on different indicators of psychological adjustment to stressful life events (Blanco et al., 2021). The findings suggest that rumination mediated the association between negative interpretation bias and anxiety. Moreover, another study investigated whether a negative interpretation bias may causally influence rumination (Hirsch et al., 2018). It was found that inducing positive interpretations through cognitive training resulted in a reduction of rumination as well as depressive symptoms. Together, these findings suggest that interpretation processes may be causally linked to some of the key emotion regulation difficulties in depression and anxiety.

Research has expanded on this work and started to investigate the role of inflexible negative interpretations in emotion dysregulation. Across two studies (Everaert et al., 2020b), researchers observed inflexibility in revising negative interpretations based on novel positive information was related to dampening positive emotions, but not rumination or positive reappraisal. Interestingly, such dampening of appraisals (e.g., thoughts such as, "I don't deserve this") mediated the relation between inflexible negative interpretations and symptoms of depression and social anxiety (even after controlling for interpretation bias). This initial work suggests that inflexibility in revising negative interpretations based on positive information may explain some of the difficulties in regulating positive emotions in depression and anxiety. However, future longitudinal research is required to establish the directional effects of interpretation inflexibility on dampening and depression and anxiety severity.

Social and Behavioral Pathways

How people interpret ambiguous social events may not only affect their regulatory attempts, but also impact how they navigate the social world. Interpretations of ambiguous situations often occur within interpersonal contexts involving close relationships and social interaction partners and within broader social networks (Alden & Taylor, 2004; Everaert, 2021; Marroquín, 2011). In these contexts, it is unclear how biased or inflexible interpretations might impact socio-affective processes to increase the risk for psychopathology. Yet it might be that individuals who tend to negatively interpret ambiguous social situations and have difficulty revising initial negative interpretations based on positive social experience also experience difficulties in socio-affective processes closely related to depression and anxiety.

Depression and anxiety are characterized by problems in forming and maintaining social relationships (Alden & Taylor, 2004; Santini et al., 2015), including difficulties in socio-affective functioning and regulating interpersonal emotional experiences (Hofmann, 2014; Marroquín, 2011; Wright et al., 2020), greater perpetuation of distorted social emotions (e.g., loneliness) over time (Elmer et al., 2020), behavior characterized by social withdrawal and interpersonal conflicts (Rappaport et al., 2017), the tendency to anxiously anticipate rejection within close relationships (Ayduk et al., 2001; Normansell & Wisco, 2017), and chronic social stress (Hames et al., 2013; Liu & Alloy, 2010; Uliaszek et al., 2012). According to the stress generation hypothesis (Hames et al., 2013; Hammen, 2006; Liu & Alloy, 2010), depressed and anxious individuals behave in ways that elicit negative reactions from others, which in turn engender these psychopathologies. Research has found extensive evidence for this hypothesis in depression and anxiety (Uliaszek et al., 2012). From a stress generation perspective (Hames et al., 2013), it seems plausible that inflexibility in revising negative interpretations after social interactions (e.g., "Others don't like me") highlights negative aspects of social experiences, thereby encouraging context-inappropriate social emotions (e.g., feeling lonely, feeling rejected). Negative interpretations of social situations and inadequate updating of negative interpretations based on subsequent experiences that cast doubt on them may elicit ineffective social behaviors (e.g., withdrawal, quarrelsomeness) that provoke negative reactions from others (e.g., conflicts with close others). Frequent occurrences of such social stress may, in turn, increase the chances of biased and/or inflexible interpretation of ambiguity, erode relationships, and reduce and trigger depression and anxiety symptoms over time.

Several studies have started to document relations between interpretation processes and socio-behavioral factors. One study examined interpersonal perceptions about biases in information processing and found an indirect pathway between negative interpretation inflexibility and suicidal ideation via perceived burdensomeness (e.g., the belief that one is a burden to others; Everaert et al., 2021). Another study on eating disorders found that inaccurate interpretations of ambiguous social situations enhance the tendency to anxiously anticipate social rejection and downregulate positive social emotions within close relationships (Bronstein et al., 2022). Finally, linking interpretation processes to social functioning, one study found that inflexibility in revising negative interpretations was related to impairment in social functioning via depressive and social anxiety symptoms (even after controlling for interpretation bias; Deng et al., 2023). These findings suggest that interpretation inflexibility not only is associated with affective symptoms but also accounts for unique variance in social functioning difficulties above and beyond biased interpretations.

Prior research on these social and behavioral pathways provides insights into how biased and inflexible interpretations might impact difficulties in socio-affective processes in depression and anxiety. However, future longitudinal studies should investigate interpretation bias and inflexibility as cognitive mechanisms that encourage maladaptive social behaviors and emotions within interpersonal relationships in people with depression and anxiety.

Implications for Clinically Applied Settings

Efforts to advance the understanding of information-processing biases, and higher-level processes such as interpretations in particular, seem integral to improving existing treatment strategies for depression and anxiety. This is because interpretation processes form a central target in many psychological treatments such as cognitive behavioral therapies (Beck & Haigh, 2014) and cognitive training programs (Fodor et al., 2020; Menne-Lothmann et al., 2014). These treatment strategies incorporate various techniques (e.g., cognitive restructuring, reappraisal) that depend on interpretation flexibility and processing of disconfirming information to modify dysfunctional beliefs about the self and others. In this respect, the increasing focus on dynamic properties of cognitive biases (i.e., inflexibility or context insensitivity; e.g., Everaert et al., 2018; Kashdan & Rottenberg, 2010; Stange et al., 2017) represents a theoretical innovation with potentially important clinical applications to improve the limited efficacy of current treatment strategies (Cuijpers et al., 2010).

One particularly interesting direction for research is to test the utility of biased and inflexible interpretations as markers of treatment success. It is plausible that individuals with more severely biased and inflexible interpretations are at risk of poor treatment response and dropout. To increase flexibility, interventions may benefit from a focus on facilitating the intake and integration of disconfirmatory positive information into existing negative beliefs (as opposed to merely providing corrective or belief-disconfirming experiences). Strategies to facilitate updating of negative interpretations may involve methods that increase awareness of attention allocation to promote the salience of belief-incongruent (positive) information (Bernstein & Zvielli, 2014; Sanchez-Lopez et al., 2019) and methods that reduce dampening appraisals of positive information that is incongruent with negative interpretations (Vanderlind et al., 2020). Future research could examine whether improvements in cognitive flexibility will lead to decreased depressive and/or anxiety symptoms. Though research is in its early stages, studying the utility of interpretation processes in predicting treatment outcomes may open up exciting lines of research that could eventually provide insights that help to reduce the burden of depression and/or anxiety.

Mental Health Communication

Communicating with people with mental health challenges, including depression and/or anxiety, requires empathy, patience, and understanding (Rogers, 1951). Going beyond these basic therapeutic conversation skills, this section offers additional pointers when communicating with people with depression and/or anxiety or persuading these people to seek help. In general, using messages to promote mental health among people afflicted with these mental health conditions presents a conundrum. We explained that people with depression or anxiety often perceive the world through gray-colored glasses, which severely impact their ability to process emotional information in an unbiased manner.

In fact, biases in information-processing highlight negative aspects of social experiences, thereby encouraging context-inappropriate social emotions (e.g., social rejection or failure). Message developers could provide positive information that disconfirms their negative initial beliefs. However, merely providing evidence that disconfirms negative beliefs may not always lead to revising initial negative interpretations. Recent work has identified certain characteristics of disconfirmatory information that facilitate updating of initial beliefs (Ferguson et al., 2019). To correct negative beliefs, messages should ideally be positive, highly diagnostic, believable, and reframing earlier experiences.

Moreover, we described that cognitive biases in depression and anxiety are particularly likely to be triggered when people with these mental health conditions engage with self-relevant information. This may imply that messages that directly ask these people to think about their own situation (e.g., "Do you feel ___?") induce cognitive biases, such as the erroneous belief that they are responsible for their mental health problems. Message developers may therefore need to be cautious in speaking directly to people with depression or anxiety about their experiences. Instead of triggering personal experiences, mass communication with people afflicted with depression or anxiety could serve psycho-educative purposes by making people aware of such self-referential negative biases and how they color affective and social experiences.

Future Research

Future research could address several limitations that currently characterize work in this area. First, current research primarily focused on interpretation processes as investigated in scenario-based cognitive tasks that have restricted ecological validity and cross-sectional designs that preclude claims about causal pathways influencing depression and anxiety (Everaert et al., 2018, 2020b, 2021). Consequently, it is unclear how biased and inflexible interpretations occur within the context of naturally occurring social environments and how they engender depressive and anxiety symptoms over time. Future studies should examine how people draw and revise negative interpretations and their causal pathways to depression and anxiety in real-world settings using longitudinal designs and/or ecological momentary assessment.

Collecting intensive longitudinal data of real-life cognitive, affective, and social factors enables opportunities for developing personalized models of depression and anxiety risk. Within-person causal relations could be identified to ascertain heterogeneity in hypothesized causal relations between interpretation bias/inflexibility and both affective and socio-behavioral mechanisms in depression and anxiety. This knowledge helps to identify actionable targets for (digital) interventions. Identifying individual differences in response to these interventions and matching clients to the most effective interventions for them might improve treatment success (Lorenzo-Luaces et al., 2021).

Finally, as pointed out previously, several important gaps in our understanding of the mechanisms underlying interpretation bias/inflexibility and how it connects to depression and anxiety remain. We identify the following as key priorities. First, future research could examine four mechanisms that may be important to understanding how biased and inflexible interpretations emerge, thereby contributing to depression and anxiety. In particular, further research could examine how specific attention-memory interactions occur in the context of interpreting ambiguity, namely, how (a) attention biases during memory encoding of interpretations modulate long-term memory biases; (b) attention biases during memory retrieval of interpretations modulate long-term memory biases; (c) long-term memory biases guide the allocation of attention and interpretations; and (d) working memory difficulties modulate the interactions between biases of attention and long-term memory during the interpretation of ambiguity. Second, while research has made significant progress in identifying biases in information processes in people with depression and anxiety, the potential pathways driving the interpretation of ambiguity in daily life situations remain understudied. Specific affective processes might be affected in depression and anxiety that influence interpretation processes that have yet to be investigated. Future research needs to establish potential causal links between biases in information processes and daily affective experiences in depression and anxiety. Finally, still little is known about how interpretation processes impact a person's ability to navigate the social world. Indeed, the social consequences of biased and inflexible interpretations may be profound and undermine a person's ability to successfully operate in social relationships. However, one's subjective experience of social relationships may be colored by inaccurate interpretations, resulting in a misconception of the relationship. To build a more comprehensive understanding of information-processing biases in social interactions in people with depression and anxiety, future research could investigate how people interpret emotional information in dyadic interactions and their social consequences using reports of both interaction partners.

Conclusion

Uncovering the nature, causes, and consequences of emotional disturbances in interpreting ambiguity may be important to understanding and treating depression and anxiety. Research has made important progress in identifying the nature of biased and inflexible interpretations in depression and anxiety, its underlying cognitive mechanisms, as well as associated difficulties in emotional responding and regulation and social relationships. Yet there remain open questions that currently challenge our understanding of how biased and inflexible interpretations operate in depression and anxiety. This chapter may help to synthesize current research and serve as a starting point for future research on interpretation processes to advance theories and treatments of depression and anxiety.

References

Alden, L. E., & Taylor, C. T. (2004). Interpersonal processes in social phobia. *Clinical Psychology Review*, *24*(7), 857–882. http://dx.doi.org/10.1016/j.cpr.2004.07.006

Armstrong, T., & Olatunji, B. O. (2012). Eye tracking of attention in the affective disorders: A meta-analytic review and synthesis. *Clinical Psychology Review*, *32*(8), 704–723. http://dx.doi.org/10.1016/j.cpr.2012.09.004

Askelund, A. D., Schweizer, S., Goodyer, I. M., & van Harmelen, A.-L. (2019). Positive memory specificity is associated with reduced vulnerability to depression. *Nature Human Behaviour*, *3*(3), 265–273. http://dx.doi.org/10.1038/s41562-018-0504-3

Ayduk, O., Downey, G., & Kim, M. (2001). Rejection sensitivity and depressive symptoms in women. *Personality and Social Psychology Bulletin*, *27*(7), 868–877. http://dx.doi.org/10.1177/0146167201277009

Bar-Haim, Y., Lamy, D., Pergamin, L., Bakermans-Kranenburg, M. J., & van Ijzendoorn, M. H. (2007). Threat-related attentional bias in anxious and nonanxious individuals: A meta-analytic study. *Psychological Bulletin*, *133*, 1–24. http://dx.doi.org/10.1037/0033-2909.133.1.1

Barry, E. S., Naus, M. J., & Rehm, L. P. (2004). Depression and implicit memory: Understanding mood congruent memory bias. *Cognitive Therapy and Research*, *28*(3), 387–414. http://dx.doi.org/10.1023/B:COTR.0000031808.00502.2e

Beck, A. T., & Haigh, E. A. P. (2014). Advances in cognitive theory and therapy: The generic cognitive model. *Annual Review of Clinical Psychology*, *10*(1), 1–24. http://dx.doi.org/10.1146/annurev-clinpsy-032813-153734

Bernstein, A., & Zvielli, A. (2014). Attention feedback awareness and control training (A-FACT): Experimental test of a novel intervention paradigm targeting attentional bias. *Behaviour Research and Therapy*, *55*, 18–26. http://dx.doi.org/10.1016/j.brat.2014.01.003

Blanchette, I., & Richards, A. (2010). The influence of affect on higher level cognition: A review of research on interpretation, judgement, decision making and reasoning. *Cognition and Emotion*, *24*(4), 561–595. http://dx.doi.org/10.1080/02699930903132496

Blanco, I., Boemo, T., & Sanchez-Lopez, A. (2021). An online assessment to evaluate the role of cognitive biases and emotion regulation strategies for mental health during the COVID-19 lockdown of 2020: Structural equation modeling study. *JMIR Mental Health*, *8*(11), e30961. http://dx.doi.org/10.2196/30961

Bronstein, M. V., Everaert, J., Kummerfeld, E., Haynos, A. F., & Vinogradov, S. (2022). Biased and inflexible interpretations of ambiguous social situations: Associations with eating disorder symptoms and socioemotional functioning. *International Journal of Eating Disorders*, *55*(4), 518–529. http://dx.doi.org/10.1002/eat.23688

Chen, J., Short, M., & Kemps, E. (2020). Interpretation bias in social anxiety: A systematic review and meta-analysis. *Journal of Affective Disorders*, *276*, 1119–1130. http://dx.doi.org/10.1016/j.jad.2020.07.121

Cisler, J. M., & Koster, E. H. W. (2010). Mechanisms of attentional biases towards threat in anxiety disorders: An integrative review. *Clinical Psychology Review*, *30*(2), 203–216. http://dx.doi.org/10.1016/j.cpr.2009.11.003

Cowden Hindash, A. H., & Rottenberg, J. A. (2017). Moving towards the benign: Automatic interpretation bias modification in dysphoria. *Behaviour Research and Therapy*, *99*, 98–107. http://dx.doi.org/10.1016/j.brat.2017.09.005

Creswell, C., & O'Connor, T. G. (2011). Interpretation bias and anxiety in childhood: Stability, specificity and longitudinal associations. *Behavioural and Cognitive Psychotherapy, 39*(2), 191–204. http://dx.doi.org/10.1017/S1352465810000494

Cuijpers, P., van Straten, A., Bohlmeijer, E., Hollon, S. D., & Andersson, G. (2010). The effects of psychotherapy for adult depression are overestimated: A meta-analysis of study quality and effect size. *Psychological Medicine, 40*(2), 211–223. http://dx.doi.org/10.1017/S0033291709006114

De Raedt, R., & Koster, E. H. W. (2010). Understanding vulnerability for depression from a cognitive neuroscience perspective: A reappraisal of attentional factors and a new conceptual framework. *Cognitive, Affective, & Behavioral Neuroscience, 10*(1), 50–70. http://dx.doi.org/10.3758/CABN.10.1.50

Deng, W., Everaert, J., Bronstein, M. V., Joormann, J., & Cannon, T. (2023). Social interpretation inflexibility and functioning: Associations with symptoms and stress. *Journal of Social and Clinical Psychology, 42*(1), 29–49. http://dx.doi.org/10.1521/jscp.2023.42.1.29

Elmer, T., Geschwind, N., Peeters, F., Wichers, M., & Bringmann, L. (2020). Getting stuck in social isolation: Solitude inertia and depressive symptoms. *Journal of Abnormal Psychology, 129*(7), 713–723. http://dx.doi.org/10.1037/abn0000588

Everaert, J. (2021). Interpretation of ambiguity in depression. *Current Opinion in Psychology, 41*, 9–14. http://dx.doi.org/10.1016/j.copsyc.2021.01.003

Everaert, J., Bernstein, A., Joormann, J., & Koster, E. H. W. (2020a). Mapping dynamic interactions among cognitive biases in depression. *Emotion Review, 12*(2), 93–110. http://dx.doi.org/10.1177/1754073919892069

Everaert, J., Bronstein, M. V., Cannon, T. D., & Joormann, J. (2018). Looking through tinted glasses: Depression and social anxiety are related to both interpretation biases and inflexible negative interpretations. *Clinical Psychological Science, 6*(4), 517–528.

Everaert, J., Bronstein, M. V., Cannon, T. D., Klonsky, E. D., & Joormann, J. (2021). Inflexible interpretations of ambiguous social situations: A novel predictor of suicidal ideation and the beliefs that inspire it. *Clinical Psychological Science, 9*(5), 879–899. http://dx.doi.org/10.1177/2167702621993867

Everaert, J., Bronstein, M. V., Castro, A. A., Cannon, T. D., & Joormann, J. (2020b). When negative interpretations persist, positive emotions don't! Inflexible negative interpretations encourage depression and social anxiety by dampening positive emotions. *Behaviour Research and Therapy, 124*, 103510. http://dx.doi.org/10.1016/j.brat.2019.103510

Everaert, J., Duyck, W., & Koster, E. H. (2014). Attention, interpretation, and memory biases in subclinical depression: A proof-of-principle test of the combined cognitive biases hypothesis. *Emotion, 14*(2), 331–340. http://dx.doi.org/10.1037/a0035250

Everaert, J., Grahek, I., Duyck, W., Buelens, J., Van den Bergh, N., & Koster, E. H. W. (2017a). Mapping the interplay among cognitive biases, emotion regulation, and depressive symptoms. *Cognition and Emotion, 31*(4), 726–735. http://dx.doi.org/10.1080/02699931.2016.1144561

Everaert, J., & Koster, E. H. W. (2020). The interplay among attention, interpretation, and memory biases in depression: Revisiting the combined cognitive bias hypothesis. In T. Aue & H. Okon-Singer (Eds.), *Cognitive biases in health and psychiatric disorders* (pp. 193–213). Academic Press. https://doi.org/10.1016/B978-0-12-816660-4.00009-X

Everaert, J., Podina, I. R., & Koster, E. H. W. (2017b). A comprehensive meta-analysis of interpretation biases in depression. *Clinical Psychology Review, 58*, 33–48. http://dx.doi.org/10.1016/j.cpr.2017.09.005

Everaert, J., Tierens, M., Uzieblo, K., & Koster, E. H. W. (2013). The indirect effect of attention bias on memory via interpretation bias: Evidence for the combined cognitive bias hypothesis in subclinical depression. *Cognition and Emotion, 27*(8), 1450–1459. http://dx.doi.org/10.1080/02699931.2013.787972

Everaert, J., Vrijsen, J. N., Martin-Willett, R., van de Kraats, L., & Joormann, J. (2022). A meta-analytic review of the relationship between explicit memory bias and depression: Depression features an explicit memory bias that persists beyond a depressive episode. *Psychological Bulletin, 148*(5–6), 435–463. http://dx.doi.org/10.1037/bul0000367

Ferguson, M. J., Mann, T. C., Cone, J., & Shen, X. (2019). When and how implicit first impressions can be updated. *Current Directions in Psychological Science, 28*(4), 331–336. http://dx.doi.org/10.1177/0963721419835206

Fodor, L. A., Georgescu, R., Cuijpers, P., Szamoskozi, Ş., David, D., Furukawa, T. A., & Cristea, I. A. (2020). Efficacy of cognitive bias modification interventions in anxiety and depressive disorders: A systematic review and network meta-analysis. *The Lancet Psychiatry, 7*(6), 506–514. http://dx.doi.org/10.1016/S2215-0366(20)30130-9

Gaddy, M. A., & Ingram, R. E. (2014). A meta-analytic review of mood-congruent implicit memory in depressed mood. *Clinical Psychology Review, 34*(5), 402–416. http://dx.doi.org/10.1016/j.cpr.2014.06.001

Hallion, L. S., & Ruscio, A. M. (2011). A meta-analysis of the effect of cognitive bias modification on anxiety and depression. *Psychological Bulletin, 137*(6), 940–958. http://dx.doi.org/10.1037/a0024355

Hames, J. L., Hagan, C. R., & Joiner, T. E. (2013). Interpersonal processes in depression. *Annual Review of Clinical Psychology, 9*(1), 355–377. http://dx.doi.org/10.1146/annurev-clinpsy-050212-185553

Hammen, C. (2006). Stress generation in depression: Reflections on origins, research, and future directions. *Journal of Clinical Psychology, 62*(9), 1065–1082. http://dx.doi.org/10.1002/jclp.20293

Herrera, S., Montorio, I., Cabrera, I., & Botella, J. (2017). Memory bias for threatening information related to anxiety: An updated meta-analytic review. *Journal of Cognitive Psychology, 29*(7), 832–854. http://dx.doi.org/10.1080/20445911.2017.1319374

Hertel, P. T., Brozovich, F., Joormann, J., & Gotlib, I. H. (2008). Biases in interpretation and memory in generalized social phobia. *Journal of Abnormal Psychology, 117*(2), 278–288. http://dx.doi.org/10.1037/0021-843X.117.2.278

Hirsch, C. R., Krahé, C., Whyte, J., Loizou, S., Bridge, L., Norton, S., & Mathews, A. (2018). Interpretation training to target repetitive negative thinking in generalized anxiety disorder and depression. *Journal of Consulting and Clinical Psychology, 86*, 1017–1030. http://dx.doi.org/10.1037/ccp0000310

Hirsch, C. R., Meeten, F., Krahé, C., & Reeder, C. (2016). Resolving ambiguity in emotional disorders: The nature and role of interpretation biases. *Annual Review of Clinical Psychology, 12*(1), 281–305. http://dx.doi.org/10.1146/annurev-clinpsy-021815-093436

Hofmann, S. G. (2014). Interpersonal emotion regulation model of mood and anxiety disorders. *Cognitive Therapy and Research, 38*(5), 483–492. http://dx.doi.org/10.1007/s10608-014-9620-1

Houben, M., Van Den Noortgate, W., & Kuppens, P. (2015). The relation between short-term emotion dynamics and psychological well-being: A meta-analysis. *Psychological Bulletin, 141*, 901–930. http://dx.doi.org/10.1037/a0038822

Ingram, R. E. (1984). Toward an information-processing analysis of depression. *Cognitive Therapy and Research, 8*(5), 443–477. http://dx.doi.org/10.1007/BF01173284

Joormann, J. (2010). Cognitive inhibition and emotion regulation in depression. *Current Directions in Psychological Science, 19*(3), 161–166. http://dx.doi.org/10.1177/0963721410370293

Joormann, J., & Stanton, C. H. (2016). Examining emotion regulation in depression: A review and future directions. *Behaviour Research and Therapy, 86*, 35–49. http://dx.doi.org/10.1016/j.brat.2016.07.007

Joormann, J., & Vanderlind, W. M. (2014). Emotion regulation in depression: The role of biased cognition and reduced cognitive control. *Clinical Psychological Science, 2*(4), 402–421. http://dx.doi.org/10.1177/2167702614536163

Joormann, J., Waugh, C. E., & Gotlib, I. H. (2015). Cognitive bias modification for interpretation in major depression: Effects on memory and stress reactivity. *Clinical Psychological Science, 3*(1), 126–139. http://dx.doi.org/10.1177/2167702614560748

Joormann, J., Yoon, K. L., & Zetsche, U. (2007). Cognitive inhibition in depression. *Applied and Preventive Psychology, 12*(3), 128–139. http://dx.doi.org/10.1016/j.appsy.2007.09.002

Kashdan, T. B., & Rottenberg, J. (2010). Psychological flexibility as a fundamental aspect of health. *Clinical Psychology Review, 30*(7), 865–878. http://dx.doi.org/10.1016/j.cpr.2010.03.001

Koster, E. H. W., De Lissnyder, E., Derakshan, N., & De Raedt, R. (2011). Understanding depressive rumination from a cognitive science perspective: The impaired disengagement hypothesis. *Clinical Psychology Review, 31*(1), 138–145. http://dx.doi.org/10.1016/j.cpr.2010.08.005

Krahé, C., Whyte, J., Bridge, L., Loizou, S., & Hirsch, C. R. (2019). Are different forms of repetitive negative thinking associated with interpretation bias in generalized anxiety disorder and depression? *Clinical Psychological Science, 7*(5), 969–981. http://dx.doi.org/10.1177/2167702619851808

Kuppens, P., & Verduyn, P. (2017). Emotion dynamics. *Current Opinion in Psychology, 17*, 22–26. http://dx.doi.org/10.1016/j.copsyc.2017.06.004

Lau, J. F., Shariff, R., & Meehan, A. (2021). Are biased interpretations of ambiguous social and non-social situations a precursor, consequence or maintenance factor of youth loneliness? *Behaviour Research and Therapy, 140*, 103829. http://dx.doi.org/10.1016/j.brat.2021.103829

LeMoult, J., & Gotlib, I. H. (2019). Depression: A cognitive perspective. *Clinical Psychology Review, 69*, 51–66. http://dx.doi.org/10.1016/j.cpr.2018.06.008

LeMoult, J., Kircanski, K., Prasad, G., & Gotlib, I. H. (2017). Negative self-referential processing predicts the recurrence of major depressive episodes. *Clinical Psychological Science, 5*(1), 174–181. http://dx.doi.org/10.1177/2167702616654898

Leung, C. J., Yiend, J., & Lee, T. M. C. (2022). The relationship between attention, interpretation, and memory bias during facial perception in social anxiety. *Behavior Therapy, 53*(4), 701–713. http://dx.doi.org/10.1016/j.beth.2022.01.011

Liu, R. T., & Alloy, L. B. (2010). Stress generation in depression: A systematic review of the empirical literature and recommendations for future study. *Clinical Psychology Review, 30*(5), 582–593. http://dx.doi.org/10.1016/j.cpr.2010.04.010

Lorenzo-Luaces, L., Peipert, A., De Jesús Romero, R., Rutter, L. A., & Rodriguez-Quintana, N. (2021). Personalized medicine and cognitive behavioral therapies for depression: Small effects, big problems, and bigger data. *International Journal of Cognitive Therapy, 14*(1), 59–85. http://dx.doi.org/10.1007/s41811-020-00094-3

MacLeod, C., & Mathews, A. (2012). Cognitive bias modification approaches to anxiety. *Annual Review of Clinical Psychology, 8*(1), 189–217. http://dx.doi.org/10.1146/annurev-clinpsy-032511-143052

Marroquín, B. (2011). Interpersonal emotion regulation as a mechanism of social support in depression. *Clinical Psychology Review*, *31*(8), 1276–1290. http://dx.doi.org/10.1016/j.cpr.2011.09.005

Matt, G. E., Vazquez, C., & Campbell, W. K. (1992). Mood-congruent recall of affectively toned stimuli—A meta-analytic review. *Clinical Psychology Review*, *12*(2), 227–255. http://dx.doi.org/10.1016/0272-7358(92)90116-P

Mehu, M., & Scherer, K. R. (2015). The appraisal bias model of cognitive vulnerability to depression. *Emotion Review*, *7*(3), 272–279. http://dx.doi.org/10.1177/1754073915575406

Menne-Lothmann, C., Viechtbauer, W., Höhn, P., Kasanova, Z., Haller, S. P., Drukker, M., van Os, J., Wichers, M., & Lau, J. Y. F. (2014). How to boost positive interpretations? A meta-analysis of the effectiveness of cognitive bias modification for interpretation. *PLoS One*, *9*(6), e100925. http://dx.doi.org/10.1371/journal.pone.0100925

Mitte, K. (2008). Memory bias for threatening information in anxiety and anxiety disorders: A meta-analytic review. *Psychological Bulletin*, *134*(6), 886–911. http://dx.doi.org/10.1037/a0013343

Mor, N., Hertel, P., Ngo, T. A., Shachar, T., & Redak, S. (2014). Interpretation bias characterizes trait rumination. *Journal of Behavior Therapy and Experimental Psychiatry*, *45*(1), 67–73. http://dx.doi.org/10.1016/j.jbtep.2013.08.002

Moran, T. P. (2016). Anxiety and working memory capacity: A meta-analysis and narrative review. *Psychological Bulletin*, *142*(8), 831–864. http://dx.doi.org/10.1037/bul0000051

Normansell, K. M., & Wisco, B. E. (2017). Negative interpretation bias as a mechanism of the relationship between rejection sensitivity and depressive symptoms. *Cognition and Emotion*, *31*(5), 950–962. http://dx.doi.org/10.1080/02699931.2016.1185395

Peckham, A. D., McHugh, R. K., & Otto, M. W. (2010). A meta-analysis of the magnitude of biased attention in depression. *Depression and Anxiety*, *27*(12), 1135–1142. https://doi.org/10.1002/da.20755

Pergamin-Hight, L., Naim, R., Bakermans-Kranenburg, M. J., van Ijzendoorn, M. H., & Bar-Haim, Y. (2015). Content specificity of attention bias to threat in anxiety disorders: A meta-analysis. *Clinical Psychology Review*, *35*, 10–18. http://dx.doi.org/10.1016/j.cpr.2014.10.005

Puccetti, N. A., Villano, W. J., Stamatis, C. A., Hall, K. A., Torrez, V. F., Neta, M., Timpano, K. R., & Heller, A. S. (2023). Negative interpretation bias connects to real-world daily affect: A multistudy approach. *Journal of Experimental Psychology: General*, *152*(6), 1690–1704. http://dx.doi.org/10.1037/xge0001351

Rappaport, L. M., Moskowitz, D. S., & D'Antono, B. (2017). Depression symptoms moderate the association between emotion and communal behavior. *Journal of Counseling Psychology*, *64*(3), 269–279. http://dx.doi.org/10.1037/cou0000194

Rogers, C. R. (1951). *Client-centered therapy: Its current practice, implications, and theory, with chapters.* Houghton Mifflin.

Romano, M., Moscovitch, D. A., Saini, P., & Huppert, J. D. (2020). The effects of positive interpretation bias on cognitive reappraisal and social performance: Implications for social anxiety disorder. *Behaviour Research and Therapy*, *131*, 103651. http://dx.doi.org/10.1016/j.brat.2020.103651

Sanchez, A., Everaert, J., De Putter, L. M. S., Mueller, S. C., & Koster, E. H. W. (2015). Life is … great! Emotional attention during instructed and uninstructed ambiguity resolution in relation to depressive symptoms. *Biological Psychology*, *109*, 67–72. http://dx.doi.org/10.1016/j.biopsycho.2015.04.007

Sanchez-Lopez, A., Everaert, J., Van Put, J., De Raedt, R., & Koster, E. H. W. (2019). Eye-gaze contingent attention training (ECAT): Examining the causal role of attention regulation in reappraisal and rumination. *Biological Psychology*, *142*, 116–125. http://dx.doi.org/10.1016/j.biopsycho.2019.01.017

Santini, Z. I., Koyanagi, A., Tyrovolas, S., Mason, C., & Haro, J. M. (2015). The association between social relationships and depression: A systematic review. *Journal of Affective Disorders*, *175*, 53–65. http://dx.doi.org/10.1016/j.jad.2014.12.049

Shi, R., Sharpe, L., & Abbott, M. (2019). A meta-analysis of the relationship between anxiety and attentional control. *Clinical Psychology Review*, *72*, 101754. http://dx.doi.org/10.1016/j.cpr.2019.101754

Songco, A., Booth, C., Spiegler, O., Parsons, S., & Fox, E. (2020). Anxiety and depressive symptom trajectories in adolescence and the co-occurring development of cognitive biases: Evidence from the CogBIAS longitudinal study. *Journal of Abnormal Child Psychology*, *48*(12), 1617–1633. http://dx.doi.org/10.1007/s10802-020-00694-9

Stange, J. P., Alloy, L. B., & Fresco, D. M. (2017). Inflexibility as a vulnerability to depression: A systematic qualitative review. *Clinical Psychology: Science and Practice*, *24*(3), 245–276. http://dx.doi.org/10.1037/h0101744

Uliaszek, A. A., Zinbarg, R. E., Mineka, S., Craske, M. G., Griffith, J. W., Sutton, J. M., Epstein, A., & Hammen, C. (2012). A longitudinal examination of stress generation in depressive and anxiety disorders. *Journal of Abnormal Psychology*, *121*(1), 4–15. http://dx.doi.org/10.1037/a0025835

Van Bockstaele, B., Verschuere, B., Tibboel, H., De Houwer, J., Crombez, G., & Koster, E. H. W. (2014). A review of current evidence for the causal impact of attentional bias on fear and anxiety. *Psychological Bulletin*, *140*(3), 682–721. http://dx.doi.org/10.1037/a0034834

Vanderlind, W. M., Millgram, Y., Baskin-Sommers, A. R., Clark, M. S., & Joormann, J. (2020). Understanding positive emotion deficits in depression: From emotion preferences to emotion regulation. *Clinical Psychology Review, 76*, 101826. http://dx.doi.org/10.1016/j.cpr.2020.101826

Watkins, P. C. (2002). Implicit memory bias in depression. *Cognition & Emotion, 16*(3), 381–402. http://dx.doi.org/10.1080/02699930143000536

Wenzlaff, R. M., & Bates, D. E. (1998). Unmasking a cognitive vulnerability to depression: How lapses in mental control reveal depressive thinking. *Journal of Personality and Social Psychology, 75*(6), 1559–1571. http://dx.doi.org/10.1037/0022-3514.75.6.1559

White, L. K., Suway, J. G., Pine, D. S., Bar-Haim, Y., & Fox, N. A. (2011). Cascading effects: The influence of attention bias to threat on the interpretation of ambiguous information. *Behaviour Research and Therapy, 49*(4), 244–251. https://doi.org/10.1016/j.brat.2011.01.004

Williams, J. M. G., Barnhofer, T., Crane, C., Hermans, D., Raes, F., Watkins, E., & Dalgleish, T. (2007). Autobiographical memory specificity and emotional disorder. *Psychological Bulletin, 133*(1), 122–148. http://dx.doi.org/10.1037/0033-2909.133.1.122

Williams, J. M. G., Watts, F. N., MacLeod, C., & Mathews, A. (1997). *Cognitive psychology and emotional disorders* (Vol. 2). Wiley.

Winer, E. S., & Salem, T. (2016). Reward devaluation: Dot-probe meta-analytic evidence of avoidance of positive information in depressed persons. *Psychological Bulletin, 142*(1), 18–78. http://dx.doi.org/10.1037/bul0000022

Wisco, B. E., Gilbert, K. E., & Marroquín, B. (2014). Maladaptive processing of maladaptive content: Rumination as a mechanism linking cognitive biases to depressive symptoms. *Journal of Experimental Psychopathology, 5*(3), 329–350. http://dx.doi.org/10.5127/jep.038213

Wittenborn, A. K., Rahmandad, H., Rick, J., & Hosseinichimeh, N. (2016). Depression as a systemic syndrome: Mapping the feedback loops of major depressive disorder. *Psychological Medicine, 46*(3), 551–562. http://dx.doi.org/10.1017/s0033291715002044

Wright, A. G., Pincus, A., & Hopwood, C. (2020). Contemporary integrative interpersonal theory: Integrating structure, dynamics, temporal scale, and levels of analysis. PsyArXiv https://doi.org/10.31234/osf.io/fknc8

Yeager, D. S., Bryan, C. J., Gross, J. J., Murray, J. S., Krettek Cobb, D., Santos, P. H. F., Gravelding, H., Johnson, M., & Jamieson, J. P. (2022). A synergistic mindsets intervention protects adolescents from stress. *Nature, 607*(7919), 512–520. http://dx.doi.org/10.1038/s41586-022-04907-7

3

Neural Correlates of Psychopathology: Implications for the Processing of Persuasive Health Messages

Caroline Ostrand and Monica Luciana
University of Minnesota

One of the challenges faced when designing behavioral health interventions, including persuasive health messages, is that not everyone will respond to an intervention in the same way. While environmental factors such as access to services or community support contribute to this variability, a great deal of research also implicates factors at the individual level. The sophisticated models resulting from such research suggest that psychological factors, including motivation, attitudes, social influence, and behavioral skills of the individual or population of interest, influence whether an individual engages in sustained behavioral change (Yzer, 2012). Given the importance of cognitive and motivational processes across many of these models, there has been a growing interest in the use of cognitive and affective neuroscience, fields of inquiry that focus on neural mechanisms that contribute to mental and behavioral processes, to investigate brain systems that are involved in health-related behaviors and persuasion (Cacioppo et al., 2018; Cascio et al., 2013). This interdisciplinary approach is known as communication neuroscience. By modeling neural mechanisms influencing human decision-making, this field has promise to provide new insights into layers of processing obscured with other forms of measurement. Critically, an integrated understanding of these mechanisms may inform the development of novel interventions that specifically target neural mechanisms to facilitate behavioral change. Just as neuroscientific approaches have already supported rapid developments in diverse fields such as economics (Camerer et al., 2005), marketing (Morin, 2011), and education (Ansari et al., 2012), it is useful to consider how this interdisciplinary approach may also inform the design of persuasive health messages.

Communication neuroscience may be particularly useful when tailoring messages to match differences in cognitive and affective processing of individuals with various conditions, including psychopathology. Psychopathology refers to a spectrum of psychological symptoms that cause distress and interfere with adaptive functioning (American Psychiatric Association & American Psychiatric Association DSM-5 Task Force, 2013). The goals of clinical scientists and practitioners who study and treat these symptoms have interestingly paralleled, if not intersected with, that of health communication given their intent to understand underlying mechanisms of cognition, emotion, and maladaptive behavior that can be targeted through interventions (Beck, 2005). There have been numerous theories regarding causal factors influencing psychological symptoms, including the functional perspective of psychodynamic theorists, behavioral theories which neglected any cognitive process at all, the cognitive approach, which resulted in therapeutic models that targeted information processing biases, and expansions of these models that include affective and motivational processes as important sources of influence. While neurobiological theories of psychopathology have been around for centuries, dating

The Handbook of Mental Health Communication, First Edition.
Edited by Marco C. Yzer and Jason T. Siegel.

back to conceptualizations of ancient philosophers (Ahonen, 2019), increasingly sophisticated technologies have significantly contributed to our understanding of how individual variations in neural circuitry at structural and functional levels may play a role in the development and maintenance of psychopathology (Cuthbert & Insel, 2013). Because these differences in neural circuitry underpin cognitive and affective processes involved in how information is perceived, evaluated, and responded to, they are crucial to consider as mechanistic targets of behavioral interventions, including persuasive messaging.

Accordingly, understanding and applying neuroscientific approaches to health messaging necessarily require integration across neuroscientific, clinical, and communication fields of inquiry (Cacioppo et al., 2018). Because assessments of neural structure and function require access to special equipment, are costly, and result in data that may be difficult to analyze and interpret, some may be reticent to embrace this methodology. However, the value of an interdisciplinary approach cannot be understated given an urgent need to use every tool available to support the health of individuals with psychopathology. The health burden in this population is devastating. A meta-analysis conducted in 2015 estimated that individuals with mental health disorders have a more than two times greater rate of mortality, with 10 years of potential life lost (Walker et al., 2015). Although a relatively small proportion of such premature mortality is due to unnatural causes such as suicide, more often the underlying cause is physical illness. Individuals with mental health disorders have an estimated 40% greater risk of developing cardiac, metabolic, or vascular conditions compared to individuals without mental health disorders. Thus, not only do individuals with mental health conditions face greater mortality, but they may also experience a poorer quality of life. If a neuroscientific approach can contribute to interventions that improve the health and well-being of those with psychopathology, the challenges of adopting these methods are clearly outweighed by the potential benefits.

Because the field's understanding of the neural correlates of effective health messaging is in a nascent stage (Cacioppo et al., 2018), how information may be perceived and neurally processed in ways that are distinct in individuals with psychopathology will require some speculation. The goals of this chapter, then, are to focus on findings from cognitive neuroscience, affective neuroscience, and clinical psychology regarding neural substrates of psychopathology and to consider possible ways in which these findings may be implicated in health messaging. An additional and crucial aspect of this discussion will be to review potential ethical implications of using neuroscience to study and supplement persuasive messaging. To accomplish these goals, the chapter is divided into three sections. In the first section, we review basic neural structures and systems involved in behavior, with a focus on circuitry implicated in the detection of salience and subsequent executive control. Next, we review neural processes implicated in persuasive health messaging. Finally, we consider how these systems may structurally or functionally vary in individuals with psychopathology and how these differences may be applied to the design of health messages Although these sections will not, by any means, provide an all-encompassing account of how brain–behavior associations may be relevant to health messaging in general or when targeted toward individuals with psychopathology, the intent is to provide a foundation for future research and continued discourse on this topic.

A Primer on Basic Neural Systems of Cognition, Affect, and Behavior

Before considering what is known about neural circuitry involved in messaging and psychopathology, it is useful to review neural systems involved in cognition and behavior at a general level. The human brain is a remarkable organ, with greater flexibility and efficiency than any machine built to date. This capacity for flexible, efficient cognition is supported by neural circuits spanning subcortical and cortical brain structures, which integrate information processed in functionally distinct brain regions via long-range neural connections (Park & Friston, 2013). By integrating information across neural processors specialized for handling the relevant computations, the brain extracts meaning from an individual's experiences to support ongoing behavior (Churchland & Sejnowski, 1992). Some of these processes are primarily sensory in nature and involve relays from sensory organs such as the eyes, ears, and skin to the brain's primary sensory cortices, situated in the occipital, temporal, and parietal lobes of the cortex These regions extract and synthesize perceptions of visual (eyes), auditory (ears), and kinesthetic (skin/touch) information, respectively, by passing information through specialized neuronal assemblies within the brain's cortex.

These information relays proceed in a hierarchical manner from primary sensory regions, where basic features are perceived, to higher level association regions that allow information from disparate sources to be integrated. Examples of higher-level association regions include the anterior temporal lobe as well as regions of the prefrontal cortex (PFC), both of which participate in abstract levels of human reasoning. Subcortical brain structures allow us to experience emotions, to encode memories, and to maintain appropriate levels of arousal. Accordingly, they are also crucially involved in automatic processing of stimulus-based and interoceptive information (MacLean, 1955). Subcortical structures that are particularly relevant to this discussion include the amygdala, which is involved in stimulus detection and the assessment of stimulus salience (LeDoux, 2007), the hippocampus, which is involved in memory encoding and retrieval, and the striatum of the basal ganglia, which is heavily implicated in reward learning, cognitive flexibility, and motivation (Schultz, 2016).

As information is extracted and integrated within the cortex, it is infused with relevance based on one's emotional state and prior experience. These perceptions and interpretations influence motor systems to guide the nature of immediate or more deliberate behavioral responses. Thus, sensory perceptions, attributions of stimulus salience, and arousal intersect with cognitive processes such as attention and memory to support appropriate and efficient responding to experiential provocations. These responses require an intact motor system as well as the ability to maintain, and assign meaning to relevant information with the guide of internal models of the world formed from past experiences (Kiefer & Pulvermüller, 2012) as well as consideration of future goals. Given the intricate nature of our environments as well as individual characteristics and personal histories, information processing at the neural level is understandably complex.

With the aid of neuroimaging technologies such as magnetic resonance imaging (MRI) and high density electrophysiological recordings, the cognitive and affective neuroscience fields have attempted to quantify and characterize information processing streams that contribute to discrete aspects of behavior. MRI allows the brain to be imaged structurally, functionally at rest, and functionally in response to task demands to describe brain structures and networks that are active during specific states (e.g., moods) and that participate in specific behaviors. Electrophysiology, which involves the use of scalp electrode recordings to measure patterns of electrical activity generated from neuronal assemblies, allows temporal aspects of information processing to be resolved at millisecond levels of precision. Psychophysiological measures of autonomic functions such as skin temperature and heart rate, both of which are neurally regulated, permit arousal levels to be discerned. Based on a plethora of research gained from the use of these and other techniques, the field has advanced from a focus on discrete brain regions and their associated behavioral functions to a network-based approach that emphasizes functional connections and interactions among spatially distinct cortical and subcortical neural regions (Park & Friston, 2013).

Although many neural networks have been described, three are often emphasized in relation to higher level aspects of behavior: the default mode network (DMN), the executive control network, and the salience network. The DMN is a set of brain regions co-activated when individuals are at rest and not engaged in a demanding task. Activity in this network is thought to represent a baseline state of cognition (Raichle et al., 2001). The core nodes, or points of connection, within this network include the angular gyrus, posteromedial cortex, inferior frontal gyrus, anterolateral middle temporal cortex, and medial prefrontal cortex (mPFC). This network supports dynamic sense-making through abstract thought and reflection and thus appears crucial for the updating of internal mental models of the self and world (Yeshurun et al., 2021). The second major network is the executive control network. Unlike the DMN, the executive control network is task-positive, meaning it is activated while an individual is engaged in attentionally demanding tasks (Fox et al., 2005). Although the regions implicated in this network vary slightly depending on method of measurement, they generally include the dorsolateral, dorsomedial, and ventromedial prefrontal cortices as well as the lateral parietal cortices (Seeley et al., 2007). This network is involved in cognitive processes required for successful goal-directed behavior including working memory and response selection. The last major network is the salience network, with core nodes including the anterior insula, amygdala, and dorsal anterior cingulate cortices (ACCs). As its name suggests, this network is involved in attending to the salience, or relevance, of internal and external stimuli. The salience network is also involved in recruiting other brain regions when a situation is deemed relevant, switching neural activation between the default mode and executive networks accordingly (Goulden et al., 2014). Together, these three networks represent a number of neural processes involved in managing behavior in response to complex environmental demands.

Neural Correlates of Persuasive Health Messaging

What, then, is known about how these processes and networks are implicated in health messaging? It has only been in the past 15 years that increasing access to technology paired with a desire to further improve the explanatory power of extant models motivated the use of tools from neuroscience to study these processes. Mirroring the general trend across scientific disciplines that were beginning to study the intricate biological mechanisms influencing cognition at a subconscious level, one of the goals of this field has been to extend the boundaries of measurement by evaluating layers of processing unobtainable by self-report or behavioral measures. The application of neuroscience to study mechanisms underpinning health messaging is known as communication neuroscience (Falk, 2012), a field that ultimately draws from diverse disciplines including psychology, neuroscience, economics, and communication to explicate the neurobiological mechanisms influencing message processing.

A common experimental paradigm applied within communication neuroscience has been to record research participants' brain activity as they view messages presented in an MRI scanner. Researchers have then assessed variations in neural activation that are associated with message features and individual characteristics. The factors addressed have often been selected based on those identified by theoretical models, which are then worked into the experimental design (messages presented or sample recruited). These factors include message sensational value (a metric of sensory intensity), argument strength, gain and loss framing, tailored messaging, and risk level of a sample (Langleben et al., 2009; Vezich et al., 2017). In addition to studying variations in brain activity during message processing, neural activation has also been tested as a predictor of relevant outcomes, including perceived message effectiveness (Kranzler et al., 2019) and actual behavioral change captured by longitudinal studies (Falk et al., 2015). Across these diverse studies, numerous brain regions have been implicated in different aspects of message processing. These include primary sensory regions such as the occipital lobe, which mediates aspects of vision, as well as cortical association regions in the inferior parietal lobule, the frontal gyrus, temporal lobe, lingual gyrus, medial and lateral prefrontal cortices (mPFC/lPFC), precuneus, insula, and the ACC. Activity within subcortical structures such as the amygdala also appears to be involved in the processing of message content (Falk et al., 2011; Kang et al., 2019; Langleben et al., 2009; Ramsay et al., 2013; Vezich et al., 2017; Wang et al., 2013; Weber et al., 2015). At a network level, these patterns indicate that brain networks involved in top-down cognitive control, including default mode, executive, and salience networks, are implicated in the processing of persuasive messages. The variety of brain regions implicated at a general level across these studies is not surprising, given that persuasive messaging is a complex phenomenon. However, considering these brain regions in aggregate, removed from their experimental context, makes it difficult to interpret their functional roles. Thus, we now consider the roles of these neural regions in the context of some of the conceptual questions addressed by this literature.

One of the major challenges faced by communication neuroscience is how to design messages that leverage limited neural resources so that a relevant message is coded as meaningful and is kept in mind. This can be done by attempting to capture attention, a cognitive process that filters and selects which information is computationally prioritized within neural processing streams (Knudsen, 2007). Attention is guided by the salience of low level sensory or affective features as well as person-specific goals and experiences (Buschman & Miller, 2007). In the context of persuasive messaging, researchers have been interested in measuring how message conditions that influence attention can support neural processes that filter and integrate complex sensory information into meaningful representations, which can then influence behavior change.

In one of the first studies to directly test this dynamic using neuroimaging, Langleben et al. (2009) measured brain activity while participants viewed anti-tobacco public service announcements (PSAs) that varied in their level of message sensational value, which in this study involved variations in visual and auditory complexity. They found that PSAs with lower sensational value (e.g., lower intensity of auditory and visual message features) recruited prefrontal, temporal, and posterior parietal cortices to a greater degree than those with higher sensational value, which primarily recruited the occipital lobe and parahippocampus. PSAs with low sensational value were also remembered better by this sample, suggesting that health messages that minimize demands on brain regions involved in low-level sensory processing and optimally engage brain regions involved in effortful cognition (e.g., the executive network) may lead to improved memory for message content.

However, this relationship appears to be moderated by factors that influence attention via alternative routes, including argument strength and individual characteristics (Ramsay et al., 2013; Wang et al., 2013; Weber et al., 2015). In a study that addressed attentional demands and message strength concurrently, Wang et al. (2013) found an interaction effect such that messages with high sensational value were effective when they also contained strong arguments. Moreover, this interaction between sensational value and argument strength was associated with neural differences including altered activation of the inferior parietal lobule, inferior frontal gyrus, fusiform gyrus, dorsal mPFC (dmPFC) and precuneus, several of which are regions involved in the DMN. Because lower dmPFC activity was associated with behavioral change one month later, and because the dmPFC is involved in the processing of personally relevant cognitive processes (Lieberman et al., 2019), the authors hypothesized that messages that reduce self-reflective processing and enhance attention directed toward external stimuli may lead to desirable longer-term outcomes. These findings reflect that the intensity of message features, as well as what these features represent (which determines which higher level cognitive processes are recruited) interact to engage differential neural systems, which ultimately influence the effectiveness of these messages.

Through various paradigms that have assessed which brain areas are involved in the processing of messages that are considered to be effective, structures within the salience, default mode, and executive networks routinely implicated (Falk & Scholz, 2018; Jovanova et al., 2022; Ramsay et al., 2013). A major focus of this research has been on the role of the mPFC, a core structure that participates in the DMN, thought to be involved in processes such as subjective valuation of information, reinforcement learning, expectancy violation, and reflections on self and others (Euston et al., 2012). In a clever study conducted by Falk et al. (2011), activity in the mPFC was measured in individuals who engaged in significant smoking but with a desire to quit as they viewed ads designed to help individuals stop smoking. Activation of the ventral portion of the mPFC significantly predicted expired carbon monoxide at follow-up. Moreover, including activation of the mPFC explained an additional 20% of the variance in this index compared to models that only included self-report. The finding that activation of the mPFC during message processing is a significant predictor of behavior change has been corroborated across a number of other studies with diverse samples and message stimuli (Cooper et al., 2018; Doré et al., 2019a; Doré et al., 2019b; Falk et al., 2010, 2012). Although there has been some disagreement as to the precise function this region serves in the message communication context, it is generally thought to be involved in value-based decision-making, such that the subjective valuation of message content via computations in the ventromedial PFC (vmPFC) influences deliberation and one's motivation to engage in behavior change (Falk & Scholz, 2018).

Consistent with the expectation that effective message processing and behavioral activation likely involve executive functions, regions implicated in the executive network appear to work alongside default mode structures as well as structures involved in affective processes (i.e., fear and reward) to influence message persuasiveness. Using functional connectivity analyses to measure co-activation of brain regions while adolescent participants viewed anti-drug PSAs with strong and weak arguments, Ramsay et al. (2013) found that network activation was associated with the strength of the argument presented. Namely, they observed that strongly persuasive PSAs were associated with greater arousal-related activity in the lateral PFC, as well as stronger co-activation between the lateral PFC and mPFC and the amygdala. Because PSAs with pre-rated stronger arguments were rated as more convincing, these findings provide evidence that the lateral PFC is recruited during processing of health messaging, particularly those that require an evaluative judgment regarding the message argument. This study also highlights the critical role of network integration during message processing, a role that has also been corroborated by Jovanova et al. (2022). Using between-person analyses of functional connectivity patterns while participants were viewing persuasive messages in a MRI scanner, they found that individuals with greater integration of the salience and default mode networks were more receptive to messages, and that activity of the default and salience networks were separately associated with behavioral outcomes. Although this study did not evaluate connectivity related to the executive network, it reflects potentially different functional roles of integrated versus isolated networks during message processing.

There are several key takeaways from these studies. The first is that numerous brain structures are involved in message processing. Given the observation that different networks and regions are involved across diverse experimental designs, this suggests that the neural mechanisms involved in message processing need to be considered relative to the type of persuasive technique being employed. Thus, their functional roles can be best understood when theory and experimental design are considered together with observed neural activity. The findings also highlight the importance of neural engagement beyond the recruitment of sensory structures, including involvement of salience, executive, and default mode networks. An integrated account of the role of these networks, supported by established research in basic neuroscience, is that sensory and affective features of message content elicit *attention*, which drives parallel processing of low-level stimulus content that is integrated and computed at higher levels by the *default and executive networks*. Importantly, the *relevance of the message content* is monitored by the salience network, which acts as a toggle to support differential engagement of executive and default systems.

Here, we may speculate on what might happen if attention is dysregulated, if one has poor levels of executive control, and/or if one is overly aroused or emotionally biased such that salience is misattributed or unduly attributed, to presented cues. While these scenarios are distinct from one another, all are likely to result in a mismatch between what is intended to be conveyed by aspects of a message's content and the actual perceptions of content based on the recipient's characteristics. For example, if a message is intended to have low sensational value but is instead perceived as having higher sensational value, it is, at a low level of processing, less likely to be remembered due to the relative lack of engagement of the executive control network. Similarly, if the salience network is underengaged, then higher-level brain regions that would otherwise be recruited to evaluate the message and its relevance in detail may be underactivated, resulting in lack of engagement with the content. As we will next describe, dysregulations of this type may be common in psychopathology as general features of illness, leading to difficulties in appropriately calibrating message content in a way that aligns well with characteristics of the intended audience.

The Structure and Neural Correlates of Psychopathology

It is a challenge to succinctly summarize all neural correlates of psychopathology, as the symptoms experienced by those with mental health conditions are diverse and implicate numerous neural regions and circuits. Accordingly, we will primarily focus on patterns that either transcend or cross diagnostic boundaries. In addition to being parsimonious, this approach coheres with recent efforts to shift away from category-based classification systems, such as the *Diagnostic and Statistical Manual of Mental Disorders*, 5th edition (DSM-5; American Psychiatric Association & American Psychiatric Association DSM-5 Task Force, 2013), toward a dimensional framework for the understanding of psychopathology that is more strongly grounded in empirical data. Rather than focusing on the types of diagnostic categories (e.g., major depressive disorder; schizophrenia) that likely come to mind when most people consider various mental health conditions, data-driven analyses of the underlying symptom structure of psychopathology suggest that psychopathology can be meaningfully described by hierarchical models that represent clusters of symptoms organized from narrow to broad levels. These models describe the structure and expression of psychopathology through fewer overarching factors that are conceptualized as dimensions rather than categories. At the narrowest level, there are the symptoms themselves (e.g., poor sleep quality, low mood, inattention). The broadest or top level is described by an overarching factor, referred to as the p-factor, representing general psychopathology (Caspi et al., 2014; Kotov et al., 2017). Individuals with high scores on the p-factor exhibit a variety of symptoms that cut across domains of function and across disorder categories. While there is some debate about how to describe the levels that lie between symptoms and the p-factor, empirical support is strongest for the dimensions of internalizing, externalizing, and thought disorder. Internalizing encompasses distress, low mood, fear, sexual problems, and eating pathology. Externalizing encompasses substance use and antisocial behavior. Thought disorder encompasses psychotic processes traditionally ascribed to the schizophrenia spectrum (Kotov et al., 2017). Thus, within this transdiagnostic framework, psychopathology can be adequately described by one's score on a p-factor and more specifically, by one's status on dimensions of internalizing, externalizing, and thought disorder. This approach is gaining traction within the field and is poised, within the near future, to influence conceptualizations of psychopathology within clinical settings.

A different type of dimensional approach was also embraced by the National Institute of Mental Health in 2009 as part of the Research Domain Criteria (RDoC) project, a research framework rationally derived through consensus of leaders in the field. Importantly, these domains link typical as well as atypical behavior to genetic and neurobiological mechanisms (Cuthbert, 2022). Many of the RDoC domains can be further linked to those that have emerged through the empirically derived transdiagnostic framework to describe the structure of psychopathology, incorporating relevant motivational and cognitive systems that are relevant (Kotov et al., 2017; Michelini et al., 2021). For instance, internalizing symptoms involve negative valence (low mood states, anxiety, and attentional biases toward negative or threatening stimuli) as well as disordered arousal.

It is important to emphasize that a dimensional approach is inherent to both the empirical and RDoC models and that research on mental health conditions is propelling the field toward a unified neurobehaviorally guided framework for understanding the cognitive and motivational mechanisms that contribute to psychopathology, how mental health conditions are expressed in behavior and how they can be treated. Thus, it is appropriate to consider neural correlates of psychopathology at the broad general level as one level of inquiry.

Given that the p-factor represents correlations observed across symptoms and clinical interview data, there have been recent attempts to identify its genetic and neural correlates. Common mental health conditions, assessed using categorical measures, are genetically correlated (Brainstorm Consortium et al., 2018). The p-factor is associated with DNA-derived single nucleotide polymorphisms in children (Neumann et al., 2016) and shows substantial heritability in twin samples with 48–80% of the variance in the factor attributable to genetic influences. Recently, Selzam et al. (2018) applied a principal components analysis to matrices of genetic correlations between major psychiatric disorders that were estimated by multiple methods, finding strong support for a genetic p-factor. Together, these studies suggest that the transdiagnostic p-factor is genetically influenced and that this genetic influence is stable over time. Thus, although the environment also exerts a measurable effect on the expression of psychopathology, biological mechanisms appear to be important.

Consistent with this view, numerous studies of children, adolescents, and adults have linked general psychopathology, quantified through factor analytic approaches, with variations in brain structure (Opel et al., 2020; Romer et al., 2021b; Romer & Pizzagalli, 2022) and function (Elliott et al., 2018; Sprooten et al., 2017). Structural variations associated with greater general psychopathology include the finding of a thinner overall cortex (Romer et al., 2021a). Structural alterations have also been observed in cortical and subcortical brain regions implicated in affective and cognitive processes. In a meta-analysis of 193 peer-reviewed articles across major DSM-based categorically defined diagnoses, Goodkind et al. (2015) found evidence that psychopathology is broadly characterized by decreased gray matter volume in core nodes of the salience network, including the bilateral anterior insula and dorsal ACC. Using a separate, healthy sample, the authors show that decreased volumes of these regions are commonly associated with deficits in executive functioning, consistent with the expectation that alterations in the salience network disrupt the brain's ability to monitor salience and to appropriately direct higher level cognitive resources in response to personally relevant stimuli.

There is also evidence that general psychopathology is associated with *functional* alterations in major neural networks (Barch, 2017). Recent meta-analyses of task-based functional MRI studies suggest that, in adults, most major categorically defined forms of psychopathology are characterized by hypoactivation in neural networks that underpin executive control (Janiri et al., 2020). Sha et al. (2019) in a large-scale meta-analysis of three large datasets that together comprised 45,760 individuals, found that intrinsic functional connectivity (functional connectivity while at rest) both within and between the default mode, executive, and salience networks, including patterns of hyper- and hypoconnectivity, were associated with executive function decrements.

It has also been proposed that general psychopathology is associated with alterations in neural circuits involved in affective processing. In a meta-analysis of studies that compared functional activity of patients with diverse psychiatric conditions to individuals without a psychiatric diagnosis while all were engaged in emotional processing tasks, McTeague et al. (2020) found common alterations in the patients in brain regions typically involved in emotional reactivity and regulation. These included regions involved in the salience network as well as supporting structures, including the insula, ventromedial PFC, and amygdala (among others). Additional research has proposed that these alterations may be functionally integrated. Using a whole brain analysis of functional circuits in a heterogenous sample of individuals with mood and psychotic disorders, Sharma et al. (2017) assessed whether individual variations in reward sensitivity were associated with differences in neural connectivity. Multiple neural regions were identified where the multivariate pattern of connectivity was dimensionally related to reward sensitivity across clinical diagnostic categories. Specifically, reward deficits were associated with hyperconnectivity within the DMN but diminished connectivity between DMN and salience network regions. Furthermore, connectivity with the nucleus accumbens, a structure that is integrally involved in reward processing, was decoupled from DMN regions and showed increased connectivity with salience network regions. Thus, individual differences in reward and cognitive processing may be interrelated in psychopathology.

While a single, unified model of the causal structure of these patterns has not yet been offered, some have hypothesized that a common, core disruption characterizes psychopathology. For example, the triple-network model of psychopathology proposed by Menon (2011, 2019) hypothesizes alterations in the mapping of environmental salience and aberrant engagement of situation-relevant internally or externally oriented networks (default mode or executive control, respectively). This model emphasizes the crucial role of the salience network in managing diverse demands and governing adaptive allocation of cognitive resources. Because the salience network is involved in the recruitment of other networks, alterations in this network may underpin the observed differences in executive and default mode network activity in individuals with psychopathology as compared to those without such conditions. These alterations may manifest in diverse behavioral differences observed across psychiatric disorders and, with more research, may partially explain apparent behavioral deficits in executive functioning (Abramovitch et al., 2021), decision-making (Goschke, 2014), and social processing (Aldridge-Waddon et al., 2020) that are commonly observed in the context of psychopathology.

Taken together, the summarized literature highlights an empirically supported perspective on the classification of psychopathology in which the diverse set of symptoms experienced across disorders can be meaningfully considered at transdiagnostic levels. At the broadest level of this classification system, there is evidence for consistent alterations in major neural networks crucial for cognitive and affective processes including the salience, default, and executive networks. While distinctions have been observed in all three networks, alterations in salience detection, informed by brain structures involved in reward and threat processing, may underpin the aberrant engagement of cognitive functions subserved by the default mode and executive networks. Thus, this transdiagnostic model of psychopathology stresses the role of the salience network as the source of other deviations at neural and behavioral levels.

Implications for Processing of Health Messages

The next question to consider is how these patterns of neural processing shape information processing and behavior change in the context of persuasive messaging.

We suggest that salience network activity may be a key feature to consider when adapting messages to better support individuals with psychopathology. Drawing from the triple network model of psychopathology, the salience network likely underlies differences in patterns observed across other networks, including the executive and default mode networks (Menon, 2011). Because it influences activity in other networks, along with having a direct role in a variety of functions including subjective feeling states, emotional processing of extrinsic motivators, self-concept, error detection, and coordination of brain network dynamics (Uddin, 2015), the salience network may influence message processing across multiple levels. At face level, we might expect that these functions will influence how individuals respond to health messaging by influencing whether or not a massage is attended to and viewed as personally relevant, the subjective emotional experience elicited by the message, how the message content fits with prior expectations, and whether or not the message content is retained and further elaborated within executive processing streams.

As described in the section on neural correlates of message processing, neural circuitry implicated in attention and value are both crucially involved in effective message processing. How does the salience network fit within this framework? Core nodes of the salience network include several structures that have been implicated in messaging, including the insula and ACC. Moreover, the salience network is tightly connected with structures involved in the processing of reward, fear, and value, which respectively include the nucleus accumbens, amygdala, and the vmPFC. Primary features of message content may be functionally integrated across these structures to determine the salience of message features, which are computed at a basic level by subcortical structures including the amygdala and nucleus accumbens, and integrated at a cortical level by the insula, ACC, and vmPFC. Drawing from a systems neuroscience perspective, this process is not unidirectional, but rather represents a continuous hierarchical integration that may change as the content of the message is further processed. For example, the initial affective features of the message may initially be computed across these regions, which elicits elaboration of the message argument in executive networks, which may then further recruit salience and affective structures to again re-evaluate the meaning of the message in relation to the elaborated content. Thus, salience network involvement may be important across multiple stages of message processing.

It is important to note that the precise mechanistic roles that this network plays in message processing in the context of psychopathology have not been well studied. However, as indicated above, there is initial evidence for aberrations in salience network activity in psychopathology as well as integral involvement of this network in message processing. Thus, messages might be tailored to accommodate the distinct patterns of salience network activity that characterize psychopathology. To this end, we suggest two general methods that health communicators might take to optimize efficacy of health communications. The first is to attempt to alter messages in such a way that optimizes engagement of the salience network based on its level of function in a given sample. For example, for individuals with some forms of internalizing psychopathology, salience network activity may be hyperactive in relation to content involving reference to personal safety (Szeszko & Yehuda, 2019). Within these individuals, this hyperactivity may result in heightened anticipated emotional relevance, leading to poorer decision-making strategies due to ineffective engagement of executive and default networks (Schimmelpfennig et al., 2023). To avoid this outcome, health messaging could be tailored to reduce emotional salience or fear-related content to a level that allows attentional resources to be allocated and decisions to be made without triggering exaggerated emotional responses in the individual (Lerner et al., 2015). Although adapting message features in consideration of the baseline salience network activity of an individual or set of individuals has not yet been tested, one strategy that may accomplish this goal is to utilize gain and loss framed messaging (Higgins, 2000).

Alternatively, messages could be designed to recruit processes and associated neural systems that are unimpaired or even enhanced in individuals with psychopathology. This approach aligns with strength-based approaches to psychopathology treatment (Tse et al., 2016). Because it may not be possible to fully circumvent the salience network, given its near constant involvement in monitoring of the environment and internal signals, health communicators may need to consider creative solutions, such as matching message content to anticipated baseline attentional tendencies (Stephenson & Palmgreen, 2001) or even encouraging adaptive salience functioning via more involved interventions, such as interpersonal message delivery. To highlight one example of how this could be implemented, individuals with certain forms of psychopathology characterized by anhedonia or blunted reward processing may experience hyperresponsivity of the salience network at rest and hyporesponsivity in the presence of positive stimuli (Pisoni et al., 2021). While these individuals may not be responsive to messages designed to elicit attention via positive motivation, they may be receptive to messages that engage neural resources through alternative processing streams, such as argument strength (logical reasoning). While further research is needed, those who design messages may also consider drawing from treatment techniques applied in individuals with psychopathology, such as behavioral activation and motivational interviewing (Dimidjian et al., 2011; Lee & Griva, 2015). These techniques support behavioral change through a recalibration of reward and salience by using strategies that meet clients where they are in terms of their levels of engagement and motivation.

Together, these examples suggest opportunities for adapting messages in consideration of patterns of activity in the salience network in individuals with psychopathology. These include techniques that design messages to align with salience network activation as well as those that rely more heavily on alternative routes of processing. Although speculative, these examples illustrate how techniques from clinical neuroscience and communication neuroscience can be integrated and applied. This integrative framework may be useful when designing research that tests these concepts and that highlights both strengths and weaknesses in processing in individuals with psychopathology.

Summary and Open Questions

This chapter presents a review of the transdiagnostic neural correlates of psychopathology, highlighting how central disruptions in the salience network may results in broader functional differences across networks implicated in cognition and affect, including the default mode and executive networks. Because these networks are also implicated in processing of persuasive health messages, neural correlates of psychopathology may contribute to unique patterns of engagement with persuasive messages in this population. Such patterns of engagement may be characterized by distinctions in attention, subjective valuation, logical reasoning, and social or self-referencing during message processing. Although further research is needed to test how messages can be tailored to unique patterns in cognitive control networks, we speculate on potential directions for future investigation. These include designing messages to match/target salience network functioning or circumvent reliance on this network by engaging alternative modes of processing.

Although the practical utility of a neurobiological approach to psychopathology has not yet been realized in the context of persuasive health messaging, we believe considering these relationships will generate expansive opportunities for interventions that have promise to alleviate the health burden in individuals with mental health conditions. We suggest major directions for future research below.

Development of an Integrated Model of Neural Circuits Involved in Persuasive Messaging

Research in communication neuroscience has primarily focused on discrete brain structures as opposed to networks implicated in effective message processing. Because individual structures may participate in multiple networks depending on task demand/cognitive context, it is crucial to develop models of networks involved in persuasion based on empirical study of these networks. Future research may consider experimentally manipulating factors of persuasive messaging in order to test functional dynamics of neural circuits through carefully controlled experiments. Such research may provide greater insight into the distinct neural components involved in persuasion, how they are integrated across networks, and how messages can be manipulated in order to engage discrete brain networks. Such knowledge will support inferences that can be made when neural profiles of unique populations, such as those with psychopathology.

Standardize Methods of Identifying/Defining Psychopathology

While the dimensional approach to psychopathology presented here is empirically supported, it is not the primary method for diagnosis in clinical settings. Future research will need to consider how neural correlates of psychopathology are represented across factor levels, including the p-factor and subdomains of internalizing and externalizing. It will be especially important to consider how levels of severity may influence patterns of neural processing, which we did not consider in this chapter. Such research may inform decisions around how modified message structures might be applied to various target samples.

Direct Evaluation of Network Activity Patterns During Message Processing in Individuals with Psychopathology

As we have emphasized throughout this chapter, there has yet to be research directly evaluating salience and other network activity in individuals with general psychopathology in the context of persuasive messaging. Further research directly testing the hypotheses presented in this chapter will be crucial. It is possible that the functional relevance of neural correlates are context-specific, meaning that functional associations observed in one context (neural correlates observed at rest) do not translate to other contexts (neural correlates while processing a message). It is possible that individuals with psychopathology engage with health messaging through alternative modes of processing not considered in this chapter or even that neural activity is not actually engaged differently in this population during message processing. These alternative possibilities require empirical testing.

Develop Techniques for Tailored Messages Based on Personalized Neural Profiles

If it is determined that the triple network model of psychopathology is relevant to persuasive messaging, techniques for adapting messages to accommodate individual differences will need to be explored. Developing these techniques may require significant effort and creativity. Novel approaches may not only incorporate variations in message content but also their modes of delivery. Interdisciplinary work that capitalizes on techniques established across other fields, including neuroeducation, neuroeconomics, and clinical psychology may all provide opportunities to explore novel strategies that are neuroscience based and clinically informed.

Test the Influence of Network Differences During Later Stages of Behavior Change

Much of the research in communication neuroscience has evaluated brain activity during immediate processing of a persuasive message. However, differences in neural circuitry likely influence later stages of behavior change (initiating a health behavior, maintaining the health behavior, seeking out additional, related information). In the context of psychopathology, it is likely that trait-based neural differences also influence behavior change beyond perception and evaluation of a given message, and so the role of these neural correlates should be considered across multiple stages. This work will require investment in longitudinal studies.

Evaluate Ethical Implications of a Communications Neuroscience Approach

While a transdiagnostic, neuroscientific framework of psychopathology may provide insight into hidden layers of processing that may inform the design of health messages, there are several ethical considerations. One question to ask is how a neuroscientific perspective of psychopathology may shape public perceptions of causal mechanisms that underpin health related decision making. When viewed out of context of psychological content (e.g., attitudes, memories) and environmental factors (access to financial or medical resources, social institutions, etc.), neuroscience-based explanations could contribute to overattributions of blame to individual variations in neurobiology. Viewed out of the context of life history and personal values, a focus on such variations may objectify and dehumanize individuals, reducing them to their component parts (neural circuitry). Such attitudes may lead some to justify tactics that are inherently manipulative, such as trying to influence behavior by appealing to emotions that are not central to the specific health-related argument (Rossi & Yudell, 2012). Techniques of persuasion that appeal to claims of faulty neural circuitry may cause unintended harms. As such, applications of a neuroscientific perspective to communication science will require integrity and bioethical oversight.

In conclusion, the nascent field of communications neuroscience has provided an initial set of studies that, when integrated, may support a unified framework to describe how messages are perceived and processed at neural levels. The hope is that this framework can be productively utilized to structure health communications that are maximally informative, persuasive, and perhaps personalized to account for individual differences in information processing strategies. More empirical work is needed to validate this approach in individuals with psychopathology with the goal of encouraging positive health outcomes and improved quality of life in this vulnerable population.

References

Abramovitch, A., Short, T., & Schweiger, A. (2021). The C factor: Cognitive dysfunction as a transdiagnostic dimension in psychopathology. *Clinical Psychology Review*, *86*, 102007. http://dx.doi.org/10.1016/j.cpr.2021.102007

Ahonen, M. (2019). Ancient philosophers on mental illness. *History of Psychiatry*, *30*(1), 3–18. http://dx.doi.org/10.1177/0957154X18803508

Aldridge-Waddon, L., Vanova, M., Munneke, J., Puzzo, I., & Kumari, V. (2020). Atypical social reward anticipation as a transdiagnostic characteristic of psychopathology: A meta-analytic review and critical evaluation of current evidence. *Clinical Psychology Review*, *82*, 101942. http://dx.doi.org/10.1016/j.cpr.2020.101942

American Psychiatric Association, & American Psychiatric Association DSM-5 Task Force. (2013). *Diagnostic and statistical manual of mental disorders: DSM-5* (5th ed.). American Psychiatric Association.

Ansari, D., De Smedt, B., & Grabner, R. H. (2012). Neuroeducation—A critical overview of an emerging field. *Neuroethics*, *5*(2), 105–117. http://dx.doi.org/10.1007/s12152-011-9119-3

Barch, D. M. (2017). The neural correlates of transdiagnostic dimensions of psychopathology. *American Journal of Psychiatry*, *174*(7), 613–615. http://dx.doi.org/10.1176/appi.ajp.2017.17030289

Beck, A. T. (2005). The current state of cognitive therapy: A 40-year retrospective. *Archives of General Psychiatry*, *62*(9), 953–959. http://dx.doi.org/10.1001/archpsyc.62.9.953

Brainstorm Consortium, Anttila, V., Bulik-Sullivan, B., Finucane, H. K., Walters, R. K., Bras, J., Duncan, L., Escott-Price, V., Falcone, G. J., Gormley, P., Malik, R., Patsopoulos, N. A., Ripke, S., Wei, Z., Yu, D., Lee, P. H., Turley, P., Grenier-Boley, B., Chouraki, V., … Murray, R. (2018). Analysis of shared heritability in common disorders of the brain. *Science*, *360*(6395), eaap8757. http://dx.doi.org/10.1126/science.aap8757

Buschman, T. J., & Miller, E. K. (2007). Top-down versus bottom-up control of attention in the prefrontal and posterior parietal cortices. *Science*, *315*(5820), 1860–1862. http://dx.doi.org/10.1126/science.1138071

Cacioppo, J. T., Cacioppo, S., & Petty, R. E. (2018). The neuroscience of persuasion: A review with an emphasis on issues and opportunities. *Social Neuroscience*, *13*(2), 129–172. http://dx.doi.org/10.1080/17470919.2016.1273851

Camerer, C., Loewenstein, G., & Prelec, D. (2005). Neuroeconomics: How neuroscience can inform economics. *Journal of Economic Literature*, *43*(1), 9–64. http://dx.doi.org/10.1257/0022051053737843

Cascio, C. N., Dal Cin, S., & Falk, E. B. (2013). Health communications: Predicting behavior change from the brain. In P. Hall (Ed.), *Social neuroscience and public health: Foundations for the science of chronic disease prevention* (pp. 57–71). Springer. http://dx.doi.org/10.1007/978-1-4614-6852-3_4

Caspi, A., Houts, R. M., Belsky, D. W., Goldman-Mellor, S. J., Harrington, H., Israel, S., Meier, M. H., Ramrakha, S., Shalev, I., Poulton, R., & Moffitt, T. E. (2014). The p factor: One general psychopathology factor in the structure of psychiatric disorders? *Clinical Psychological Science*, *2*(2), 119–137. http://dx.doi.org/10.1177/2167702613497473

Churchland, P. S., & Sejnowski, T. J. (1992). *The computational brain*. MIT Press.

Cooper, N., Garcia, J. O., Tompson, S. H., O'Donnell, M. B., Falk, E. B., & Vettel, J. M. (2018). Time-evolving dynamics in brain networks forecast responses to health messaging. *Network Neuroscience*, *3*(1), 138–156. http://dx.doi.org/10.1162/netn_a_00058

Cuthbert, B. N. (2022). Research domain criteria (RDoC): Progress and potential. *Current Directions in Psychological Science*, *31*(2), 107–114. http://dx.doi.org/10.1177/09637214211051363

Cuthbert, B. N., & Insel, T. R. (2013). Toward the future of psychiatric diagnosis: The seven pillars of RDoC. *BMC Medicine*, *11*(1), 126. http://dx.doi.org/10.1186/1741-7015-11-126

Dimidjian, S., Barrera, M., Martell, C., Muñoz, R. F., & Lewinsohn, P. M. (2011). The origins and current status of behavioral activation treatments for depression. *Annual Review of Clinical Psychology*, *7*(1), 1–38. http://dx.doi.org/10.1146/annurev-clinpsy-032210-104535

Doré, B. P., Cooper, N., Scholz, C., O'Donnell, M. B., & Falk, E. B. (2019a). Cognitive regulation of ventromedial prefrontal activity evokes lasting change in the perceived self-relevance of persuasive messaging. *Human Brain Mapping*, *40*(9), 2571–2580. http://dx.doi.org/10.1002/hbm.24545

Doré, B. P., Tompson, S. H., O'Donnell, M. B., An, L. C., Strecher, V., & Falk, E. B. (2019b). Neural mechanisms of emotion regulation moderate the predictive value of affective and value-related brain responses to persuasive messages. *Journal of Neuroscience*, *39*(7), 1293–1300. http://dx.doi.org/10.1523/JNEUROSCI.1651-18.2018

Elliott, M. L., Romer, A., Knodt, A. R., & Hariri, A. R. (2018). A connectome-wide functional signature of transdiagnostic risk for mental illness. *Biological Psychiatry*, *84*(6), 452–459. http://dx.doi.org/10.1016/j.biopsych.2018.03.012

Euston, D. R., Gruber, A. J., & McNaughton, B. L. (2012). The role of medial prefrontal cortex in memory and decision making. *Neuron*, *76*(6), 1057–1070. http://dx.doi.org/10.1016/j.neuron.2012.12.002

Falk, E., & Scholz, C. (2018). Persuasion, influence, and value: Perspectives from communication and social neuroscience. *Annual Review of Psychology*, *69*(1), 329–356. http://dx.doi.org/10.1146/annurev-psych-122216-011821

Falk, E. B. (2012). Can neuroscience advance our understanding of core questions in communication studies? An overview of communication neuroscience. In S. Jones (Ed.), *Communication @ the center* (pp. 77–94). Hampton Press.

Falk, E. B., Berkman, E. T., & Lieberman, M. D. (2012). From neural responses to population behavior: Neural focus group predicts population-level media effects. *Psychological Science*, *23*(5), 439–445. http://dx.doi.org/10.1177/0956797611434964

Falk, E. B., Berkman, E. T., Mann, T., Harrison, B., & Lieberman, M. D. (2010). Predicting persuasion-induced behavior change from the brain. *Journal of Neuroscience*, *30*(25), 8421–8424. http://dx.doi.org/10.1523/JNEUROSCI.0063-10.2010

Falk, E. B., Berkman, E. T., Whalen, D., & Lieberman, M. D. (2011). Neural activity during health messaging predicts reductions in smoking above and beyond self-report. *Health Psychology*, *30*(2), 177–185. http://dx.doi.org/10.1037/a0022259

Falk, E. B., O'Donnell, M. B., Cascio, C. N., Tinney, F., Kang, Y., Lieberman, M. D., Taylor, S. E., An, L., Resnicow, K., & Strecher, V. J. (2015). Self-affirmation alters the brain's response to health messages and subsequent behavior change. *Proceedings of the National Academy of Sciences*, *112*(7), 1977–1982. http://dx.doi.org/10.1073/pnas.1500247112

Fox, M. D., Snyder, A. Z., Vincent, J. L., Corbetta, M., Van Essen, D. C., & Raichle, M. E. (2005). The human brain is intrinsically organized into dynamic, anticorrelated functional networks. *Proceedings of the National Academy of Sciences*, *102*(27), 9673–9678. http://dx.doi.org/10.1073/pnas.0504136102

Goodkind, M., Eickhoff, S. B., Oathes, D. J., Jiang, Y., Chang, A., Jones-Hagata, L. B., Ortega, B. N., Zaiko, Y. V., Roach, E. L., Korgaonkar, M. S., Grieve, S. M., Galatzer-Levy, I., Fox, P. T., & Etkin, A. (2015). Identification of a common neurobiological substrate for mental illness. *JAMA Psychiatry*, *72*(4), 305–315. http://dx.doi.org/10.1001/jamapsychiatry.2014.2206

Goschke, T. (2014). Dysfunctions of decision-making and cognitive control as transdiagnostic mechanisms of mental disorders: Advances, gaps, and needs in current research. *International Journal of Methods in Psychiatric Research*, *23*(S1), 41–57. http://dx.doi.org/10.1002/mpr.1410

Goulden, N., Khusnulina, A., Davis, N. J., Bracewell, R. M., Bokde, A. L., McNulty, J. P., & Mullins, P. G. (2014). The salience network is responsible for switching between the default mode network and the central executive network: Replication from DCM. *NeuroImage*, *99*, 180–190. http://dx.doi.org/10.1016/j.neuroimage.2014.05.052

Higgins, E. T. (2000). Making a good decision: Value from fit. *American Psychologist*, *55*(11), 1217–1230. http://dx.doi.org/10.1037/0003-066X.55.11.1217

Janiri, D., Moser, D. A., Doucet, G. E., Luber, M. J., Rasgon, A., Lee, W. H., Murrough, J. W., Sani, G., Eickhoff, S. B., & Frangou, S. (2020). Shared neural phenotypes for mood and anxiety disorders. *JAMA Psychiatry*, *77*(2), 172–179. http://dx.doi.org/10.1001/jamapsychiatry.2019.3351

Jovanova, M., Falk, E. B., Pearl, J. M., Pandey, P., Brook O'Donnell, M., Kang, Y., Bassett, D. S., & Lydon-Staley, D. M. (2022). Brain system integration and message consistent health behavior change. *Health Psychology*, *41*(9), 611–620. http://dx.doi.org/10.1037/hea0001201

Kang, Y., Strecher, V. J., Kim, E., & Falk, E. B. (2019). Purpose in life and conflict-related neural responses during health decision-making. *Health Psychology*, *38*(6), 545–552. http://dx.doi.org/10.1037/hea0000729

Kiefer, M., & Pulvermüller, F. (2012). Conceptual representations in mind and brain: Theoretical developments, current evidence and future directions. *Cortex*, *48*(7), 805–825. http://dx.doi.org/10.1016/j.cortex.2011.04.006

Knudsen, E. I. (2007). Fundamental components of attention. *Annual Review of Neuroscience*, *30*(1), 57–78. http://dx.doi.org/10.1146/annurev.neuro.30.051606.094256

Kotov, R., Krueger, R. F., Watson, D., Achenbach, T. M., Althoff, R. R., Bagby, R. M., Brown, T. A., Carpenter, W. T., Caspi, A., Clark, L. A., Eaton, N. R., Forbes, M. K., Forbush, K. T., Goldberg, D., Hasin, D., Hyman, S. E., Ivanova, M. Y., Lynam, D. R., Markon, K., … Zimmerman, M. (2017). The hierarchical taxonomy of psychopathology (HiTOP): A dimensional alternative to traditional nosologies. *Journal of Abnormal Psychology, 126*(4), 454–477. http://dx.doi.org/10.1037/abn0000258

Kranzler, E. C., Schmälzle, R., O'Donnell, M. B., Pei, R., & Falk, E. B. (2019). Adolescent neural responses to antismoking messages, perceived effectiveness, and sharing intention. *Media Psychology, 22*(2), 323–349. http://dx.doi.org/10.1080/15213269.2018.1476158

Langleben, D. D., Loughead, J. W., Ruparel, K., Hakun, J. G., Busch-Winokur, S., Holloway, M. B., Strasser, A. A., Cappella, J. N., & Lerman, C. (2009). Reduced prefrontal and temporal processing and recall of high "sensation value" ads. *NeuroImage, 46*(1), 219–225. http://dx.doi.org/10.1016/j.neuroimage.2008.12.062

LeDoux, J. (2007). The amygdala. *Current Biology: CB, 17*(20), R868–R874. http://dx.doi.org/10.1016/j.cub.2007.08.005

Lee, A., & Griva, K. (2015). Motivational interviewing and neuroscience: Moving forward while looking deeper. *European Health Psychologist, 17*(3), 111–114.

Lerner, J. S., Li, Y., Valdesolo, P., & Kassam, K. S. (2015). Emotion and decision making. *Annual Review of Psychology, 66*(1), 799–823. http://dx.doi.org/10.1146/annurev-psych-010213-115043

Lieberman, M. D., Straccia, M. A., Meyer, M. L., Du, M., & Tan, K. M. (2019). Social, self, (situational), and affective processes in medial prefrontal cortex (MPFC): Causal, multivariate, and reverse inference evidence. *Neuroscience & Biobehavioral Reviews, 99*, 311–328. http://dx.doi.org/10.1016/j.neubiorev.2018.12.021

MacLean, P. D. (1955). The limbic system (visceral brain) and behavior. *A.M.A. Archives of Neurology and Psychiatry, 73*(2), 130–134. http://dx.doi.org/10.1001/archneurpsyc.1955.02330080008004

McTeague, L. M., Rosenberg, B. M., Lopez, J. W., Carreon, D. M., Huemer, J., Jiang, Y., Chick, C. F., Eickhoff, S. B., & Etkin, A. (2020). Identification of common neural circuit disruptions in emotional processing across psychiatric disorders. *American Journal of Psychiatry, 177*(5), 411–421. http://dx.doi.org/10.1176/appi.ajp.2019.18111271

Menon, B. (2019). Towards a new model of understanding—The triple network, psychopathology and the structure of the mind. *Medical Hypotheses, 133*, 109385. http://dx.doi.org/10.1016/j.mehy.2019.109385

Menon, V. (2011). Large-scale brain networks and psychopathology: A unifying triple network model. *Trends in Cognitive Sciences, 15*(10), 483–506. http://dx.doi.org/10.1016/j.tics.2011.08.003

Michelini, G., Palumbo, I. M., DeYoung, C. G., Latzman, R. D., & Kotov, R. (2021). Linking RDoC and HiTOP: A new interface for advancing psychiatric nosology and neuroscience. *Clinical Psychology Review, 86*, 102025. http://dx.doi.org/10.1016/j.cpr.2021.102025

Morin, C. (2011). Neuromarketing: The new science of consumer behavior. *Society, 48*(2), 131–135. http://dx.doi.org/10.1007/s12115-010-9408-1

Neumann, A., Pappa, I., Lahey, B. B., Verhulst, F. C., Medina-Gomez, C., Jaddoe, V. W., Bakermans-Kranenburg, M. J., Moffitt, T. E., van IJzendoorn, M. H., & Tiemeier, H. (2016). Single nucleotide polymorphism heritability of a general psychopathology factor in children. *Journal of the American Academy of Child & Adolescent Psychiatry, 55*(12), 1038–1045.e4. http://dx.doi.org/10.1016/j.jaac.2016.09.498

Opel, N., Goltermann, J., Hermesdorf, M., Berger, K., Baune, B. T., & Dannlowski, U. (2020). Cross-disorder analysis of brain structural abnormalities in six major psychiatric disorders: A secondary analysis of mega-and meta-analytical findings from the ENIGMA consortium. *Biological Psychiatry, 88*(9), 678–686. http://dx.doi.org/10.1016/j.biopsych.2020.04.027

Park, H.-J., & Friston, K. (2013). Structural and functional brain networks: From connections to cognition. *Science, 342*(6158), 1238411. http://dx.doi.org/10.1126/science.1238411

Pisoni, A., Davis, S. W., & Smoski, M. (2021). Neural signatures of saliency-mapping in anhedonia: A narrative review. *Psychiatry Research, 304*, 114123. http://dx.doi.org/10.1016/j.psychres.2021.114123

Raichle, M. E., MacLeod, A. M., Snyder, A. Z., Powers, W. J., Gusnard, D. A., & Shulman, G. L. (2001). A default mode of brain function. *Proceedings of the National Academy of Sciences, 98*(2), 676–682. http://dx.doi.org/10.1073/pnas.98.2.676

Ramsay, I. S., Yzer, M. C., Luciana, M., Vohs, K. D., & MacDonald, A. W., III (2013). Affective and executive network processing associated with persuasive antidrug messages. *Journal of Cognitive Neuroscience, 25*(7), 1136–1147.

Romer, A. L., Elliott, M. L., Knodt, A. R., Sison, M. L., Ireland, D., Houts, R., Ramrakha, S., Poulton, R., Keenan, R., Melzer, T. R., Moffitt, T. E., Caspi, A., & Hariri, A. R. (2021a). Pervasively thinner neocortex as a transdiagnostic feature of general psychopathology. *American Journal of Psychiatry, 178*(2), 174–182. http://dx.doi.org/10.1176/appi.ajp.2020.19090934

Romer, A. L., Knodt, A. R., Sison, M. L., Ireland, D., Houts, R., Ramrakha, S., Poulton, R., Keenan, R., Melzer, T. R., Moffitt, T. E., Caspi, A., & Hariri, A. R. (2021b). Replicability of structural brain alterations associated with general psychopathology: Evidence from a population-representative birth cohort. *Molecular Psychiatry, 26*(8), 3839–3846. http://dx.doi.org/10.1038/s41380-019-0621-z

Romer, A. L., & Pizzagalli, D. A. (2022). Associations between brain structural alterations, executive dysfunction, and general psychopathology in a healthy and cross-diagnostic adult patient sample. *Biological Psychiatry Global Open Science, 2*(1), 17–27. http://dx.doi.org/10.1016/j.bpsgos.2021.06.002

Rossi, J., & Yudell, M. (2012). The use of persuasion in public health communication: An ethical critique. *Public Health Ethics, 5*(2), 192–205. http://dx.doi.org/10.1093/phe/phs019

Schimmelpfennig, J., Topczewski, J., Zajkowski, W., & Jankowiak-Siuda, K. (2023). The role of the salience network in cognitive and affective deficits. *Frontiers in Human Neuroscience*, *17*, 1133367. http://dx.doi.org/10.3389/fnhum.2023.1133367

Schultz, W. (2016). Dopamine reward prediction error coding. *Dialogues in Clinical Neuroscience*, *18*(1), 23–32. https://doi.org/10.31887/DCNS.2016.18.1/wschultz

Seeley, W. W., Menon, V., Schatzberg, A. F., Keller, J., Glover, G. H., Kenna, H., Reiss, A. L., & Greicius, M. D. (2007). Dissociable intrinsic connectivity networks for salience processing and executive control. *Journal of Neuroscience*, *27*(9), 2349–2356. http://dx.doi.org/10.3389/fnhum.2023.1133367

Selzam, S., Coleman, J. R., Caspi, A., Moffitt, T. E., & Plomin, R. (2018). A polygenic p factor for major psychiatric disorders. *Translational Psychiatry*, *8*(1), 205. http://dx.doi.org/10.1038/s41398-018-0217-4

Sha, Z., Wager, T. D., Mechelli, A., & He, Y. (2019). Common dysfunction of large-scale neurocognitive networks across psychiatric disorders. *Biological Psychiatry*, *85*(5), 379–388. http://dx.doi.org/10.1016/j.biopsych.2018.11.011

Sharma, A., Wolf, D. H., Ciric, R., Kable, J. W., Moore, T. M., Vandekar, S. N., Katchmar, N., Daldal, A., Ruparel, K., Davatzikos, C., Elliott, M. A., Calkins, M. E., Shinohara, R. T., Bassett, D. S., & Satterthwaite, T. D. (2017). Common dimensional reward deficits across mood and psychotic disorders: A connectome-wide association study. *The American Journal of Psychiatry*, *174*(7), 657–666. http://dx.doi.org/10.1176/appi.ajp.2016.16070774

Sprooten, E., Rasgon, A., Goodman, M., Carlin, A., Leibu, E., Lee, W. H., & Frangou, S. (2017). Addressing reverse inference in psychiatric neuroimaging: Meta-analyses of task-related brain activation in common mental disorders. *Human Brain Mapping*, *38*(4), 1846–1864. http://dx.doi.org/10.1002/hbm.23486

Stephenson, M., & Palmgreen, P. (2001). Sensation seeking, perceived message sensation value, personal involvement, and processing of anti-marijuana PSAs. *Communication Monographs*, *68*(1), 49–71. http://dx.doi.org/10.1080/03637750128051

Szeszko, P. R., & Yehuda, R. (2019). Magnetic resonance imaging predictors of psychotherapy treatment response in post-traumatic stress disorder: A role for the salience network. *Psychiatry Research*, *277*, 52–57. http://dx.doi.org/10.1016/j.psychres.2019.02.005

Tse, S., Tsoi, E. W., Hamilton, B., O'Hagan, M., Shepherd, G., Slade, M., Whitley, R., & Petrakis, M. (2016). Uses of strength-based interventions for people with serious mental illness: A critical review. *International Journal of Social Psychiatry*, *62*(3), 281–291. http://dx.doi.org/10.1177/0020764015623970

Uddin, L. Q. (2015). Salience processing and insular cortical function and dysfunction. *Nature Reviews. Neuroscience*, *16*(1), 55–61. http://dx.doi.org/10.1038/nrn3857

Vezich, I. S., Katzman, P. L., Ames, D. L., Falk, E. B., & Lieberman, M. D. (2017). Modulating the neural bases of persuasion: Why/how, gain/loss, and users/non-users. *Social Cognitive and Affective Neuroscience*, *12*(2), 283–297. http://dx.doi.org/10.1093/scan/nsw113

Walker, E. R., McGee, R. E., & Druss, B. G. (2015). Mortality in mental disorders and global disease burden implications: A systematic review and meta-analysis. *JAMA Psychiatry*, *72*(4), 334–341. http://dx.doi.org/10.1001/jamapsychiatry.2014.2502

Wang, A.-L., Ruparel, K., Loughead, J. W., Strasser, A. A., Blady, S. J., Lynch, K. G., Romer, D., Cappella, J. N., Lerman, C., & Langleben, D. D. (2013). Content matters: Neuroimaging investigation of brain and behavioral impact of televised anti-tobacco public service announcements. *The Journal of Neuroscience: The Official Journal of the Society for Neuroscience*, *33*(17), 7420–7427. http://dx.doi.org/10.1523/JNEUROSCI.3840-12.2013

Weber, R., Huskey, R., Mangus, J. M., Westcott-Baker, A., & Turner, B. O. (2015). Neural predictors of message effectiveness during counterarguing in antidrug campaigns. *Communication Monographs*, *82*(1), 4–30. http://dx.doi.org/10.1080/03637751.2014.971414

Yeshurun, Y., Nguyen, M., & Hasson, U. (2021). The default mode network: Where the idiosyncratic self meets the shared social world. *Nature Reviews Neuroscience*, *22*(3), 181–192. http://dx.doi.org/10.1038/s41583-020-00420-w

Yzer, M. (2012). The integrative model of behavioral prediction as a tool for designing health messages. In H. Cho (Ed.), *Health communication message design: Theory and practice* (pp. 21–40). Sage.

4

Cognitive Deficits in Major Depression: Characteristics, Role, and Relevance

Elayne Ahern
University of Limerick

Major depressive disorder (MDD) is a prevalent and debilitating condition, with reports that between 280 to almost 300 million individuals are affected globally (Ferrari et al., 2013; World Health Organization, 2023). The experience of depressive symptoms can be a normal occurrence. MDD, on the other hand, is typically understood as a mood disorder that is characterized by sadness or decreased interest or pleasure in activities for a minimum two-week period, and accompanied by a collection of at least five symptoms across behavioral, somatic, and cognitive domains (American Psychiatric Association, 2013). The experience of depression and associated symptoms for the two-week period (episode) can be followed by a period of wellness (remission) and then subsequently marked by another episode (relapse) to form the cycle of MDD. The emotional aspects of MDD, such as the sadness and feelings of guilt or worthlessness, have been central to the public understanding of this mental health condition. Nonetheless, the cognitive aspects of MDD relevant to how an individual perceives, processes, and utilizes information are of great interest within research and therapeutic fields. This is due to the role that cognitive functions hold in the vulnerability for MDD onset (MacKenzie et al., 2019), maintenance of the depressive cycle following onset (Ahern et al., 2019), risk of relapse following treatment (Majer et al., 2004), and as a prominent contributor to the impairment in social and occupational domains during and following MDD (Cambridge et al., 2018). It is estimated that by 2030, MDD will be the leading cause of disability (World Health Organization, 2012).

This chapter discusses cognitive functions in MDD and how insights garnered from this field of work can be applied to persuasion and communication literature for mental health messaging. The cognitive functions that will be discussed are somewhat differentiated from the higher-order, negative cognitive biases introduced in early cognitive models of depression (Beck, 1967), which drew focus to the preferential processing of negative material. Specifically, the cognitive functions that will be the focus of this chapter are the general abilities of processing speed, attention, learning, memory, problem-solving, and planning engaged in by the individual. These cognitive functions will be discussed in terms of their characteristics in MDD; the role they serve in information processing, alongside the negative, cognitive biases, as well as the broader implications of cognitive functions in MDD for treatment help-seeking. Throughout, recommendations for the design and evaluation of mental health messages will be provided.

The Handbook of Mental Health Communication, First Edition.
Edited by Marco C. Yzer and Jason T. Siegel.

The Neuropsychological Profile in MDD

Understanding the Characteristics of Cognitive Deficits in MDD

Cognitive function is complex as a concept, with little consensus in the definitions used across the literature and contributory disciplines; this is an issue more generally within the field of neuropsychology, but particularly in the case of MDD (Hammar et al., 2022; Pan et al., 2019). This is due to complementary fields of theory and research that have largely developed independently despite both drawing on cognitive function in MDD, either in terms of general cognitive deficits, as is the case in neuropsychology, or affective (emotional) cognitive deficits in response to valenced (positive, negative) material, cognitive biases, or negative self-referent thought, as is the case in clinical psychology, cognitive psychology and the neurosciences. The distinctions and interactions between these fields will be elucidated further throughout this chapter, with focus primarily on the neuropsychological approach.

Broadly, cognitive function relates to the mental processes of acquiring information, working with this information, storing, retrieving, and then applying to guide decisions and behavior. This consists of interrelated domains of component abilities, such as attention, learning, memory, and executive function. For example, the executive function domain, relevant to control and direction of basic processing in order to execute a task, can consist of a number of component abilities such as the ability to shift focus, inhibit a response, update material, and plan (Harvey, 2022). Cognitive deficits, then, simply put, relate to a diminished ability to think, concentrate, or make decisions (American Psychiatric Association, 2013). Significant cognitive deficits of small-large magnitude have been observed across the domains of processing speed, attention, visual/verbal learning and memory, executive function, and planning by individuals currently experiencing a depressive episode (Rock et al., 2014) and even between episodes during a period of wellness known as remission (Semkovska et al., 2019). This finding has been consistently observed in meta-analytical investigations of cognitive function in MDD relative to healthy controls (e.g., Ahern & Semkovska, 2017; Nuño et al., 2021; Snyder, 2013).

As mentioned, the symptomatology of MDD is multifaceted and by virtue of this, not all individuals with MDD may experience cognitive deficits. Nonetheless, findings suggest that up to 94% of individuals self-report the experience of such cognitive deficits ($N = 267$; Conradi et al., 2011), with estimates that between 25.2% ($N = 111$; Tran et al., 2021) to 45.3% ($N = 58$ inpatients; Douglas et al., 2018) of individuals with MDD show global cognitive deficit as per objective neuropsychological test assessments (≥1SD below norm). Such estimates vary to quite an extent dependent on several considerations, such as the severity of depressive symptoms (Douglas et al., 2018; Petersen et al., 2019) and whether cognitive deficits are based on self-report or objective performance-based neuropsychological tests (Srisurapanont et al., 2017), as self-reported, perceived deficits tend to be overestimated (Rnic et al., 2021).

Furthermore, even with objective assessments, differences in the rate and extent of deficit are dependent on the criteria applied to establish the deficit. Cognitive deficit can be established on the basis of population norms, such as performing 1SD below the population average, or idiosyncratically in accordance with premorbid performance estimates. Idiosyncratic assessments tend to be more sensitive to capturing indices of deficit particularly when an individual would otherwise typically perform above the norm and could present as within the norm despite experiencing deficit (Tran et al., 2021). In addition to assessment approaches, the degree to which an individual experiences cognitive deficits has been associated with several neurobiological (e.g., hippocampal volume, neuroinflammation, fronto-subcortical circuity; Pan et al., 2019), demographic (e.g., age, education level; Vicent-Gil et al., 2021), and clinical features of illness (depressive symptom severity, hospitalization, number of past episodes; Douglas et al., 2018; Petersen et al., 2019; Semkovska et al., 2019). The cognitive profile of MDD is therefore understood to be quite heterogeneous which can make it difficult to draw generalized conclusions regarding the pattern, extent, and persistence of these deficits throughout the course of illness.

In order to better understand the characteristics of cognitive deficits throughout the course of MDD, the temporal relationship between the cognitive deficits and the major depressive episode have been investigated (Hammar et al., 2022). *State*-like cognitive deficits are considered to be an epiphenomenon of mood state, only present during the depressive episode, and alleviating then in accordance with depressive symptom improvement. State-like qualities have been observed for the cognitive functions of processing speed and attention, meaning that these select cognitive deficits are observed only during the episode, not thereafter. *Trait*-like cognitive deficits are present before, during, and persist following a depressive episode, thus indicative of a vulnerability factor for MDD onset. Executive functions such as set shifting have tended to show trait-like characteristics, with significant deficits observed right from the first depressive episode, with evidence of some persistence thereafter (Ahern & Semkovska, 2017). Similarly, *scar*-like cognitive deficits present as a vulnerability factor for MDD, or more specifically, MDD relapse, as residual deficits accumulate as a neurotoxic scar of past depressive episodes. Scarring effects have been observed for psychomotor processing speed, as the extent of deficit has been observed to be greater with each recurrent number of past episodes (Gorwood et al., 2014). Of course, this is further complicated as select cognitive functions often show characteristics of several competing mechanisms. This, in part, can be brought back to the ability of different study designs to efficiently elucidate these mechanisms unless prospective, longitudinal approaches are taken to appropriately disentangle possible mechanisms (Allott et al., 2016).

Explanatory Hypotheses for Cognitive Deficits in MDD

The state, trait, and scar classifications of cognitive deficits in MDD provide a useful framework to understand the interactions between cognition and affect (depressive mood state) throughout the course of illness, but does not necessarily offer much insight into how exactly cognitive deficits materialize in MDD. Several hypotheses have been proposed to support our understanding of these underlying mechanisms. This section provides a summary of the two prominent hypotheses as relevant to cognitive–affective perspectives: the resource allocation (Ellis & Ashbrook, 1988) and affective interference (Siegle et al., 2002) hypotheses.

We know that humans are limited capacity processors (Ingram, 1984). Put simply, we cannot attend to all information within our environment; as such, other than what is processed automatically, we need to allocate a certain amount of our limited cognitive resources to process select pieces of information. Ellis and Ashbrook (1988) introduced the *resource allocation* hypothesis, which proposes that cognitive capacity is inherently reduced due to the depressive disorder itself and in addition is reduced due to depression-relevant processing such as thinking about the negative mood state (e.g., rumination), mood-congruent preferential processing of negative content (e.g., enhanced recall of negative memories), or directing attention to task-irrelevant information (e.g., emotional distractors). In a mutually reinforcing manner, the limited cognitive resources that are available are used up by processing that aligns with the depressive mood state; that is, it is mood-congruent and serves to reinforce the mood state, but this is at the expense of other general cognitive functions.

When examining this hypothesis at a neurobiological level, structural brain changes such as reduced gray matter volume have been observed among individuals with MDD relative to healthy controls; although gray matter structural changes are likely to be a common transdiagnostic factor with other conditions such as anxiety, MDD-specific functional changes have nonetheless also been observed (Brandl et al., 2022). These functional changes tend to be observed in the resting state networks which are relevant to self-referential processing (default mode network); the detection of emotionally relevant stimuli (salience network), alongside top-down regulation via attention and executive control, involved in directing cognitive resources to internal and external environments, respectively (frontoparietal networks; Menon, 2011). Indeed, MDD is thought to be associated with distinct functional patterns. These are characterized by hyperactivity in the frontoparietal-default mode network, which is indicative of impaired top-down regulation as cognitive resources likely fail to be directed away from internally oriented and self-referent thought, as well as hypoactivity in limbic-salience network connections, which suggests dysfunctional processing of salience for internal and external stimuli (Brandl et al., 2022). Resultantly, cognitive resources may remain directed internally, at the expense of actively engaging in the external world around us. The implication of this is that individuals with MDD have fewer available resources to support the efficient carrying out of cognitive tasks in everyday life such as memorizing details of a shopping list, coordinating tasks at work, and directing attention to public health messages.

Competing with the resource allocation hypothesis is the proposition of *affective interference* (Siegle et al., 2002). The proposition is that, due to automatic processing of negative material in MDD, priority will be given to the processing of affective material in instances where affective and nonaffective processing occur in parallel. For example, in a valence task where individuals were asked to determine the valence of a word (e.g., *hopeless* as negative/positive/neutral; affective processing), individuals with dysphoria responded faster to the identification of negative relative to neutral words. However, when completing a lexical decision task that required a decision on whether a string of letters was a word or nonword (nonaffective processing), individuals with dysphoria took longer to determine the status of negative words (vs. neutral), compared with nondysphoric controls. When tasks require that emotional content is ignored, as was the case in the lexical decision task, the preferential processing of negative content can interfere and ultimately contribute to cognitive deficits in what otherwise would be considered a neutral task (Is it a word or nonword?). Similarly, on average, individuals with MDD have been observed to perform slower relative to healthy controls when asked to correctly identify whether facial responses (positive, negative, neutral) were previously presented or not (Lin et al., 2021). This again converges to suggest that nonaffective processing is impaired in the context of affective material.

The preferential processing of negative content is relevant to both the resource allocation and affective interference hypotheses for cognitive deficits in MDD. Nonetheless, it is important to note that the symptomatology of MDD encapsulates cognitive, emotional, behavioral, somatic, as well as motivational factors. Therefore, it is plausible that cognitive deficits in MDD may manifest as a result of a set of symptoms beyond just the emotional state. Indeed, anhedonic features, or the loss of interest and/or pleasure, is oftentimes a key feature of MDD and is specified as one of the core symptoms in the diagnostic criteria (Su & Si, 2022). Anhedonia is multifaceted, composed of aspects of desire, anticipatory and consummatory pleasure, and effort/decision-making or motivation (Rizvi et al., 2016). Specifically, motivational deficits can also offer a compelling explanation for the cognitive profile of MDD. It has been proposed that motivation underpins the allocation of cognitive control during MDD (Grahek et al., 2019). Notably, only very few studies ($k = 7$, $N = 409$ MDD patients) include performance validity tests so it is difficult to ascertain whether the cognitive deficits observed during neuropsychological testing are indicative of deficit, or indeed, an epiphenomenon of emotion and motivation-related factors (Legemaat et al., 2022). There is some evidence to suggest that when additional, goal-directed instructions are provided for neuropsychological tasks (e.g., goal to achieve 20% more in the following task), complex visual processing and psychomotor speed, as well as verbal learning and memory, can significantly improve among individuals hospitalized with MDD ($N = 60$) so that they no longer show deficient performance, relative to controls (Scheurich et al., 2008). Of course, it is plausible that the findings are not the product of increased motivation. The provision of instructions may have helped orient attention to task-relevant information so that cognitive resources are effectively allocated (resource allocation hypothesis).

Although several hypotheses have been proposed to account for the presence of cognitive deficits in MDD, a few of which we have discussed here, no clear indication has been found to suggest that one, of any, may be best situated to consistently explain this phenomenon. The cognitive profile of MDD is heterogeneous, which again attests to the complex affect–cognition interaction. Although the origin of cognitive deficits may be contended, what is clear, however, is that cognitive deficits are present throughout the course of MDD for many individuals, for those at risk, during initial onset, throughout depressive episodes, and through to periods of clinical remission. As such, cognitive deficits necessitate consideration alongside the traditional focus on the negatively biased cognitive profile in MDD.

The Role of MDD Cognitive Deficits in Information Processing

Interacting Hot and Cold Cognitive Processes

Traditionally, dysfunctional cognition in MDD has been understood from the seminal work by Beck in the 1960s on the cognitive theory of depression. Beck (1967) proposed that individuals with MDD have deeply held representations about themselves, others, and the world known as schemas. These tend to be characterized by negative themes and in the context of self-schemas may contribute to beliefs about being unlovable, unworthy, or a failure. Following stress, these schemas can be activated and underlie the biased cognition toward the preferential processing, attending to, and memory recall of negative content consistent with the depressive mood state. Indeed, evidence converges to indicate that individuals with MDD tend to interpret ambiguous situations negatively, have difficulty disengaging attention from negative content, have better recall of negative content, and increased elaboration of negative content (LeMoult & Gotlib, 2019). All of these are likely reinforced by a difficulty exerting cognitive control over negative material, encompassing the ability to inhibit negative thoughts, shift away from these negative thoughts and then update the contents of working memory (Joormann & Vanderlind, 2014; Quigley et al., 2022), ultimately resulting in the extended processing and maintenance of negative material. This has been core to our understanding of the cognitive aspects of MDD and, with this, oriented focus to cognitive function in the context of emotionally relevant material.

Accumulating evidence on the cognitive profile in MDD over recent decades has tended to develop somewhat separately, although complementary to each other, across the respective fields of neuropsychology, cognitive psychology and the neurosciences. Specifically, cognitive control processes, also known as executive function and the component abilities of inhibition, shifting, and updating working memory, set the stage for the interaction between these fields. Within cognitive psychology and the cognitive neurosciences, cognitive control has been examined as the mechanism linking cognitive biases to the dysregulation of emotion in MDD (LeMoult & Gotlib, 2019). Individuals with MDD have difficulty exerting control over the processing of negative material, coupled with difficulty disengaging from negative material to effectively override the cognitive bias, which makes negative content more available (Gotlib & Joormann, 2010; Joormann & Vanderlind, 2014). Rumination, a style of thinking characterized by repetitive thought regarding, or in response to, the negative affect (Nolen-Hoeksema et al., 2008) ultimately reinforces the depressive mood state and in a reciprocal fashion both results from and contributes to, dysfunctional attentional control in MDD (Koster et al., 2011). Computerized experimental paradigms that are borne from the cognitive psychology literature are typically used in investigations of affective cognitive control, such as incorporating emotional material into the go/no go or stop–signal tasks, Stroop test, and shifting tasks (Paulus, 2015).

Within the neuropsychological domain, cognitive control, more commonly referred to as executive function, and broader domains of processing speed, attention, visual/verbal learning and memory, and complex executive functions (e.g., planning) are typically examined using neuropsychological testing batteries. These can be in the traditional paper–pencil format, such as the Delis Kaplan Executive Function System Test (Delis et al. 2001), or computerized, such as the Cambridge Automated Neuropsychological Test Battery (CANTAB; Smith et al., 2013). The contents of these tests are non-affective, or neutral. As previously outlined, a broad array of cognitive deficits are observed in MDD (Ahern & Semkovska, 2017; Nuño et al., 2021; Rock et al., 2014; Snyder, 2013) and during clinical remission (Semkovska et al., 2019). While cognitive psychology and the cognitive neurosciences predominantly explore cognitive control in the context of emotion and emotion regulation, the neuropsychological approach further orients toward bridging cognitive function with application to psychosocial and occupational functioning (Trivedi, 2006).

To best conceptualize cognitive function in affective and nonaffective contexts, indices of hot and cold have been applied (Roiser & Sahakian, 2013). Cold cognition occurs in the absence of affective material, thus, cognitive performance in response to otherwise neutral content. For example, processing speed, attention, memory, and executive functions assessed using neuropsychological test batteries—the aforementioned general cognitive deficits. Hot cognition refers to function in the presence of affective material such as valenced (positive, negative) test stimuli, music, or task feedback that induces an affective state such as disappointment. For example, performance on emotional versions of traditional neuropsychological tests such as the Stroop, attentional bias toward negative content, rumination, and value-based decision-making for risk or reward would be examples of hot cognitive function.

Individuals with MDD may show different facets of hot and cold cognitive dysfunction. An investigation of antidepressant-free individuals with MDD ($N = 98$) relative to controls evidenced three cognitive profile clusters characterized by strong negative biases (hot cognition) but no significant deficits across cold cognitive tasks ($N = 38$); positive biases in emotion processing and moderate deficits across all cold cognitive tasks ($N = 28$); or large deficits across both hot and cold cognition ($N = 26$). These cognitive clusters were associated with depression severity with large deficits across hot and cold cognition more likely a function of severe MDD, whereas a cluster profile of deficits in just hot cognition with relatively intact cold cognition would not be typical of a severe MDD presentation (Dam et al., 2021). It is important to clarify that although the dichotomy of hot and cold cognition suggests distinct processes, they are best understood as dynamic and interacting (Ahern et al., 2019; Roiser & Sahakian, 2013).

A classic illustration of the interplay between hot and cold cognition can be drawn from the work of Beats et al. (1996) on the catastrophic response to perceived failure. In the Tower of London task, a measure of spatial planning ability, elderly individuals with MDD ($N = 24$) did not significantly differ from controls ($N = 15$) in the number of trials completed successfully (minimum number of moves). However, a significant difference was observed in the number of moves subsequently taken following initial failed attempts, which became more pronounced at the latter trials when the difficulty level increased. Further, Elliott et al. (1996) examined a group of middle-aged individuals with MDD ($N = 28$) across a battery of neuropsychological tests, relative to healthy controls ($N = 22$); following the Tower of London as well as the Delayed Matching to Sample task, measures of spatial planning and visuospatial memory recognition respectively, explicit and immediate computerized feedback was provided on performance in the form of a green tick or red cross, accompanied with a high or low tone. Again, it was found that following failure on the preceding trial, individuals with MDD were more likely to fail the subsequent trial on the task. These findings converge to suggest that although the individuals with MDD evidence what appears to be nonaffective, cold cognitive deficits, these deficits may otherwise be best accounted for by hot cognition resulting from sensitivity to negative performance feedback. Activated hot cognition may be a negative failure schema (e.g., "I have failed, I will fail, I am a failure") or a ruminative style of thinking that dwells on the failure. Notably, this catastrophic response is irrespective of whether the feedback was explicit or perceived, as illustrated through the work by Beats et al. (1996) and Elliott et al. (1996) previously described. Seemingly nonaffective contexts (i.e., neuropsychological testing) can be superimposed with affective relevance due to cognitive processing during MDD (i.e., activation of negative schema).

A novel hot–cold cognitive model of MDD was proposed by Ahern et al. (2019) to bridge the work on cognition borne out Beck's (1967) seminal theory and accumulating evidence on cold cognitive deficits in MDD. Specifically, the model proposes that to understand cognition in MDD, both hot and cold aspects demand consideration. Specifically, cold deficits may *become hot,* acting as a gateway to contribute to the onset and maintenance of negative cognitive biases and mood state. In this way, general attention abilities may facilitate the expression of negative biases whereby the basic deficits in attention underpin the difficulty in disengaging from negative content. Similar can be applied to the negative biases of interpretation (general processing speed deficits) and memory (general learning and memory deficits). Conversely, hot can *become cold,* when cognitive deficits become exacerbated in the context of emotional processing, whether this be explicit or implicit, as is the case with affective interference from performance (self-)feedback, for example. The impact of this model is that it can be applied as a framework to help reconcile some of the debates in the field regarding cognition in MDD—such as the relevance of cold, cognitive deficits in the depressive cycle alongside the characteristic hot cognitions—as well as unifying complementary fields of research in an endeavor to optimize efforts in the prevention and treatment of MDD.

In a similar way, the hot–cold cognitive model can be applied to mental health messaging to understand that although individuals with MDD may preferentially process negative content (hot cognition), general cognitive deficits (cold cognition) may already impair one's ability to effectively attend to, remember, and coordinate action in response to any health care message among the competing demands in day-to-day life.

In sum, cognition in MDD is multifaceted, impacting the processing of emotional as well as nonemotional content in a mutually reinforcing manner. Hot and cold processing deficits serve to perpetuate the depressive cycle. Therefore, to consider just the traditional, hot facet of cognition in MDD (negative cognitive biases) would not sufficiently capture the dysfunctional information processing and day-to-day functional impairment that is associated with MDD. From this, health messaging could consider how cognition in MDD is not just relevant to the processing of valenced message content but also how deficient general (cold) cognitive functions might otherwise impact the intended behavior (i.e., help-seeking) following the message. These considerations, with recommendations for mental health communication research, are discussed in further detail over the subsequent sections.

Limited Availability of Cognitive Resources

As mentioned, limited cognitive resources are available to direct to all processing needs. In the case of MDD, the hot cognitive profile including cognitive biases and emotion dysregulation strategies mean that additional demands are already placed on these limited resources. When hot cognition is activated, fewer resources may be available to direct to other day-to-day cognitive tasks. This in turn can result in broader cognitive deficits that impact how well an individual engages in and interacts with their environment (Ahern et al., 2019). Cognitive load, or the demands placed on cognitive processes, inevitably will affect one's ability to recruit the required resources for the purposes of attention, learning and memory, as well as executive function and problem-solving. Experimentally, the impact of cognitive load is typically examined in cognitive tasks of varying difficulty or effort level, in parallel with investigations of the effortful processing hypothesis.

The effortful processing hypothesis (Hasher & Zacks, 1979) proposes that information processing is primarily dependent on whether the processing requirements are effortful or automatic. Automatic processing can be described as nonintentional, not requiring the direction of attention, and not distracting from any ongoing operations of the cognitive system. Effortful processing, on the other hand, requires the conscious direction of attention ("effort") and therefore can interfere with other ongoing cognitive operations (Hartlage et al., 1993). For example, Hammar et al. (2003) compared individuals with MDD to healthy controls ($N = 21$, MDD and healthy controls, respectively) on a series of automatic and effortful tasks based on a visual search paradigm with one (black, horizontal rectangles) or two types of distractors (black, horizontal rectangle and gray, upright rectangle) presented. Individuals with MDD performed comparably to controls when only one distractor was present, with the target easily recognized (black, upright rectangle); however, when a more effortful attentive search strategy was required, individuals with MDD required more time to locate the target than controls. These deficits in effortful processing were resolved at 10-year follow-up when the sample with MDD were in remission (Hammar & Årdal, 2012).

It can be postulated that both hot and cold cognition are activated in effortful processing. For example, the added task complexity may stimulate negative self-referent schemas (e.g., "I am not capable," "I am a failure") alongside the demands on basic cold cognitive processes of attention, learning and memory, or executive function. Due to this cognitive loading, insufficient resources result in a deficient ability to engage with the task at hand. Bowie et al. (2017) investigated the association between depressive symptom severity and performance across high and low cognitive loadings of the Paced Auditory Serial Addition Task (PASAT; Gronwall, 1977), which requires participants to add a given number to the one presented immediately prior. The more demanding high-cognitive loading trials presented a digit every 1.6 s, while the low-cognitive loading trial presented a digit every 2.4 s. Across 235 participants, findings indicated that more correct responses were provided on the low-cognitive load than the high-cognitive load task. Moreso, elevated depressive symptom severity (moderate-severe) was associated with more consecutively skipped items on the high-cognitive load relative to the low-cognitive load task, more so than that observed across lower symptom severity profiles (minimal, mild-moderate). It is important to note that these findings remained consistent even when controlling for general processing speed abilities, assessed using the Digit Symbol Coding neuropsychological test. Given that performance was worse on high-cognitive load trials, it is possible that this performance on the task served to activate a negative, self-referent cognition (e.g., feelings of failure, worthlessness) among those with more severe depressive symptom severity. With less cognitive resources then available to efficiently engage in the high demand task, resulting in disengagement.

The inverse is also something to consider: When cognitive resources are directed to several demands, less resources are subsequently available for emotion-congruent processing. Van Dillen and

Koole (2007) proposed a working memory model of distraction from emotion where cognitive load attenuates negative mood and emotion-congruent negative processing. In a series of experiments, the authors varied the demands placed on working memory through the presence of a math task, task complexity, and task predictability (no task, announced task, sudden task). Findings indicated that working memory load moderated the impact of viewing a negative image on mood state among a sample of student volunteers. Following high working memory load, relative to low working memory load, less emotion-congruent processing occurred, resulting in a self-report of less negative mood in response to negative pictures. Mood was not affected by working memory load in neutral trials. However, given that this sample were not explicitly recruited from a population with a risk of depression, it is possible that these findings would not hold up in a subclinical/clinical sample as there may be more difficulty to overturn the preferential processing of negative content. However, when considered in the context of subthreshold depression, Hu et al. (2021) produced similar findings: Negative material was more easily forgotten by individuals with subthreshold depression ($N = 53$) under the condition of high cognitive load, relative to low, and compared with controls. Therefore, due to current cognitive demands, less resources are subsequently available for extra-task processing that typically would be emotion-congruent (hot) in nature, serving to reinforce the negative mood state.

The concept of cognitive loading can be applied to mental health messaging. Indeed, according to resource-matching theory (Anand & Sternthal, 1989), persuasive effects are likely to best occur when there is a match between the cognitive demands of the message and the available cognitive resources of the recipient. Thus, if the demands are greater than the available cognitive resources, processing of the message is likely to be suboptimal. By one such example, messages that contain visual and narrative cues place competing demands on cognitive processes, which can be further depleted by contextual factors such as the experience of stress or negative mood state when presented with health information (Wilson & Wolf, 2009). This can be further exacerbated in the context of gain- and loss-framed messages that promote hot processing relevant to risk and reward. Gain and loss-framing are well explored in the persuasion literature, with varying levels of effect observed (Gallagher & Updegraff, 2011). This has cast interest to the exploration of individual factors in framing effects such as current mood state, which may somewhat account for the variable findings across the persuasion literature (Nabi et al., 2020).

Framing effects can be of interest in help-seeking for depression given that individuals with MDD tend to have impairments in reward-related processing (Cléry-Melin et al., 2019), which is a feature of gain-framing, while the loss- or risk-framing is consistent with the negative cognitive style in MDD and thus supports preferential processing of this negative risk frame (Beck, 1967). Nonetheless, message framing effects may not be clearly observed among competing demands for attention within a given environment as well as within the health message itself with competing visual and textual components. When there is competition for limited resources, extra-task processing may not be viable to evidence classic gain- and loss-framed effects. In an examination of attention patterns to gain- and loss-framed depression messages using eye tracking technology, Lueck (2017) found that the total time spent viewing; the number of times components were viewed (facial visuals, heading, textual information), and the time spent viewing the components were largely comparable across gain- and loss-framed messages as well as across levels of depressive symptom severity. These findings are of interest given that literature suggests that the orientation of attention to negative material is likely not an automatic bias in MDD but more so represents an inability to disengage following the direction of attention (Hartlage et al., 1993; Joormann, 2004). This would suggest that the time spent viewing the gain- and loss-framed messages would differ, with significantly more time spent on the loss-framed messages. Nonetheless, if there are numerous components vying for attention, the conditions for hot cognitive processing in response to loss-framing may not be consistently evidenced.

Recommendation: Brief, Clear Messaging to Avoid Overwhelming Available Cognitive Resources

We are limited capacity processors. Due to depressive, negative cognition in MDD, this is even more the case (Ahern et al., 2019; Ellis & Ashbrook, 1988). Multiple elements to messaging in the form of visuals, health information, action cues, as well as extraneous factors such as stress related to the health context, can demand many cognitive resources (Wilson & Wolf, 2009). For individuals with elevated depressive symptoms or MDD, high cognitive demands that require effort can often result in disengagement (e.g., Bowie et al., 2017). When basic cold cognitive demands are largely recruited to attend to visuals, text, and action cues in messaging, the boomerang effects of message framing can be understood in terms of high cognitive loading. These demands detract resources from emotional processing and constrain elaborative processing or rumination in response to negative material (Hu et al., 2021; Songco et al., 2023). All in all, framing effects with the intention that negatively-framed content would result in emotion-congruent facilitative processing may not be clearly evidenced if individuals with elevated depressive symptoms tend to show cognitive effort avoidance in response to high cognitive loads, which may be the case when presented with multiple message features. Therefore, it would be incumbent to provide brief, clear instructions in messaging.

Cold Cognitive Deficits: What Do they Contribute?

It is difficult to disentangle the effects of hot and cold cognition in the MDD cycle due to their interactive nature. Consideration of cold cognitive deficits alongside the established hot cognitive biases in MDD offers a framework to better understand the onset and maintenance of dysfunctional information processing but also facilitates a movement beyond the mood-central focus in MDD toward broader functioning in MDD.

In the context of depressive mood onset and maintenance, executive functions, including the ability to inhibit, shift, and update contents of working memory, have been closely linked with the regulation of emotion through what is described as cognitive control (Joormann & Vanderlind, 2014; LeMoult & Gotlib, 2019). It is not wholly clear whether depressive symptoms are associated with a generalized deficit in executive functions or a select deficit in cognitive control over affective contents. When investigating task switching (single, repeat, switch trials), Dell'Acqua et al. (2022) observed cognitive control difficulties across both emotional and nonemotional versions of the paradigm during switch trials. In addition to this, difficulties in simple processing occurred during the single trial blocks for emotional material relative to nonemotional but not during the more complex task blocks. This indicates both a general cognitive deficit, as well as a deficit in basic affective processing. In experimental work where cognitive control training is undertaken, such as that based on the PASAT (Gronwall, 1977), positive effects have been observed even when nonemotional material (numerical digits) is the basis of the training; this includes reductions in rumination, stress reactivity, and depressive symptom severity, albeit these findings are not consistently observed across the literature (Koster et al., 2017). Although typically examined in a hot cognitive framework, cold cognitive control is still somewhat relevant to the maintenance and/or reduction of ruminative processes during MDD. This is not to say that cold cognitive processes should take precedence over investigations of hot cognition but more so that consideration of both will help to elucidate potential mechanisms by which effective preventative, treatment, and health communication strategies can be developed.

When considering information processing in everyday contexts, there is an advantage to extending focus beyond the cognitive control processes that have been implicated in the onset and maintenance of negative depressive cognition. Indeed, cold cognitive function, assessed using neuropsychological tests (neutral material) has been associated with everyday function in MDD across domains relevant to quality of life, social interaction, work, and global function. In a meta-analysis of 28 studies by Cambridge et al. (2018), broad associations between cognitive deficits and impaired functioning were observed in cross-sectional literature, with select cognitive deficits in domains such as verbal learning and executive function also prospectively linked to impaired functioning. Of course, it could be argued that concurrent depressive mood symptoms could better explain these findings. However, during periods of remission when depressive mood symptoms have resided, cognitive deficits still remain an important mediator of functional impairment (Bortolato et al., 2016). In particular, pronounced difficulties in workplace environments continue to be reported during remission from MDD (Papalexi et al., 2022; Woo et al., 2016), possibly due to the extent of cognitive demands and higher-order coordination of tasks in accordance with schedules. Equally, cognitive factors could interact with motivational factors (Grahek et al., 2019) to account for deficient performance. Nonetheless, it remains that functional abilities in MDD are impacted. When applying these insights to health communication research, a general difficulty in coordinating tasks suggests that the evaluation of health message efficacy in terms of intended or actual help-seeking behavior could be confounded by deficient motivational–cognitive–functional abilities among individuals with severe presentations of MDD.

Recommendation: The Evaluation of Health Message Efficacy (e.g., in Terms of Intentions to Engage in Help-Seeking Behavior) Should Consider Barriers to Intended or Actual Behavior

General cognitive abilities to attend to, process, coordinate, and execute goal-directed behavior mean that individuals with more severe presentations of MDD may have difficulty in planning how they will go about seeking treatment. If messaging efficacy is determined by the likelihood of seeking treatment (e.g., How likely are you to seek help with a mental health care professional/general practitioner?), self-reports may be confounded by general motivational–cognitive–functional difficulties in planning and executing this goal-directed behavior (e.g., difficulty in prioritizing goals, forgetting scheduled appointments). Intentions in help-seeking behavior can include a conscious plan and to exert effort (White et al., 2018). Thus, capturing possible motivational–cognitive–functional barriers would be informative to health message efficacy (e.g., "I am not likely to engage in help-seeking because it requires too much cognitive effort").

Alongside the potential impact of cognitive deficits on planning help-seeking behavior, cognitive deficits may also influence treatment attitudes, expectations, and engagement. Young people already seeking treatment for MDD have reported that the experience of cognitive deficits impacts on depressive symptoms, negative self-attributions, everyday function, and engagement with therapy (Ferguson et al., 2023; Morey-Nase et al., 2019). Thus, even among those that are treatment-seeking for depression, cognitive deficits can remain a barrier to engagement. In a survey of 2,008 individuals with self-reported MDD and 1,046 healthcare providers across eight countries, individuals with MDD reported that mood, physical, and cognitive symptoms were inadequately addressed with current treatment, significantly more so than the perceived treatment inadequacy by health care providers (Baune & Christensen, 2019). In a further multinational survey, patients currently experiencing MDD reported that only the cognitive symptom domain was associated with functioning and therefore a priority for treatment. For health care providers, the cognitive and mood domains were identified to explain impaired functioning (Christensen et al., 2020). The promotion of help-seeking inevitably is impacted by expectations or attitudes toward treatment (e.g., Lueck, 2018; Yzer et al., 2022). Nonetheless, there is a degree of discordance between patient and health care provider perspectives on how well cognitive symptoms are addressed in treatment and their role in supporting a more complete, functional recovery following MDD.

Recommendation: To Promote Help-seeking, Messages Should Be Developed in Accordance with the Experiences and Concerns of Individuals with Depression

Communication efforts in health care messaging should reflect the experiences and concerns of individuals with depressive symptoms to best encourage help-seeking (Bell et al., 2010). These experiences will differ for everyone, so careful consideration should be given to the stage of depression. For example, mental health messaging could incorporate some of these lesser-known cognitive features of elevated depressive symptoms or MDD to help validate lived experiences. For a proportion of individuals with elevated depressive symptom severity or MDD, self-reported experiences of cognitive deficits are likely (Conradi et al., 2011; Douglas et al., 2018). Specifically, concentration/attention, executive function, and memory difficulties tend to be most frequently reported among individuals with MDD (Kriesche et al., 2023).

If health messages clarify that depression can be multifaceted, which for example includes difficulties with attention, memory, and the ability to plan or coordinate multiple tasks, then individuals may feel validated in their experiences, recognize the condition, and subsequently seek help—for example, "Depression can affect anyone and in a variety of ways such as low mood or lack of interest, disturbances in sleep or appetite, physical aches and pains, and/or difficulties with thinking such as concentration, attention, memory, and planning abilities." Likewise, if there is an expectation that current treatment options are suboptimal in addressing patient preferred outcomes (e.g., functioning as a treatment target; Christensen et al., 2020), then self-reports on the intention or actual help-seeking behavior may be impacted by such negative outcome expectations. Thus, health messages should also clarify that multiple treatment options are available to explore with a healthcare professional to determine how best to address the presenting symptoms—for example, "Many treatment options are available depending on your experiences of depression."

Conclusion

In conclusion, cognitive deficits in MDD are relevant, albeit complicated by the nuanced interaction with depressive mood states. Not everyone will experience significant cognitive deficits, but for a proportion of individuals with moderate-severe MDD, (cold) cognitive deficits are a pertinent consideration for their experience during, as well as in between, depressive episodes. Cognition in MDD cannot be summed up exclusively as negatively biased; it also broadly encompasses deficits across the domains of processing speed, attention, learning, memory, executive function, and problem-solving, which further extends to deficits in day-to-day functioning. The oft overshadowed cold cognitive deficits are now considered a transdiagnostic C factor (Abramovitch et al., 2021), implicated across many psychiatric conditions. This growing interest in cold cognitive deficits maps on to how their consideration can optimize our approach to disrupt the MDD cycle and support a more complete functional recovery following treatment—a call to action that is echoed from patient perspectives. Following the insights provided in this chapter, perhaps a consideration of cognitive deficits in MDD may now also be applied to augment approaches in the persuasion and communication literature and, ultimately, optimize help-seeking for depression.

References

Abramovitch, A., Short, T., & Schweiger, A. (2021). The C factor: Cognitive dysfunction as a transdiagnostic dimension in psychopathology. *Clinical Psychology Review*, *86*, 102007. http://dx.doi.org/10.1016/j.cpr.2021.102007

Ahern, E., Bockting, C. L., & Semkovska, M. (2019). A hot-cold cognitive model of depression: Integrating the neuropsychological approach into the cognitive theory framework. *Clinical Psychology in Europe*, *1*(3), 1–35. http://dx.doi.org/10.32872/cpe.v1i3.34396

Ahern, E., & Semkovska, M. (2017). Cognitive functioning in the first-episode of major depressive disorder: A systematic review and meta-analysis. *Neuropsychology*, *31*(1), 52–72. http://dx.doi.org/10.1037/neu0000319

Allott, K., Fisher, C. A., Amminger, G. P., Goodall, J., & Hetrick, S. (2016). Characterizing neurocognitive impairment in young people with major depression: State, trait, or scar? *Brain and Behavior*, *6*(10), e00527. http://dx.doi.org/10.1002/brb3.527

American Psychiatric Association. (2013). *Diagnostic and statistical manual of mental disorders* (5th ed.). https://doi.org/10.1176/appi.books.9780890425596

Anand, P., & Sternthal, B. (1989). Strategies for designing persuasive messages: Deductions from the resource matching hypothesis. In P. Cafferata & A. M. Tybout (Eds.), *Cognitive and affective responses to advertising* (pp. 135–159). Lexington Books/D. C. Heath and Com.

Baune, B. T., & Christensen, M. C. (2019). Differences in perceptions of major depressive disorder symptoms and treatment priorities between patients and health care providers across the acute, post-acute, and remission phases of depression. *Frontiers in Psychiatry*, *10*, 335. http://dx.doi.org/10.3389/fpsyt.2019.00335

Beats, B., Sahakian, B. J., & Levy, R. (1996). Cognitive performance in tests sensitive to frontal lobe dysfunction in the elderly depressed. *Psychological Medicine*, *26*(3), 591–603. http://dx.doi.org/10.1017/s0033291700035662

Beck, A. T. (1967). *Depression: Clinical, experimental and theoretical aspects*. Harper & Row.

Bell, R. A., Paterniti, D. A., Azari, R., Duberstein, P. R., Epstein, R. M., Rochlen, A. B., Johnson, M. D., Orrange, S. E., Slee, C., & Kravitz, R. L. (2010). Encouraging patients with depressive symptoms to seek care: A mixed methods approach to message development. *Patient Education and Counseling*, *78*(2), 198–205. http://dx.doi.org/10.1016/j.pec.2009.07.007

Bortolato, B., Miskowiak, K. W., Köhler, C. A., Maes, M., Fernandes, B. S., Berk, M., & Carvalho, A. F. (2016). Cognitive remission: A novel objective for the treatment of major depression? *BMC Medicine*, *14*(1), 1–18. http://dx.doi.org/10.1186/s12916-016-0560-3

Bowie, C. R., Milanovic, M., Tran, T., & Cassidy, S. (2017). Disengagement from tasks as a function of cognitive load and depressive symptom severity. *Cognitive Neuropsychiatry, 22*(1), 83–94. http://dx.doi.org/10.1080/13546805.2016.1267617

Brandl, F., Weise, B., Mulej Bratec, S., Jassim, N., Hoffmann Ayala, D., Bertram, T., Ploner, M., & Sorg, C. (2022). Common and specific large-scale brain changes in major depressive disorder, anxiety disorders, and chronic pain: A transdiagnostic multimodal meta-analysis of structural and functional MRI studies. *Neuropsychopharmacology, 47*(5), 1071–1080. http://dx.doi.org/10.1038/s41386-022-01271-y

Cambridge, O. R., Knight, M. J., Mills, N., & Baune, B. T. (2018). The clinical relationship between cognitive impairment and psychosocial functioning in major depressive disorder: A systematic review. *Psychiatry Research, 269*, 157–171. http://dx.doi.org/10.1016/j.psychres.2018.08.033

Christensen, M. C., Wong, C. M. J., & Baune, B. T. (2020). Symptoms of major depressive disorder and their impact on psychosocial functioning in the different phases of the disease: Do the perspectives of patients and healthcare providers differ? *Frontiers in Psychiatry, 11*, 280. http://dx.doi.org/10.3389/fpsyt.2020.00280

Cléry-Melin, M.-L., Jollant, F., & Gorwood, P. (2019). Reward systems and cognitions in major depressive disorder. *CNS Spectrums, 24*(1), 64–77. http://dx.doi.org/10.1017/S1092852918001335

Conradi, H. J., Ormel, J., & de Jonge, P. (2011). Presence of individual (residual) symptoms during depressive episodes and periods of remission: A 3-year prospective study. *Psychological Medicine, 41*(6), 1165–1174. http://dx.doi.org/10.1017/S0033291710001911

Dam, V., Stenbæk, D. S., Köhler-Forsberg, K., Ip, C., Ozenne, B., Sahakian, B., Knudsen, G., Jørgensen, M., & Frokjaer, V. (2021). Hot and cold cognitive disturbances in antidepressant-free patients with major depressive disorder: A NeuroPharm study. *Psychological Medicine, 51*(14), 2347–2356. http://dx.doi.org/10.1017/S0033291720000938

Delis, D. C., Kaplan, E., & Kramer, J. H. (2001). *Delis-Kaplan executive function system (D–KEFS)*. APA PsycTests.

Dell'Acqua, C., Messerotti Benvenuti, S., Vallesi, A., Palomba, D., & Ambrosini, E. (2022). Depressive symptoms and cognitive control: The role of affective interference. *Cognition and Emotion, 36*(7), 1389–1403. http://dx.doi.org/10.1080/02699931.2022.2128065

Douglas, K. M., Gallagher, P., Robinson, L. J., Carter, J. D., McIntosh, V. V., Frampton, C. M., Watson, S., Young, A. H., Ferrier, I. N., & Porter, R. J. (2018). Prevalence of cognitive impairment in major depression and bipolar disorder. *Bipolar Disorders, 20*(3), 260–274. http://dx.doi.org/10.1111/bdi.12602

Elliott, R., Sahakian, B. J., McKay, A., Herrod, J., Robbins, T. W., & Paykel, E. (1996). Neuropsychological impairments in unipolar depression: The influence of perceived failure on subsequent performance. *Psychological Medicine, 26*(5), 975–989. http://dx.doi.org/10.1017/S0033291700035303

Ellis, H. C., & Ashbrook, P. W. (1988). Resource allocation model of the effects of depressed mood states on memory. In K. Fiedler & J. F. Forgas (Eds.), *Affect, cognition and social behavior* (pp. 25–43). Hogrefe.

Ferguson, N., Rice, S., Gleeson, J., Davey, C. G., & Hetrick, S. E. (2023). The experience of young people receiving cognitive behavioural therapy for major depression: A qualitative study. *Early Intervention in Psychiatry, 17*(1), 47–56. http://dx.doi.org/10.1111/eip.13290

Ferrari, A. J., Charlson, F. J., Norman, R. E., Patten, S. B., Freedman, G., Murray, C. J., Vos, T., & Whiteford, H. A. (2013). Burden of depressive disorders by country, sex, age, and year: Findings from the global burden of disease study 2010. *PLoS Medicine, 10*(11), e1001547. http://dx.doi.org/10.1371/journal.pmed.1001547

Gallagher, K. M., & Updegraff, J. A. (2011). Health message framing effects on attitudes, intentions, and behavior: A meta-analytic review. *Annals of Behavioral Medicine, 43*(1), 101–116. http://dx.doi.org/10.1007/s12160-011-9308-7

Gorwood, P., Richard-Devantoy, S., Baylé, F., & Cléry-Melun, M.-L. (2014). Psychomotor retardation is a scar of past depressive episodes, revealed by simple cognitive tests. *European Neuropsychopharmacology, 24*(10), 1630–1640. http://dx.doi.org/10.1016/j.euroneuro.2014.07.013

Gotlib, I. H., & Joormann, J. (2010). Cognition and depression: Current status and future directions. *Annual Review of Clinical Psychology, 6*, 285–312. http://dx.doi.org/10.1146/annurev.clinpsy.121208.131305

Grahek, I., Shenhav, A., Musslick, S., Krebs, R. M., & Koster, E. H. (2019). Motivation and cognitive control in depression. *Neuroscience & Biobehavioral Reviews, 102*, 371–381. http://dx.doi.org/10.1016/j.neubiorev.2019.04.011

Gronwall, D. M. A. (1977). Paced auditory serial-addition task: A measure of recovery from concussion. *Perceptual and Motor Skills, 44*(2), 367–373. http://dx.doi.org/10.2466/pms.1977.44.2.367

Hammar, Å., & Årdal, G. (2012). Effortful information processing in patients with major depression—A 10-year follow-up study. *Psychiatry Research, 198*(3), 420–423. http://dx.doi.org/10.1016/j.psychres.2011.11.020

Hammar, Å., Lund, A., & Hugdahl, K. (2003). Selective impairment in effortful information processing in major depression. *Journal of the International Neuropsychological Society, 9*(6), 954–959. http://dx.doi.org/10.1017/S1355617703960152

Hammar, Å., Ronold, E. H., & Rekkedal, G. Å. (2022). Cognitive impairment and neurocognitive profiles in major depression—A clinical perspective. *Frontiers in Psychiatry, 13*, 764374. http://dx.doi.org/10.3389/fpsyt.2022.764374

Hartlage, S., Alloy, L. B., Vázquez, C., & Dykman, B. (1993). Automatic and effortful processing in depression. *Psychological Bulletin, 113*(2), 247–278. http://dx.doi.org/10.1037/0033-2909.113.2.247

Harvey, P. D. (2022). Domains of cognition and their assessment. *Dialogues in Clinical Neuroscience, 21*(3), 227–237. https://doi.org/10.31887/DCNS.2019.21.3/pharvey

Hasher, L., & Zacks, R. T. (1979). Automatic and effortful processes in memory. *Journal of Experimental Psychology, 108*(3), 356–388. http://dx.doi.org/10.1037/0096-3445.108.3.356

Hu, Y., Wu, X., Chen, X., Maguire, P., & Wang, D. (2021). Can increased cognitive load help people with subthreshold depression to forget negative information? *Journal of Affective Disorders, 283*, 384–394. http://dx.doi.org/10.1016/j.jad.2021.01.062

Ingram, R. E. (1984). Toward an information-processing analysis of depression. *Cognitive Therapy and Research, 8*, 443–477. http://dx.doi.org/10.1007/BF01173284

Joormann, J. (2004). Attentional bias in dysphoria: The role of inhibitory processes. *Cognition and Emotion, 18*(1), 125–147. http://dx.doi.org/10.1080/02699930244000480

Joormann, J., & Vanderlind, W. M. (2014). Emotion regulation in depression: The role of biased cognition and reduced cognitive control. *Clinical Psychological Science, 2*(4), 402–421. http://dx.doi.org/10.1177/2167702614536163

Koster, E. H., De Lissnyder, E., Derakshan, N., & De Raedt, R. (2011). Understanding depressive rumination from a cognitive science perspective: The impaired disengagement hypothesis. *Clinical Psychology Review, 31*(1), 138–145. http://dx.doi.org/10.1016/j.cpr.2010.08.005

Koster, E. H. W., Hoorelbeke, K., Onraedt, T., Owens, M., & Derakshan, N. (2017). Cognitive control interventions for depression: A systematic review of findings from training studies. *Clinical Psychology Review, 53*, 79–92. http://dx.doi.org/10.1016/j.cpr.2017.02.002

Kriesche, D., Woll, C. F. J., Tschentscher, N., Engel, R. R., & Karch, S. (2023). Neurocognitive deficits in depression: A systematic review of cognitive impairment in the acute and remitted state. *European Archives of Psychiatry and Clinical Neuroscience, 273*(5), 1105–1128. http://dx.doi.org/10.1007/s00406-022-01479-5

Legemaat, A. M., Haagedoorn, M. A., Burger, H., Denys, D., Bockting, C. L., & Geurtsen, G. J. (2022). Is suboptimal effort an issue? A systematic review on neuropsychological performance validity in major depressive disorder. *Journal of Affective Disorders, 323*(15), 731–740. http://dx.doi.org/10.1016/j.jad.2022.12.043

LeMoult, J., & Gotlib, I. H. (2019). Depression: A cognitive perspective. *Clinical Psychology Review, 69*, 51–66. http://dx.doi.org/10.1016/j.cpr.2018.06.008

Lin, W., Lin, J., Cai, X., Deng, J., Gao, Y., & Mo, L. (2021). Effects of two different emotion-inducing methods on the emotional memory of non-clinically depressed individuals. *PLoS One, 16*(5), e0249863. http://dx.doi.org/10.1371/journal.pone.0249863

Lueck, J. A. (2017). Matching message design and depressed cognition: An exploration of attention patterns for gain-and loss-framed depression help-seeking messages. *Journal of Health Communication, 22*(7), 593–603. http://dx.doi.org/10.1080/10810730.2017.1324538

Lueck, J. A. (2018). Examining determinants of seeking help for depression: Implications for effective health promotion messages. *Journal of Communication in Healthcare, 11*(1), 19–29. http://dx.doi.org/10.1080/17538068.2017.1417957

MacKenzie, L. E., Uher, R., & Pavlova, B. (2019). Cognitive performance in first-degree relatives of individuals with vs without major depressive disorder: A meta-analysis. *JAMA Psychiatry, 76*(3), 297–305. http://dx.doi.org/10.1001/jamapsychiatry.2018.3672

Majer, M., Ising, M., Künzel, H., Binder, E., Holsboer, F., Modell, S., & Zihl, J. (2004). Impaired divided attention predicts delayed response and risk to relapse in subjects with depressive disorders. *Psychological Medicine, 34*(8), 1453–1463. http://dx.doi.org/10.1017/S0033291704002697

Menon, V. (2011). Large-scale brain networks and psychopathology: A unifying triple network model. *Trends in Cognitive Sciences, 15*(10), 483–506. http://dx.doi.org/10.1016/j.tics.2011.08.003

Morey-Nase, C., Phillips, L. J., Bryce, S., Hetrick, S., Wright, A. L., Caruana, E., & Allott, K. (2019). Subjective experiences of neurocognitive functioning in young people with major depression. *BMC Psychiatry, 19*(1), 209. http://dx.doi.org/10.1186/s12888-019-2197-1

Nabi, R. L., Walter, N., Oshidary, N., Endacott, C. G., Love-Nichols, J., Lew, Z. J., & Aune, A. (2020). Can emotions capture the elusive gain-loss framing effect? A meta-analysis. *Communication Research, 47*(8), 1107–1130. http://dx.doi.org/10.1177/0093650219861256

Nolen-Hoeksema, S., Wisco, B. E., & Lyubomirsky, S. (2008). Rethinking rumination. *Perspectives on Psychological Science, 3*(5), 400–424. http://dx.doi.org/10.1111/j.1745-6924.2008.00088.x

Nuño, L., Gómez-Benito, J., Carmona, V. R., & Pino, O. (2021). A systematic review of executive function and information processing speed in major depression disorder. *Brain Sciences, 11*(2), 147. http://dx.doi.org/10.3390/brainsci11020147

Pan, Z., Park, C., Brietzke, E., Zuckerman, H., Rong, C., Mansur, R. B., Fus, D., Subramaniapillai, M., Lee, Y., & McIntyre, R. S. (2019). Cognitive impairment in major depressive disorder. *CNS Spectrums, 24*(1), 22–29. http://dx.doi.org/10.1017/S1092852918001207

Papalexi, E., Galanopoulos, A., Roukas, D., Argyropoulos, I., Michopoulos, I., Douzenis, A., Gkolia, I., Fotiadis, P., Kontis, D., & Zervas, I. M. (2022). Residual cognitive and psychosocial functional impairment in outpatients in

Greece who responded to conventional antidepressant monotherapy treatments for major depressive disorder (MDD). *Journal of Affective Disorders, 314*, 185–192. http://dx.doi.org/10.1016/j.jad.2022.07.009

Paulus, M. P. (2015). Cognitive control in depression and anxiety: Out of control? *Current Opinion in Behavioral Sciences, 1*, 113–120. http://dx.doi.org/10.1016/j.cobeha.2014.12.003

Petersen, J. Z., Porter, R. J., & Miskowiak, K. W. (2019). Clinical characteristics associated with the discrepancy between subjective and objective cognitive impairment in depression. *Journal of Affective Disorders, 246*, 763–774. http://dx.doi.org/10.1080/23279095.2021.1969398

Quigley, L., Thiruchselvam, T., & Quilty, L. C. (2022). Cognitive control biases in depression: A systematic review and meta-analysis. *Psychological Bulletin, 148*(9–10), 662–709. http://dx.doi.org/10.1037/bul0000372

Rizvi, S. J., Pizzagalli, D. A., Sproule, B. A., & Kennedy, S. H. (2016). Assessing anhedonia in depression: Potentials and pitfalls. *Neuroscience & Biobehavioral Reviews, 65*, 21–35. https://doi.org/10.1016/j.neubiorev.2016.03.004

Rnic, K., Jung, Y.-E., Torres, I., Chakrabarty, T., LeMoult, J., Vaccarino, A. L., Morton, E., Bhat, V., Giacobbe, P., McInerney, S., Frey, B. N., Milev, R. V., Müller, D., Ravindran, A. V., Rotzinger, S., Kennedy, S. H., & Lam, R. W. (2021). Association between discrepancy in objective and subjective cognitive abilities and treatment response in patients with major depressive disorder: A CAN-BIND-1 study report. *Journal of Affective Disorders, 295*, 1095–1101. http://dx.doi.org/10.1016/j.jad.2021.09.002

Rock, P. L., Roiser, J. P., Riedel, W. J., & Blackwell, A. D. (2014). Cognitive impairment in depression: A systematic review and meta-analysis. *Psychological Medicine, 44*(10), 2029–2040. http://dx.doi.org/10.1017/S0033291713002535

Roiser, J. P., & Sahakian, B. J. (2013). Hot and cold cognition in depression. *CNS Spectrums, 18*(3), 139–149. http://dx.doi.org/10.1017/S1092852913000072

Scheurich, A., Fellgiebel, A., Schermuly, I., Bauer, S., Wölfges, R., & Müller, M. (2008). Experimental evidence for a motivational origin of cognitive impairment in major depression. *Psychological Medicine, 38*(2), 237–246. http://dx.doi.org/10.1017/S0033291707002206

Semkovska, M., Quinlivan, L., O'Grady, T., Johnson, R., Collins, A., O'Connor, J., Knittle, H., Ahern, E., & Gload, T. (2019). Cognitive function following a major depressive episode: A systematic review and meta-analysis. *The Lancet Psychiatry, 6*(10), 851–861. http://dx.doi.org/10.1016/S2215-0366(19)30291-3

Siegle, G. J., Ingram, R. E., & Matt, G. E. (2002). Affective interference: An explanation for negative attention biases in dysphoria? *Cognitive Therapy and Research, 26*, 73–87. http://dx.doi.org/10.1023/A:1013893705009

Smith, P. J., Need, A. C., Cirulli, E. T., Chiba-Falek, O., & Attix, D. K. (2013). A comparison of the Cambridge automated neuropsychological test battery (CANTAB) with "traditional" neuropsychological testing instruments. *Journal of Clinical and Experimental Neuropsychology, 35*(3), 319–328. http://dx.doi.org/10.1080/13803395.2013.771618

Snyder, H. R. (2013). Major depressive disorder is associated with broad impairments on neuropsychological measures of executive function: A meta-analysis and review. *Psychological Bulletin, 139*(1), 81–132. http://dx.doi.org/10.1037/a0028727

Songco, A., Patel, S. D., Dawes, K., Rodrigues, E., O'Leary, C., Hitchcock, C., Dalgleish, T., & Schweizer, S. (2023). Affective working memory in depression. *Emotion, 23*(6), 1802–1807. http://dx.doi.org/10.1037/emo0001130

Srisurapanont, M., Suttajit, S., Eurviriyanukul, K., & Varnado, P. (2017). Discrepancy between objective and subjective cognition in adults with major depressive disorder. *Scientific Reports, 7*(1), 3901. http://dx.doi.org/10.1038/s41598-017-04353-w

Su, Y.-A., & Si, T. (2022). Progress and challenges in research of the mechanisms of anhedonia in major depressive disorder. *General Psychiatry, 35*(1), e100724. http://dx.doi.org/10.1136/gpsych-2021-100724

Tran, T., Milanovic, M., Holshausen, K., & Bowie, C. R. (2021). What is normal cognition in depression? Prevalence and functional correlates of normative versus idiographic cognitive impairment. *Neuropsychology, 35*(1), 33–41. http://dx.doi.org/10.1037/neu0000717

Trivedi, J. K. (2006). Cognitive deficits in psychiatric disorders: Current status. *Indian Journal of Psychiatry, 48*(1), 10–20. http://dx.doi.org/10.4103/0019-5545.31613

Van Dillen, L. F., & Koole, S. L. (2007). Clearing the mind: A working memory model of distraction from negative mood. *Emotion, 7*(4), 715–723. http://dx.doi.org/10.1037/1528-3542.7.4.715

Vicent-Gil, M., Portella, M. J., Serra-Blasco, M., Navarra-Ventura, G., Crivillés, S., Aguilar, E., Palao, D., & Cardoner, N. (2021). Dealing with heterogeneity of cognitive dysfunction in acute depression: A clustering approach. *Psychological Medicine, 51*(16), 2886–2894. http://dx.doi.org/10.1017/S0033291720001567

White, M. M., Clough, B. A., & Casey, L. M. (2018). What do help-seeking measures assess? Building a conceptualization framework for help-seeking intentions through a systematic review of measure content. *Clinical Psychology Review, 59*, 61–77. http://dx.doi.org/10.1016/j.cpr.2017.11.001

Wilson, E. A. H., & Wolf, M. S. (2009). Working memory and the design of health materials: A cognitive factors perspective. *Patient Education and Counseling, 74*(3), 318–322. http://dx.doi.org/10.1016/j.pec.2008.11.005

Woo, Y. S., Rosenblat, J. D., Kakar, R., Bahk, W.-M., & McIntyre, R. S. (2016). Cognitive deficits as a mediator of poor occupational function in remitted major depressive disorder patients. *Clinical Psychopharmacology and Neuroscience, 14*(1), 1–16. http://dx.doi.org/10.9758/cpn.2016.14.1.1

World Health Organization. (2012). *Global burden of mental disorders and the need for a comprehensive, coordinated response from health and social sectors at the country level: Report by the secretariat. 65th world health assembly.* World Health Organization. https://apps.who.int/iris/handle/10665/78898

World Health Organization. (2023). Depressive disorder. https://www.who.int/news-room/fact-sheets/detail/depression

Yzer, M., Kinzer, H., & Malone, M. (2022). A reasoned action approach to depression help-seeking messaging for college students: Implications of cognitive biases in depression. *Health Communication, 37*(14), 1731–1739. http://dx.doi.org/10.1080/10410236.2021.1917744

5

The Impact of Self- and Partner Schemas on Information Processing and Treatment Seeking in Depression

Fei Ying*, Gabriela C. M. Murphy*, and David J. A. Dozois
Western University

Globally, depression affects 322 million individuals each year and has severe consequences for all aspects of life, ranging from physical and psychological well-being to employment to suicidal ideation (World Health Organization, 2017). Given its pervasiveness, multifaceted approaches and models are needed to improve our understanding of depression and its underlying vulnerabilities. Of particular relevance to mental health communication are cognitive theories and models of depression, which help elucidate how individuals with depression understand and respond to messaging in their day-to-day lives. This chapter adopts a cognitive view of depression, focusing on how schemas impact information processing and interpersonal processes for individuals with the disorder. Following a theoretical overview, we turn to potential applications and discuss how schemas can be addressed to enhance the treatment of depression and impact the course of help-seeking behaviors. We conclude by discussing how researchers and clinicians might utilize the information highlighted in this chapter to improve mental health communication.

Cognitive Schemas in Depression

Many contemporary cognitive theories of depression have evolved from A. T. Beck's (1967) cognitive model of depression. Beck's theory, and other cognitive models of depression (Abramson et al., 2002; Ingram, 1984), contend that maladaptive thinking and negative appraisals of life events contribute to the onset and maintenance of the disorder. Like many models of psychopathology, cognitive theories of depression are largely diathesis-stress models, whereby cognitive vulnerabilities are thought to increase the likelihood of developing depression following stressful life events (Dozois & Beck, 2008). Beck (1967) proposed that these vulnerabilities occur at different levels of cognition, ranging from more surface-level automatic thoughts to intermediate thought processes (e.g., memory, attention, or interpretation biases), to deeper cognitive structures. How these deeper cognitive structures, which Beck (1967) referred to as *schemas*, impact information processing, particularly in the context of depression, is the focus of this chapter.

Although schemas have been defined in a variety of ways, for the purposes of this chapter they can be described as "the basic structural components of cognitive organization through which humans come to identify, interpret, categorize, and evaluate their experiences" (Schmidt et al., 1999, p. 129). We develop schemas because they allow us to process the constant flow of information from the world around us (and within ourselves) quickly and effortlessly. However, there is a cost of using schemas to

*Fei Ying and Gabriela C. M. Murphy contributed equally to this work.

The Handbook of Mental Health Communication, First Edition.
Edited by Marco C. Yzer and Jason T. Siegel.

interpret our experiences—filtering information through an individual lens is, naturally, subject to personal biases (Dozois & Beck, 2008). For example, we frequently stereotype others based on our perception of their membership in a certain group (Linville, 1982). The internal representations we form of the external world may not wholly reflect reality and have the potential to be negatively biased, inflexible, and self-perpetuating (Dozois & Beck, 2011). For individuals with depression, such is the case for the schemas that they form about themselves and others.

Self-Schemas

To date, most research on schemas in depression has focused on the beliefs an individual holds about themselves (i.e., self-schemas). Individuals with depression tend to hold highly negative beliefs centered around views of the self as unlovable, incompetent, defective, or worthless (Dozois & Beck, 2008). Thus, their cognitions often revolve around feelings of loss, failure, or hopelessness (Beck et al., 1979). Because of these negative biases, individuals with depression tend to focus on negative information and devalue positive or neutral information (Collins et al., 2023). Indeed, although depression shares features of negative affect with anxiety, low positive affect appears to differentiate depression from other psychiatric conditions (Brown et al., 1998). Notably, schemas are composed not simply of core beliefs but also of how those beliefs are organized (i.e., schema structure; Ingram et al., 1998). Schema structure refers to the degree of interconnection between internal representations of beliefs and related memories or emotional experiences that are organized as nodes in a cognitive network (Bower, 1981). When activated by internal or external experiences, content purportedly spreads more quickly across more closely interconnected nodes (Ingram et al., 1998; Segal et al., 1988). Studies assessing schema structure have found that adults and youth with depression consistently exhibit self-schema structures with highly interconnected negative content and loosely interconnected positive content compared with nonpsychiatric controls (Diehl et al., 2017; Dozois et al., 2012; Dozois & Dobson, 2001b; Lumley et al., 2012). These highly consolidated negative schema structures have been shown to remain stable across time, even in individuals who have remitted from depression (Dozois, 2007; Dozois & Dobson, 2001a).

Beck (1967) theorized that the highly negative and interconnected schema structures observed in individuals experiencing depression form early in life due to a variety of adverse childhood experiences. Childhood maltreatment, for example, has been found to contribute to the development of early maladaptive schemas, which in turn increases the risk for depression. Lumley and Harkness (2007) found that the development of schemas centered around loss or worthlessness mediated the link between childhood adversity and a depressive symptom profile. Importantly, although depressive self-schemas may develop early in life, they are thought to remain dormant until activated by negative life events (Beck et al., 1979). Indeed, numerous longitudinal studies have supported Beck's theory that the interaction of cognitive vulnerabilities and life stress predicts the onset of depression (Alloy et al., 2006; Evans et al., 2005; Lewinsohn et al., 2001; Seeds & Dozois, 2010).

Once activated by stressful life events, negative self-schemas influence information processing in depression in numerous ways (Dozois & Hayden, 2022). For example, an individual who views themself as incompetent may develop dysfunctional beliefs that center their self-worth on performance at work or the opinions of others. These dysfunctional beliefs often take the form of if–then statements such as "*If* I fail at work, *then* I am a failure as a person" (Kuiper & Olinger, 1986). To avoid the emotional distress that occurs when these stringent criteria for self-worth are not met, individuals may develop and engage in compensatory or coping strategies such as striving for perfection (Dozois & Beck, 2008). At the level of intermediate beliefs, activated schemas impact what information is attended to and how information is interpreted or encoded (i.e., attention, memory, and interpretational biases; Dozois & Beck, 2011). For example, an individual with depression may selectively process information that implies they are unlovable and disregard information that suggests otherwise. This type of thinking is an example of *selective abstraction* and *disqualifying the positive*, which are common information processing biases that Beck termed *cognitive errors.* Other cognitive errors relevant to depression include *catastrophizing* (i.e., viewing negative events as intolerable), *dichotomous thinking* (i.e., seeing things in mutually exclusive categories), and *overgeneralization* (i.e., viewing events as reflective of life in general; Dozois & Beck, 2008). Cognitive errors and other information processing biases are also evident in automatic thoughts, which are the streams of consciousness we experience in our everyday lives that arise as reactions to internal or external cues, rather than through deliberate contemplation (Dozois & Beck, 2011). In depression, automatic thoughts often take the form of negative views of the self, the world, and the future (i.e., the *cognitive triad*; Beck, 1967). Taken together, these findings highlight the importance of considering the impact of negative self-schemas on various levels of information processing in depression.

Partner Schemas

Although cognitive theory has historically focused on intrapsychic, rather than interpersonal events (Dobson et al., 2014), depressive experiences do not occur in isolation. Indeed, decades of literature have demonstrated strong connections between romantic relationships and depression (Schneider, 2014), which can occur through a variety of paths. As noted by Davila (2001), negative relationship events (e.g., conflict, divorce) can lead to depressive symptoms, and depressive symptoms can lead to relationship distress. Whether depression causes relationship distress or vice versa remains contested, but it is clear that the association between romantic relationships and depression is ever present and self-sustaining (Whisman et al., 2021). Given the inextricable linkages between romantic relationships and experiences of depression, self-schemas should not be the exclusive focus of cognitive research attempting to increase our understanding of depression. Indeed, as an individual engages in information processing throughout their quotidian life, they form and use not only self-schemas but also schemas about others. Considering that negative thinking about interpersonal themes has been noted as a particular risk factor for depression (Dozois, 2007), schemas concerning beliefs about others—though historically neglected in the literature—are equally paramount to examine. One type of interpersonal schema that has received recent attention are partner schemas.

Partner schemas can be defined as "conceptualizations of one's romantic partner, derived from past experience, which organize and guide the processing of partner-related information" (Chatav & Whisman, 2009, p. 51). Partner schemas are conceptually related to self-schemas in that both their content and structure can be assessed (Wilde & Dozois, 2019). For example, an individual may possess a highly interconnected positive partner schema and a loosely interconnected negative partner schema. Theoretically, an individual with this schema structure about their partner would likely recall and process positive information about their partner more quickly than negative information. Unlike self-schemas, however, partner schemas involve mental representations of one's partner—rather than oneself or even the relationship—with previous work suggesting that, though related, the two constructs are indeed separable (Murphy et al., 2024; Wilde & Dozois, 2018). In other words, it is possible for an individual to have a loosely organized positive self-schema but highly consolidated positive partner schema.

Preliminary work examining partner schemas suggests that they are instrumental in shaping mental and relational well-being. Indeed, Baldwin (1992, 1995) proposed that relational schemas (a broad term encompassing schemas of interpersonal relatedness) play an influential role in information processing through multiple pathways. For example, like self-schemas, relational schemas may shape interpersonal expectancies, thus increasing the likelihood that individuals preferentially notice and remember everyday events in their relationship that are consistent with their partner schemas (Baldwin, 1992). Moreover, when the information presented is ambiguous, individuals should, in theory, rely on their relational schemas to infer missing information. To illustrate, consider an individual whose partner mentions, "I like your outfit today." This comment can be interpreted in several ways, and according to Baldwin (1992), relational schemas would impact the interpretation of this statement. Was this statement, for example, a sincere compliment, an attempt to make up for a fight yesterday, or an implication that on most days your partner does not like your outfit? Taken together, Baldwin's (1992, 1995) works underscore the need to move beyond exclusively examining self-schemas and highlight the role of relational schemas in shaping both personal and relationship well-being.

Literature specifically examining partner schemas supports their purported influence on well-being. Whisman and Delinsky (2002) found that partner schemas are correlated with marital satisfaction, even after controlling for depressive symptoms. Further, these researchers found dyadic effects such that the partner schema of one individual impacted the marital satisfaction of their partner and vice versa. Moreover, Chatav and Whisman (2009) found that these types of relationship-oriented cognitions extended to dating couples. This work also revealed that relationship-oriented cognitions impact the distress-maintaining attributions an individual may form regarding their partner's negative behaviors, in addition to affecting overall relationship satisfaction.

More recent work on partner schemas and their role in information processing has focused specifically on the structure of partner schemas—that is, the cognitive organization of the beliefs an individual has about their partner. Wilde and Dozois (2018), for example, found that partner schema structures are associated with various facets of relationship health, such as romantic relationship adjustment, satisfaction, and commitment, a finding that has since been replicated across different samples (Murphy et al., 2024). Research with couples has also found dyadic effects of partner schema structures. Specifically, Hicks (2023) found that the partner schema structure of one member of the dyad had a significant impact on the relationship well-being of their partner, in addition to a significant impact on oneself. In other words, the structure of the beliefs an individual has about their partner can shape their partner's relationship well-being. Beyond relationship well-being, an individual's partner schema structures are also associated with their own symptoms of depression, stress, and anxiety (Murphy et al., 2024). Together, this work provides preliminary evidence that the beliefs one has about themselves and their partner, though related, exert separable and quantifiable impacts on one's own personal and relationship well-being, and the well-being of their partner.

To integrate research highlighting linkages between self-schemas and depression (see Dozois & Beck, 2023, for review), partner schemas and relationship health (Hicks, 2023; Murphy et al., 2024; Wilde & Dozois, 2018), and depression and relationship health (Schneider, 2014), Wilde and Dozois (2019) proposed the Dyadic Partner-Schema Model (DPSM). The DPSM provides a theoretical framework for the processes believed to underlie how self- and partner schemas affect information processing about oneself and intimate partners and how this, in turn, may contribute to maladaptive behaviors and mental health outcomes (e.g., depression). Specifically, the DPSM proposes that underlying self- and partner schemas interact to bias cognitions about partner behaviors (e.g., blame and responsibility attributions) and, consequently, each partner's responses toward one another (e.g., withdrawal or demand behavior). The DPSM also posits that these cognitions and behaviors occur in a dyadic context and interact to contribute to the mutual reinforcement of relationship dissatisfaction and depressive symptoms, both concurrently and longitudinally. Finally, according to the DPSM, relationship dissatisfaction and depressive symptoms serve to reinforce underlying self- and partner schemas, creating a cyclical process.

Several tenets of this model have been supported by the current literature (e.g., the mutual reinforcement of relationship dissatisfaction and depressive symptoms). However, many processes both within and beyond this model remain unexplored. For example, the exact mechanisms through which self- and partner schemas interact to impact relationship distress and depression are unclear. Future work could also examine whether positive partner schemas might buffer the depressive experiences of one's partner. Lastly, previous research has implicated self-schemas in a variety of other disorders beyond depression, such as paranoia (Mihić et al., 2019), social anxiety (Dozois & Frewen, 2006), and personality disorders (Kunst et al., 2020). Although beyond the scope of this chapter, future research may elucidate how disorders beyond depression are impacted by partner and self-schemas. Notwithstanding these future directions, research on the DPSM, and schemas more generally, offers several implications for treatment, help seeking, and mental health communication, as discussed in the subsequent section.

Applications of Schemas to Mental Health Treatment and Communication

Treatment

Given the pervasive role of negative schemas in depression, it is important that mental health care providers consider how to target schemas when treating individuals with depression. Although addressing schemas may not be necessary for all patients (Dobson & Dobson, 2017) and not all individuals are ready to change their core beliefs, the following techniques from cognitive behavior therapy (CBT) may be helpful for modifying negative schemas in depression. To begin, psychoeducation about the interaction between conscious thoughts, early life events, and deeper levels of cognition can be used to help patients learn how their negative beliefs developed and understand that, although they may have been functional in their early life, they are no longer adaptive in their current environment (Dozois & Bieling, 2010). For patients who are struggling to identify their core beliefs, the downward arrow technique can help bring underlying conditional assumptions to their conscious awareness (Greenberger & Padesky, 2016). The downward arrow technique is used to reveal schema content by having the patient identify recurring automatic thoughts, probing what the thought means to the patient, and what the thought might mean about them or what the consequences would be if it were true. Once core beliefs and schemas are revealed, they can be modified over time through the continual use of thought records, behavioral experiments, and Socratic questioning (see Dozois & Beck, 2023, for a full description of these techniques). Various other strategies for modifying core beliefs and schemas (e.g., strengthening new beliefs, therapy role plays, and cognitive continuum) are described in Dobson and Dobson (2017) and J. S. Beck (2021). When using these techniques, it is key that the therapist helps the patient form a narrative about the development of their core beliefs, view their experiences more objectively and sympathetically, and foster hope that their schemas can be changed over the course of therapy (Dozois & Bieling, 2010). Ultimately, the goal of CBT is to help patients form alternative beliefs and thought processes that are adaptive and can be applied to subsequent experiences.

The efficacy and effectiveness of CBT for depression have been extensively studied and well established. A meta-analysis of 91 randomized controlled trials, for instance, demonstrated that CBT is superior to placebo and equivalent to antidepressant medication and other evidence-based psychotherapies (López-López et al., 2019). CBT appears to be particularly effective for relapse prevention, with individuals treated with short-term CBT showing a lower risk of relapse than those treated with short-term medication (DeRubeis et al., 2005, 2019) and equivalent risk of relapse to those treated with continuance medication (Hollon et al., 2005). However, researchers have only recently begun to gather empirical evidence for whether and how schemas are changed through CBT. A review of the evidence surrounding cognitive restructuring (i.e., schematic change mechanisms in CBT) concluded that CBT indeed produces cognitive change and is an effective strategy for treating depression, but that more research is needed to determine how it compares to other interventions (Clark, 2013). Other studies on schema structure have shown that CBT increases the interconnectedness of positive self-schema content and decreases the interconnectedness of negative content (Dozois et al., 2009; Quilty et al., 2014), but so does pharmacotherapy (Quilty et al., 2014). Although some studies have found that changes in cognition mediate treatment improvement, overall evidence of a direct causal relationship has been equivocal or inconclusive (Crits-Christoph et al., 2017). Thus, more research is needed to test whether CBT indeed promotes changes in schemas and whether these cognitive changes explain the benefits of CBT for depression.

Given the paucity of literature surrounding partner schemas in specific, it is unknown whether targeting partner schemas in treatment for depression will be helpful. However, considering the linkages between self- and partner schemas as well as between depression and relationship distress, addressing negative partner schemas may help alleviate relationship distress and depressive symptoms. Indeed, a preliminary study on problem-focused couples therapy for depression found that changes in illness-related attitudes helped improve patients' marital satisfaction, reduce depressive symptoms, and mitigate partners' perceived burden (Cohen et al., 2014). Additionally, Christensen et al. (2021) found that adding an acceptance component to traditional couples therapy (which focuses primarily on changing behaviors) increased effect sizes. Learning to accept a partner's flaws can be conceptualized as a belief shift, and as such Christensen et al.'s (2021) findings suggest that integrating partner schemas into existing couples therapy frameworks could be a promising avenue for future research and possibly improve treatment outcomes for couples. Finally, it may be helpful to consider Beck's (1989) proposition that the negatively biased belief systems we develop about our partners can be changed through evidence-based thinking. If indeed true, then many of the cognitive restructuring strategies developed for depression may also be applicable to shifting partner schemas.

Help Seeking

Unfortunately, despite the promise of targeting schemas in mental health treatment, many individuals who experience depression or other forms of distress—whether personal or relational—do not seek treatment (Henderson et al., 2013; Hubbard & Anderson, 2021; Parnell & Hammer, 2018; Thornicroft et al., 2017; Waitzfelder et al., 2018). There are many reasons for this, spanning from individual factors to broader societal barriers, many of which have been previously highlighted in the literature. For example, many individuals do not seek treatment as a result of mental health stigma (Barney et al., 2006), gendered socialization experiences (Hubbard & Anderson, 2021; Möller-Leimkühler, 2002), duration of symptoms (Boerema et al., 2016), and/or a lack of culturally sensitive health care (Rastogi et al., 2012). Factors unique to depression, such as feelings of hopelessness and motivational deficits (Eddington et al., 2014) may also impede the likelihood of seeking help. Although the barriers to seeking treatment are numerous, the role of schemas in help-seeking behaviors is particularly relevant to this chapter.

As previously discussed, individuals experiencing depression often possess a tightly interconnected negative schema structure and loosely interconnected positive schema structure, resulting in biased information processing. Therefore, when processing messaging regarding mental health, schemas may play a role in what researchers have labeled the *boomerang effect*, a term generally applied to instances in which communication influences the targeted recipient in the opposite direction advocated by the message (Cho & Salmon, 2007). Lienemann et al. (2013) provide useful insight into boomerang effects within the context of depression and the bias produced by negative self-schemas. Specifically, they illustrate how a public service announcement targeting individuals with depression may be misinterpreted, noting how the message, "Many people have overcome depression," could be interpreted as, "I am weak since so many other people have been able to overcome depression" (p. 719). In support of this example, Lienemann et al. (2013) found that, compared with a control advertisement, viewing an advertisement targeted at individuals with depression increased self-stigma and that this self-stigma mediated the association between depressive symptoms and help-seeking intentions. In other words, despite positive intentions, the negative bias in information processing commonly observed among individuals experiencing depression may result in messaging having the opposite effect as intended.

Although not yet empirically investigated, the boomerang effect may also hold true for partner schemas. To illustrate, consider a romantic partner who, although hoping to motivate their loved one to seek treatment for their depressive symptoms, says, "Why have you not gotten help yet? When my friend was depressed, treatment really helped them." Despite the encouraging intent, this statement may result in a boomerang effect through the activation of both self- and partner schemas. The recipient of this message may process the statement through a negative lens and deduce that they themself are a burden in their relationship (self-schemas) and that their partner is being bossy or overbearing (partner schemas). This example is supported indirectly by previous research suggesting that one's romantic partner can play an influential role in either increasing or impeding the likelihood of seeking mental health treatment (Muscari & Fleming, 2019). Moreover, the potential for boomerang effects in dyadic interactions aligns closely with the propositions of the DPSM, which purports that relationship dissatisfaction and depressive symptoms are mutually reinforcing and both serve to reinforce underlying partner and self-schemas.

In addition to schemas impacting how mental health communication is received, it is important to caution that mental health communication may also result in inadvertent consequences that further impede the likelihood of help seeking. Thus, schemas not only affect how an individual processes the information in mental health messages but may also play a role in shaping the behavioral consequences that result from mental health communication. For example, mental health messaging received by individuals with highly interconnected negative self- and partner schemas may increase their likelihood of negative feedback seeking to confirm their self- and partner conceptions (Evraire & Dozois, 2011, for review). Indeed, previous research suggests that when an individual experiencing depressive symptoms receives a favorable evaluation (e.g., a positive comment from a physician), this information is interpreted as being discrepant with their own beliefs. To resolve this discrepancy, these individuals will often seek negative information to reaffirm their negative self-beliefs (Swann et al., 1992). Thus, an individual with depression whose partner notes, "You can beat this; you are a strong person," may interpret the message as highly discordant with their own self-view. It is also possible that this positive comment may be incongruent with the negative partner schemas held by the individual experiencing depressive symptoms. As a consequence, such a statement may inadvertently trigger the individual to seek negative feedback to reaffirm their negative partner schemas. Thus, the negative schemas held by individuals with depression could play an important role in how messaging is interpreted and its impact on behavior.

Advice for Mental Health Communication

Before considering how and when to apply cognitive theories to mental health communication, it is paramount to bear in mind that many individual and societal factors shape one's schemas, interpretation of messaging, treatment, and help-seeking behaviors. Schemas, particularly self-schemas, have largely been investigated in WEIRD (i.e., Western, educated, industrialized, rich, and democratic) populations, and this work often neglects how more collective belief systems may shape schematic structures (Dozois & Hayden, 2022). For example, inaccessibility of services, acculturative difficulties, stigma, fear of judgment by healthcare providers, and cultural beliefs are some of the many factors that impact help-seeking behaviors and treatment (Callister et al., 2011; Chung, 2010; Recto & Champion, 2018). As researchers, we must continue to investigate and engage in global discourse on diversity by, for example, seeking research from non-Western sources. Health care providers and individuals who communicate about mental health must also support open channels of communication and ensure that the messages relayed are sensitive to their audiences' intersecting identities.

Furthermore, mental health care researchers and clinicians should be cognizant of their own schemas, belief systems, and susceptibility to information processing biases. Yager et al. (2021) conducted a selective review of biases pertinent to psychotherapy and found that therapists are prone to anchoring (i.e., fixating on their initial impression of the patient and failing to adjust in light of later information), being influenced by visceral reactions (i.e., positive or negative gut feelings toward the patient), and many other biases. Indeed, several studies have demonstrated that clinicians rely on their intuition and experience—which is typically not as sound as believed—rather than empirical evidence to make clinical decisions (Stewart et al., 2018). For example, Schulte and Eifert (2002) found that clinicians change their therapeutic direction based on anticipation of failure versus success, which correlates more with clinician mood rather than actual treatment progress. Additionally, most individuals are more likely to believe that others, not themselves, are biased with regard to social stigmas (Wang & Jeon, 2020). However, it is essential that mental health care providers recognize their own beliefs and biases because implicit racial, ethnic, gender, and age-based biases are associated with lower quality of care (see FitzGerald & Hurst, 2017, for a review of physicians and nurses). Recognizing that everyone, including mental health care providers, is prone to biases can help reduce our tendency to attribute biases to others but not ourselves (Wang & Jeon, 2020). Other strategies to mitigate cognitive biases include educating mental health care providers about common biases and/or countertransference, along with regularly reviewing therapy sessions (Yager et al., 2021). Lastly, clinicians should rely on outcome monitoring and form falsifiable hypotheses about their own treatment plans to ensure they are practicing in an evidence-based manner (Dozois, 2013).

Considering the issues discussed in this chapter, we recommend that mental health care providers and individuals promoting treatments for depression remain aware of their own schemas and biases as well as the schemas of those around them. It is important to recognize that individuals process information through personal filters and belief systems and that consequently there may be a disconnect between the intended message and how it is received (e.g., boomerang effects). Thus, it is essential that we verify whether mental health campaigns are received as intended and that we adapt based on the ever evolving theory and evidence concerning information processing in depression. The impact of schemas on mental health messaging should be investigated with diverse samples, allowing us to make data-informed adjustments to increase the efficacy of our messaging across a broad range of populations. Further investigation of the role that partner schemas play in depression treatment and messaging is also needed. Finally, mental health providers working directly with patients should be especially cognizant of the negative self-schemas held by individuals with depression and account for how their words or actions may be interpreted.

Conclusion

In this chapter, we provided a conceptual and empirical review of self- and partner schemas in depression and proposed that modifying schemas and being aware of these belief systems can enhance treatment, increase help-seeking behaviors, and improve mental health communication strategies. Additionally, being aware of our own schemas and using strategies (e.g., outcome monitoring, evidence-based practice; see Dozois, 2013) to minimize biases can enhance clinical decision-making, improve outcomes, and promote more effective mental health communication. Understanding our patients' belief systems, and communicating with this in mind, may help to bolster help seeking and maximize communication between providers and their intended recipients.

References

Abramson, L. Y., Alloy, L. B., Hankin, B. L., Haeffel, G. J., MacCoon, D. G., & Gibb, B. E. (2002). Cognitive vulnerability-stress models of depression in a self-regulatory and psychobiological context. In I. H. Gotlib & C. L. Hammen (Eds.), *Handbook of depression* (pp. 268–294). Guildford Press.

Alloy, L. B., Abramson, L. Y., Whitehouse, W. G., Hogan, M. E., Panzarella, C., & Rose, D. T. (2006). Prospective incidence of first onsets and recurrences of depression in individuals at high and low cognitive risk for depression. *Journal of Abnormal Psychology, 115*(1), 145–156. https://doi.org/10.1037/0021-843X.115.1.145

Baldwin, M. W. (1992). Relational schemas and the processing of social information. *Psychological Bulletin, 112*(3), 461–484. https://doi.org/10.1037/0033-2909.112.3.461

Baldwin, M. W. (1995). Relational schemas and cognition in close relationships. *Journal of Social and Personal Relationships, 12*(4), 547–552. https://doi.org/10.1177/0265407595124008

Barney, L. J., Griffiths, K. M., Jorm, A. F., & Christensen, H. (2006). Stigma about depression and its impact on help-seeking intentions. *Australian & New Zealand Journal of Psychiatry, 40*(1), 51–54. https://doi.org/10.1080/j.1440-1614.2006.01741.x

Beck, A. T. (1967). *Depression: Causes and treatment.* University of Pennsylvania Press.

Beck, A. T. (1989). *Love is never enough: How couples can overcome misunderstandings, resolve conflicts, and solve relationship problems through cognitive therapy.* Harper Perennial.

Beck, A. T., Rush, A. J., Shaw, B. F., & Emery, G. (1979). *Cognitive therapy of depression.* Guilford Press.

Beck, J. S. (2021). *Cognitive behavior therapy: Basics and beyond* (3rd ed.). Guilford Press.

Boerema, A. M., Kleiboer, A., Beekman, A. T. F., Van Zoonen, K., Dijkshoorn, H., & Cuijpers, P. (2016). Determinants of help-seeking behavior in depression: A cross-sectional study. *BMC Psychiatry, 16*(1), 78. https://doi.org/10.1186/s12888-016-0790-0

Bower, G. H. (1981). Mood and memory. *American Psychologist, 36*(2), 129–148. https://doi.org/10.1037/0003-066X.36.2.129

Brown, T. A., Chorpita, B. F., & Barlow, D. H. (1998). Structural relationships among dimensions of the DSM-IV anxiety and mood disorders and dimensions of negative affect, positive affect, and autonomic arousal. *Journal of Abnormal Psychology, 107*(2), 179–192. https://doi.org/10.1037/0021-843X.107.2.179

Callister, L. C., Beckstrand, R. L., & Corbett, C. (2011). Postpartum depression and help-seeking behaviors in immigrant Hispanic women. *Journal of Obstetric, Gynecologic & Neonatal Nursing, 40*(4), 440–449. https://doi.org/10.1111/j.1552-6909.2011.01254.x

Chatav, Y., & Whisman, M. A. (2009). Partner schemas and relationship functioning: A states of mind analysis. *Behavior Therapy, 40*(1), 50–56. https://doi.org/10.1016/j.beth.2007.12.005

Cho, H., & Salmon, C. T. (2007). Unintended effects of health communication campaigns. *Journal of Communication, 57*(2), 293–317. https://doi.org/10.1111/j.1460-2466.2007.00344.x

Christensen, A., Wheeler, J. G., Doss, B. D., & Jacobson, N. S. (2021). Couple distress. In D. H. Barlow (Ed.), *Clinical handbook of psychological disorders: A step-by-step treatment manual* (6th ed., pp. 742–772). Guilford Press.

Chung, I. (2010). Changes in the sociocultural reality of Chinese immigrants: Challenges and opportunities in help-seeking behaviour. *International Journal of Social Psychiatry, 56*(4), 436–447. https://doi.org/10.1177/0020764009105647

Clark, D. A. (2013). Cognitive restructuring. In S. G. Hofmann (Ed.), *The Wiley handbook of cognitive behavioral therapy* (pp. 1–22). Wiley. https://doi.org/10.1002/9781118528563.wbcbt02

Cohen, S., Daniel O'Leary, K., Foran, H. M., & Kliem, S. (2014). Mechanisms of change in brief couple therapy for depression. *Behavior Therapy, 45*(3), 402–417. https://doi.org/10.1016/j.beth.2014.01.003

Collins, A. C., Lass, A. N. S., & Winer, E. S. (2023). Negative self-schemas and devaluation of positivity in depressed individuals: A moderated network analysis. *Current Psychology*. https://doi.org/10.1007/s12144-023-04262-4

Crits-Christoph, P., Gallop, R., Diehl, C. K., Yin, S., & Gibbons, M. B. C. (2017). Mechanisms of change in cognitive therapy for major depressive disorder in the community mental health setting. *Journal of Consulting and Clinical Psychology, 85*(6), 550–561. https://doi.org/10.1037/ccp0000198

Davila, J. (2001). Paths to unhappiness: The overlapping courses of depression and romantic dysfunction. In S. R. H. Beach (Ed.), *Marital and family processes in depression: A scientific foundation for clinical practice* (pp. 71–87). American Psychological Association. https://doi.org/10.1037/10350-004

DeRubeis, R. J., Hollon, S. D., Amsterdam, J. D., Shelton, R. C., Young, P. R., Salomon, R. M., O'Reardon, J. P., Lovett, M. L., Gladis, M. M., Brown, L. L., & Gallop, R. (2005). Cognitive therapy vs medications in the treatment of moderate to severe depression. *Archives of General Psychiatry, 62*(4), 409–416. https://doi.org/10.1001/archpsyc.62.4.409

DeRubeis, R. J., Keefe, J. R., & Beck, A. T. (2019). Cognitive therapy. In K. S. Dobson & D. J. A. Dozois (Eds.), *Handbook of cognitive-behavioral therapies* (pp. 218–248). Guilford Press.

Diehl, C., Yin, S., Markell, H., Gallop, R., Gibbons, M. B. C., & Crits-Christoph, P. (2017). The measurement of cognitive schemas: Validation of the Psychological Distance Scaling Task in a community mental health sample. *International Journal of Cognitive Therapy, 10*(1), 17–33. https://doi.org/10.1521/ijct_2016_09_18

Dobson, D. J. G., & Dobson, K. S. (2017). *Evidence-based practice of cognitive-behavioral therapy* (2nd ed.). Guilford Press.

Dobson, K. S., Quigley, L., & Dozois, D. J. (2014). Toward an integration of interpersonal risk models of depression and cognitive-behaviour therapy. *Australian Psychologist, 49*(6), 328–336. https://doi.org/10.1111/ap.12079

Dozois, D. J. A. (2007). Stability of negative self-structures: A longitudinal comparison of depressed, remitted, and nonpsychiatric controls. *Journal of Clinical Psychology, 63*(4), 319–338. https://doi.org/10.1002/jclp.20349

Dozois, D. J. A. (2013). Psychological treatments: Putting evidence into practice and practice into evidence. *Canadian Psychology, 54*(1), 1–11. https://doi.org/10.1037/a0031125

Dozois, D. J. A., & Beck, A. T. (2008). Cognitive schemas, beliefs and assumptions. In K. S. Dobson & D. J. A. Dozois (Eds.), *Risk factors in depression* (pp. 121–143). Elsevier Academic Press. https://doi.org/10.1016/B978-0-08-045078-0.00006-X

Dozois, D. J. A., & Beck, A. T. (2011). Cognitive therapy. In J. D. Herbert & E. M. Forman (Eds.), *Acceptance and mindfulness in cognitive behavior therapy* (pp. 26–56). Wiley. https://doi.org/10.1002/9781118001851.ch2

Dozois, D. J. A., & Beck, A. T. (2023). Negative thinking: Cognitive products and schema structures. In D. J. A. Dozois & K. S. Dobson (Eds.), *Treatment of psychosocial risk factors in depression* (pp. 207–232). American Psychological Association. https://doi.org/10.1037/0000332-010

Dozois, D. J. A., & Bieling, P. J. (2010). Cognitive therapy for depression. In S. Hofmann & M. Reinecke (Eds.), *Cognitive-behavioral therapy with adults* (1st ed., pp. 1–17). Cambridge University Press. https://doi.org/10.1017/CBO9780511781919.003

Dozois, D. J. A., Bieling, P. J., Patelis-Siotis, I., Hoar, L., Chudzik, S., McCabe, K., & Westra, H. A. (2009). Changes in self-schema structure in cognitive therapy for major depressive disorder: A randomized clinical trial. *Journal of Consulting and Clinical Psychology, 77*(6), 1078–1088. https://doi.org/10.1037/a0016886

Dozois, D. J. A., & Dobson, K. S. (2001a). A longitudinal investigation of information processing and cognitive organization in clinical depression: Stability of schematic interconnectedness. *Journal of Consulting and Clinical Psychology, 69*(6), 914–925. https://doi.org/10.1037/0022-006X.69.6.914

Dozois, D. J. A., & Dobson, K. S. (2001b). Information processing and cognitive organization in unipolar depression: Specificity and comorbidity issues. *Journal of Abnormal Psychology, 110*(2), 236–246. https://doi.org/10.1037/0021-843X.110.2.236

Dozois, D. J. A., Eichstedt, J. A., Collins, K. A., Phoenix, E., & Harris, K. (2012). Core beliefs, self-perception, and cognitive organization in depressed adolescents. *International Journal of Cognitive Therapy, 5*(1), 99–112. https://doi.org/10.1521/ijct.2012.5.1.99

Dozois, D. J. A., & Frewen, P. A. (2006). Specificity of cognitive structure in depression and social phobia: A comparison of interpersonal and achievement content. *Journal of Affective Disorders, 90*(2–3), 101–109. https://doi.org/10.1016/j.jad.2005.09.008

Dozois, D. J. A., & Hayden, E. P. (2022). Exceptional Canadian contributions to research on cognitive vulnerability to depression. *Canadian Journal of Behavioural Science, 54*(2), 96–106. https://doi.org/10.1037/cbs0000301

Eddington, K. M., Dozois, D. J. A., & Backs-Dermott, B. J. (2014). Evaluation of the internal consistency, factor structure, and validity of the depression change expectancy scale. *Assessment, 21*(5), 607–617. https://doi.org/10.1177/1073191113517929

Evans, J., Heron, J., Lewis, G., Araya, R., & Wolke, D. (2005). Negative self-schemas and the onset of depression in women: Longitudinal study. *British Journal of Psychiatry*, *186*(4), 302–307. https://doi.org/10.1192/bjp.186.4.302

Evraire, L. E., & Dozois, D. J. A. (2011). An integrative model of excessive reassurance seeking and negative feedback seeking in the development and maintenance of depression. *Clinical Psychology Review*, *31*(8), 1291–1303. https://doi.org/10.1016/j.cpr.2011.07.014

FitzGerald, C., & Hurst, S. (2017). Implicit bias in healthcare professionals: A systematic review. *BMC Medical Ethics*, *18*(1), 19. https://doi.org/10.1186/s12910-017-0179-8

Greenberger, D., & Padesky, C. A. (2016). *Mind over mood: Change how you feel by changing the way you think* (2nd ed.). Guilford Press.

Henderson, C., Evans-Lacko, S., & Thornicroft, G. (2013). Mental illness stigma, help seeking, and public health programs. *American Journal of Public Health*, *103*(5), 777–780. https://doi.org/10.2105/AJPH.2012.301056

Hicks, O. (2023). *The effects of self- and partner-schemas on relationship quality and depression in romantic dyads* [University of Western Ontario]. Electronic Thesis and Dissertation Repository. https://ir.lib.uwo.ca/etd/9386

Hollon, S. D., DeRubeis, R. J., Shelton, R. C., Amsterdam, J. D., Salomon, R. M., O'Reardon, J. P., Lovett, M. L., Young, P. R., Haman, K. L., Freeman, B. B., & Gallop, R. (2005). Prevention of relapse following cognitive therapy vs medications in moderate to severe depression. *Archives of General Psychiatry*, *62*(4), 417. https://doi.org/10.1001/archpsyc.62.4.417

Hubbard, A. K., & Anderson, J. R. (2021). The moderating effect of gender on expectations and threats related to relationship help-seeking. *Journal of Couple & Relationship Therapy*, *20*(1), 76–98. https://doi.org/10.1080/15332691.2020.1757546

Ingram, R. E. (1984). Toward an information-processing analysis of depression. *Cognitive Therapy and Research*, *8*(5), 443–477. https://doi.org/10.1007/BF01173284

Ingram, R. E., Miranda, J., & Segal, Z. V. (1998). *Cognitive vulnerability to depression*. Guilford Press.

Kuiper, N. A., & Olinger, L. J. (1986). Dysfunctional attitudes and a self-worth contingency model of depression. In P. C. Kendall (Ed.), *Advances in cognitive-behavioral research and therapy* (Vol. 5, pp. 115–142). Academic Press.

Kunst, H., Lobbestael, J., Candel, I., & Batink, T. (2020). Early maladaptive schemas and their relation to personality disorders: A correlational examination in a clinical population. *Clinical Psychology & Psychotherapy*, *27*(6), 837–846. https://doi.org/10.1002/cpp.2467

Lewinsohn, P. M., Joiner, T. E., & Rohde, P. (2001). Evaluation of cognitive diathesis-stress models in predicting major depressive disorder in adolescents. *Journal of Abnormal Psychology*, *110*(2), 203–215. https://doi.org/10.1037/0021-843X.110.2.203

Lienemann, B. A., Siegel, J. T., & Crano, W. D. (2013). Persuading people with depression to seek help: Respect the boomerang. *Health Communication*, *28*(7), 718–728. https://doi.org/10.1080/10410236.2012.712091

Linville, P. W. (1982). The complexity–extremity effect and age-based stereotyping. *Journal of Personality and Social Psychology*, *42*(2), 193–211. https://doi.org/10.1037/0022-3514.42.2.193

López-López, J. A., Davies, S. R., Caldwell, D. M., Churchill, R., Peters, T. J., Tallon, D., Dawson, S., Wu, Q., Li, J., Taylor, A., Lewis, G., Kessler, D. S., Wiles, N., & Welton, N. J. (2019). The process and delivery of CBT for depression in adults: A systematic review and network meta-analysis. *Psychological Medicine*, *49*(12), 1937–1947. https://doi.org/10.1017/S003329171900120X

Lumley, M. N., Dozois, D. J. A., Hennig, K. H., & Marsh, A. (2012). Cognitive organization, perceptions of parenting and depression symptoms in early adolescence. *Cognitive Therapy and Research*, *36*(4), 300–310. https://doi.org/10.1007/s10608-011-9365-z

Lumley, M. N., & Harkness, K. L. (2007). Specificity in the relations among childhood adversity, early maladaptive schemas, and symptom profiles in adolescent depression. *Cognitive Therapy and Research*, *31*(5), 639–657. https://doi.org/10.1007/s10608-006-9100-3

Mihić, L. J., Novović, Z., Dozois, D. J. A., Bentall, R. P., & Bošković, T. (2019). Structure of self-schemas in patients with paranoia. *Psihologija*, *52*(1), 21–33. https://doi.org/10.2298/PSI171120026M

Möller-Leimkühler, A. M. (2002). Barriers to help-seeking by men: A review of sociocultural and clinical literature with particular reference to depression. *Journal of Affective Disorders*, *71*(1–3), 1–9. https://doi.org/10.1016/S0165-0327(01)00379-2

Murphy, G. C. M., Ying, F., Wilde, J. L., Hicks, O., Sivakumar, P., Maxwell, J. A., & Dozois, D. J. A. (2024). *Assessing the psychometric properties of the Psychological Distance Scaling Task* [Manuscript submitted for publication]. Department of Psychology, Western University.

Muscari, E. C., & Fleming, C. E. (2019). Help-seeking for mental health concerns: The role of partner influence. *Couple and Family Psychology: Research and Practice*, *8*(4), 181–196. https://doi.org/10.1037/cfp0000125

Parnell, K. J., & Hammer, J. H. (2018). Deciding on couple therapy: The role of masculinity in relationship help-seeking. *Psychology of Men & Masculinity*, *19*(2), 212–222. https://doi.org/10.1037/men0000098

Quilty, L. C., Dozois, D. J. A., Lobo, D. S. S., Ravindran, L. N., & Bagby, R. M. (2014). Cognitive structure and processing during cognitive behavioral therapy vs. pharmacotherapy for depression. *Therapy*, *7*(3), 235–250. https://doi.org/10.1521/ijct.2014.7.3.235

Rastogi, M., Massey-Hastings, N., & Wieling, E. (2012). Barriers to seeking mental health services in the Latino/a community: A qualitative analysis. *Journal of Systemic Therapies, 31*(4), 1–17. https://doi.org/10.1521/jsyt.2012.31.4.1

Recto, P., & Champion, J. D. (2018). "We don't want to be judged": Perceptions about professional help and attitudes towards help-seeking among pregnant and postpartum Mexican-American adolescents. *Journal of Pediatric Nursing, 42*, 111–117. https://doi.org/10.1016/j.pedn.2018.04.010

Schmidt, N. B., Schmidt, K. L., & Young, J. E. (1999). Schematic and interpersonal conceptualizations of depression: An integration. In T. Joiner & J. C. Coyne (Eds.), *The interactional nature of depression: Advances in interpersonal approaches* (pp. 127–148). American Psychological Association. https://doi.org/10.1037/10311-005

Schneider, B. (2014). *Interpersonal distress and interpersonal problems associated with depression* [Columbia University]. Columbia Academic Commons. https://doi.org/10.7916/D8707ZH5

Schulte, D., & Eifert, G. H. (2002). What to do when manuals fail? The dual model of psychotherapy. *Clinical Psychology: Science and Practice, 9*(3), 312–328. https://doi.org/10.1093/clipsy.9.3.312

Seeds, P. M., & Dozois, D. J. A. (2010). Prospective evaluation of a cognitive vulnerability-stress model for depression: The interaction of schema self-structures and negative life events. *Journal of Clinical Psychology, 66*(12), 1307–1323. https://doi.org/10.1002/jclp.20723

Segal, Z. V., Hood, J. E., Shaw, B. F., & Higgins, E. T. (1988). A structural analysis of the self-schema construct in major depression. *Cognitive Therapy and Research, 12*(5), 471–485. https://doi.org/10.1007/BF01173414

Stewart, R. E., Chambless, D. L., & Stirman, S. W. (2018). Decision making and the use of evidence-based practice: Is the three-legged stool balanced? *Practice Innovations, 3*(1), 56–67. https://doi.org/10.1037/pri0000063

Swann, W. B., Wenzlaff, R. M., & Tafarodi, R. W. (1992). Depression and the search for negative evaluations: More evidence of the role of self-verification strivings. *Journal of Abnormal Psychology, 101*(2), 314–317. https://doi.org/10.1037/0021-843X.101.2.314

Thornicroft, G., Chatterji, S., Evans-Lacko, S., Gruber, M., Sampson, N., Aguilar-Gaxiola, S., Al-Hamzawi, A., Alonso, J., Andrade, L., Borges, G., Bruffaerts, R., Bunting, B., De Almeida, J. M. C., Florescu, S., De Girolamo, G., Gureje, O., Haro, J. M., He, Y., Hinkov, H., ... Kessler, R. C. (2017). Undertreatment of people with major depressive disorder in 21 countries. *British Journal of Psychiatry, 210*(2), 119–124. https://doi.org/10.1192/bjp.bp.116.188078

Waitzfelder, B., Stewart, C., Coleman, K. J., Rossom, R., Ahmedani, B. K., Beck, A. T., Zeber, J. E., Daida, Y. G., Trinacty, C., Hubley, S., & Simon, G. E. (2018). Treatment initiation for new episodes of depression in primary care settings. *Journal of General Internal Medicine, 33*(8), 1283–1291. https://doi.org/10.1007/s11606-017-4297-2

Wang, Q., & Jeon, H. J. (2020). Bias in bias recognition: People view others but not themselves as biased by preexisting beliefs and social stigmas. *PLoS One, 15*(10), e0240232. https://doi.org/10.1371/journal.pone.0240232

Whisman, M. A., & Delinsky, S. S. (2002). Marital satisfaction and an information-processing measure of partner-schemas. *Cognitive Therapy and Research, 26*(5), 617–627. https://doi.org/10.1023/A:1020305226067

Whisman, M. A., Sbarra, D. A., & Beach, S. R. H. (2021). Intimate relationships and depression: Searching for causation in the sea of association. *Annual Review of Clinical Psychology, 17*(1), 233–258. https://doi.org/10.1146/annurev-clinpsy-081219-103323

Wilde, J. L., & Dozois, D. J. A. (2018). It's not me, It's you: Self- and partner-schemas, depressive symptoms, and relationship quality. *Journal of Social and Clinical Psychology, 37*(5), 356–380. https://doi.org/10.1521/jscp.2018.37.5.356

Wilde, J. L., & Dozois, D. J. A. (2019). A dyadic partner-schema model of relationship distress and depression: Conceptual integration of interpersonal theory and cognitive-behavioral models. *Clinical Psychology Review, 70*, 13–25. https://doi.org/10.1016/j.cpr.2019.03.003

World Health Organization. (2017). *Depression and other common mental disorders: Global health estimates.* World Health Organization.

Yager, J., Kay, J., & Kelsay, K. (2021). Clinicians' cognitive and affective biases and the practice of psychotherapy. *American Journal of Psychotherapy, 74*(3), 119–126. https://doi.org/10.1176/appi.psychotherapy.20200025

Part II

Conceptualization and Measurement of Primary Variables

6

A Typology of Health Communication Variables Relevant for Mental Health

Romy RW[1], Xingman Wu[2], Rudy Sunrin Kim[2], and Xiaoli Nan[2]

[1] Loyola Marymount University
[2] University of Maryland, College Park

Mental health messaging plays a vital role in addressing and alleviating mental health crises (Smith-Frigerio, 2020). Despite the effectiveness of health messaging in many health domains other than mental health, how and when mental health messaging works to improve outcomes remains unclear given the lack of a systematic approach to the research on its effects. It may therefore be useful for those who want to use messaging to promote mental health but who may not be familiar with health communication science to learn more about the communication and persuasion variables that are commonly tested in this research. To this end, in this chapter, we introduce a framework based on the prominent communication/persuasion model (Berlo, 1960; McGuire, 1989). The communication/persuasion model proves to be a promising framework for understanding how communication and persuasion variables function in the design of mental health messages. By applying the principles of effective communication in mental health messaging, we enhance our ability to succeed in crucial interventions aimed at addressing mental health challenges in the United States and worldwide.

Developed and refined by psychologists and communication scholars over the years, the communication/persuasion model outlines principal input variables that influence communication outcomes (Berlo, 1960; McGuire, 1989). The most common principal input variables include source, message, channel, receiver, and destination, which are especially relevant in the context of communication. The source is the originator of the communication, the person or group that intends to convey a message or induce change. Message is the content or information that the source wants to communicate. Channel refers to the medium through which the message is delivered. The receiver is the person or group that receives the message. The final variable in the model, destination, refers to the kind of outcomes at which a message is aimed (e.g., beliefs vs. attitudes, short-term vs. long-term changes, increasing acceptance vs. inducing resistance). The communication/persuasion model provides a typology of input as well as output variables for understanding the communication process, roughly mirroring Lasswell's (1948) classic description of the communication process as "who," "says what," "through which channel," "to whom," and "with what effect" (Nan et al., 2022). The communication/persuasion model helps us intuitively make sense of not only the process of communication such as how information flows from the source to the receiver but also the forces that shape communication outcomes in various contexts. The model suggests that communication outcomes (e.g., change in some mental state or behavior) may be understood as being shaped by the characteristics of the source, message, channel, receiver, and destination. In communication research,

The Handbook of Mental Health Communication, First Edition.
Edited by Marco C. Yzer and Jason T. Siegel.

especially in the field of persuasion, these characteristics and their impact on communication or persuasion outcomes have been extensively studied.

Input Variables

Sources

Characteristics of the message source play an important role in determining communication outcomes, encompassing dimensions such as credibility, including expertise and trustworthiness, likability, similarity, and physical attractiveness (O'Keefe, 2016). Generally, sources with heightened expertise, trustworthiness, likability, perceived similarity to the audience, and physical attractiveness tend to wield greater persuasive influence (Dillard & Shen, 2012; Pornpitakpan, 2004; Wilson & Sherrell, 1993).

In the realm of health communication, researchers conduct a thorough examination to elucidate the impact of various factors on source credibility. For instance, a scoping review delved into the influence of source credibility factors, such as trustworthiness and expertise, on the efficacy of nutrition communication. The findings indicated that factors like language usage (e.g., personalization), expertise heuristics (e.g., author credentials), and bandwagon heuristics (e.g., social media metrics) significantly shaped the effects of source credibility (Jenkins et al., 2020). The assessment of credibility commonly relies on established scales and instruments. Validated scales like McCroskey and Teven's (1999) Source Credibility Scale, which encompasses goodwill, trustworthiness, and competence constructs, and Ohanian's Scale (1990), including attractiveness, trustworthiness, and expertise constructs, are frequently employed. Utilizing message sources effectively not only strengthens the validity and applicability of research findings but also provides essential insights crucial in crafting health communication messages.

Messages

While a message is the content or information that the source wants to communicate, the way or format in which a message is delivered can be impactful on communication outcomes. Therefore, key characteristics of a message that influence communication outcomes are best conceptualized as including both message content (i.e., what to communicate) and executions (i.e., how to communicate). In terms of message content, the current literature has considered content based on utilitarian appeals, normative appeals, and value appeals (Nan et al., 2022). Utilitarian appeals accentuate the benefits or costs of an idea or action to evoke cost–benefit analysis that often underlies decision-making. Utilitarian appeals can be effective if the highlighted benefits and costs are considered significant by the message receiver (O'Keefe, 2016). Normative appeals, in contrast, highlight descriptive or injunctive norms for an idea or action (e.g., how prevalent are a particular action and what is the level of societal approval for this action). Normative appeals are often quite effective as humans are highly tuned to social information (Chung & Rimal, 2016; Rhodes et al., 2020). Lastly, value appeals emphasize how performing a recommended behavior upholds or violates one's values or other high-level goals. Attaching values to an idea or action can have a surprisingly strong impact on persuasive outcomes as values are deeply held, highly regarded beliefs shaping other thoughts and behavior (Nan et al., 2022). Value appeals have demonstrated effectiveness across diverse domains. Notably, a meta-analysis revealed a modest persuasive effect when cultural values (e.g., individualism, collectivism) were aligned with those of the audience (Hornikx & O'Keefe, 2009). Another meta-analysis focusing on climate change messages found heightened persuasive effects on attitudes and behavioral intentions when messages centered on moral values (Li & Su, 2018). Individuals exhibited a higher likelihood of persuasion when the message about COVID-19 vaccination aligned with their political values (Nan et al., 2022).

In terms of message executions, the current literature offers a rich set of message strategies that can significantly shape communication outcomes. These message features include the use of narratives (Green & Brock, 2000; Slater & Rouner, 2002), visuals (Garcia-Retamero & Cokely, 2017; Lipkus, 2007), and emotional appeals (Dillard & Peck, 2000; Nabi, 1999). Consistent evidence, as indicated by Braddock and Dillard's (2016) meta-analysis, suggests that narrative messages or stories tend to outperform didactic messages in motivating actions. For instance, Shen et al.'s (2017) experiment, utilizing video clips on sexual health topics as narrative messages, resulted in significant effects on persuasive outcomes (e.g., increased behavioral intention to get tested for sexually transmitted diseases). Visuals, when used to communicate health risks, are more persuasive than texts alone (Clarke et al., 2020; Noar et al., 2020). For instance, a meta-analysis by Clarke et al. (2020) revealed that health warning labels incorporating both images and text were more effective in reducing harmful consumption of food and alcoholic drinks compared with text-only messages. Finally, strategic use of emotional appeals—especially fear, guilt, hope, and compassion appeals—are important communication strategies that amplify persuasive effects (Myrick & Oliver, 2015; Reichard et al., 2013; Tannenbaum et al., 2015; Xu & Guo, 2018). For example, Becheur and Valette-Florence (2014) crafted three health messages employing shame, fear, and guilt to combat alcohol abuse among young people and found that the use of these emotions resulted in significant persuasive outcomes.

Receiver

In crafting impactful communication, beyond considering source and message factors, the attributes of the messages themselves play a crucial role. Recognizing the significance of receiver characteristics is paramount, as the impact of a message can vary widely among different individuals or groups. Moreover, within a specific audience, certain messages may prove more persuasive than others. The imperative of attending to receiver characteristics finds strong support in the extensive literature on message targeting and tailoring, as highlighted by Nan et al. (2022). Both message targeting and tailoring share the common goal of aligning messages with receiver characteristics to enhance persuasive outcomes. Notably, meta-analytic reviews conducted by Noar et al. (2007) and Joyal-Desmarais et al. (2022) underscore that message matching, whether through targeting or tailoring, significantly amplifies persuasion.

Within the domain of mental health, a crucial aspect of audience characteristics that demands consideration is the severity of mental health conditions among message recipients. Individuals grappling with mental health issues, such as depression, exhibit cognitive biases during message processing, influencing their reception, interpretation, and retention of information (Yzer & Siegel, 2024). Specifically, individuals contending with depression tend to harbor negative biases in their memory, making it more accessible for them to retrieve negative memories. When individuals with depression are exposed to interventions, negative attitudes are more likely to be elicited, whether these attitudes were preexisting memories or formed anew after accessing negative information in their memory (Siegel et al., 2017). Importantly, these negative attitudes persist as a filtering mechanism when encountering subsequent messages in the future.

Channel

According to the communication/persuasion model, the medium through which a message is delivered (i.e., channel) can have a significant impact on communicative outcomes. Generally, there are two primary channels utilized: the traditional face-to-face and the mediated e-health channels.

Traditional mental health interventions involve direct face-to-face communication between mental health providers and patients, typically taking place in a mental health provider's office or a clinical setting. Utilizing a face-to-face communication channel in mental health interventions offers many advantages. It enables mental health professionals to establish rapport, receive verbal and nonverbal cues, and provide immediate support and feedback. This traditional approach has been widely utilized and is an important component of effective mental health interventions.

E-health channels encompass a wide array of mental health intervention types that cater to diverse needs and preferences. Videoconferencing facilitates live and visual communication between mental health providers and patients, allowing for effective interaction and the exchange of verbal and nonverbal cues (Holmes & Foster, 2012). Telephone helplines provide immediate mental health support and crisis interventions through phone calls, offering a lifeline for individuals in distress. Online synchronous chat platforms enable real-time communication between mental health professionals and patients through text-based messages, fostering timely and responsive support. Mobile applications provide patients with direct access to guided mental health interventions on their smartphones or tablets. These apps offer a range of features including mood tracking, meditation exercises, cognitive behavior therapy techniques, and self-help modules. Furthermore, virtual reality interventions utilize immersive virtual environments to simulate therapeutic scenarios or experiences, aiding individuals in confronting phobias, addressing posttraumatic stress disorder, practicing social skills in virtual social situations, and exploring relaxation and mindfulness exercises. To communicate effectively, we need to choose appropriate channels that are aligned with our communication goals. The traditional face-to-face channel allows for direct and immediate interaction and the interpretation of nonverbal cues between mental health providers and patients. On the other hand, most mediated e-health channels provide flexibility, convenience, and accessibility. Given their diverse features, using different channels can accomplish unique goals associated with mental health outcomes.

Destination

The last variable in the communication/persuasion model, within the category of input communication factors, is the destination, which consists of variables related to the kind of target outcome (e.g., beliefs versus attitudes versus behaviors; short-term versus long-term outcomes; increasing acceptance versus inducing resistance).

In the realm of health communication research, researchers and practitioners alike are most intrigued by the outcomes of beliefs, attitudes, and behaviors. The theory of reasoned action, introduced by Martin Fishbein and Icek Ajzen in 1975, posits that behavior is significantly shaped by an individual's attitudes toward a specific behavior, with this influence predominantly mediated by their intention. Consequently, in most instances, there exists a consistency and positive correlation among individuals' beliefs, attitudes, and behaviors. Any alteration in one of these variables often leads to corresponding variations in the other two. It is noteworthy that while these three variables are generally aligned, the effectiveness of a message can fluctuate based on the specific outcome variable it addresses. Owing to practical constraints such as time, financial resources, and the accessibility of medical facilities, it is plausible that a single message might bring about substantial changes in respondents' beliefs and attitudes. However, the translation of these changes into behaviors may be subtle or challenging to detect.

The persuasive influence of a message can also be contingent upon the endurance of the outcome variables that captivate scholars' interest. While many studies have concentrated on scrutinizing the short-term effects of message framings on respondents' beliefs and attitudes, assuming that the most substantial changes occur immediately post-exposure, a broader examination considering long-term outcomes reveals a nuanced persuasive landscape. A pertinent example is the sleeper effect in persuasion. Messages linked to noncredible sources typically yield negative impacts on short-term outcomes (Tormala et al., 2006). However, the persuasiveness of such messages can amplify over time as the discounting cue becomes unavailable in respondents' memory (Kumkale & Albarracín, 2004). Moreover, theories like cultivation theory, agenda-setting theory, and social learning theory posit that individuals' perceptions undergo gradual cultivation and shaping through prolonged exposure to media.

In addition to fostering individuals' receptivity to positive changes, bolstering the capacity to resist persuasion emerges as a crucial focus in health communication. This is particularly evident in endeavors to empower individuals, such as those experiencing depression, to recognize and withstand stigmatizing messages prevalent in society. One effective strategy in this context is inoculation, as proposed by McGuire (1964). By exposing individuals to a persuasive message that incorporates both a threat and refutational preemption, a form of "immunity" is cultivated, rendering them more resilient to subsequent, stronger persuasion attempts. Another viable approach is rooted in the concept of prior commitment, as outlined by Greenwald (1965). Individuals can fortify their resistance by openly or privately articulating their initial positions before encountering persuasive influences. This proactive commitment serves as a protective shield, contributing to a heightened ability to resist external pressures and maintain steadfastness in one's convictions.

Summary

The communication/persuasion model highlights key input variables shaping communication outcomes. Source characteristics like credibility dimensions impact persuasive influence, especially in health communication. Messages, influenced by content and executions, leverage appeals and strategic features. Aligning messages with receiver characteristics enhances persuasion, particularly in mental health contexts. Channels, traditional or e-health, offer distinct advantages based on communication goals. The destination, focusing on beliefs, attitudes, and behaviors, considers short-term versus long-term effects.

Crafting effective mental health messages requires understanding persuasion as a multifaceted process that encompasses various variables. It is essential to recognize that some message features are more effective in impacting some specific outcomes than others and that the more distal an outcome variable is, the less likely direct message effects are to occur. Hence, by focusing on how messages can influence output variables such as attention and awareness, comprehension, elaboration, memory, beliefs, attitudes, and behaviors, mental health message designers can efficiently enhance communication effectiveness and audience engagement.

Output Variables

Attention and Awareness

The initial exposure of individuals to health messages, capturing their attention and raising awareness, constitutes a crucial step in the persuasive process. This exposure, guided by attitude and mediated through repeated instances, holds the potential to instigate behavioral changes (Petty et al., 2009). Examining consumer behavior, research by Fazio (1990) reveals that repeated exposure to a product name can cultivate feelings of favorability, heightening the likelihood of eventual purchase. Depending on the nature of the message, this repeated exposure becomes a key factor in enhancing the overall effectiveness of the communication.

The extent of attention devoted to a stimulus hinges on both the content and form of the message, considering factors such as novelty, intensity, and complexity—especially pertinent in the realm of health campaigns (Donohew et al., 1994). Attention plays a dual role in governing the automatic processing of individuals engaging with the message and, concurrently as well as contribute to the sustained exposure to that message (Donohew et al., 1994). Recognizing that numerous health messages go unnoticed, research endeavors have been dedicated to uncovering strategies to capture audience attention in health communications. For example, Houts et al. (2006) delve into the impact of incorporating pictures in health communication, discovering that both pictures and text-only messages heighten attention, with pictures proving particularly effective in drawing attention compared with text-only messages.

However, awareness alone of a health issue or topic is deemed "a necessary, but not sufficient, condition" for effecting changes in behavior or garnering policy support (Niederdeppe et al., 2008, p. 502). Previous research suggests diverse message strategies for amplifying public awareness. Notably, expository language (providing straightforward information) emerged as more effective in heightening awareness of aquatic conservation compared to narrative messages (Kolandai-Matchett et al., 2021). Additionally, the use of narratives, normative appeals, and visual images is recommended as effective strategies for elevating public awareness regarding social determinants of health and population health disparities (Niederdeppe et al., 2008).

Comprehension

The effectiveness of persuasive messages in shaping attitudes and inducing behavior change is intricately tied to individuals' comprehension of the messages. Comprehension involves the process through which individuals interpret the meaning of linguistic or visual elements to derive a comprehensive understanding (Houts et al., 2006).

This understanding is closely intertwined with personal abilities and message characteristics. In the realm of health communication, cognitive abilities crucial for comprehension encompass processing capacity and domain-specific knowledge, including health-related knowledge (Morrow et al., 2012). Specifically, processing capacity, such as working memory, facilitates the temporary storage and manipulation of information. This enables individuals to grasp complex messages by integrating new information with their existing knowledge (Baddeley, 1992). In this process, relevant knowledge plays a pivotal role, aiding individuals in comprehending text more efficiently (O'Reilly et al., 2019). Additionally, features like the use of pictures and interactivity significantly contribute to enhancing comprehension. In many cases, supplementing text with simple, pertinent images, such as matchstick figures, proves more effective in aiding comprehension than text alone (Houts et al., 2006). Advanced technology further supports this by significantly improving individuals' comprehension through increased message interactivity (Lustria, 2007).

However, individuals tend to process information in a manner aligned with their desires, emotions, and preexisting beliefs. Motivated reasoning suggests that individuals, instead of objectively analyzing information, tend to interpret and comprehend it in ways that reinforce their existing attitudes and preferences (Kunda, 1990). It is crucial to note that for those holding incorrect preexisting beliefs and attitudes, repeating accurate information does not guarantee acceptance; instead, it may trigger reactance and reinforce their original beliefs (Baekgaard et al., 2017; Rains, 2012). To mitigate this barrier, leveraging narratives (storytelling) and emphasizing the shared identity between message senders (source) and the audience (receiver) in the message can be effective (Chu et al., 2021; Chen et al., 2024).

Elaboration

When individuals encounter new or relevant information in persuasive messages, two modes of elaboration, or issue-relevant thinking, come into play. The elaboration likelihood model (ELM; Petty & Wegener, 1999) asserts that individuals engage in information processing through either the peripheral or central routes of persuasion. The choice between these routes depends on the level of thinking about the information on the given topic: the central route is taken when elaboration is relatively high, while the peripheral route is adopted when elaboration is low (O'Keefe, 2012). Similarly, the heuristic–systematic model of information processing posits that systematic and heuristic processing differ in the mental effort and ability required to contemplate the given topic (Chaiken & Ledgerwood, 2012). Systematic processing involves deep, thoughtful deliberation, while heuristic processing relies on cues or shortcuts for making decisions based on limited information and mental resources. O'Keefe (2012) identifies two factors influencing the degree of elaboration. Elaboration motivation hinges on personal relevance and the need for cognition. Individuals with high personal relevance to the message and a strong need for cognition are more motivated to process information with greater elaboration. Elaboration ability, on the other hand, depends on distraction and prior knowledge. Higher distraction and lower prior knowledge diminish individuals' elaboration ability. The effectiveness of persuasion and message processing is shaped by thought generation and the depth of elaboration. Information has the most persuasive impact when individuals are both motivated and able to process the provided information. This cognitive processing leads to positive and enduring thoughts about the presented agenda, as emphasized by O'Keefe (2012).

Memory

Memory or recall of a message is another important outcome in the realm of persuasion. Additionally, message features and issue involvement influence message recall. For instance, the incorporation of simple, congruent images alongside health education text has been shown to enhance individuals' ability to recall the message compared with text alone (Houts et al., 2006; Lochbuehler et al., 2017). Moreover, individuals with high issue involvement tend to recollect more message arguments than their low-issue-involved counterparts (Leippe & Elkin, 1987). Within the context of memory as a persuasion outcome, two predominant approaches elucidate the process from encountering a message to the formation of attitudes: online processing and memory-based processing. Online processing suggests that upon encountering a message, audiences concurrently form a judgment, which is then stored in their memory. When queried about their attitude toward the object described in the message, they access their memory and report it directly. In contrast, memory-based processing entails messages being directly placed into individuals' working memory, circumventing the initial step of forming a judgment (Carpenter & Boster, 2013; Hastie & Park, 1986). Research indicates that memory-based processing yields short-term persuasion effects, while online processing results in more enduring persuasion effects (Hill et al., 2013).

Beliefs and Attitudes

Understanding the impact of mental health messages on individuals' beliefs is important. Belief is defined as "the subjective probability of a relation between the object of the belief and some other object, value, concept, or attribute" (Fishbein & Ajzen, 1975, p. 131). An effective strategy for crafting persuasive mental health messages involves altering the set of salient beliefs, a mechanism outlined by O'Keefe (2016). This can be achieved through introducing new salient beliefs or adjusting the relative salience of existing beliefs. However, careful evaluation of the compatibility of these candidate beliefs with the existing set is crucial (O'Keefe, 2012). Emphasizing positive attributes in the audience's beliefs during message crafting enhances overall attitude, making the approach of altering the relative salience of beliefs potentially more effective than directly influencing belief evaluation.

Beliefs serve as the foundation for attitude, another outcome influenced by health messages. Attitude is defined as "a psychological tendency that is expressed by evaluating a particular entity with some degree of favor or disfavor" (Eagly & Chaiken, 1993, p. 1). The expectancy–value approach breaks down attitude into cognitive (thoughts about the attitude object) and affective aspects (emotions related to the attitude object) (O'Keefe, 2016). Fishbein and Ajzen (1975) offer a formula decomposing attitude into the multiplicative combination of one's beliefs or expectations about an object and how one evaluates these expectations, providing a clearer method for attitude assessment. The symbolic attitude approach suggests that emotion and symbols, rather than beliefs, are central to attitude formation. Individuals develop strong attitudes toward symbols such as nation, religion, culture, and race, which are instilled from a young age by parents, peers, and mass media (Sears & Funk, 1991). The symbolic approach is particularly relevant to political beliefs, positing that strong ideological viewpoints influence attitude development.

Despite the diverse ways audiences form attitudes, a general strategy for designing persuasive messages to change attitudes is functional matching (Katz, 1960). The functional matching effect emphasizes that tailoring persuasive appeals to the receiver's attitude function is more effective than using mismatched appeals (Carpenter, 2012; Katz, 1960). This effectiveness is rooted in the fact that functionally matched appeals directly address the receiver's psychological needs. Two crucial considerations in this context are the quality of arguments, with functionally matched messages perceived as containing better arguments, and the distinction between symbolic and instrumental attitude functions. Symbolic functions involve expressing moral beliefs, symbolizing values, and projecting self-images, while instrumental functions encompass summarizing intrinsic properties and appraising an object based on specific consequences or attributes (O'Keefe, 2016). Optimal design of health communication messages involves leveraging both symbolic and instrumental attitude functions, recognizing that individuals' attitudes may have a combination of these underpinnings.

Behaviors

Behaviors stand out as a significant variable in the realm of persuasive outcomes, particularly within the context of health communication. Although attitudes play a pivotal role in shaping behaviors, motivating individuals to engage in a specific behavior remains challenging, even when they already hold a positive attitude toward it. Beyond attitude, several factors influence behavior. According to the theory of planned behavior (Fishbein & Ajzen, 1975), attitude, subjective norms (perceived expectations from others), perceived behavioral control (individuals' belief in the ease of performing a specific behavior), and behavioral intentions collectively predict a person's behavior. In a meta-analysis of health behaviors (Godin & Kok, 1996), attitudes, subjective norms, perceived behavioral control, and intentions collectively explained 34 percent of the variance in behavior, a notably high value in the social sciences. In the domain of mental health, help-seeking behavior is a commonly investigated key behavior. This behavior involves seeking professional mental health services, such as visiting a counselor, therapist, or psychiatrist. For college students' help-seeking behavior related to depression, attitude, norms, and control contributed to 42 percent of the variance in the intention to seek professional help (Lueck & Yzer, 2018).

Addressing certain health behaviors proves to be intricate due to the need for sustained behavior change. To prolong behavioral modifications beyond the initial phase, a comprehensive understanding of the contextual background of the behavior change process becomes imperative. This includes identifying factors that either facilitate or impede the behavior, delineating specifics of the target behaviors, understanding the intervention environment, and grasping the overall change mechanisms involved (Ory et al., 2010). For instance, a study on exercise maintenance and well-being revealed that sustaining health-promoting behavior necessitates self-regulation skills, with social media engagement emerging as a tool that can foster and support these skills effectively (Zhou & Krishnan, 2019).

When targeting help-seeking behavior, the intended behavior involves distinct stages, starting with prompting individuals to seek mental health services and attend intake appointments. Subsequently, fostering continued attendance at counseling sessions becomes crucial. Research indicates that varying vignettes modeling an initial counseling session not only impact help-seeking attitudes but also influence willingness to continue counseling (Ægisdóttir et al., 2011). Exploring factors contributing to continuous engagement in mental health services, Wilson and Deane (2012) found that maintaining a therapeutic relationship with the mental health provider, perceived utility of counseling, and autonomy about the counseling process were crucial aspects influencing individuals to persist in counseling.

Summary

The communication/persuasion model has been widely used to inform research in areas such as advertising, marketing, public health communication, media effects, and political communication. It offers a useful framework for understanding the effects or effectiveness of communication stimuli or interventions by highlighting the key components of communication and how they shape communication outcomes.

In sum, focusing on strengthening key output variables such as attention, awareness, comprehension, elaboration, memory, beliefs, attitudes, and behaviors is essential for crafting effective mental health messages. Attention and awareness, critical for persuasion, require strategic exposure to drive behavioral change. Comprehension, influenced by cognitive abilities and message features, plays a pivotal role, with efforts to address motivated reasoning. Tailoring messages to individuals' cognitive processing style, known as elaboration, is crucial. Memory, influencing persuasiveness, benefits from image incorporation for better recall. Prioritizing belief change through altering the salience of existing beliefs enhances overall attitude. Finally, behavioral change hinges on attitudes, subjective norms, perceived behavioral control, and intentions. Understanding these elements enhances the impact of mental health messages in broader health communication discussions.

Mental Health Implications

The implications drawn from the examination of input and output variables in the communication/persuasion process underscore the significance of strategic message design for optimal impact. Currently, there is limited research examining the impact of source credibility on mental health messages. Emphasizing factors such as expertise and trustworthiness in message sources can guide the selection and presentation of sources, offering mental health communicators a valuable framework for developing messages that resonate authentically with their audience and contribute to positive mental health outcomes. In the realm of mental health messages research, the effectiveness of communication hinges not only on the content of the message but also on how it is delivered. For example, when designing a mental health message, normative appeals can be integrated (e.g., "Many individuals join a mental health support community") or value appeals emphasizing how performing a recommended behavior upholds or violates one's values or other high-level goals (e.g., "Embrace self-compassion as a core value"). Tailoring mental health messages to individual characteristics is a crucial communication principle. Considering factors like age, health conditions, race, gender, and more enhances the effectiveness of persuasion. The choice of channels plays a vital role in achieving specific mental health goals, considering the diverse features each channel provides. Traditional face-to-face interactions enable direct engagement and interpretation of nonverbal cues between mental health providers and patients. In contrast, mediated e-health channels offer flexibility and convenience, enhancing accessibility.

Applying these insights to mental health messages research allows for the development of communication strategies that are not only informative but also tailored to effectively engage and motivate individuals toward positive mental health outcomes. Finally, considering the type of target outcome (i.e., destination) is crucial for effective communication. Health messages most frequently aim to elicit a change in belief, attitude, and behavioral intention. As discussed in the reasoned action approach (Fishbein & Ajzen, 2011), beliefs constitute attitudes, which in turn lead to behavioral intention. Thus, understanding specific beliefs the target population holds toward help-seeking behavior can guide what needs to be targeted within messages. As positive attitudes lead to behavioral intention, it is possible to create change in behavior by changing beliefs and attitudes toward mental health services. For example, specific beliefs that are found to hinder the target populations' intention to seek help such as, "What I share during my counseling sessions will not remain confidential," or "Counseling will not help me," can be identified and targeted to change negative or incorrect beliefs individuals hold about counseling.

We end with a cautionary note. Our illustrative recommendations served to highlight the usefulness of the communication/persuasion matrix for systematically considering options for effective message design. These recommendations were based on what we have learned in domains other than mental health. As depression affects information processing and other variables that are relevant for message effects (Yzer & Siegel, 2024), we stress the need to carefully test the effects of input variables among people affected by mental illness.

Summary

The examination of input and output variables in the communication/persuasion process underscores the crucial role of strategic message design for optimal impact. While limited research explores source impact, factors like expertise and trustworthiness guide authentic message development. Effective mental health messages consider not just content but also delivery and channel choice. Applying these insights develops informative, tailored strategies that engage and motivate for positive mental health outcomes, targeting specific beliefs to change attitudes and behaviors effectively. Acknowledging the central role of health messages in various outputs, including attention, awareness, comprehension, elaboration, memory, belief, attitude, and behaviors, underscores the need to understand the specific beliefs held by the target population. Applying these insights to mental health messages research facilitates the creation of customized communication strategies that inform, engage, and motivate individuals toward positive mental health outcomes.

Conclusion

The communication/persuasion model outlines principal input and output variables in the communication process and provides a useful framework for understanding mental health message designs. The principal input variables include source, message, channel, receiver, and destination. The key output variables include awareness, comprehension, elaboration, memory, and beliefs, attitudes, and behaviors. Theory-based mental health communication messaging offers a systematic approach to understanding, addressing, and treating mental health conditions, thereby enhancing mental healthcare. The current literature lacks sufficient exploration of the application of communication theory in mental health messaging contexts, despite communication and persuasion variables playing important roles in designing such messages. This chapter bridges this gap by incorporating the communication/persuasion model to understand mental health communication. The integration of the communication/persuasion model into mental health messaging offers a range of practical benefits. By addressing elements such as source, channel, message, receiver, and destination, and distinguishing between different outcomes, significant improvements can be made in the effectiveness and quality of mental health messages. According to a report by the National Institutes of Mental Health (2023), more than one in five adults in the United States, approximately 57.8 million individuals, live with a mental illness. This highlights the urgency and importance of addressing mental health issues. The communication/persuasion model offers valuable insights for guiding future directions in research and practice within mental health messaging. Future research should explore the specific communication variables that influence mental health message designs. As technology continues to advance, social media plays a significant role in promoting mental health messages. The importance of understanding and leveraging e-mental health is underscored by a White House report (2023) that prioritizes this area in mental health research. Future studies should focus on investigating the effectiveness of mental health messages across various mental health conditions and populations. Mental health conditions disproportionately afflict disadvantaged communities, an additional obstacle in promoting inclusivity within mental health research. It is crucial to prioritize equity in promoting mental health and understanding, preventing, identifying, and treating mental health conditions (The White House, 2023). Therefore, future research efforts should examine how receiver characteristics, including age, gender, cultural background, and socioeconomic status, interact with communication processes in mental health message designs.

References

Ægisdóttir, S., O'Heron, M., Hartong, J., Haynes, S., & Linville, M. (2011). Enhancing attitudes and reducing fears about mental health counseling: An analogue study. *Journal of Mental Health Counseling, 33*(4), 327–346. http://dx.doi.org/10.17744/mehc.33.4.a5673mh711w3g441

Baddeley, A. (1992). Working memory. *Science, 255*(5044), 556–559. http://dx.doi.org/10.1126/science.1736359

Baekgaard, M., Christensen, J., Dahlmann, C. M., Mathiasen, A., & Petersen, N. B. (2017). The role of evidence in politics: Motivated reasoning and persuasion among politicians. *British Journal of Political Science, 49*(3), 1117–1140. http://dx.doi.org/10.1017/s0007123417000084

Becheur, I., & Valette-Florence, P. (2014). The use of negative emotions in health communication messages: Study of the effects of fear, guilt, and shame. *Recherche et Applications en Marketing (English Edition), 29*(4), 89–109. http://dx.doi.org/10.1177/2051570714552620

Berlo, D. K. (1960). *The process of communication; an introduction to theory and practice.* Holt, Rinehart and Winston.

Braddock, K., & Dillard, J. P. (2016). Meta-analytic evidence for the persuasive effect of narratives on beliefs, attitudes, intentions, and behaviors. *Communication Monographs, 83*(4), 446–467. http://dx.doi.org/10.1080/03637751.2015.1128555

Carpenter, C. J. (2012). A meta-analysis of the functional matching effect based on functional attitude theory. *Southern Communication Journal, 77*(5), 438–451. http://dx.doi.org/10.1080/1041794x.2012.699989

Carpenter, C. J., & Boster, F. J. (2013). The relationship between message recall and persuasion: More complex than it seems. *Journal of Communication, 63*(4), 661–681. http://dx.doi.org/10.1111/jcom.12042

Chaiken, S., & Ledgerwood, A. (2012). A theory of heuristic and systematic information processing. In P. A. M. Van Lange, A. W. Kruglanski, & E. T. Higgins (Eds.), *Handbook of theories of social psychology* (pp. 246–266). Sage. http://dx.doi.org/10.4135/9781446249215.n13

Chen, M., Dong, Y., & Wang, J. (2024). A meta-analysis examining the role of character-recipient similarity in narrative persuasion. *Communication Research, 51*(1), 56–82. http://dx.doi.org/10.1177/00936502231204834

Chu, J., Pink, S. L., & Willer, R. (2021). Religious identity cues increase vaccination intentions and trust in medical experts among American Christians. *Proceedings of the National Academy of Sciences, 118*(49), e2106481118. http://dx.doi.org/10.1073/pnas.2106481118

Chung, A., & Rimal, R. N. (2016). Social norms: A review. *Review of Communication Research, 4*, 1–28. https://doi.org/10.12840/issn.2255-4165.2016.04.01.008

Clarke, N., Pechey, E., Kosīte, D., König, L. M., Mantzari, E., Blackwell, A. K., Marteau, T. M., & Hollands, G. J. (2020). Impact of health warning labels on selection and consumption of food and alcohol products: Systematic review with meta-analysis. *Health Psychology Review, 15*(3), 1–24. http://dx.doi.org/10.1080/17437199.2020.1780147

Dillard, J. P., & Peck, E. (2000). Affect and persuasion: Emotional responses to public service announcements. *Communication Research, 27*(4), 461–495. http://dx.doi.org/10.1177/009365000027004003

Dillard, J. P., & Shen, L. (2012). *The SAGE handbook of persuasion: Developments in theory and practice*. Sage. http://dx.doi.org/10.4135/9781452218410

Donohew, L., Palmgreen, P., & Lorch, E. P. (1994). Attention, need for sensation, and health communication campaigns. *American Behavioral Scientist, 38*(2), 310–322. http://dx.doi.org/10.1177/0002764294038002011

Eagly, A. H., & Chaiken, S. (1993). *The psychology of attitudes*. Harcourt Brace Jovanovich College Publishers.

Fazio, R. H. (1990). Multiple processes by which attitudes guide behavior: The MODE model as an integrative framework. In M. Zanna (Ed.), *Advances in experimental social psychology* (pp. 75–109). Academic Press.

Fishbein, M., & Ajzen, I. (1975). *Belief, attitude, intention, and behavior: An introduction to theory and research*. Addison-Wesley.

Fishbein, M., & Ajzen, I. (2011). *Predicting and changing behavior: The reasoned action approach*. Psychology Press. http://dx.doi.org/10.4324/9780203838020

Garcia-Retamero, R., & Cokely, E. T. (2017). Designing visual aids that promote risk literacy: A systematic review of health research and evidence-based design heuristics. *Human Factors, 59*(4), 582–627. http://dx.doi.org/10.1177/0018720817690634

Godin, G., & Kok, G. (1996). The theory of planned behavior: A review of its applications to health-related behaviors. *American Journal of Health Promotion, 11*(2), 87–98. http://dx.doi.org/10.4278/0890-1171-11.2.8

Green, M. C., & Brock, T. C. (2000). The role of transportation in the persuasiveness of public narratives. *Journal of Personality and Social Psychology, 79*(5), 701. http://dx.doi.org/10.1037/0022-3514.79.5.701

Greenwald, A. G. (1965). Effects of prior commitment on behavior change after a persuasive communication. *Public Opinion Quarterly, 29*(4), 595–601. http://dx.doi.org/10.1086/267362

Hastie, R., & Park, B. (1986). The relationship between memory and judgment depends on whether the judgment task is memory-based or on-line. *Psychological Review, 93*(3), 258–268. http://dx.doi.org/10.1037/0033-295x.93.3.258

Hill, S. J., Lo, J., Vavreck, L., & Zaller, J. (2013). How quickly we forget: The duration of persuasion effects from mass communication. *Political Communication, 30*(4), 521–547. http://dx.doi.org/10.1080/10584609.2013.828143

Holmes, C., & Foster, V. (2012). A preliminary comparison study of online and face-to-face counseling: Client perceptions of three factors. *Journal of Technology in Human Services, 30*(1), 14–31. http://dx.doi.org/10.1080/15228835.2012.662848

Hornikx, J., & O'Keefe, D. J. (2009). Adapting consumer advertising appeals to cultural values: A meta-analytic review of effects on persuasiveness and ad liking. *Annals of the International Communication Association, 33*(1), 39–71. http://dx.doi.org/10.1080/23808985.2009.11679084

Houts, P. S., Doak, C. C., Doak, L. G., & Loscalzo, M. J. (2006). The role of pictures in improving health communication: A review of research on attention, comprehension, recall, and adherence. *Patient Education and Counseling, 61*(2), 173–190. http://dx.doi.org/10.1016/j.pec.2005.05.004

Jenkins, E. L., Ilicic, J., Barklamb, A. M., & McCaffrey, T. A. (2020). Assessing the credibility and authenticity of social media content for applications in health communication: Scoping review. *Journal of Medical Internet Research, 22*(7), e17296. http://dx.doi.org/10.2196/17296

Joyal-Desmarais, K., Scharmer, A. K., Madzelan, M. K., See, J. V., Rothman, A. J., & Snyder, M. (2022). Appealing to motivation to change attitudes, intentions, and behavior: A systematic review and meta-analysis of 702 experimental tests of the effects of motivational message matching on persuasion. *Psychological Bulletin, 148*(7–8), 465–517. http://dx.doi.org/10.1037/bul0000377

Katz, D. (1960). The functional approach to the study of attitudes. *Public Opinion Quarterly, 24*(2), 163–204. http://dx.doi.org/10.1086/266945

Kolandai-Matchett, K., Armoudian, M., & Li, E. (2021). Communicating complex ocean issues: How strategically framed messages affect awareness and motivation when conveyed using narrative vs. expository language. *Aquatic Conservation: Marine and Freshwater Ecosystems, 31*(4), 870–887. http://dx.doi.org/10.1002/aqc.3484

Kumkale, G. T., & Albarracín, D. (2004). The sleeper effect in persuasion: A meta-analytic review. *Psychological Bulletin, 130*(1), 143–172. http://dx.doi.org/10.1037/0033-2909.130.1.143

Kunda, Z. (1990). The case for motivated reasoning. *Psychological Bulletin, 108*(3), 480–498. http://dx.doi.org/10.1037/0033-2909.108.3.480

Lasswell, H. D. (1948). The structure and function of communication in society. In L. Bryson (Ed.), *The communication of ideas* (pp. 37–51). Harper and Row.

Leippe, M. R., & Elkin, R. A. (1987). When motives clash: Issue involvement and response involvement as determinants of persuasion. *Journal of Personality and Social Psychology, 52*(2), 269–278. http://dx.doi.org/10.1037/0022-3514.52.2.269

Li, N., & Su, L. Y.-F. (2018). Message framing and climate change communication: A meta-analytical review. *Journal of Applied Communications, 102*(3), 1–16. http://dx.doi.org/10.4148/1051-0834.2189

Lipkus, I. M. (2007). Numeric, verbal, and visual formats of conveying health risks: Suggested best practices and future recommendations. *Medical Decision Making, 27*(5), 696–713. http://dx.doi.org/10.1177/0272989X07307271

Lochbuehler, K., Mercincavage, M., Tang, K. Z., Dana Tomlin, C., Cappella, J. N., & Strasser, A. A. (2017). Effect of message congruency on attention and recall in pictorial health warning labels. *Tobacco Control, 27*(3), 266–271. http://dx.doi.org/10.1136/tobaccocontrol-2016-053615

Lueck, J., & Yzer, M. (2018). Explaining intentions to seek help for depressive symptoms in the context of responsibility message framing. *Health Communication, 33*(8), 946–953. http://dx.doi.org/10.1080/10410236.2017.1322857

Lustria, M. L. (2007). Can interactivity make a difference? Effects of interactivity on the comprehension of and attitudes toward online health content. *Journal of the American Society for Information Science and Technology, 58*(6), 766–776. http://dx.doi.org/10.1002/asi.20557

McCroskey, J. C., & Teven, J. J. (1999). Goodwill: A reexamination of the construct and its measurement. *Communications Monographs, 66*(1), 90–103. http://dx.doi.org/10.1080/03637759909376464

McGuire, W. J. (1964). Some contemporary approaches. *Advances in Experimental Social Psychology, 1*, 191–229. http://dx.doi.org/10.1016/s0065-2601(08)60052-0

McGuire, W. J. (1989). Theoretical foundations of campaigns. In R. E. Rice & C. K. Atkin (Eds.), *Public communication campaigns.* Sage.

Morrow, D., D'andrea, L., Stine-Morrow, E. A. L., Shake, M., Bertel, S., Chin, J., Kopren, K., Gao, X., Conner-Garcia, T., Graumlich, J., & Murray, M. (2012). Comprehension of multimedia health information among older adults with chronic illness. *Visual Communication, 11*(3), 347–362. http://dx.doi.org/10.1177/1470357212446413

Myrick, J. G., & Oliver, M. B. (2015). Laughing and crying: Mixed emotions, compassion, and the effectiveness of a YouTube PSA about skin cancer. *Health Communication, 30*(8), 820–829. http://dx.doi.org/10.1080/10410236.2013.845729

Nabi, R. L. (1999). A cognitive-functional model for the effects of discrete negative emotions on information processing, attitude change, and recall. *Communication Theory, 9*(3), 292–320. http://dx.doi.org/10.1111/j.1468-2885.1999.tb00172.x

Nan, X., Iles, I. A., Yang, B., & Ma, Z. (2022). Public health messaging during the COVID-19 pandemic and beyond: Lessons from communication science. *Health Communication, 37*(1), 1–19. http://dx.doi.org/10.1080/10410236.2021.1994910

National Institutes of Mental Health. (2023). *Mental illness.* https://www.nimh.nih.gov/health/statistics/mental-illness

Niederdeppe, J., Bu, Q. L., Borah, P., Kindig, D. A., & Robert, S. A. (2008). Message design strategies to raise public awareness of social determinants of health and population health disparities. *The Milbank Quarterly, 86*(3), 481–513. http://dx.doi.org/10.1111/j.1468-0009.2008.00530.x

Noar, S. M., Benac, C. N., & Harris, M. S. (2007). Does tailoring matter? Meta-analytic review of tailored print health behavior change interventions. *Psychological Bulletin, 133*(4), 673–693. http://dx.doi.org/10.1037/0033-2909.133.4.673

Noar, S. M., Rohde, J. A., Barker, J. O., Hall, M. G., & Brewer, N. T. (2020). Pictorial cigarette pack warnings increase some risk appraisals but not risk beliefs: A meta-analysis. *Human Communication Research, 46*(2–3), 250–272. http://dx.doi.org/10.1093/hcr/hqz016

Ohanian, R. (1990). Construction and validation of a scale to measure celebrity endorsers' perceived expertise, trustworthiness, and attractiveness. *Journal of Advertising*, 39–52. http://dx.doi.org/10.1080/00913367.1990.10673191

O'Keefe, D. J. (2012). The elaboration likelihood model. In *The SAGE handbook of persuasion: Developments in theory and practice* (pp. 137–149). Sage. http://dx.doi.org/10.4135/9781452218410.n9

O'Keefe, D. J. (2016). *Persuasion: Theory and research* (3rd ed.). Sage.

O'Reilly, T., Wang, Z., & Sabatini, J. (2019). How much knowledge is too little? When a lack of knowledge becomes a barrier to comprehension. *Psychological Science, 30*(9), 1344–1351. http://dx.doi.org/10.1177/0956797619862276

Ory, M. G., Lee Smith, M., Mier, N., & Wernicke, M. M. (2010). The science of sustaining health behavior change: The health maintenance consortium. *American Journal of Health Behavior, 34*(6), 647–659. http://dx.doi.org/10.5993/AJHB.34.6.2

Petty, R. E., Brinol, P., & Priester, J. R. (2009). Mass media attitude change: Implications of the elaboration likelihood model of persuasion. In J. Bryant & M. B. Oliver (Eds.), *Media effects: Advances in theory and research* (pp. 125–164). Routledge.

Petty, R. E., & Wegener, D. T. (1999). The elaboration likelihood model: Current status and controversies. In S. Chaiken & Y. Trope (Eds.), *Dual process theories in social psychology* (pp. 37–72). Guilford.

Pornpitakpan, C. (2004). The persuasiveness of source credibility: A critical review of five decades' evidence. *Journal of Applied Social Psychology, 34*(2), 243–281. http://dx.doi.org/10.1111/j.1559-1816.2004.tb02547.x

Rains, S. A. (2012). The nature of psychological reactance revisited: A meta-analytic review. *Human Communication Research, 39*(1), 47–73. http://dx.doi.org/10.1111/j.1468-2958.2012.01443.x

Reichard, R. J., Avey, J. B., Lopez, S., & Dollwet, M. (2013). Having the will and finding the way: A review and meta-analysis of hope at work. *The Journal of Positive Psychology, 8*(4), 292–304. http://dx.doi.org/10.1080/17439760.2013.800903

Rhodes, N., Shulman, H. C., & McClaran, N. (2020). Changing norms: A meta-analytic integration of research on social norms appeals. *Human Communication Research, 46*(2–3), 161–191. http://dx.doi.org/10.1093/hcr/hqz023

Sears, D. O., & Funk, C. L. (1991). The role of self-interest in social and political attitudes. *Advances in Experimental Social Psychology*, *24*, 1–91. http://dx.doi.org/10.1016/S0065-2601(08)60327-5

Shen, L., Seung, S., Andersen, K. K., & McNeal, D. (2017). The psychological mechanisms of persuasive impact from narrative communication. *Studies in Communication Sciences*, *17*(2), 165–181. https://doi.org/10.24434/j.scoms.2017.02.003

Siegel, J. T., Lienemann, B. A., & Rosenberg, B. D. (2017). Resistance, reactance, and misinterpretation: Highlighting the challenge of persuading people with depression to seek help. *Social and Personality Psychology Compass*, *11*(6), e12322. http://dx.doi.org/10.1111/spc3.12322

Slater, M. D., & Rouner, D. (2002). Entertainment—Education and elaboration likelihood: Understanding the processing of narrative persuasion. *Communication Theory*, *12*(2), 173–191. http://dx.doi.org/10.1111/j.1468-2885.2002.tb00265.x

Smith-Frigerio, S. (2020). Grassroots mental health groups' use of advocacy strategies in social media messaging. *Qualitative Health Research*, *30*(14), 2205–2216. http://dx.doi.org/10.1177/1049732320951532

Tannenbaum, M. B., Hepler, J., Zimmerman, R. S., Saul, L., Jacobs, S., Wilson, K., & Albarracín, D. (2015). Appealing to fear: A meta-analysis of fear appeal effectiveness and theories. *Psychological Bulletin*, *141*(6), 1178–1204. http://dx.doi.org/10.1037/a0039729

The White House. (2023). *White House report on mental health research priorities*. https://www.whitehouse.gov/wp-content/uploads/2023/02/White-House-Report-on-Mental-Health-Research-Priorities.pdf

Tormala, Z. L., Briñol, P., & Petty, R. E. (2006). When credibility attacks: The reverse impact of source credibility on persuasion. *Journal of Experimental Social Psychology*, *42*(5), 684–691. http://dx.doi.org/10.1016/j.jesp.2005.10.005

Wilson, C. J., & Deane, F. P. (2012). Brief report: Need for autonomy and other perceived barriers relating to adolescents' intentions to seek professional mental health care. *Journal of Adolescence*, *35*(1), 233–237. http://dx.doi.org/10.1016/j.adolescence.2010.06.011

Wilson, E. J., & Sherrell, D. L. (1993). Source effects in communication and persuasion research: A meta-analysis of effect size. *Journal of the Academy of Marketing Science*, *21*, 101–112. http://dx.doi.org/10.1007/BF02894421

Xu, Z., & Guo, H. (2018). A meta-analysis of the effectiveness of guilt on health-related attitudes and intentions. *Health Communication*, *33*(5), 519–525. http://dx.doi.org/10.1080/10410236.2017.1278633

Yzer, M., & Siegel, J. (2024). Recipient-focused research on depression help-seeking messaging. In G. De Bruijn & H. Vandebosch (Eds.), *Handbook of communication science: Health, media, and communication*. De Gruyter Mouton.

Zhou, X., & Krishnan, A. (2019). What predicts exercise maintenance and well-being? Examining the influence of health-related psychographic factors and social media communication. *Health Communication*, *34*(6), 589–597. http://dx.doi.org/10.1080/10410236.2018.1428851

7

Introducing Health Communication Science to Mental Health Researchers: An Examination of Information Seeking, Processing, and Dissemination Frameworks

Brian Quick, Sarah Caban, Minhey Chung, and Jia Yan
University of Illinois Urbana-Champaign

Mental health encompasses our emotional, psychological, and social well-being (Centers for Disease Control and Prevention, 2023). The World Health Organization (2022) refers to mental health as a psychological state of mental well-being, which allows individuals to cope with life stress, realize their abilities, and contribute to their community. Approximately 20% of adults in the United States live with a mental illness such as schizophrenia, bipolar disorder, or major depression, among many others (Centers for Disease Control and Prevention, 2023). Furthermore, research indicates that some populations are affected by mental illness more heavily than others. For instance, suicide is the fourth leading cause of death among 15- to 29-year-olds (World Health Organization, 2022). Additionally, compared to men, women are more likely to report experiences with mental disorders (Patalay & Demkowicz, 2023). Even if the prevalence of some mental disorders varies by population, mental health challenges are a public health issue that is relevant for everyone (Gao et al., 2020; O'Reilly et al., 2018).

In response to numerous public health issues, communication principles have informed the design of promotional messages sought to abate mental health issues. The application to message-based mental health promotion is emerging. Therefore, we believe it will be useful for those who want to use messaging to promote mental health but who may be unfamiliar with health communication science to learn more about some of the foci in health communication scholarship, as revealed throughout this volume. A strength of the study of health communication is found in its diversity with respect to context, methods, and analytic strategies. Health communication is diverse in that it transcends various contexts including intrapersonal, interpersonal, intergroup, organizational, and mass communication (McCullock et al., 2021; Thompson & Harrington, 2021). Additionally, health communication research is diverse in the methods employed, with researchers employing computational methods, conversation analysis, surveys, interviews, experiments, focus groups, and content analysis to answer a range of questions (Kim et al., 2010; McCullock et al., 2021). Health communication scientists test and apply a host of theories to predict and explain individual behavior and it stands to help the mental health field (for a review, see Thompson & Harrington, 2021).

The Handbook of Mental Health Communication, First Edition.
Edited by Marco C. Yzer and Jason T. Siegel.

Health communication refers to "the way we seek, process, and share health information" (Kreps & Thornton, 1992, p. 2). Communication theory is evaluated by its scope, appropriateness, heuristic value, validity, parsimony, and openness to diverse applications and address a myriad of questions asked by health communication researchers (Littlejohn, 1999). The theories introduced in this chapter meet these criteria. Here, we present how health communication researchers can offer both theoretical and pragmatic advice for mental health scholars and practitioners by giving attention to the leading frameworks of how individuals seek, process, and disseminate information. We begin with a discussion of information seeking.

Information Seeking

Health information seeking behavior is generally conceptualized as the process by which individuals purposively obtain the type and amount of information to actively engage in medical decision making, using either online or offline sources (Lambert & Loiselle, 2007). Information seeking serves as a vital tool for improving public health literacy, reducing stigma, promoting help-seeking behaviors, and empowering individuals to be a part of the health decision-making process (Brashers et al., 2002; Lambert & Loiselle, 2007; Moorman & Matulich, 1993; Nicholson et al., 2005). Information seeking is characterized by the type and volume of health-related information sought, the specific actions taken to acquire the information, and the sources individuals use (Lambert & Loiselle, 2007). Communication scholars studying information seeking often center their research on answering the questions of whether, how, and why people engage in information seeking and what the subsequent outcomes are (Brashers et al., 2002; Chang & Huang, 2020; Ou & Ho, 2022).

Many communication research and theories inform and guide the explorations of these questions. For example, the comprehensive model of information seeking (Johnson & Meischke, 1993) explains why, how, and when people seek information. The model identifies two primary determinants: demographics and personal characteristics (i.e. individual's age, gender, knowledge, and personal experiences), and information-carrying channels (i.e. resources or avenues through which people seek and receive information, including interpersonal networks, mass media, online sources), that determine various information seeking actions (i.e. active search, ongoing search, and scanning). Similarly, the risk information seeking and processing (RISP) model (Griffin et al., 1999, 2004) also seeks to understand how individuals search for and process information, especially related to risks. The RISP model highlights the roles of perceived risk characteristics (e.g. severity and likelihood), perceived information gathering capacity, and perceived information sufficiency (i.e. amount of information individuals believe they need to deal with a risk adequately) in determining information seeking behaviors. The factors highlighted in these theories provide valuable perspectives for public health researchers and mental health practitioners to better understand the process by which people seek information about mental health, through identifying the potential barriers and challenges arising from this process. This, in turn, enhances coping strategies for mental health conditions by fostering health information seeking. In a meta-analysis that examined 89 studies to explore factors related to information seeking (Ou & Ho, 2022), researchers pinpointed sociocultural and information carrier factors as having the most pronounced correlation with information seeking. Specifically, social norms largely shape health information seeking behaviors. Moreover, compared to online platforms, offline channels—primarily represented by individuals' social networks—more effectively encourage health information seeking. This enhanced engagement is likely because family, friends, and healthcare professionals can increase patients' comprehension of and trust in health information (Peng et al., 2019). It is noticeable that the roles of social networks and interactions in association with information seeking stand out from the meta-analysis. In fact, another communication theory, the theory of motivated information management (TMIM), theorizes the factors associated with information seeking behaviors within interpersonal relationships.

Theory of Motivated Information Management

TMIM is a communication theory that explains how individuals seek and manage information in response to uncertainties related to important matters (Afifi & Morse, 2015; Afifi & Weiner, 2004). The theory focuses on psychological factors and proposes a three-phase process: interpretation, evaluation, and decision, associated with information management behaviors. During the interpretation phase, people notice a discrepancy between the level of uncertainty they are comfortable with (desired uncertainty individuals identify) and the level of uncertainty they currently experience (experienced uncertainty). The discrepancy often triggers anxiety and other negative emotions (Morse et al., 2009). These reactions stem from an appraisal mechanism, which is also influenced by individual traits such as personality and perceived control (Chaiken et al., 1996). After the interpretation phase is the evaluation phase. During the evaluation phase, individuals assess the potential outcomes of seeking information and their self-efficacy in finding and understanding the necessary information. For example, the costs and benefits of information seeking related to a health condition, as well as the communication, target, and coping efficacy toward the information seeking process, are evaluated (Afifi & Morse, 2015; Afifi & Weiner, 2004). Finally, individuals determine whether to seek information, known as the decision-making phase. Typically, when the anticipated benefits surpass the costs and individuals are confident in their ability to obtain and understand the information (i.e., demonstrating high efficacy), they exhibit a stronger intention toward information seeking (Kuang & Wilson, 2021).

TMIM was first developed in the context of sexual health and has been used to predict information management strategies, especially information seeking, across a spectrum of health subjects (e.g. organ donation, family health history, cancer; Afifi & Weiner, 2006; Hovick, 2014; Lewis & Martinez, 2014) within different close relationships (Kuang & Wilson, 2021) and has seen increasing application in online support groups (Kanter et al., 2019). A meta-analysis of TMIM (Kuang & Wilson, 2021) posits that people are indeed more likely to seek health information when they experience higher uncertainty discrepancy, anticipate positive outcomes, and perceive themselves as having a high level of efficacy. Further, uncertainty discrepancy was found to have a positive, direct effect on information seeking. This association was also moderated by factors including health contexts and demographic characteristics.

The conclusions from the meta-analysis gained further backing from a subsequent study applied to the context of mental health information seeking (Kuang & Wang, 2022). This longitudinal research confirmed the predictive power of these antecedent factors in determining direct information seeking about mental health, with such direct information seeking leading to improved coping and health outcomes. In their study, Kuang and Wang adopted a three-wave longitudinal design to track changes in uncertainty discrepancy associated with mental illness over a span of 4 weeks. Aside from information seeking, individuals with mental illness also tend to concurrently seek support when interacting with close others, such as family and friends, but not with online support group members. And yet, information seeking and direct support seeking did not lead to a change in uncertainty discrepancy over time, but indirect support seeking resulted in maladaptive outcomes. The inclusion of outcomes of information seeking in this study applying TMIM to mental illness highlights the uniqueness of this highly stigmatized health context, noting that certain information and support seeking behaviors (e.g. indirect) may backfire. Therefore, more contextualized considerations that take relational and individual experience into account are needed to fully unfold how information seeking may alter mental illness experiences.

Theory of Motivated Information Management Within the Context of Mental Health

Research on information seeking reveals important implications in the realm of mental health. Grasping the stages outlined by TMIM can guide mental health professionals in crafting communication strategies accounting for individuals' needs at different stages. This spans from navigating uncertainty and anxiety to enhancing self-efficacy, fostering positive outcome expectations, and aiding informed decision-making. First, recognizing negative emotions arising from the uncertainty surrounding mental health conditions and addressing them empathetically, while providing additional resources, explanations, or support, may help better assist people in their information seeking journey (Kuang & Wilson, 2021). Second, emphasizing the benefits of seeking information and equipping individuals with the necessary resources can boost their confidence and motivation to engage in health information seeking behavior. In addition, the role of close relationships, such as family, friends, and coworkers, is pivotal in this journey, as they can facilitate or hinder information seeking efforts (Taniguchi-Dorios et al., 2022; Thompson et al., 2020). Furthermore, mental health professionals should recognize online support groups, given their rising prominence, as invaluable platforms for information exchange and support (Pan et al., 2019; Wright, 2016). By ensuring these platforms provide accurate and beneficial information, mental health practitioners may contribute further to proactive information seeking and improving mental health outcomes.

However, we should also note that the one study applying TMIM to the mental health context revealed nuanced differences in how mental illness information seeking takes place and is associated with various outcomes. To obtain further insights into ways to design message-based mental health promotion strategies, more research is needed to examine the utility of mental health information associated with different mental health conditions, in combination with people's inherent needs to maintain social image when facing this stigmatized health topic. With a brief overview of information seeking as well as one of the leading information seeking frameworks, we turn our attention to information processing.

Information Processing

The valence, strength, and nature of communication effect, as an outcome of information sought and/or received, can vary depending on how the information is processed. Relatedly, the information processing perspective has significantly contributed to advancing our knowledge of communication phenomena (Greene, 2012). In line with this trend, information processing has been important in advancing health communication research across multiple topics (e.g. body image interventions, Davies et al., 2023; cancer communication, Lang, 2006; healthy diet interventions, Ko et al., 2011; organ donation campaigns, Quick et al., 2016). The information processing model (McGuire, 1985, 2001) describes the varying effects of input factors, source (i.e. who delivers the message), characteristics of the message (i.e. what information is included in the message and how it is presented), channel or medium of information delivery (i.e. characteristics of the medium the message is presented on), or receiver or audience (i.e. individual characteristics of the audience), on output factors. These output factors include attitudes and behaviors, behavioral change being the higher-order outcome that can be achieved after those appearing earlier in the sequence have been achieved (McGuire, 1985). By exploring the effects of one or more of the input factors on outcomes, information processing research can illuminate effective communication strategies to elicit intended persuasive outcomes.

Input factors, such as source, message, channel or medium, and receiver or audience factors can be further broken down to answer specific questions of the researcher. For instance, those interested in the differential impact of a message depending on the *messenger* can examine if and how varying degrees of perceived source credibility—such as credibility, authority, or likeability—shape outcomes. Furthermore, health communication researchers interested in *message type* could explore how messages written in rational language (e.g. factual approach, see Holbrook, 1978), those that elicit discrete emotions (e.g. fear, see Tannenbaum et al., 2015), those including exemplars (see Zillmann, 1999) versus statistics (see Allen & Preiss, 1997), or in the form of narratives (see Green, 2006) affect information processing and its respective persuasive outcomes. Still, further information processing research can investigate if a message elicits different responses depending on *receiver characteristics* such as media literacy (see Jeong et al., 2012), or how tailoring a message to the receiver (see Rimer & Kreuter, 2006) or crafting different messages by grouping receivers based on their demographics and psychographics (i.e. targeting) affect communication outcomes in the health topic of interest. Some specific health topics that have been studied extensively in health communication include tobacco use and safe sex.

Parallel to information seeking and dissemination research, an essential element of information processing research is theory, which can be used to generate testable predictions, raise questions, and explain or describe phenomena. Multiple theories have proven to be useful in this endeavor, including those focused on emotional processing (affect, Dillard & Seo, 2012; discrete emotions, Nabi, 2015; Nabi et al., 2019) and those dedicated to understanding how emotional and cognitive trajectories can accompany each other during message processing (e.g. the limited capacity model of motivated mediated message processing, Lang, 2000, 2006). Mindful of the purview of this chapter (for a review of information processing theories in persuasion, see Dillard & Shen, 2012), the following section introduces one exemplary framework, the elaboration likelihood model (ELM) (Petty & Cacioppo, 1986). After explicating the central tenets of this framework, we review relevant studies, focusing on their implications for mental health communication researchers and practitioners.

Elaboration Likelihood Model

The ELM (Petty & Cacioppo, 1986) is a psychological theory that explains attitude change in response to a persuasive message as a function of how the information in that message is processed. The ELM posits that information processing involves two routes, central to which is the idea that message recipients engage in different degrees of systematic thinking about relevant information (O'Keefe, 2013). When elaboration is relatively high, message recipients engage in thoughtful examination of issue-relevant considerations (e.g. quality of arguments in the message), activating the central route (Petty & Cacioppo, 1986). Conversely, the peripheral route is activated when messages are processed using mental shortcuts, often relying on heuristic cues (e.g. communicator credibility, norms) rather than engaging in thorough examination of the messages' arguments and evidence.

According to the ELM, the degree of elaboration recipients engage in is dependent on the ***desire*** to undertake issue-relevant thinking (referred to as elaboration motivation) as well as the ***capability*** to undertake it (referred to as elaboration ability). O'Keefe (2013) illustrates that elaboration motivation can vary as a result of message recipients' involvement level and need for cognition, whereas elaboration ability can be influenced by prior knowledge about the topic, the medium used to disseminate the message, as well as the presence of an environmental distraction. For instance, Tam and Ho (2005), in their study on the topic of web personalization, found that preference matching influences elaboration motivation. In a similar vein, Cao et al. (2017) found that prior knowledge influences a patient's elaboration ability while selecting which physician to consult online. In essence, the amount of elaboration message recipients engage in is a joint result of elaboration motivation and ability (e.g. prior knowledge, ease of understanding, text-only versus infographic presentation format; Lam et al., 2022).

Persuasion can occur at any point along the continuum from high to little or no elaboration, granted that the nature of persuasion varies (Petty & Wegener, 1999). Driven by high amounts of issue-relevant and effortful thinking, attitudes formed through central processing generally tend to be stronger than those from peripheral processing (Petty et al., 2009). Attitude strength in this context is analogous to how consequential it is. Research has found that attitude change through central route processing is generally more stable over time, resistant to counterarguments, and more likely to lead to behavioral change (O'Keefe, 2013; Petty & Cacioppo, 1986). Thus, the general takeaway for communicators is that central route processing produces long-term benefits, although it is more difficult to achieve (O'Keefe, 2013). With that said, it is imperative to note that central route processing is not exempt from unintended consequences, such as the persuasive message resulting in enduring negative attitude change, and could affect individuals with psychological vulnerabilities (e.g. depression) differentially from their less vulnerable counterparts. Therefore, communication research is key to unlocking effective message strategies.

The ELM has been popularly utilized in health communication research that seeks to understand how different types of health messages are processed, the results from which aid the improvement of existing intervention and campaign messages as well as the development of effective strategies for communicating about health (for a review, see Petty et al., 2009). One specific area the ELM has been useful for is promoting attitude and behavior change for the betterment of public health. For example, Flynn and associates (2011), in their research on improving smoking prevention messaging strategies, found that messages emphasizing explicit factual arguments for avoiding negative consequences of smoking (versus messages focusing on peer modeling arguments such as social norms) could be useful for reaching higher risk youth. In their study, students who were at higher risk of smoking initiation (i.e. higher involvement) indicated having cognitively processed messages focused on factual arguments more than messages with fewer or no direct arguments. Moreover, the ELM has also been employed in evaluating the effectiveness of messages in preventative and clinical interventions and social marketing campaigns. For instance, Willoughby and Liu (2018) studied how the use of narrative messages and emojis in a health text message intervention affects message processing and attention of young adults. Their study indicated that nonnarrative messages without emojis led to more message elaboration and higher perceptions of credibility. Highlighting the fact that their study shows mixed results beyond this finding, the authors recommend that message creators consider message format and features depending on the goal and content of intervention messages. Still further, the model has also been applied in conjunction with other information processing theories for a comprehensive examination of individuals' health-related behaviors. To illustrate, Zhang et al. (2023) found that individual motivation and information richness can serve as central processing cues, whereas trust in information sources can serve as peripheral processing cues, to positively affect sharing intention.

The Elaboration Likelihood Model Within the Context of Mental Health

Congruent to past health communication research, there exist endless application opportunities for the ELM within the context of mental health. For example, Neimeyer and fellow researchers (1989) applied the ELM to pretreatment attitudes toward a therapy for treating eating disorders to examine what drives intervention effects. Largely consistent with the model's assumptions, they found that intervention quality (i.e. central route characteristics) was the primary determinant of attitude change and that it interacted with source credibility (i.e. peripheral route features) to predict measures of behavioral compliance. Beyond examining outcomes of persuasion in the context of mental health interventions, the ELM has guided communication efforts to combat biased and inaccurate views about specific mental health conditions, stigmatized populations, and treatment methods. For instance, Yeh and Jewell (2015) utilized the ELM to explore how myth/fact message frames are processed in messages designed to change misconceptions about mental illnesses. More recently, Jin and Hashim (2021) applied the model to examine the effects of utilizing a dual-process method to promote stigmatized attitude changes about depression among Malaysian college students. The authors evaluated how different depression public service announcements (high- versus low-quality messages) were processed and found that the high-quality message with strong arguments, developed from an existing public social announcement from of the World Health Organization, was more effective in changing stigmatized attitudes by eliciting higher elaboration, compared to the low-quality message, which had poor argument quality.

Future research could examine how the channel through which information about mental health is delivered influences message processing and respective persuasive outcomes, the implications from which would be a steppingstone for research on interface features (e.g. interactivity, anonymity) that drive intended effects in mental health messaging. Information processing research for mental health communication is open to many more doors and expanding knowledge about one type of effect—source, message, channel or medium, or receiver or audience—can ignite insightful explorations of another, or multiple effects in tandem. With an overview of implications of information processing research for the research and practice of mental health communication, we turn our attention to information dissemination.

Information Dissemination

Health communication scholarship continues to contribute to the literature around how best to communicate specialized, scientific information to public audiences and other fields of study. Various types of health communication scholarship (i.e. mass media, risk, interpersonal) has been used to unpack *how* to communicate the information to audiences and provide further recommendations on the operationalization of communication efforts (e.g. Noar, 2012; Pope et al., 2017). Although the dissemination literature can span many topics and concepts, most can be described as understanding one of three questions: What *channels* provide the most opportunity for health information? What *messages* about the health topic resonate the best? Who is the best *messenger* to communicate on this topic? This has led to a breadth of literature on topics related impact of various messaging channels (e.g. mass media channels, the role of social media in disseminating; Hoffner & Cohen, 2015; Latha et al., 2020), assessing certain message characteristics (e.g. framing mental health from a loss or gain perspective, appealing emotional appeals, narrative versus argumentation style messaging; Chang, 2008; Yap et al., 2019), and characteristics of the messenger (e.g. credible, trustworthiness; Hocevar et al., 2017) on health outcomes and behaviors.

Yet, only one theory, the diffusion of innovation theory (Rogers, 1995, 2003), routinely demonstrates how best to disseminate health information because it is a theory that provides insights to each of these questions. The diffusion of innovation theory is an ideal theory to guide dissemination efforts because the theory combines behavior change logic with communication and marketing principles to describe how information diffuses through communities and fosters behavior adoption (Oldenburg & Glanz, 2008). Yet, this theory is seldom mentioned within the mental health context. Thus, this section provides an overview of the diffusion of innovation theory and its current uses within the health field to date.

The Diffusion of Innovation Theory

The diffusion of innovation theory posits that diffusion is the outcome of dissemination efforts. Rogers (1995) argues that diffusion is the "process by which an innovation is communicated through certain channels over time among members of a social system" (p. 10). Thus, health communicators must consider (a) how the innovation is communicated, (b) the time it takes to diffuse an innovation, (c) the channels used to diffuse information about the innovation, and (d) how to best implement the innovation based on the community's social system. In addition to providing insights into the key components of diffusion, the diffusion of innovation theory underscores the importance of understanding audiences. The theory posits that innovation is adopted by, and passes through, different members within a community. For instance, Rogers (1983, 2003) notes that each of the five adopter categories (i.e. innovators, early adopters, early majority adopters, late majority adopters, and laggards) requires a unique set of messages that aligns with their attitudes toward adopting new products (Table 7.1).

The first component for communicators to consider in the diffusion of innovation is the characteristics of the innovation. Rogers (1983) defines *innovation* as any tangible or intangible product (e.g. ideas, behaviors, items) that is perceived to be new and argues that the way an innovation is communicated is pivotal to the use of an innovation. The author suggests that communicators must create messages that highlight the innovation to be relatively advantageous compared to previously known products (relative advantage), be compatible to their lifestyle (compatibility), be easy to implement or use (complexity), be easily tested and modified (trialability), and have measurable outcomes after implementation (observability). The second component is time. Although innovations that have the outlined characteristics are likely to diffuse quicker than those that do not, diffusion requires *time* because individuals must cycle through the innovation-decision process (Rogers, 1995), which includes (a) acquiring knowledge, (b) being persuaded that the innovation is positive, (c) making the decision to try the innovation, (d) trialing (or initially adopting) the innovation, and (e) confirming that they would like to sustain the innovation long term (i.e. fully adopting an innovation). Conversely, when these innovation messages fail to show advantage, compatibility, lack of complexity, ability to trial, and observability, they are less

Table 7.1 Adopter Categories and Characteristics

Category	*Common characteristics*
Innovators	• Require the shortest adoption period • Adventurous, risk takers
Early adopters	• Opinion leaders • Trend setters • Serve as role models • Attracted to high risk and high reward activities
Early Majority	• Interact frequently with others • Can serve as second tier opinion leaders (e.g. later in the process) • Do not like complexity • Risk averse • Cost conscious • Progress to adoption slowly
Late Majority	• Responds to peer pressure and economic necessity • Skeptical • Cost sensitive • Requires well-established solutions • Easily influenced by laggards
Laggards	• Suspicious of innovation • Compares innovations to past innovations • Wants to maintain status quo • Will adopt only if alternatives are worse

Note. Adapted from Kaminski (2011).

likely to move people through the innovation-decision process (Afraz et al., 2021). For instance, when considering whether to implement integrated care using a Global Treatment Budget (i.e. the innovation), leaders at psychiatric and medical facilities indicated that issues related to trying and reversing the innovation if needed (triability) and the lack of compatibility with regular care structures hindered their ability to be persuaded to use the innovation—even after becoming more knowledgeable about the innovation. In a study assessing antecedents to adopting mobile health (mHealth) applications in Indonesia, Octavius and Antonio (2021) found that customers' perceptions of compatibility in (a) adoption intention (trialability), (b) expected performance (relative advantage), and (c) expected effort (complexity) predicted customers' decision to try the innovation (i.e. mHealth application).

The third component to consider are the channels of promotion. *Channels* refer to the mechanism in which messages spread throughout a community, including mass media (e.g. television, social media) and interpersonal communication (e.g. Rogers, 1995, 2003). Each channel has a unique purpose in the diffusion of innovation process and the decision of which channel to utilized should align with the type of knowledge need by the community to continue through the knowledge acquisition phase of the innovation-decision process: (a) awareness knowledge (i.e. awareness that the innovation exists), (b) procedural knowledge (i.e. how to use the innovation), or (c) principles knowledge (i.e. understanding how the innovation works). According to the theory, when determining the best channel for diffusion, communicators should consider what type of knowledge they are trying to improve in their process to diffuse information. For instance, when attempting to improve awareness knowledge, mass media channels are necessary because they allow the innovation to be promoted to a large group at once; however, interpersonal (or interactive) mechanisms (i.e. face-to-face, online discussion platforms) may be more useful for understanding how to use and implement an innovation. As such, Rogers (2003) argues, although that communicators and practitioners should utilize multiple types of channels when promoting information, it is important to consider interpersonal avenues (e.g. doctor–patient communication, peer discussions) because they are more strongly associated with adoption of the innovation (e.g. Arthars & Liu, 2020).

Fourth, the diffusion of innovation theory suggests that communicators must consider the social systems surrounding the innovation and community. In line with much of the behavior change literature logic that highlights social networks as a primary motivator of behavior, the diffusion of innovation theory assumes that people are social beings that are influenced by others (e.g. Crosby et al., 2013; Rogers, 1995, 2003). As such, this theory posits that diffusion of innovation is a process that is contingent on social considerations. Understanding the norms of a community and the communication structure (i.e. established patterns of communication) is important, as they guide how and to whom to draft the messages about the innovation (Crosby et al., 2013; Dearing, 2009). In addition, Rogers (1995, 2003) indicates that gaining insight into how individuals fit into the community is also pivotal in understanding the social system. The diffusion of innovation theory notes that every community has individuals that fall into one of the five adoption categories (Table 7.1) and the percentage of the population with each category tends to follow a bell curve. The theory notes that although innovators may be the first to implement behavior, it is the early adopters who are often the thought leaders (i.e. change agents) and help to spread information to people in the early and late majority. Thus, it is imperative that communicators and practitioners understand individual preferences within a community (e.g. differences between audience segments) to best identify the change agents and utilize the social system as a part of their diffusion efforts (see Quick et al., 2021).

The premise of diffusion of innovation has received support across various health contexts, including diffusion of physical activity behaviors (Glowacki et al., 2016; Owen et al., 2006), diabetes management programs (Chen et al., 2022; De Civita & Dasgupta, 2007), and vaccination intentions (Mo et al., 2021; Pinariya et al., 2020). For instance, when assessing the diffusion of wearing activity trackers for type 2 diabetes management, scholars found that adoption intentions increased when the benefits of the tracker were perceived to meet three of the five innovation characteristics (i.e. observable, compatible/not complex, relative advantage). Owen et al.'s (2006) review of the diffusion of physical activity programs suggests that the school-based CATCH program, aimed at improving moderate to vigorous physical activity (MVPA) in children's physical education classes, successfully diffused across the state of Texas (i.e. MVPA was included in up to 65% of their physical education class activities) because of the successful inclusion of top-ranked physical education teachers as the change agents (i.e. early adopter). A study on COVID-19 vaccination intentions also provides support for the role that compatible innovations, interactive communication channels, social systems, and individual innovation attitudes influenced intentions to get free or self-paid vaccinations (Mo et al., 2021). More specifically, their study concluded that perceived self-efficacy, use of social media, openness to the vaccine, and perceptions about whether others are getting vaccinated were significant predictors of behavioral intentions to get vaccinated, regardless of whether it was self-pay or free.

Diffusion of Innovation Theory Within the Context of Mental Health

Despite the support for the diffusion of innovation theory in other health contexts (e.g. De Civita & Dasgupta, 2007; Pinariya et al., 2020) and calls from scholars to utilize this theory as a guide for mental health communication (e.g. Albright et al., 2022; Gotham, 2004; Kelly et al., 2007), it has not been widely assessed within the context of mental health and is specifically lacking literature about diffusion within nonclinical populations. Moreover, when used within a mental health context, much of the focus has been on understanding audience features to encourage behavior change (e.g. assessing digital healthcare tools to improve access and adherence to mental health treatment) to the relative neglect of understanding communication preferences (i.e. channels, messages, messengers). For example, Haun et al. (2020) assessed the diffusion of a mental health service tool (i.e. video consultation implementation software) to general practitioners. The authors examined different general practitioner perceptions of a video consultation implementation software, noting that general practitioners were well characterized by the adoption categories laid out in the diffusion of innovation theory (Table 7.1); yet, their article provides relatively little insight into the communication channels, characteristics of the message, or community messengers that may help diffuse the tool. When assessing the adoption and implementation of a computer-assisted therapy (CAT) for substance use disorders, Elison et al.'s (2014) findings attend to describing the level of understanding about the innovation, characteristics of the social system and those that have adopted the CAT, and decisions to adopt or not adopt the innovation. Their findings highlight important factors related to the social system's needs and suggest that messages that speak to a lack of complexity and ease of use may resonate more with members in their intended community. However, their article provides little information on key messengers and communication channels needed to promote these messages.

Although the application of the diffusion of innovation is scarce in the broader research on mental health communication (particularly to nonclinical audiences), scholarship suggests that the diffusion of innovation may be fruitful for interpreting the success of some communication efforts, particularly as they pertain to the message, messenger, and channels. For instance, the application of the diffusion of innovation theory may help to explain why some efforts using interpersonal promotion channels have continued success and others waiver in their findings. For instance, the success of many gatekeeper-based mental health literacy programs, programs that teach peer leaders how to identify poor mental health and promote help-seeking actions (e.g. Choi, 2017; Story et al., 2016), suggests having community leaders as health messengers are likely instrumental in encouraging people to seek help for poor mental health. Conversely, the lack of identifying the correct health messenger could be a reason why contact-based interventions, which include interpersonal messaging, tend to lack long-term results (Caban et al., 2022; Thornicroft et al., 2016). Further, the diffusion of innovation research may also help to better understand why social media disclosures of mental health often act as both a promotional tool and a deterrent to mental health help-seeking actions. For instance, the diffusion of innovation theory can provide insights into whether/how the message, messenger, and/or channel characteristics influence the reception of celebrity mental health disclosures, such as Carrie Fisher's and Demi Lovato's disclosure about bipolar disorder (Park & Hoffner, 2020; Wong et al., 2017) and Kid Cudi's disclosure of depression (Francis, 2018), beyond general statements that celebrities are with ideal or not ideal promoters and social media is solely positive or negative to mental health promotion efforts.

Taken together, the diffusion of innovation theory may be a useful theory to utilize in the context of health behavior because it describes the importance of the message, messenger, and communication channel in persuading both clinical and non-clinical audiences to take on beneficial health practices (e.g. implementing tools for more therapeutic accessibility, encouraging help-seeking). As such, many health researchers have utilized the theory to help guide the success of their health promotion efforts. Although the theory is still in its infancy within the context of mental health, the continued support for this theory, along with the alignment with results from the broader mental health scholarship, makes this theory an ideal theory for communicators and practitioners to consider as they continue to disseminate their mental health information.

Conclusion

In closing, the theoretical and applied contributions produced from a health communication perspective have much to offer mental health practitioners and researchers in the search for contributing to the mental health communication scholarship. It was our goal to demonstrate how a careful look at how individuals seek, process, and disseminate health information will better inform our efforts to improve the overall mental health of society. Across these three important phases of information seeking, processing, and dissemination, health communication scholarship prioritizes theories that place importance on the message, the messenger of the message, as well as the channel in which the message is disseminated (Thompson & Harrington, 2021). We believe the theories described throughout this chapter represent just a few of the novel approaches guiding the questions we ask regarding mental illness and these frameworks provide a road map for future work. As alluded to throughout this chapter, the epistemological, theoretical, and contextual breadth offered from a health communication standpoint will continue to add diversity to the mental health scholarship. As the severity and susceptibility of experiencing the outcomes of negative mental health continue to rise (Leeb et al., 2020), the opportunities for health communication researchers are endless. The research addressing the mental health crisis has only begun to scratch the surface. Health communication researchers are poised to contribute to this important literature in the discovery of answers to these pressing issues.

References

Afifi, W. A., & Morse, C. R. (2015). Expanding the role of emotion in the theory of motivated information management. In T. D. Afifi & W. A. Afifi (Eds.), *Uncertainty, information management, and disclosure decisions* (pp. 87–105). Routledge.

Afifi, W. A., & Weiner, J. L. (2004). Toward a theory of motivated information management. *Communication Theory, 14*(2), 167–190. https://doi.org/10.1111/j.1468-2885.2004.tb00310.x

Afifi, W. A., & Weiner, J. L. (2006). Seeking information about sexual health: Applying the theory of motivated information management. *Human Communication Research, 32*(1), 35–57. https://doi.org/10.1111/j.1468-2958.2006.00002.x

Afraz, F. C., Vogel, A., Dreher, C., & Berghöfer, A. (2021). Promoting integrated care through a global treatment budget: A qualitative study in German mental health care using Rogers' diffusion of innovation theory. *International Journal of Integrated Care, 21*(4), 27. https://doi-org/10.5334/ijic.5940

Albright, K., Navarro, E. I., Jarad, I., Boyd, M. R., Powell, B. J., & Lewis, C. C. (2022). Communication strategies to facilitate the implementation of new clinical practices: A qualitative study of community mental health therapists. *Translational Behavioral Medicine, 12*(2), 324–334. https://doi.org/10.1093/tbm/ibab139

Allen, M., & Preiss, R. W. (1997). Comparing the persuasiveness of narrative and statistical evidence using meta-analysis. *Communication Research Reports, 14*(2), 125–131. https://doi.org/10.1080/08824099709388654

Arthars, N., & Liu, D. Y.-T. (2020). How and why faculty adopt learning analytics. In D. Ifenthaler & D. Gibson (Eds.), *Adoption of data analytics in higher education learning and teaching* (pp. 201–220). Springer International Publishing. https://doi.org/10.1007/978-3-030-47392-1_11

Brashers, D. E., Goldsmith, D. J., & Hsieh, E. (2002). Information seeking and avoiding in health contexts. *Human Communication Research, 28*(2), 258–271. https://doi.org/10.1111/j.1468-2958.2002.tb00807.x

Caban, S., Makos, S., & Thompson, C. M. (2022). The role of interpersonal communication in mental health literacy interventions for young people: A theoretical review. *Health Communication, 38*(13), 1–15. https://doi.org/10.1080/10410236.2022.2121473

Cao, X., Liu, Y., Zhu, Z., Hu, J., & Chen, X. (2017). Online selection of a physician by patients: Empirical study from elaboration likelihood perspective. *Computers in Human Behavior, 73*, 403–412. https://doi.org/10.1016/j.chb.2017.03.060

Centers for Disease Control and Prevention. (2023). *Mental health*. https://www.cdc.gov/mentalhealth/index.htm

Chaiken, S., Giner-Sorolla, R., & Chen, S. (1996). Beyond accuracy: Defense and impression motives in heuristic and systematic information processing. In P. M. Gollwitzer & J. A. Bargh (Eds.), *The psychology of action: Linking cognition and motivation to behavior* (pp. 553–578). Guilford Press.

Chang, C. (2008). Increasing mental health literacy via narrative advertising. *Journal of Health Communication, 13*(1), 37–55. https://doi.org/10.1080/10810730701807027

Chang, C.-C., & Huang, M.-H. (2020). Antecedents predicting health information seeking: A systematic review and meta-analysis. *International Journal of Information Management, 54*, 102115. https://doi.org/10.1016/j.ijinfomgt.2020.102115

Chen, P., Shen, Y., Li, Z., Sun, X., Feng, X. L., & Fisher, E. B. (2022). What factors predict the adoption of type 2 diabetes patients to wearable activity trackers—Application of diffusion of innovation theory. *Frontiers in Public Health, 9*, 773293. https://doi.org/10.3389/fpubh.2021.773293

Choi, Y.-J. (2017). Effects of a program to improve mental health literacy for married immigrant women in Korea. *Archives of Psychiatric Nursing, 31*(4), 394–398. https://doi.org/10.1016/j.apnu.2017.04.012

Crosby, R. A., DiClemente, R. J., & Salazar, L. F. (2013). Diffusion of innovations theory. In R. J. DiClemente, L. F. Salazar, & R. A. Crosby (Eds.), *Health behavior theory for public health: Principles, foundations, and applications* (pp. 211–230). Jones & Bartlett Learning.

Davies, B., Turner, M., & Udell, J. (2023). Are humorous or distractor images more effective than self-compassion messages for combatting the negative body image consequences of social media? An experimental test of possible micro-intervention stimuli. *Body Image, 46*, 356–371. https://doi.org/10.1016/j.bodyim.2023.07.003

De Civita, M., & Dasgupta, K. (2007). Using diffusion of innovations theory to guide diabetes management program development: An illustrative example. *Journal of Public Health, 29*(3), 263–268. https://doi.org/10.1093/pubmed/fdm033

Dearing, J. W. (2009). Applying diffusion of innovation theory to intervention development. *Research on Social Work Practice, 19*(5), 503–518. https://doi.org/10.1177/1049731509335569

Dillard, J. P., & Seo, K. (2012). Affect and persuasion. In J. Dillard & L. Shen (Eds.), *The SAGE handbook of persuasion: Developments in theory and practice* (2nd ed., pp. 150–166). Sage.

Dillard, J. P., & Shen, L. (2012). *The SAGE handbook of persuasion: Developments in theory and practice* (2nd ed.). Sage. https://doi.org/10.4135/9781452218410

Elison, S., Ward, J., Davies, G., & Moody, M. (2014). Implementation of computer-assisted therapy for substance misuse: A qualitative study of breaking free online using Roger's diffusion of innovation theory. *Drugs and Alcohol Today, 14*(4), 207–218. https://doi.org/10.1108/DAT-05-2014-0025

Flynn, B. S., Worden, J. K., Yanushka, B. J., Connolly, S. W., & Dorwaldt, A. L. (2011). Evaluation of smoking prevention television messages based on the elaboration likelihood model. *Health Education Research, 26*(6), 976–987. https://doi-org/10.1093/her/cyr082

Francis, D. B. (2018). Young black men's information seeking following celebrity depression disclosure: Implications for mental health communication. *Journal of Health Communication, 23*(7), 687–694. https://doi.org/10.1080/10810730.2018.1506837

Gao, J., Zheng, P., Jia, Y., Chen, H., Mao, Y., Chen, S., Wang, Y., Fu, H., & Dai, J. (2020). Mental health problems and social media exposure during COVID-19 outbreak. *PLoS One, 15*(4), 1–10. https://doi.org/10.1371/journal.pone.0231924

Glowacki, E. M., Centeio, E. E., Van Dongen, D. J., Carson, R. L., & Castelli, D. M. (2016). Health promotion efforts as predictors of physical activity in schools: An application of the diffusion of innovations model. *Journal of School Health, 86*(6), 399–406. https://doi.org/10.1111/josh.12390

Gotham, H. J. (2004). Diffusion of mental health and substance abuse treatments: Development dissemination, and implementation. *Clinical Psychology: Science and Practice, 11*(2), 160–176. https://doi.org/10.1093/clipsy.bph067

Green, M. C. (2006). Narratives and cancer communication. *Journal of Communication, 56*(Suppl. 1), S163–S183. https://doi.org/10.1111/j.1460-2466.2006.00288.x

Greene, J. O. (2012). Information processing. In W. Donsbach (Ed.), *The international encyclopedia of communication.* Blackwell. https://doi.org/10.1002/9781405186407.wbieci023.pub2

Griffin, R. J., Dunwoody, S., & Neuwirth, K. (1999). Proposed model of the relationship of risk information seeking and processing to the development of preventive behaviors. *Environmental Research, 80*(2), S230–S245. https://doi.org/10.1006/enrs.1998.3940

Griffin, R. J., Neuwirth, K., Dunwoody, S., & Giese, J. (2004). Information sufficiency and risk communication. *Media Psychology, 6*(1), 23–61. https://doi.org/10.1207/s1532785xmep0601_2

Haun, M. W., Stephan, I., Wensing, M., Hartmann, M., Hoffmann, M., & Friederich, H.-C. (2020). Intent to adopt video-based integrated mental health care and the characteristics of its supporters: Mixed methods study among general practitioners applying diffusion of innovations theory. *JMIR Mental Health, 7*(10), e23660. https://doi.org/10.2196/23660

Hocevar, K. P., Metzger, M., & Flanagin, A. J. (2017). Source credibility, expertise, and trust in health and risk messaging. In M. Powers (Ed.), *Oxford research encyclopedia of communication.* https://doi.org/10.1093/acrefore/9780190228613.013.287

Hoffner, C. A., & Cohen, E. L. (2015). Portrayal of mental illness on the TV series Monk: Presumed influence and consequences of exposure. *Health Communication, 30*(10), 1046–1054. https://doi.org/10.1080/10410236.2014.917840

Holbrook, M. B. (1978). Beyond attitude structure: Toward the informational determinants of attitude. *Journal of Marketing Research, 15*(4), 545–556. https://doi.org/10.2307/3150624

Hovick, S. R. (2014). Understanding family health information seeking: A test of the theory of motivated information management. *Journal of Health Communication, 19*(1), 6–23. https://doi.org/10.1080/10810730.2013.778369

Jeong, S. H., Cho, H., & Hwang, Y. (2012). Media literacy interventions: A meta-analytic review. *Journal of Communication, 62*(3), 454–472. https://doi.org/10.1111/j.1460-2466.2012.01643.x

Jin, Y. F., & Hashim, N. (2021). Applying the elaboration likelihood model to analyze the effects of depression public service announcements among Malaysian college students. *International Journal of Modern Trends in Social Sciences, 4*(17), 54–73. https://doi.org/10.35631/IJMTSS.417006

Johnson, J. D., & Meischke, H. (1993). A comprehensive model of cancer-related information seeking applied to magazines. *Human Communication Research, 19*(3), 343–367. https://doi.org/10.1111/j.1468-2958.1993.tb00305.x

Kaminski, J. (2011). Diffusion of innovation theory. *Canadian Journal of Nursing Informatics, 6*(2), 1–6. https://cjni.net/journal/?p=1444

Kanter, E., Bevan, J. L., & Dorros, S. M. (2019). The use of online support groups to seek information about chronic illness: Applying the theory of motivated information management. *Communication Quarterly, 67*(1), 100–121. https://doi.org/10.1080/01463373.2018.1539406

Kelly, C. M., Jorm, A. F., & Wright, A. (2007). Improving mental health literacy as a strategy to facilitate early intervention for mental disorders. *Medical Journal of Australia, 187*(S7), S26–S30. https://doi.org/10.5694/j.1326-5377.2007.tb01332.x

Kim, J.-N., Park, S.-C., Yoo, S.-W., & Shen, H. (2010). Mapping health communication scholarship: Breadth, depth, and agenda of published research in health communication. *Health Communication, 25*(6), 487–503. https://doi.org/10.1080/10410236.2010.507160

Ko, L. K., Campbell, M. K., Lewis, M. A., Earp, J. A., & DeVellis, B. (2011). Information processes mediate the effect of a health communication intervention on fruit and vegetable consumption. *Journal of Health Communication, 16*(3), 282–299. https://doi.org/10.1080/10810730.2010.532294

Kreps, G. L., & Thornton, B. C. (1992). *Health communication: Theory & practice* (2nd ed.). Waveland Press.

Kuang, K., & Wang, N. (2022). A longitudinal investigation of information and support seeking processes that alter the uncertainty experiences of mental illness. *Communication Monographs, 89*(4), 470–492. https://doi.org/10.1080/03637751.2021.2022736

Kuang, K., & Wilson, S. R. (2021). Theory of motivated information management: A meta-analytic review. *Communication Theory, 31*(3), 463–490. https://doi.org/10.1093/ct/qtz025

Lam, C., Huang, Z., & Shen, L. (2022). Infographics and the elaboration likelihood model (ELM): Differences between visual and textual health messages. *Journal of Health Communication, 27*(10), 737–745. https://doi.org/10.1080/10810730.2022.2157909

Lambert, S. D., & Loiselle, C. G. (2007). Health information-seeking behavior. *Qualitative Health Research, 17*(8), 1006–1019. https://doi.org/10.1177/1049732307305199

Lang, A. (2000). The limited capacity model of mediated message processing. *Journal of Communication, 50*(1), 46–70. https://doi.org/10.1093/joc/50.1.46

Lang, A. (2006). Motivated cognition (LC4MP): The influence of appetitive and aversive activation on the processing of video games. In P. Messarsis & L. Humphries (Eds.), *Digital media: Transformation in human communication* (pp. 237–256). Peter Lang. https://doi.org/10.1080/23808985.2018.1534552

Latha, K., Meena, K. S., Pravitha, M. R., Dasgupta, M., & Chaturvedi, S. K. (2020). Effective use of social media platforms for promotion of mental health awareness. *Journal of Education and Health Promotion, 9*(124), 1–6. https://doi.org/10.4103/jehp.jehp_90_20

Leeb, R. T., Bitsko, R. H., Radhakrishnan, L., Martinez, P., Njai, R., & Holland, K. M. (2020). Mental health-related emergency department visits among children aged <18 years during the COVID-19 pandemic—United States, January 1–October 17, 2020. *Morbidity and Mortality Weekly Report, 69*(45), 1675–1680. http://dx.doi.org/10.15585/mmwr.mm6945a3

Lewis, N., & Martinez, L. S. (2014). Does the number of cancer patients' close social ties affect cancer-related information seeking through communication efficacy? Testing a mediation model. *Journal of Health Communication, 19*(9), 1076–1097. https://doi.org/10.1080/10810730.2013.872724

Littlejohn, S. W. (1999). *Theories of human communication* (6th ed.). Wadsworth Publishing Company.

McCullock, S. P., Hildenbrand, G. M., Schmitz, K. J., & Perrault, E. K. (2021). The state of health communication research: A content analysis of articles published in *Journal of Health Communication* and *Health Communication* (2010–2019). *Journal of Health Communication, 26*(1), 28–38. https://doi.org/10.1080/10810730.2021.1879320

McGuire, W. J. (1985). Attitudes and attitude change. In L. Gardner & A. Elliot (Eds.), *The handbook of social psychology* (3rd ed., pp. 233–346). Erlbaum.

McGuire, W. J. (2001). Input and output variables currently promising for constructing persuasive communications. In R. Rice & C. Atkin (Eds.), *Public communication campaigns* (3rd ed., pp. 22–48). Sage. https://doi.org/10.4135/9781452233260.n2

Mo, P. K., Luo, S., Wang, S., Zhao, J., Zhang, G., Li, L., Li, L., Xie, L., & Lau, J. T. F. (2021). Intention to receive the COVID-19 vaccination in China: Application of the diffusion of innovations theory and the moderating role of openness to experience. *Vaccines, 9*(2), 129. https://doi.org/10.3390/vaccines9020129

Moorman, C., & Matulich, E. (1993). A model of consumers' preventive health behaviors: The role of health motivation and health ability. *Journal of Consumer Research, 20*(2), 208–228. http://dx.doi.org/10.1086/209344

Morse, C. R., Afifi, W. A., Morgan, S. E., Stephenson, M. T., Reichert, T., Harrison, T. R., & Long, S. D. (2009). Religiosity, anxiety, and discussions about organ donation: Understanding a complex system of associations. *Health Communication, 24*(2), 156–164. https://doi.org/10.1080/10410230802676755

Nabi, R. L. (2015). Emotional flow in persuasive health messages. *Health Communication, 30*(2), 114–124. https://doi.org/10.1080/10410236.2014.974129

Nabi, R. L., Walter, N., Oshidary, N., Endacott, C. G., Love-Nichols, J., Lew, Z. J., & Aune, A. (2019). Can emotions capture the elusive gain-loss framing effect? A meta-analysis. *Communication Research, 47*(8), 1107–1130. https://doi.org/10.1177/0093650219861256

Neimeyer, G. J., Guy, J., & Metzler, A. (1989). Changing attitudes regarding the treatment of disordered eating: An application of the elaboration likelihood model. *Journal of Social and Clinical Psychology, 8*(1), 70–86. https://doi.org/10.1521/jscp.1989.8.1.70

Nicholson, W., Gardner, B., Grason, H. A., & Powe, N. R. (2005). The association between women's health information use and health care visits. *Women's Health Issues, 15*(6), 240–248. https://doi.org/10.1016/j.whi.2005.05.004

Noar, S. M. (2012). An Audience–Channel–Message–Evaluation (ACME) framework for health communication campaigns. *Health Promotion Practice, 13*(4), 481–488. https://doi.org/10.1177/1524839910386901

Octavius, G. S., & Antonio, F. (2021). Antecedents of intention to adopt mobile health (mHealth) application and its impact on intention to recommend: An evidence from Indonesian customers. *International Journal of Telemedicine and Applications, 2021*, 1–24. https://doi.org/10.1155/2021/6698627

O'Keefe, D. J. (2013). The elaboration likelihood model. In J. P. Dillard & L. Shen (Eds.), *The SAGE handbook of persuasion: Developments in theory and practice* (2nd ed., pp. 137–149). Sage.

Oldenburg, B., & Glanz, K. (2008). Diffusion of innovations. In B. Oldenburg & K. Glanz (Eds.), *Health behavior and health education: Theory, research, and practice* (4th ed., pp. 313–333). John Wiley & Sons.

O'Reilly, M., Dogra, N., Whiteman, N., Hughes, J., Eruyar, S., & Reilly, P. (2018). Is social media bad for mental health and wellbeing? Exploring the perspectives of adolescents. *Clinical Child Psychology Psychiatry, 23*(4), 601–613. https://doi.org/10.1177/135910451877515

Ou, M., & Ho, S. S. (2022). A meta-analysis of factors related to health information seeking: An integration from six theoretical frameworks. *Communication Research*, *49*(4), 567–593. https://doi.org/10.1177/00936502211043024

Owen, N., Glanz, K., Sallis, J. F., & Kelder, S. H. (2006). Evidence-based approaches to dissemination and diffusion of physical activity interventions. *American Journal of Preventive Medicine*, *31*(4), 35–44. https://doi.org/10.1016/j.amepre.2006.06.008

Pan, W., Feng, B., & Wingate, V. S. (2019). What you say is what you get: How self-disclosure in support seeking affects language use in support provision in online support forums. *Journal of Language and Social Psychology*, *37*(1), 3–27. https://doi.org/10.1177/0261927X17706983

Park, S., & Hoffner, C. A. (2020). Tweeting about mental health to honor Carrie Fisher: How #InHonorOfCarrie reinforced the social influence of celebrity advocacy. *Computers in Human Behavior*, *110*, 1–11. https://doi.org/10.1016/j.chb.2020.106353

Patalay, P., & Demkowicz, O. (2023). Debate: Don't mind the gap—why do we not care about the gender gap in common mental health difficulties? *Child and Adolescent Mental Health*, *28*(2), 341–343. https://doi.org/10.1111/camh.12647

Peng, Y., Yin, P., Deng, Z., & Wang, R. (2019). Patient–physician interaction and trust in online health community: The role of perceived usefulness of health information and services. *International Journal of Environmental Research and Public Health*, *17*(1), 139. https://doi.org/10.3390/ijerph17010139

Petty, R. E., Barden, J., & Wheeler, S. C. (2009). The elaboration likelihood model of persuasion: Developing health promotions for sustained behavioral change. In R. J. DiClemente, R. A. Crosby, & M. C. Kegler (Eds.), *Emerging theories in health promotion practice and research* (pp. 185–214). Jossey-Bass/Wiley.

Petty, R. E., & Cacioppo, J. T. (1986). *Communication and persuasion: Central and peripheral routes to attitude change.* Springer-Verlag. http://doi.org/10.1007/978-1-4612-4964-1

Petty, R. E., & Wegener, D. T. (1999). The elaboration likelihood model: Current status and controversies. In S. Chaiken & Y. Trope (Eds.), *Dual-process models in social psychology* (pp. 32–48). Guilford.

Pinariya, J. M., Ikhsano, A. N. D. R. E., & Sutjipto, A. M. (2020). Accelerating diffusion innovation using celebrities as opinion leader millennials: HPV vaccines in Indonesia. *Malaysian Journal of Communication*, *36*(3), 32–48. https://doi.org/10.17576/JKMJC-2020-3603-03

Pope, J. P., Pelletier, L., & Guertin, C. (2017). Starting off on the best foot: A review of message framing and message tailoring, and recommendations for the comprehensive messaging strategy for sustained behavior change. *Health Communication*, *33*(9), 1068–1077. https://doi.org/10.1080/10410236.2017.1331305

Quick, B. L., Reynolds-Tylus, T., Fico, A. E., & Feeley, T. H. (2016). Source and message framing considerations for recruiting mature adults as organ donors through direct mail campaigns. *Progress in Transplantation*, *26*(4), 309–313. https://doi.org/10.1177/1526924816663518

Quick, B. L., Reynolds-Tylus, T., Martinez, A., Gonzalez, S. H., & Mackert, M. (2021). Segmenting priority audiences employing individual difference variables to improve health promotion efforts. In T. Thompson & P. Schultz (Eds.), *Health communication theory: Foundations of communication theory* (pp. 19–41). Wiley Blackwell.

Rimer, B. K., & Kreuter, M. W. (2006). Advancing tailored health communication: A persuasion and message effects perspective. *Journal of Communication*, *56*(Suppl. 1), S184–S201. https://doi.org/10.1111/j.1460-2466.2006.00289.x

Rogers, E. M. (1983). *Diffusion of innovations* (3rd ed.). Free Press.

Rogers, E. M. (1995). *Diffusion of innovations* (4th ed.). Free Press.

Rogers, E. M. (2003). *Diffusion of innovations* (5th ed.). Free Press.

Story, C. R., Kirkwood, A. D., Parker, S., & Weller, B. E. (2016). Evaluation of the better todays/better tomorrows youth suicide prevention program: Increasing mental health literacy in rural communities. *Best Practices in Mental Health: An International Journal*, *12*(1), 14–25.

Tam, K. Y., & Ho, S. Y. (2005). Web personalization as a persuasion strategy: An elaboration likelihood model perspective. *Information Systems Research*, *16*(3), 271–291. https://doi.org/10.1287/isre.1050.0058

Taniguchi-Dorios, E., Thompson, C., & Reid, T. (2022). Testing a model of disclosure, perceived support quality, and well-being in the college student mental illness context: A weekly diary study. *Health Communication*, *38*(11), 1–11. https://doi.org/10.1080/10410236.2022.2086841

Tannenbaum, M. B., Hepler, J., Zimmerman, R. S., Saul, L., Jacobs, S., Wilson, K., & Albarracín, D. (2015). Appealing to fear: A meta-analysis of fear appeal effectiveness and theories. *Psychological Bulletin*, *141*(6), 1178–1204. https://doi.org/10.1037/a0039729

Thompson, C. M., Pulido, M. D., & Caban, S. (2020). Why is it difficult for social network members to support people living with mental illnesses? Linking mental illness uncertainty to support provision. *Health Communication*, *37*(2), 202–213. https://doi.org/10.1080/10410236.2020.1831166

Thompson, T. L., & Harrington, N. G. (2021). *The Routledge handbook of health communication* (3rd ed.). Routledge.

Thornicroft, G., Mehta, N., Clement, S., Evans-Lacko, S., Doherty, M., Rose, D., Koschorke, M., Shidhaye, R., O'Reilly, C., & Henderson, C. (2016). Evidence for effective interventions to reduce mental-health-related stigma and discrimination. *Lancet*, *387*(10023), 1123–1132. https://doi.org/10.1016/S0140-6736(15)00298-6

Willoughby, J. F., & Liu, S. (2018). Do pictures help tell the story? An experimental test of narrative and emojis in a health text message intervention. *Computers in Human Behavior*, *79*, 75–82. https://doi.org/10.1016/j.chb.2017.10.031

Wong, N. C., Lookadoo, K. L., & Nisbett, G. S. (2017). "I'm Demi and I have bipolar disorder": Effect of parasocial contact on reducing stigma toward people with bipolar disorder. *Communication Studies*, *68*(3), 314–333. https://doi.org/10.1080/10510974.2017.1331928

World Health Organization. (2022). *Mental health.* https://www.who.int/news-room/fact-sheets/detail/mental-health-strengthening-our-response.

Wright, K. B. (2016). Communication in health-related online social support groups/communities: A review of research on predictors of participation, applications of social support theory, and health outcomes. *Review of Communication Research*, *4*, 65–87. https://doi.org/10.12840/issn.2255-4165.2016.04.01.010

Yap, J. E., Zubcevic-Basic, N., Johnson, L. W., & Lodewyckx, M. A. (2019). Mental health message appeals and audience engagement: Evidence from Australia. *Health Promotion International*, *34*(1), 28–37. https://doi.org/10.1093/heapro/dax062

Yeh, M. A., & Jewell, R. D. (2015). The myth/fact message frame and persuasion in advertising: Enhancing attitudes toward the mentally ill. *Journal of Advertising*, *44*(2), 161–172. https://doi.org/10.1080/00913367.2015.1018466

Zhang, M., Lin, W., Ma, Z., Yang, J., & Zhang, Y. (2023). Users' health information sharing intention in strong ties social media: Context of emerging markets. *Library Hi Tech*, *41*(3), 853–876. https://doi.org/10.1108/LHT-02-2020-0024

Zillmann, D. (1999). Exemplification theory: Judging the whole by some of its parts. *Media Psychology*, *1*(1), 69–94. https://doi.org/10.1207/s1532785xmep0101_5

8

Pretesting and Selecting Messages Using Perceived Message Effectiveness Ratings

Seth M. Noar[1], Haijing Ma[2], and Jacob A. Rohde[3]

[1] University of North Carolina at Chapel Hill
[2] University of Houston-Victoria
[3] RTI International

Health communication campaigns are an effective behavior change tool that can impact a broad range of outcomes (Noar, 2006; Snyder & LaCroix, 2013; Wakefield et al., 2010), including mental health. During the process of campaign development, a critical decision involves which message(s) to use in a campaign. Given the universe of possible messages to choose from, how can campaign designers confidently develop and select messages to achieve their goals?

One common approach is the use of target audience message ratings, or what is referred to as perceived message effectiveness (PME) (Bigsby et al., 2013; Dillard et al., 2007b; Yzer et al., 2015). In this approach, target audience members rate messages on PME, and those data are then used to inform message selection for the campaign. While communication researchers have historically used a myriad of different constructs and measures to assess PME (Dillard & Ye, 2008; Noar et al., 2018b; Yzer et al., 2015), this literature has advanced over the past two decades, giving campaign designers evidence-based guidance and tools for how to best apply PME to the message selection process. The purpose of this chapter is to (a) introduce and define PME; (b) describe the relationship between PME and actual message effectiveness (AME); (c) describe a protocol for applying PME; (d) share two case studies that used PME for message selection; (e) discuss critiques and limitations of PME; and (f) discuss implications for mental health campaign designers.

Defining PME

A campaign is effective if it achieves its intended goal. In many campaigns, this goal is to change mediators of behavior—such as attitudes, beliefs, and intentions—and perhaps behavior itself. Message effectiveness is thus the extent to which message exposure leads to changes in the chosen outcomes of interest. In field trials and experimental work, this is often referred to as AME (Bigsby et al., 2013). For example, a test of messages designed to increase intentions to engage in help-seeking behavior (e.g., seek therapy) would examine whether the messages did exactly that (i.e., increased participants' intentions to contact a mental health therapist). Importantly, such an effectiveness test would *not* be concerned with whether participants *perceived* the messages as increasing their intentions but only whether participants' intentions actually increased as a result of message exposure.

While AME refers to changes in intended campaign outcomes, PME is concerned with *perceptions* of the likely effectiveness of messages. Formally, we define PME as an "estimate of the degree to which a persuasive message will be favorably evaluated by recipients of that message" (Dillard & Ye, 2008,

The Handbook of Mental Health Communication, First Edition.
Edited by Marco C. Yzer and Jason T. Siegel.

p. 150). This definition clarifies that PME (a) is assessed on a continuous scale (i.e., degree); (b) is applied to persuasive messages advocating a particular action; and (c) involves message recipients making judgments about the message (i.e., evaluations). Next, we discuss conceptual and measurement issues identified in the PME literature.

Message Versus Effects Perceptions

Traditionally, there has been substantial heterogeneity in how researchers assess and apply PME (Brennan et al., 2014; Cappella, 2018; Dillard et al., 2007a; Noar et al., 2018a, 2018b; O'Keefe, 2018; Pechmann et al., 2003; Yzer et al., 2015). A systematic review of the literature (in the tobacco prevention and control realm) revealed that diverse PME measures generally tap two broad constructs: message perceptions and effects perceptions. *Message perceptions* are evaluations of a message in terms of its ability to promote further processing that can lead to persuasion (Baig et al., 2021), and have also been referred to as message attributes (Dillard & Ye, 2008) or ad-directed perceived effectiveness (Brennan et al., 2014). An example message perceptions PME item is, "This message is compelling" (Davis et al., 2013). *Effects perceptions*, on the other hand, refer to the potential of a message to change key precursors of behavior or behavior itself (Baig et al., 2021) and have also been referred to as message impact (Dillard & Ye, 2008) or personalized perceived effectiveness (Brennan et al., 2014). An example effects perception PME item is, "This message discourages me from vaping" (Noar et al., 2023). As we discuss later in this chapter, while there is evidence to support both types of PME, existing evidence demonstrates effects perceptions to be more strongly related to behavior-oriented outcomes than message perceptions. Thus, using effects perceptions ratings to select messages may be most useful if the goal of a campaign is to change behavior.

Use of Personal and Behavioral Referents

A referent has to do with *who* and *what* the message being evaluated refers to. By their very nature, message perceptions are less likely to contain personal or behavioral referents than effects perceptions. For example, the item, "This message is compelling," may provide useful information, but it does not specify *who* it refers to (e.g., compelling to me or someone else?). Some studies have found that in the absence of specifying a personal referent, participants may consider themselves, someone else, or a combination of people as the referent, thus engendering measurement error (Baig et al., 2019; Dillard & Ye, 2008). In addition, this example item does not tell us *what* about the message is compelling, meaning if participants find some idiosyncratic feature of the message compelling or interpret the message with a different meaning than what was intended, the resulting data may similarly contain measurement error.

In contrast, effects perceptions tend to contain both personal and behavioral referents. Take for example, "This message encourages me to seek therapy," which contains the personal referent "me," clarifying that I evaluate the message about myself, not others. It also contains a behavioral action (i.e., to seek therapy), ensuring that participants are evaluating the intended purpose of the message. In addition, we would expect that PME ratings for this message would be associated with peoples' perceptions toward therapy-seeking behavior, whereas message perceptions are less likely to be associated with such behavioral-oriented outcomes (Baig et al., 2021).

Correspondence

Prior work applying PME measures has not always been conducted in a way that properly aligns PME with AME. For example, if the goal of a campaign is to increase the number of people who seek therapy, then AME may focus on help-seeking behavioral outcomes, such as the number of people who seek therapy as a result of the campaign. Thus, it would make little sense for PME measures to focus on how much participants like the messages, yet some prior studies have used similar unrelated constructs that have little or no correspondence with what the messages are trying to achieve (Noar et al., 2018a, 2018b).

Instead, PME measures should reflect message goals, and in that sense PME can be viewed simply as the perception that the messages will result in the corresponding AME (Noar et al. 2018b; Yzer et al., 2015). Thus, instead of, "How much do you like this message," a PME item with outcome correspondence might be, "How much does this message encourage you to contact a therapist?" By using outcome-relevant PME items, researchers can increase the chances that participants are evaluating the messages on the very elements intended by the message.

Relationship of PME and AME

More than two decades of research on PME suggest that it may be a valuable proxy for attitude or behavior change elicited by a message, and researchers have used several approaches to examine the relationship between PME and AME (Ma et al., 2023a; Noar et al., 2020a). One approach is *experimental correspondence*, which examines the direction of the experimental effects of message conditions on PME and AME. For instance, Noar et al. (2020c) examined effects of *The Real Cost* vaping prevention ads, a US Food and Drug Administration (FDA)–funded communication campaign designed for youth tobacco prevention, in a sample of adolescents. They found that, compared with control videos (i.e., educational facts provided by a scientific expert), *The Real Cost* ads were rated higher on PME (both effects and message perceptions) and had better AME effects (i.e., increased negative attitudes toward vaping, higher beliefs about the harms of vaping, and lower intentions to vape) compared with control ads. Ma et al. (2023a) conducted a similar study but in the form of a longitudinal randomized controlled trial (RCT). In this study, PME ratings (both effects and message perceptions) of *The Real Cost* vaping prevention ads at Visit 1 anticipated the impact of ads on susceptibility to vaping three weeks later, compared with control videos (Ma et al., 2023a). In another experiment, Rayala et al. (2022) found that environment- and health-focused messages advocating for lower meat consumption were rated higher on PME and led to greater intentions to reduce meat consumption compared with control messages. Together, these studies show experimental correspondence—both in terms of statistical significance and direction of effect—between PME and AME.

A second approach is *prediction*, which examines the association between PME and AME. For instance, in a longitudinal study, Brennan et al. (2014) found that perceived personalized effectiveness (similar to effects perceptions) of antismoking ads predicted smoking behavior at three-week follow-up. By contrast, ad-directed effectiveness (similar to message perceptions) was not associated with behavior change at follow-up. In another study, Davis et al. (2017) examined the validity of PME ratings of *Tips From Former Smokers* campaign messages and found that higher PME (message perceptions) at baseline was positively associated with participants' odds of making a quit attempt at four-month follow-up. In addition, a meta-analysis of the correlation between PME and attitudes revealed associations across diverse topics (Dillard et al., 2007b), while another on tobacco education messages found longitudinal associations between PME ratings and message recall, beliefs about smoking, and intentions to quit smoking (Noar et al., 2020a). Although these findings provide strong evidence to support an association between PME and AME, correlational analyses alone lack the ability to demonstrate a causal link between these constructs (O'Keefe, 2020).

A third approach is *aggregate prediction*, which is similar to *prediction* but with added rigor since it uses aggregate PME ratings rather than individual PME ratings (Bigsby et al., 2013; Kim & Cappella, 2019b). In this approach, participants rate several randomly assigned messages (from a larger pool of messages) on PME and then fill out AME measures. Researchers then compute an average PME score for each message from the individual ratings and then replace each individual PME score with the aggregate score. This avoids the possible confound of reverse causation (i.e., AME affecting PME), since it is not possible for an individual's AME to cause or affect aggregate-level PME. Using this approach, studies have shown PME to predict participants' intentions to quit tobacco products (Bigsby et al., 2013) and smoking quit attempts (Kim & Cappella, 2019b). This work provides evidence suggesting that PME causally impacts AME and that the causal direction from PME to AME is preserved, as "individual's intention to quit could not predict the group's aggregate evaluation of the [public service announcement's] PSAs' persuasiveness" (Kim & Cappella, 2019b, p. 119).

A fourth approach is ***mediation***, which examines the role of PME as a mediator between messages and AME outcomes in experiments (Baig et al., 2021; Brewer et al., 2019; Popova & Li, 2022). Baig et al. (2021) found that effects perceptions mediated the impact of messages about toxic chemicals in cigarettes on butting out, forgoing, and attempts to quit smoking cigarettes; however, message perceptions did ***not*** mediate the effects of message conditions on any of these behavioral outcomes. In another study, Popova and Li (2022) showed that PME (measured as negative message perceptions) mediated the relationship between emotions elicited by e-cigarette prevention messages and intentions to use e-cigarettes. Finally, Ma et al. (2023a) found effects perceptions to fully mediate the impact of vaping prevention ads on susceptibility to vaping in a longitudinal RCT, while message perceptions only partially mediated the effect.

In conclusion, the literature reviewed above provides evidence that there is a meaningful relationship between PME and AME, suggesting that such ratings can provide valuable information about the likely effectiveness of messages.

Protocol for Applying PME

In this section, we describe a protocol for message testing that is based on the PME literature (Kim & Cappella, 2019b) as well as our own experience conducting message testing studies (Boynton et al., 2022; Galper et al., 2024). The protocol involves the following steps: (a) determine the study goal and experimental design; (b) specify the goal of the messages and develop a message pool; (c) identify valid and reliable measures, including PME; (d) gather message ratings from the target population; and (e) analyze data and make conclusions.

Determine the Study Goal and Experimental Design

First, researchers need to know what they are trying to achieve with their message testing study. Typically, there are two types of such studies. One type involves isolating message features that are most promising, such as examining whether gain- or loss-framed messages are more effective for depression help-seeking (Lueck, 2017, 2018) or examining what visual frames (Sontag, 2018) or metaphors (Lazard et al., 2016) are most effective for mental health messages. These kinds of studies generally use a between-subjects design where participants are randomly assigned to message conditions that are identical except for the factor being manipulated (e.g., message frame). The goal here is to contribute to generalizable knowledge by discovering a message principle that leads to more effective messages.

A second type involves testing messages to identify which are most promising to then make decisions about which messages to use in a campaign or intervention. This involves identifying or creating a pool of messages to test, and these kinds of studies tend to use within-subject designs in which participants rate a series of messages that may vary on many features (Boynton et al., 2022; Galper et al., 2024; Kim & Cappella, 2019a). The goal here is more practical in the sense that the results inform evidence-based decisions regarding which messages to use in a campaign.

In some cases, both goals can be achieved in the context of a single study. This will be illustrated in the following case studies.

Specify the Goal of the Messages and Develop a Message Pool

Before messages can be developed or collected, the goal of the messages must be decided. For instance, is the goal of messages to increase general mental health help-seeking behavior (Pace et al., 2018), increase depression help-seeking (Lienemann et al., 2013), reduce the stigma of mental illness (Subramanian & Santo, 2021), or something else? All messages tested should clearly reflect the goal that is decided on. Once a goal is identified, a message pool can be created. This can be achieved by collecting existing messages, creating new messages, or both. Existing messages from prior campaigns and interventions (Senanayake et al., 2019; Sevilla-Llewellyn-Jones et al., 2018; Shalaby et al., 2022) can provide ideas and information for the development of new messages or can be amended for use in a study. During this process, qualitative work can be incredibly useful in understanding nuanced responding to messages and message features (Atkin & Freimuth, 2001; Pace et al., 2018; Pettigrew & Donovan, 2009).

As mentioned already, between-subject studies are typically applied when the goal is to isolate key message features, which are manipulated in experimental conditions. In this case, multiple messages per condition are recommended (rather than a single message) to avoid the case category confound that can take place when single messages are used to represent broad constructs (Jackson, 1992; O'Keefe, 2015). Within-subjects designs are useful for message selection studies, as each participant can rate a series of messages. If the message pool is large, participants can be randomly assigned to a smaller selection of messages (e.g., 5–10) from the larger pool (e.g., 100+) (Boynton et al., 2022; Galper et al., 2024; Kim & Cappella, 2019b).

Identify Valid and Reliable Measures, Including PME

Regardless of the study design and the types of messages to be tested, researchers need to identify valid and reliable measures for their study. The core measure is PME, and as discussed earlier, it is important for PME measures to show correspondence to the intended goal or outcome that the messages are trying to impact. A literature search may identify existing PME measures that can be used or adapted. If there are no existing or useful measures, researchers will need to create their own PME scale. Guidance for designing a PME measure can be informed by the approaches taken in prior studies (Kurtzman et al., 2021; Noar et al., 2018b, 2023) as well as the case studies discussed in this chapter.

Depending on the goals of the study and the nature of the messages being tested, researchers may also wish to include other measures in their data collection, such as emotional reactions or psychological reactance (Leshner et al., 2009; Ma & Miller, 2022). For instance, in the domain of graphic or pictorial warnings for cigarette packs, negative emotions such as fear, disgust, and sadness are key constructs often assessed in such studies (Noar et al., 2020b), as is reactance to such messages (Hall et al., 2016). Additional measures should be informed by the study goals, design, and context.

Gather Message Ratings from the Target Population

Gathering PME ratings (and potentially data on other constructs) from the target audience is critical to understanding the extent to which messages are or are not promising among the target population. Individuals respond differently to messages based on various factors, including demographic and psychological characteristics. Thus, a well-designed message that works for a particular target population may not affect another population similarly or could even cause unintended effects (e.g., increasing individuals' anxiety). Therefore, it is critical to evaluate messages among members of the target population. If recruitment results in a broader sample (e.g., those with and without mental health conditions), research should—at minimum—conduct subgroup analyses with the target population. If possible, researchers should aim to collect at least $N = 25$ ratings per message (Kim & Cappella, 2019a).

There is evidence that those suffering from mental health conditions may substantively differ from those without such mental health conditions. For example, studies suggest that individuals with depression may perceive help-seeking behaviors differently than those without depression (Lueck & Yzer, 2018; Yzer et al., 2022). Moreover, there is evidence that individuals with depression may respond to depression help-seeking messages in ways that differ from those without depression (Lienemann et al., 2013; Lueck, 2017). Thus, all efforts should be made to test the messages with the precise target population when possible, as even those who are demographically similar to the target population but do not suffer from the mental health condition may respond to messages differently.

Analyze Data and Make Conclusions

Once data are collected, they can be analyzed in light of the study design, message goals, and measures collected. Researchers may examine mean PME levels of the messages tested and may conduct significance tests to look for differences across study conditions. Decisions about message selection can be guided heavily by PME; however, other factors may also be important to consider, such as any unintended effects of messages (e.g., increasing stigma) or any real-world constraints to implementing particular messages.

Case Studies Applying PME

Next, we present two case studies that have applied PME for message selection. The first was a study pretesting messages for an inflammatory bowel disease (IBD) social support and disease self-management text messaging intervention among adults with IBD. The second was a study testing messages about e-cigarette and vaping harms among youth.

Inflammatory Bowel Disease Self-Management Message Pretesting Study

In this first example, we developed and pretested 20 unique disease self-management support text messages (~40–50 words per message) designed to reduce distress among people with IBD. The statements were informed by our prior empirical findings identifying topics that people with IBD and distress frequently acknowledge (e.g., concerns with nutrition, medications) (Rohde et al., 2021) as well as IBD self-management literature (Keefer & Kane, 2016). Messages were grouped into four distinct disease management themes: (a) symptoms, (b) nutrition, (c) social, and (d) other topics, including medication management. There were five different text messages per theme. The study stimuli were static images designed to look like text messages sent to a smartphone, which was the medium used in the final intervention (Rohde et al., 2022a). Messages were reviewed by several subject matter experts to ensure message content was accurate for people with IBD. Experts included a gastroenterologist who treats people with IBD and an individual diagnosed with IBD.

Participants ($N = 44$) in this pretest study were adults (aged 18+) in the United States with a self-reported IBD diagnosis (e.g., Crohn's disease). The study sample was recruited from various social media platforms (e.g., Reddit) in fall 2020. After providing informed consent, participants were randomly assigned in an online survey to view and evaluate five different support messages in a single disease management theme. Participants evaluated messages one at a time on a PME scale that began with the stem, "How much does this message…," and included the following five items: (a) give you important information about IBD; (b) make you feel more confident in managing your IBD; (c) make you feel supported about your IBD; (d) give you ideas about how to better cope with your IBD; and (e) make you think that better managing IBD can improve your symptoms. Each PME item tapped into a different theoretical area related to the evaluation of the support messages (e.g., self-efficacy, perceived support). Items were assessed on a 5-point scale that ranged from 1 = *not at all* to 5 = *a great deal,* and coefficient alpha for the scale was high ($\alpha = 0.91$). Participants also provided open-ended assessments about what they liked and what could be improved about each message. We used rank-ordered PME ratings paired with open-ended message feedback to select and improve the content of the messages prior to the final intervention.

Figure 8.1 shows the PME means of all messages grouped by IBD management message theme, ordered from highest to lowest. On average, messages in the symptoms management theme scored the highest on PME ($M = 3.31$), followed by messages in the nutrition ($M = 3.01$), other topics ($M = 2.68$), and social ($M = 2.46$) themes. Table 8.1 shows evaluations of example support messages from each of the four disease management themes. Message 1 was from the symptoms management theme and provided a resource to help people track their IBD symptoms, while Message 2 was from the nutrition management theme and provided information about what foods to eat when experiencing an IBD-related flare. Moderately high PME ratings for Messages 1 ($M = 3.80$) and 2 ($M = 3.22$) indicated that people who have IBD and distress perceived support on these topics as important. This was partly supported by open-ended feedback, as participants noted that messages felt relatable and offered valuable information. We partly modified the content of Messages 1 and 2 based on feedback and included them in the final intervention.

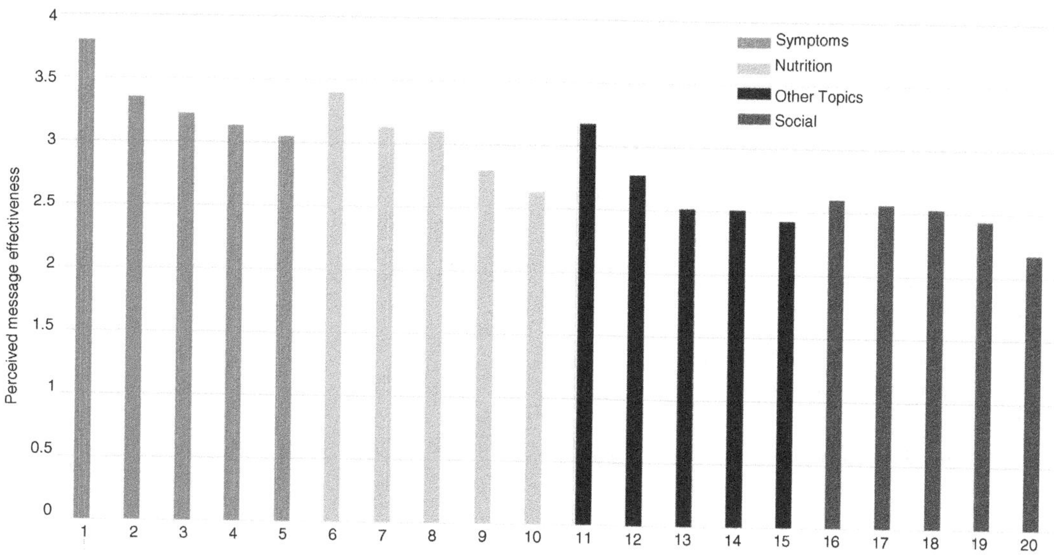

Figure 8.1 Perceived message effectiveness ratings of IBD support messages. Each bar on the X-axis represents a different message. The order of the message themes (left to right) is the same as the order in the legend (top to bottom).

Messages 3 and 4, on the other hand, were not rated favorably by our study sample. Message 3 concerned IBD medication management (part of the other topics theme), and many participants noted the patronizing tone of the message. Message 4 was from the social management theme and tapped into issues concerning finding public restrooms during symptom flares. Although participants found Message 4 helpful, several acknowledged that the information was too obvious. The low PME ratings of both Message 3 ($M = 2.51$) and Message 4 ($M = 2.18$)—paired with the negative open-ended feedback—prompted us to exclude these messages from the final intervention.

While the procedures in this study represent a snapshot of a larger message evaluation process, they illustrate how to develop and utilize a study-specific PME measure. The messages we pretested were designed to change key theoretical constructs linked to IBD self-management behavior, such as self-efficacy, knowledge, and outcome expectations. Thus, we created a PME measure with items tapping into those constructs. This process emphasizes outcome correspondence with scale items, which can maximize effects when using PME to evaluate messages. Our study findings also highlight how PME ratings and rankings can be used to identify high-quality health communication messages—particularly when paired with other message evaluation tools such as open-ended participant feedback. Similar procedures could be integrated in other health communication contexts, such as designing support messages for improving mental health.

E-Cigarette and Vaping Prevention

In this study, we developed and tested a series of messages for a text-messaging e-cigarette and vaping prevention intervention for youth (Galper et al., 2024). Guided by formative research with adolescents, including a seven-member youth advisory board, in-depth interviews with adolescents, and existing literature, we settled on a message strategy focused on how vaping negatively affects youth. That is, our formative research suggested message content related to the negative consequences of vaping was perceived as most relevant to youth and most discouraged e-cigarette use (Boynton et al., 2022; Ma et al., 2023b). We next wrote messages based upon the following vaping harm themes: (a) nicotine addiction; (b) chemical harms; (c) health symptoms; (d) mental health; (e) health effects on organs; (f) cosmetic effects; and (g) monetary cost. The process of writing messages for each theme was iterative and included several rounds of feedback from our research team.

Table 8.1 PME Ratings and Open-Ended Evaluations of Inflammatory Bowel Disease Self-Management Support Messages

Example messages (IBD management theme)	*PME score M (SD)*	*n*	*What was liked?*	*What could be improved?*
Message 1 (symptom management): IBD flares aren't easy to handle, especially when they come out of nowhere. A good way to manage flares is to keep track of symptom activity using a phone app such as "MyGut." Being aware of symptom changes can also help doctors recommend different treatment options. For more info about MyGut, click here: (URL here)	3.80 (1.01)	12	• Offers resource (*n* = 7) • Useful reminder (*n* = 2) • Encouraging tone (*n* = 1)	• Make clear that message is not an ad (*n* = 2) • Less cluttered text (*n* = 1)
Message 2 (nutrition management): Knowing what foods to eat during IBD flares isn't easy. Certain nutritious foods, such as low-fiber fruits (bananas) and lean proteins (white meat chicken), can be easier to digest when experiencing symptoms. For more advice, take a look at this webpage: (URL here)	3.40 (0.97)	8	• Offered suggestions (*n* = 4) • Relatable (*n* = 3)	• Food choices can be subjective (*n* = 1) • Do not use http://bit.ly URL (*n* = 1)
Message 3 (other management—e.g., medication): Regularly taking IBD medication can seem like a nuisance, especially when symptoms aren't present. Most IBD medication is intended for long-term use. Because of this, it's important for people with IBD to keep taking medication they were prescribed for it to be most effective	2.51 (1.06)	13	• Useful information and reminder (*n* = 5) • To the point (*n* = 2) • Encouraging message (*n* = 1)	• Patronizing/not relatable (*n* = 5) • More support (*n* = 2) • Add information about specific medications (*n* = 1)
Message 4 (social management): It can be stressful going to some events because of IBD. A helpful way to manage IBD in public, such as at a restaurant or when shopping, is to keep track of where the nearest restrooms are. That way, you can stay on top of certain symptoms if they come out of nowhere.	2.18 (0.84)	11	• Helpful tone (*n* = 4) • Useful information for newly diagnosed (*n* = 2)	• Too obvious (*n* = 6) • Add resource to additional support, such as managing accidents (*n* = 2)

Note. PME = perceived message effectiveness; *M* = mean; *SD* = standard deviation; *n* = participant sample size.

Once we had a broad set of messages across themes, we convened a panel of four experts in toxicology and addiction science. This expert panel provided both verbal and written feedback on the messages. Feedback from this panel resulted in some messages being revised and others being discarded. We also elicited input from our youth advisory board on both message wording and perceived impact of the messages, which we used to further refine the messages. Our final set of messages consisted of 43 unique statements across the seven themes. We also included three neutral control messages about e-cigarette and vape litter to compare against our intervention messages. We chose littering as our control category because prior studies have shown that this topic is not particularly persuasive in discouraging vaping (Brewer et al., 2019; Rohde et al., 2022b).

Next, we conducted a large study using PME ratings. Participants were a nationally representative sample of 1,603 US adolescents aged 13–17 years, recruited in summer 2022. Adolescents were randomly assigned to view seven vaping prevention messages (one from each of the seven harms themes) and one control message (vape litter theme) from the larger pool of 46 messages. Messages were presented as text statements, and adolescents rated each statement on PME using the University of North Carolina Perceived Message Effectiveness Scale for Youth (Kurtzman et al., 2021; Noar et al., 2023). After each message, participants were asked, "How much does this message…" (a) make you worry about what vaping will do to you? (b) make you think vaping is a bad idea? and (c) discourage you from vaping? Items were assessed on a 5-point scale that ranged from 1 = ***not at all*** to 5 = ***a great deal***, and coefficient alpha for the scale was high ($\alpha = 0.95$).

We used the PME data from this study in two ways. First, we examined whether the vaping prevention themes outperformed the vaping litter control theme. Results of linear mixed models indicated that all vaping prevention message themes outperformed control on PME, indicating that each of the seven message themes had some level of promise (Galper et al., 2024). However, some message themes had larger effects than others. We applied these findings to the final intervention by including messages from all themes but using more messages from themes that exhibited larger PME effects, such as health effects on organs and chemical harms.

Second, we used the PME means to choose specific messages to use in the text-messaging intervention, with higher means indicating more potentially effective messages. To accomplish this, we looked at the means for each individual message and its respective theme. Given that our intervention was being designed for youth who vape or are susceptible to vaping in the future, we focused on the means from those at-risk sub-groups when making message selection decisions.

Table 8.2 shows the number of messages that we tested in each harms theme, as well as example messages and their corresponding PME scores. Figure 8.2 displays the means of all messages for youth susceptible to vaping and youth who currently vape, respectively. Several observations can be made

Table 8.2 Vaping Prevention Themes and Example Messages Tested in the Study

Theme	*Description*	*Messages tested*	*Messages retained*	*Example message*	*PME M (SD)*
Health effects on organs	Potential effects of vaping on the body, including lungs, heart, and brain development	6	5	"Vaping could lead to lung diseases."	Susceptible: 4.28 (0.90) User: 3.41 (1.85)
Chemical harms	Chemicals found in e-cigarette aerosol that the user inhales while vaping	7	5	"E-cigarette vapor can contain formaldehyde, a known cause of cancer."	Susceptible: 4.11 (0.88) User: 3.67 (1.92)
Nicotine addiction	The addictive nature of nicotine found in vapes	7	4	"Some vapes deliver as much addictive nicotine as a pack of 20 cigarettes."	Susceptible: 4.09 (1.00) User: 3.51 (1.87)
Health symptoms	Potential symptoms of vaping, such as coughing, wheezing, and headaches	5	4	"Vaping can make you cough and wheeze."	Susceptible: 4.03 (0.90) User: 2.82 (1.68)
Mental health	Potential effects of vaping in worsening mental health	6	2	"Vaping could lead to more days feeling down."	Susceptible: 3.38 (1.03) User: 2.61 (1.62)
Cosmetic effects	Potential effects of vaping on physical appearance	6	3	"E-cigarette vapor could harm your skin."	Susceptible: 3.45 (1.10) User: 2.64 (1.63)
Monetary costs	Monetary cost of vapes	6	3	"Money spent on vaping means less money to spend with friends."	Susceptible: 3.24 (1.08) User: 2.27 (1.51)
Control	Vape litter	3	0	"Please refrain from littering vapes."	Susceptible: 2.66 (1.31) User: 2.14 (1.46)

Note. Table shows means and standard deviations for example messages for susceptible (at-risk) non-users of e-cigarettes ($n = 656$) and past 30-day e-cigarette users ($n = 107$); PME = perceived message effectiveness; M = mean; SD = standard deviation.

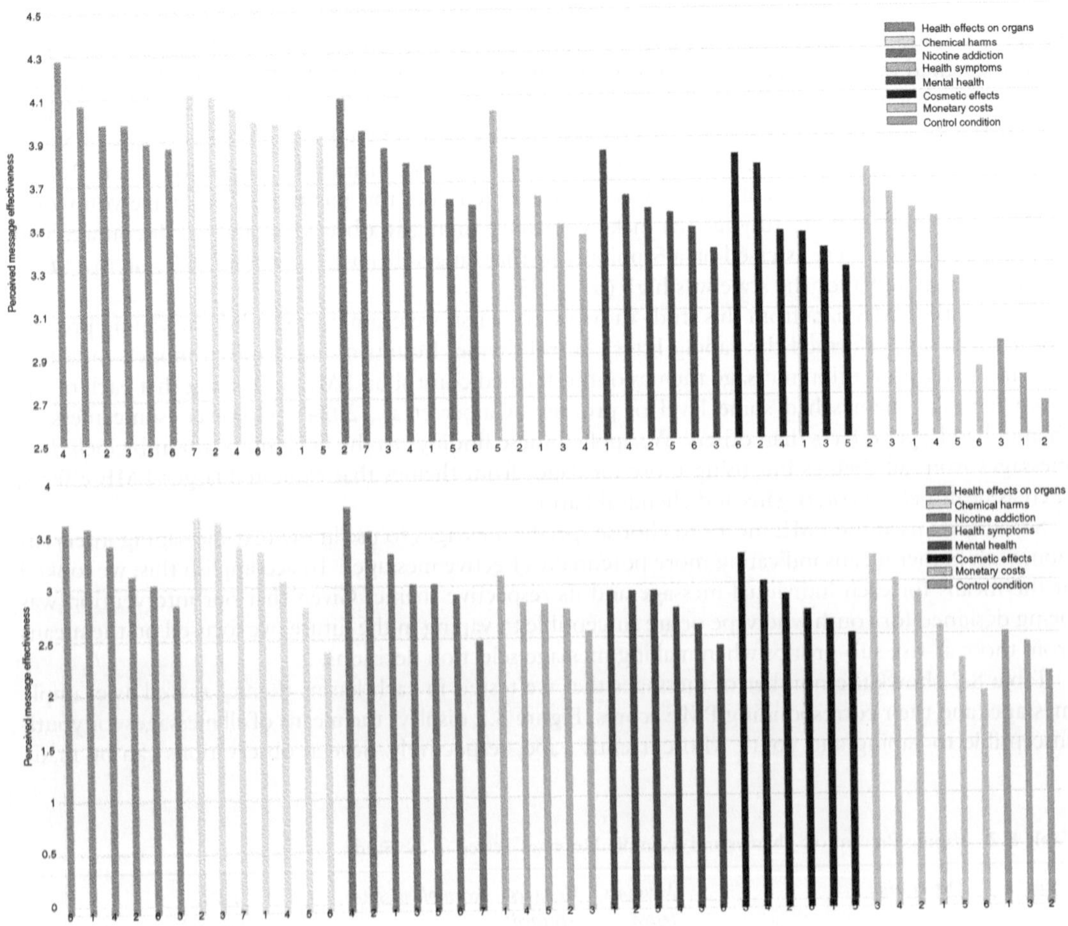

Figure 8.2 Perceived message effectiveness ratings among youth susceptible to vaping (top panel) and past 30-day users (bottom panel). Each bar on the X-axis represents a different message (numbers refer to specific messages). The order of the message themes (left to right) is the same as the order in the legend (top to bottom).

from these data: (a) messages from some themes tended to have higher means than those from other themes, with Figure 8.2 generally showing the themes in order from most to least promising; (b) messages varied on PME *within* theme, indicating that some messages within themes were more promising than others; and (c) users generally rated the messages as lower on PME than susceptible nonusers, which is not surprising given that users are more likely to be critical of messages than nonusers. Our focus was less on this difference and more on which messages both target audiences viewed as promising (and not promising). Of the 43 intervention messages tested, we discarded 17 messages and retained 26, based on PME ratings. Thus, these ratings provided invaluable data for selecting messages that these target audiences perceived as more persuasive and helped us select the most promising messages for reducing openness to vaping and discouraging vaping behaviors.

In conclusion, both case studies demonstrate how PME can be fruitfully applied in message testing to efficiently evaluate the potential of a pool of messages. In both cases, messages were developed with qualitative input from experts and the target audience (through the youth advisory board) and were tested using experiments with the target audience that involved the use of PME ratings. Both case studies generated generalizable knowledge about what message themes were most promising, and the data from both studies allowed the researchers to select (and in some cases refine) specific messages for the intervention. Thus, these case studies illustrate how PME ratings can be used to guide message selection in ways that help message designers select the most promising messages for their communication interventions, thereby increasing the likelihood of impact.

Critiques and Limitations of PME

It is important to acknowledge some critiques raised about PME in the literature. One set of critiques focuses on the use of correlational data as evidence for the validity of PME (O'Keefe, 2020), discussed already as *prediction*. This is a well-documented concern (Dillard et al., 2007a; Noar et al., 2018b), as those who are predisposed to more favorable AME outcomes may be more likely to rate messages as highly effective, giving the illusion that PME ratings drive AME (when it could be that AME drives PME ratings). However, other evidence presented earlier in this chapter, such as experimental correspondence and aggregate PME ratings, are not subject to this critique yet still support the notion that PME provides meaningful information about AME.

A second set of critiques is mostly conceptual and is based on the assertion that people rely on faulty beliefs as to what types of messages may be persuasive. This line of reasoning suggests that PME ratings are misleading guesses more than meaningful information (O'Keefe, 1993). Building on this idea, a meta-analysis looked at PME ratings across extant messages and found little evidence to suggest that these ratings helped researchers select better messages (O'Keefe, 2018). However, there were several limitations to this meta-analysis, including that many of the so-called PME constructs and measures went beyond what many researchers would consider to be well-conceived PME measures. Also, many of the studies included were not designed to test the relationship between PME and AME (Noar et al. 2018a). Thus, the conclusion of this work—namely, that PME ratings are not useful—is premature. This line of work also seems to largely ignore the increasing accumulation of evidence supporting PME ratings, including meaningful applications from both researchers (Cappella, 2018) and practitioners (Davis & Duke, 2018).

There are some limitations, however, to applying PME ratings in message testing and selection studies. Most centrally, there is no known cutoff on PME scales as to what makes a given message effective. Therefore, message designers should select messages with higher PME scores, knowing that there is no guarantee that because a message achieves a particular score that it *will* be effective. Related to this, it is important to note that many factors influence effectiveness in the real world beyond the message itself, most notably message exposure. Thus, it is critical that the target audience has a high frequency of exposure to the messages, as even highly effective messages are unlikely to have impact if exposure is low (Hornik, 2002; Noar, 2006).

Relatedly, evidence also seems to suggest that large differences between PME ratings translate into smaller differences in AME (Ma et al., 2023a). This is not unlike the empirical observation that a large change in behavioral intentions is needed to produce a small change in behavior (Webb & Sheeran, 2006). Thus, if messages exhibit very small differences in PME, then PME may not offer much guidance as to which messages to select, and in fact it may matter little what message is selected with regard to its promise in impacting AME.

Conclusion and Implications for Mental Health Campaigns

In this chapter, we introduced and defined PME as a tool that message designers can use to help identify the most promising messages to use in a campaign or intervention. We provided conceptual and measurement recommendations for PME and presented evidence that PME is meaningfully related to the actual impact of messages. We further described a protocol for applying PME and provided case studies that demonstrate applications of the PME protocol to two diverse topics. Finally, we discussed critiques and limitations of PME.

Those tasked with developing messages and campaigns to improve mental health can apply the knowledge discussed in this chapter to identify the most promising messages to use in their communication efforts. The process of developing high-quality messages is taxing and may include discussions with content experts, qualitative research, and quantitative studies. However, this effort is well worth it given the ability of careful message development and pretesting to contribute not only to increased confidence in the selected messages but also to generalizable knowledge in the field. Moreover, such careful work can help avoid unintended negative consequences of messages, such as the possibility of well-intended mental health messages having *negative* effects among individuals with depression (Lienemann et al., 2013; Siegel et al., 2019).

Those developing mental health messages should clearly specify the goal of their messages and should undertake studies with the target audience to advance an understanding of message effects prior to the implementation of such messages. Such work may examine myriad outcomes in the mental health field, such as increasing help-seeking (Siegel et al., 2015), enhancing mental health empathy (Kresovich, 2022), and reducing mental health stigma (Kroska & Harkness, 2021), and may apply diverse theoretical perspectives, such as gain-and-loss framing (Gilbert et al., 2021), visual framing (Sontag, 2018), mistargeting (Siegel et al., 2015), and fear appeals (Lueck, 2019). By applying practices from the field of communication, those focused on mental health communication efforts can advance scientific knowledge and increase the chances of impact, thereby achieving their goals and improving mental health outcomes for diverse populations.

References

Atkin, C. K., & Freimuth, V. S. (2001). Formative evaluation research in campaign design. In R. E. Rice & C. K. Atkin (Eds.), *Public communication campaigns* (3rd ed., pp. 125–145). Sage Publications.

Baig, S. A., Noar, S. M., Gottfredson, N. C., Boynton, M. H., Ribisl, K. M., & Brewer, N. T. (2019). UNC perceived message effectiveness: Validation of a brief scale. *Annals of Behavioral Medicine, 53*(8), 732–742. http://dx.doi.org/10.1093/abm/kay080

Baig, S. A., Noar, S. M., Gottfredson, N. C., Lazard, A. J., Ribisl, K. M., & Brewer, N. T. (2021). Message perceptions and effects perceptions as proxies for behavioral impact in the context of anti-smoking messages. *Preventive Medicine Reports, 23*, 101434. http://dx.doi.org/10.1016/j.pmedr.2021.101434

Bigsby, E., Cappella, J. N., & Seitz, H. H. (2013). Efficiently and effectively evaluating public service announcements: Additional evidence for the utility of perceived effectiveness. *Communication Monographs, 80*(1), 1–23. https://doi.org/10.1080%2F03637751.2012.739706

Boynton, M., Sanzo, N., Brothers, W., Kresovich, A., Sutfin, E. L., Sheeran, P., & Noar, S. M. (2022). Perceived effectiveness of objective elements of vaping prevention messages among adolescents. *Tobacco Control, 32*, e228–e235. http://dx.doi.org/10.1186/s12889-016-3151-5

Brennan, E., Durkin, S. J., Wakefield, M. A., & Kashima, Y. (2014). Assessing the effectiveness of antismoking television advertisements: Do audience ratings of perceived effectiveness predict changes in quitting intentions and smoking behaviours? *Tobacco Control, 23*(5), 412–418. http://dx.doi.org/10.1136/tobaccocontrol-2012-050949

Brewer, N. T., Jeong, M., Hall, M. G., Baig, S. A., Mendel, J. R., Lazard, A. J., Noar, S. M., Kameny, M. R., & Ribisl, K. M. (2019). Impact of e-cigarette health warnings on motivation to vape and smoke. *Tobacco Control, 28*(e1), e64–e70. http://dx.doi.org/10.1136/tobaccocontrol-2018-054878

Cappella, J. N. (2018). Perceived message effectiveness meets the requirements of a reliable, valid, and efficient measure of persuasiveness. *Journal of Communication, 68*(5), 994–997. http://dx.doi.org/10.1093/joc/jqy044

Davis, K. C., Duke, J., Shafer, P., Patel, D., Rodes, R., & Beistle, D. (2017). Perceived effectiveness of antismoking ads and association with quit attempts among smokers: Evidence from the tips from former smokers campaign. *Health Communication, 32*(8), 931–938. https://doi.org/10.1080/10410236.2016.1196413

Davis, K. C., & Duke, J. C. (2018). Evidence of the real-world effectiveness of public health media campaigns reinforces the value of perceived message effectiveness in campaign planning. *Journal of Communication, 68*(5), 998–1000. http://dx.doi.org/10.1093/joc/jqy045

Davis, K. C., Nonnemaker, J., Duke, J., & Farrelly, M. C. (2013). Perceived effectiveness of cessation advertisements: The importance of audience reactions and practical implications for media campaign planning. *Health Communication, 28*(5), 461–472. https://doi.org/10.1080/10410236.2012.696535

Dillard, J. P., Shen, L., & Vail, R. G. (2007a). Does perceived message effectiveness cause persuasion or vice versa? Seventeen consistent answers. *Human Communication Research, 33*(4), 467–488. http://dx.doi.org/10.1111/j.1468-2958.2007.00308.x

Dillard, J. P., Weber, K. M., & Vail, R. G. (2007b). The relationship between the perceived and actual effectiveness of persuasive messages: A meta-analysis with implications for formative campaign research. *Journal of Communication, 57*(4), 613–631. http://dx.doi.org/10.1111/j.1460-2466.2007.00360.x

Dillard, J. P., & Ye, S. (2008). The perceived effectiveness of persuasive messages: Questions of structure, referent, and bias. *Journal of Health Communication, 13*(2), 149–168. http://dx.doi.org/10.1080/10810730701854060

Galper, E. F., Gottfredson O'Shea, N., Ritchie, C., Kresovich, A., Ma, H., Sutfin, E. L., Sheeran, P., & Noar, S. M. (2024). Identifying promising themes and messages for youth vaping prevention: A national study. *Social Science & Medicine, 348*, 116864.

Gilbert, G., Williamson, C., Richards, J., Collyer, T. A., & Kelly, P. (2021). Do framed mental health messages on social media influence university students' motivation for physical activity? *International Journal of Environmental Research and Public Health, 18*(16), 8671. http://dx.doi.org/10.3390/ijerph18168671

Hall, M. G., Sheeran, P., Noar, S. M., Ribisl, K. M., Bach, L. E., & Brewer, N. T. (2016). Reactance to health warnings scale: Development and validation. *Annals of Behavioral Medicine, 50*(5), 736–750. http://dx.doi.org/10.1007/s12160-016-9799-3

Hornik, R. (2002). *Public health communication: Evidence for behavior change*. Routledge.

Jackson, S. (1992). *Message effects research: Principles of design and analysis*. Guilford Press.

Keefer, L., & Kane, S. (2016). Self-management techniques in IBD. In R. K. Cross & A. R. Watson (Eds.), *Telemanagement of inflammatory bowel disease* (pp. 55–70). Springer. http://dx.doi.org/10.1007/978-3-319-22285-1_5

Kim, M., & Cappella, J. N. (2019a). An efficient message evaluation protocol: Two empirical analyses on positional effects and optimal sample size. *Journal of Health Communication, 24*(10), 761–769. http://dx.doi.org/10.1080/10810730.2019.1668090

Kim, M., & Cappella, J. N. (2019b). Reliable, valid and efficient evaluation of media messages: Developing a message testing protocol. *Journal of Communication Management, 23*(3), 179–197. http://dx.doi.org/10.1108/JCOM-12-2018-0132

Kresovich, A. (2022). An experimental test of pop music lyrics referencing anxiety on female college students' audience involvement and peer mental health empathy. *Journal of Health Communication, 27*(3), 192–200. http://dx.doi.org/10.1080/10810730.2022.2078910

Kroska, A., & Harkness, S. K. (2021). Information vs. inspiration: Evaluating the effectiveness of mental illness stigma-reduction messages. *Social Science Research, 96*, 102543. http://dx.doi.org/10.1016/j.ssresearch.2021.102543

Kurtzman, R. T., Vereen, R., Mendel Sheldon, J., Adams, E., Hall, M. G., Brewer, N. T., Gottfredson, N. C., & Noar, S. M. (2021). Cognitive interviews with adolescents: Understanding smoking and vaping risk language to inform scale development. *Nicotine & Tobacco Research, 24*(11), 1741–1747. http://dx.doi.org/10.1093/ntr/ntac127

Lazard, A. J., Bamgbade, B. A., Sontag, J. M., & Brown, C. (2016). Using visual metaphors in health messages: A strategy to increase effectiveness for mental illness communication. *Journal of Health Communication, 21*(12), 1260–1268. http://dx.doi.org/10.1080/10810730.2016.1245374

Leshner, G., Bolls, P., & Thomas, E. (2009). Scare 'em or disgust 'em: The effects of graphic health promotion messages. *Health Communication, 24*(5), 447–458. https://doi.org/10.1080/10410230903023493

Lienemann, B. A., Siegel, J. T., & Crano, W. D. (2013). Persuading people with depression to seek help: Respect the boomerang. *Health Communication, 28*(7), 718–728. http://dx.doi.org/10.1080/10410236.2012.712091

Lueck, J., & Yzer, M. (2018). Explaining intentions to seek help for depressive symptoms in the context of responsibility message framing. *Health Communication, 33*(8), 946–953. http://dx.doi.org/10.1080/10410236.2017.1322857

Lueck, J. A. (2017). Matching message design and depressed cognition: An exploration of attention patterns for gain-and loss-framed depression help-seeking messages. *Journal of Health Communication, 22*(7), 593–603. http://dx.doi.org/10.1080/10810730.2017.1324538

Lueck, J. A. (2018). Respecting the 'stages' of depression: Considering depression severity and readiness to seek help. *Patient Education and Counseling, 101*(7), 1276–1282. http://dx.doi.org/10.1016/j.pec.2018.02.007

Lueck, J. A. (2019). Should we activate risk perceptions in the context of suicide prevention? Examining fear appeals, help-seeking determinants, and help-seeking sources among university employees who suffer from depression. *Prevention Science, 20*(6), 884–893. http://dx.doi.org/10.1007/s11121-019-0979-9

Ma, H., Gottfredson O'Shea, N., Kieu, T., Rohde, J. A., Hall, M. G., Brewer, N. T., & Noar, S. M. (2023a). Examining the longitudinal relationship between perceived and actual message effectiveness: A randomized trial. *Health Communication*. Advance online publication. https://doi.org/10.1080/10410236.2023.2222459

Ma, H., Kieu, T. K., Ribisl, K. M., & Noar, S. M. (2023b). Do vaping prevention messages impact adolescents and young adults? A meta-analysis of experimental studies. *Health Communication, 38*(8), 1–14. http://dx.doi.org/10.1080/10410236.2023.2185578

Ma, H., & Miller, C. H. (2022). "I felt completely turned off by the message": The effects of controlling language, fear, and disgust appeals on responses to COVID-19 vaccination messages. *Journal of Health Communication, 27*(6), 427–438. http://dx.doi.org/10.1080/10810730.2022.2119311

Noar, S. M. (2006). A 10-year retrospective of research in health mass media campaigns: Where do we go from here? *Journal of Health Communication*, *11*(1), 21–42. http://dx.doi.org/10.1080/10810730500461059

Noar, S. M., Barker, J., Bell, T., & Yzer, M. (2020a). Does perceived message effectiveness predict the actual effectiveness of tobacco education messages? A systematic review and meta-analysis. *Health Communication*, *35*(2), 148–157. http://dx.doi.org/10.1080/10410236.2018.1547675

Noar, S. M., Barker, J., & Yzer, M. (2018a). Measurement and design heterogeneity in perceived message effectiveness studies: A call for research. *Journal of Communication*, *68*(5), 990–993. http://dx.doi.org/10.1093/joc/jqy047

Noar, S. M., Bell, T., Kelley, D., Barker, J., & Yzer, M. (2018b). Perceived message effectiveness measures in tobacco education campaigns: A systematic review. *Communication Methods and Measures*, *12*(4), 295–313. http://dx.doi.org/10.1080/19312458.2018.1483017

Noar, S. M., Gottfredson, N. C., Vereen, R., Kurtzman, R., Mendel Sheldon, J., Adams, E., Hall, M. G., & Brewer, N. T. (2023). Development of the UNC perceived message effectiveness scale for youth. *Tobacco Control*, *32*(5), 553–558. http://dx.doi.org/10.1136/tobaccocontrol-2021-056929

Noar, S. M., Rohde, J. A., Barker, J. O., Hall, M. G., & Brewer, N. T. (2020b). Pictorial cigarette pack warnings increase some risk appraisals but not risk beliefs: A meta-analysis. *Human Communication Research*, *46*(2–3), 250–272. http://dx.doi.org/10.1093/hcr/hqz016

Noar, S. M., Rohde, J. A., Prentice-Dunn, H., Kresovich, A., Hall, M. G., & Brewer, N. T. (2020c). Evaluating the actual and perceived effectiveness of e-cigarette prevention advertisements among adolescents. *Addictive Behaviors*, *109*, 106473. https://doi.org/10.1016/j.addbeh.2020.106473

O'Keefe, D. J. (1993). Understanding social influence: Relations between lay and technical perspectives. *Communication Studies*, *44*(3–4), 228–238. http://dx.doi.org/10.1080/10510979309368397

O'Keefe, D. J. (2015). Message generalizations that support evidence-based persuasive message design: Specifying the evidentiary requirements. *Health Communication*, *30*(2), 106–113. http://dx.doi.org/10.1080/10410236.2014.974123

O'Keefe, D. J. (2018). Message pretesting using assessments of expected or perceived persuasiveness: Evidence about diagnosticity of relative actual persuasiveness. *Journal of Communication*, *68*(1), 120–142. http://dx.doi.org/10.1093/joc/jqx009

O'Keefe, D. J. (2020). Message pretesting using perceived persuasiveness measures: Reconsidering the correlational evidence. *Communication Methods and Measures*, *14*(1), 25–37. http://dx.doi.org/10.1080/19312458.2019.1620711

Pace, K., Silk, K., Nazione, S., Fournier, L., & Collins-Eaglin, J. (2018). Promoting mental health help-seeking behavior among first-year college students. *Health Communication*, *33*(2), 102–110. http://dx.doi.org/10.1080/10410236.2016.1250065

Pechmann, C., Zhao, G., Goldberg, M. E., & Reibling, E. T. (2003). What to convey in antismoking advertisements for adolescents: The use of protection motivation theory to identify effective message themes. *Journal of Marketing*, *67*, 1–18. https://doi.org/10.1509/jmkg.67.2.1.18607

Pettigrew, S., & Donovan, R. (2009). Older audiences' responses to mental health promotion messages. *International Journal of Mental Health Promotion*, *11*(1), 23–31. http://dx.doi.org/10.1080/14623730.2009.9721779

Popova, L., & Li, Y. (2022). Perceived message effectiveness: Do people need to think about message effectiveness to report the message as effective? *Health Education & Behavior*, 1–9. https://doi.org/doi.org/10.1177%2F10901981211068412

Rayala, H. T., Rebolledo, N., Hall, M. G., & Taillie, L. S. (2022). Perceived message effectiveness of the meatless Monday campaign: An experiment with US adults. *American Journal of Public Health*, *112*(5), 724–727. https://doi.org/10.2105/AJPH.2022.306766

Rohde, J. A., Fisher, E. B., Boynton, M. H., Freelon, D., Frohlich, D. O., Barnes, E. L., & Noar, S. M. (2022a). A self-management SMS text messaging intervention for people with inflammatory bowel disease: Feasibility and acceptability study. *JMIR Formative Research*, *6*(5), e34960. http://dx.doi.org/10.2196/34960

Rohde, J. A., Noar, S. M., Mendel, J., Hall, M. G., & Brewer, N. T. (2022b). Identifying promising themes for adolescent vaping warnings: A national experiment. *Nicotine & Tobacco Research*, *24*(9), 1379–1385. http://dx.doi.org/10.1093/ntr/ntac093

Rohde, J. A., Sibley, A. L., & Noar, S. M. (2021). Topics analysis of Reddit and Twitter posts discussing inflammatory bowel disease and distress from 2017 to 2019. *Crohn's & Colitis 360*, *3*((3)). http://dx.doi.org/10.1093/crocol/otab044

Senanayake, B., Wickramasinghe, S. I., Chatfield, M. D., Hansen, J., Edirippulige, S., & Smith, A. C. (2019). Effectiveness of text messaging interventions for the management of depression: A systematic review and meta-analysis. *Journal of Telemedicine and Telecare*, *25*(9), 513–523. http://dx.doi.org/10.1177/1357633x19875852

Sevilla-Llewellyn-Jones, J., Santesteban-Echarri, O., Pryor, I., McGorry, P., & Alvarez-Jimenez, M. (2018). Web-based mindfulness interventions for mental health treatment: Systematic review and meta-analysis. *JMIR Mental Health*, *5*(3), e10278. http://dx.doi.org/10.2196/10278

Shalaby, R., Adu, M. K., El Gindi, H. M., & Agyapong, V. I. O. (2022). Text messages in the field of mental health: Rapid review of the reviews. *Frontiers in Psychiatry*, *13*, 921982. http://dx.doi.org/10.3389/fpsyt.2022.921982

Siegel, J. T., Flores-Medel, E., Martinez, D. A., & Berger, D. E. (2019). Can mental health anti-stigma messages have untoward effects on some people with depression?: An exploratory study. *Journal of Health Communication, 24*(11), 821–828. http://dx.doi.org/10.1080/10810730.2019.1672838

Siegel, J. T., Lienemann, B. A., & Tan, C. N. (2015). Influencing help-seeking among people with elevated depressive symptomatology: Mistargeting as a persuasive technique. *Clinical Psychological Science, 3*(2), 242–255. http://dx.doi.org/10.1177/2167702614542846

Snyder, L. B., & LaCroix, J. M. (2013). How effective are mediated health campaigns? A synthesis of meta-analyses. In R. E. Rice & C. K. Atkin (Eds.), *Public communication campaigns* (Vol. 4, pp. 113–129). Sage.

Sontag, J. M. (2018). Visual framing effects on emotion and mental health message effectiveness. *Journal of Communication in Healthcare, 11*(1), 30–47. http://dx.doi.org/10.1080/17538068.2018.1435017

Subramanian, R., & Santo, J. B. (2021). Reducing mental illness stigma: What types of images are most effective? *Journal of Visual Communication in Medicine, 44*(2), 52–61. http://dx.doi.org/10.1080/17453054.2021.1901561

Wakefield, M., Loken, B., & Hornik, R. C. (2010). Use of mass media campaigns to change health behaviour. *The Lancet, 376*(9748), 1261–1271. http://dx.doi.org/10.1016/S0140-6736(10)60809-4

Webb, T. L., & Sheeran, P. (2006). Does changing behavioral intentions engender behavior change? A meta-analysis of the experimental evidence. *Psychological Bulletin, 132*(2), 249–268. http://dx.doi.org/10.1037/0033-2909.132.2.249

Yzer, M., Kinzer, H., & Malone, M. (2022). A reasoned action approach to depression help-seeking messaging for college students: Implications of cognitive biases in depression. *Health Communication, 37*(14), 1731–1739. http://dx.doi.org/10.1080/10410236.2021.1917744

Yzer, M., LoRusso, S., & Nagler, R. H. (2015). On the conceptual ambiguity surrounding perceived message effectiveness. *Health Communication, 30*(2), 125–134. http://dx.doi.org/10.1080/10410236.2014.974131

9

The Conceptualization, Measurement, and Reduction of Self-Stigma of Seeking Help

David L. Vogel[1], Patrick J. Heath[2], Rachel E. Brenner[3], Daniel G. Lannin[4], and Nan Zhao[1]

[1] Iowa State University
[2] Gustavus Adolphus College
[3] Twilio
[4] Illinois State University

Mental health concerns affect 13% of the global population and will cost the world economy approximately $6 trillion by 2030—more than the projected costs of cancer, diabetes, and chronic respiratory disease combined (World Health Organization, 2022). These rates of mental health problems increased in recent years (Richter et al., 2019) and may have been exacerbated by the COVID-19 pandemic (Santomauro et al., 2021). Yet, according to the National Center for Health Statistics, less than 10% of those experiencing a diagnosable problem seek therapy each year (Terlizzi & Norris, 2021), and those who do seek help often wait years before doing so or drop out of treatment early (Wang et al., 2004). The most often cited psychological reason for why someone does not seek treatment is mental health stigma (Corrigan, 2004).

Self-stigma of seeking help is one type of mental health stigma that describes the reduction in self-worth an individual anticipates experiencing should they seek mental health treatment. This form of stigma has been found to be a primary deterrent in the decision to seek mental health services and continue treatment (Lannin et al., 2015). In fact, the self-stigma of seeking help is the strongest predictor of attitudes toward, and intent to, seek mental health services (see meta-analyses; Lannin & Bible, 2022; Yu et al., 2023) and has been related to lower rates of accessing online information about mental health and treatment (Lannin et al., 2016) and decreased use of services over a two-year period (Seidman et al., 2019b). Self-stigma of seeking help has also been linked with a weaker client–therapist working alliance (Owen et al., 2013) and decreased willingness to return for subsequent counseling sessions (Wade et al., 2011). Meta-analyses show that self-stigma is an important barrier for at least one-quarter to one-third of participants (Clement et al., 2015), while other forms of stigma (e.g., public stigma) are inconsistently linked with help seeking (Schnyder et al., 2017). Accordingly, there is a clear need to better understand the theoretical differentiation between self-stigma of seeking help and other types of stigma, as well as its role in help-seeking outcomes to inform the development of interventions designed to effectively reduce this type of stigma. To address this need, the subsequent chapter reviews the conceptualization of the self-stigma of seeking help and its measurement, reports on the current state of the science, and explores new research findings, promising interventions, and future directions.

The Handbook of Mental Health Communication, First Edition.
Edited by Marco C. Yzer and Jason T. Siegel.

Mental Health Stigma

Mental health stigma is a major obstacle to health and wellness (Mejia-Lancheros et al., 2021). Corrigan (1998, 2004) first asserted that two separate yet related types of mental health stigma affect the decision to seek treatment. The first, *public stigma*, is the perception held by others (i.e., by society) that an individual is socially unacceptable (Corrigan, 1998). The second, *self-stigma*, is the perception held by the individual that they are socially unacceptable (Corrigan, 1998). The existence of public stigma surrounding mental illness and the seeking of psychological services is clear. The public often describes people with a mental illness in negative terms (Angermeyer & Dietrich, 2006), and while there are some improvements in recent years, ongoing negative perceptions of mental health disorders persist, particularly for severe mental illness (Pescosolido et al., 2021). A systematic review found that people in the United States view those with mental illnesses as violent, dangerous, and incompetent—and these beliefs are tied to the desire to keep social distanced from individuals with mental illnesses (Parcesepe & Cabassa, 2013). Beyond having a disorder, the act of seeking mental health services is also stigmatized by the public. People who use mental health services are rated less favorably and treated more negatively than those who do not (Sibicky & Dovidio, 1986), with stereotyped labels such as unstable, needy, incompetent, and inadequate (Hammer & Vogel, 2017). This type of public stigma associated with seeking therapy is linked with more negative attitudes and intentions to seek treatment (Vogel et al., 2006, 2009) and decreased likelihood of having sought therapy for those with mental health concerns (Jennings et al., 2017).

Although much of the early mental health stigma research focused on the effects of public stigma of mental illness and seeking mental health treatment, over the last 20 years increased attention has been paid to the role of self-stigma, with over 1,400 references to self-stigma from 2000 to 2023 (retrieved from PsycINFO on June 1, 2023). Link et al. (1989) first applied *modified labeling theory* to discuss a process by which societal devaluation and discrimination toward the mentally ill could directly lead to negative consequences for a person's self-esteem if they are labeled—by themselves or others—as having a mental illness and that people may avoid treatment to try to avoid these consequences. Subsequently, Corrigan (1998, 2004) introduced the *social-cognitive model of stigma* and the term self-stigma to describe how negative external perceptions toward those with a mental illness (i.e., public stigma) can be internalized and seeing oneself as inferior, inadequate, or weak.

This theorized internalization of public stigma as self-stigma is one of the most studied stigma processes examined in the help-seeking literature with meta-analyses showing that public stigma shares a strong positive association with self-stigma (Yu et al., 2023), though the strength of the relationship may vary across demographic groups such as age, gender, and race/ethnicity (Mackenzie et al., 2019b) and across samples from many parts of the world (Vogel et al., 2017; Yu et al., 2021). While fewer studies have examined the links longitudinally, Chan et al. (2023) recently showed that experienced discrimination exacerbated self-stigma and in turn impeded recovery and well-being over two years. In turn, Vogel et al. (2013b) conducted a longitudinal cross-panel analysis showing that the internalization process of time 1 public stigma to time 2 self-stigma, demonstrated the best, most parsimonious fit to the data.

Accordingly, there is a need to continue to understand the role of self-stigma of seeking help. This chapter discusses the conceptualization of self-stigma and its role in the help-seeking process across diverse groups and then discusses self-stigma's measurement in more detail before discussing ways to reduce it.

Conceptualizing Self-Stigma of Seeking Help

Rooted in the prior theories (e.g., Corrigan, 1998; Link et al., 1989), Vogel et al. (2006, 2009) identified the potential impact of two distinct self-stigmas—one associated *with mental illness* and one associated with *seeking help*—that could uniquely influence help-seeking outcomes. Extending upon this work, Lannin et al. (2015) proposed the *internalized stigma model* (ISM; see Figure 9.1) to depict how the two self-stigmas might uniquely relate to self-esteem and help seeking. Specifically, ISM posits that both self-stigmas are uniquely linked to lower self-esteem because self-stigma operates by eliciting

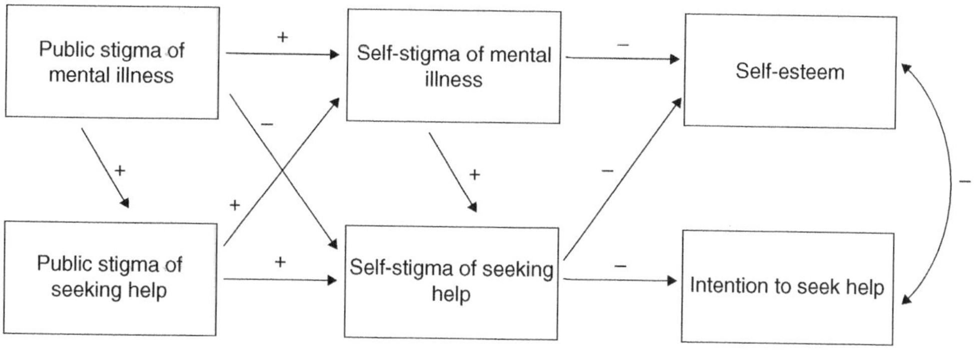

Figure 9.1 The internalized stigma model. Lannin et al. (2015)/with permission of American Psychological Association.

negative self-evaluations; however, the self-stigma of seeking help would show stronger relationships with intentions to seek help than the self-stigma of mental illness because the self-stigma of seeking help directly devalues seeking psychological services. Consistent with this, Brenner et al. (2019) and others (e.g., Tucker et al., 2013) have found that the self-stigma of seeking help was uniquely associated with lower intention to seek help and with an unwillingness to receive feedback on current levels of psychological distress.

As a result of the unique and potentially greater salience of the self-stigma of seeking help on treatment seeking, it has become a major area of research focus. Research has shown consistent a moderate to strong links between self-stigma of seeking help and negative attitudes toward and lower intentions to seek psychological help—see meta-analysis in Lannin and Bible (2022) and Yu et al. (2023). The self-stigma of seeking help has also shown a robust ability to mediate the relationships between public stigma of seeking help and clinically relevant outcome variables (e.g., self-esteem and intent to seek psychological help; Yu et al., 2023). This mediation model has also received cross-sectional support across the world (Vogel et al., 2017). Self-stigma of seeking help has also been associated with help-seeking–related behavior and can even interfere with the likelihood of accepting information about counseling when given the option (Lannin et al., 2016), and spending less time reading a brochure designed to decrease self-stigma (Cornish et al., 2019). Self-stigma of seeking help has predicted a lower likelihood of electing to receive results from a mental health screening measure (Brenner et al., 2019). Furthermore, while direct longitudinal examination of self-stigma to behavioral outcomes is limited, a recent meta-analysis by Lannin and Bible (2022) found a moderate negative relationship between self-stigma and help-seeking behaviors (at two months and two years later).

Even after seeking therapy, self-stigma associated with seeking help can impact the clinical process and willingness to continue treatment. For example, self-stigma of seeking help was associated with lower perceived benefits and greater perceived risk of disclosing to a counselor as assessed prior to an intake session (Seidman et al., 2019a). In turn, three studies have directly examined the relationship between the self-stigma of seeking therapy and the working alliance. First, Wade et al. (2011) found that self-stigma of seeking therapy predicted intentions and interest in continuing group therapy. Second, Owen et al. (2013) found that higher self-stigma of seeking therapy was associated with lower ratings of the working alliance and indirectly affected session outcomes through the working alliance. Third, Seidman et al. (2022) found that self-stigma negatively impacted the working alliance and its effects became more pronounced as symptoms of distress increased, a state in which clients are simultaneously most likely to need help yet least likely to feel allied with their therapist.

Self-Stigma of Seeking Help and Sociocultural Diversity

Of particular concern is that some groups seek psychological help even less frequently than others. For example, researchers have found that Asian Americans, African Americans, and Latino Americans are all less receptive to psychological help than European Americans (Sun et al., 2016; Whaley & Dubose, 2018). Similarly, older men also seek professional help at lower rates than younger men

(Crabb & Hunsley, 2006). However, only limited research has focused on sociocultural diversity factors and the role they play in the stigma associated with seeking help. Therefore, this section reviews the work that has been done across gender, race/ethnicity, age, global/region, and the role of intersectional identities.

Gender

The most researched factor in relation to group status is gender, with a particular focus on understanding why men seek help less than women. It has been argued that self-stigma of seeking help may be particularly salient for men because the emphasis of the traditional male gender role on being independent and in control may lead men to believe that needing therapy means they are a failure (Addis & Mahalik, 2003). Consistent with this, men have been found to experience greater self-stigma than women (Sigal & Plunkett, 2023; Vogel et al., 2006). The link between self-stigma and having an undiagnosed disorder is also higher for men than women (Griffiths et al., 2015). Subsequently, studies have shown that traditional masculine gender role norms are linked to attitudes and intentions to seek help via self-stigma (Levant et al., 2013). Heath et al. (2017b) also found that there was an interaction between the traditional masculine norm of restrictive emotionality (i.e., proscribed norm to be stoic and in control of one's emotions) such that when distress symptoms are severe enough masculine gender role factors might be less important in predicting stigma but that when the symptoms are less clear self-stigma might be likely influenced by masculine norm.

Most of this research has focused on cisgender men and largely ignored the transgender/gender nonconforming community. This is an important omission, as transgender individuals are at great risk for mental health issues and suicidal thoughts and attempts (Avery et al., 2001), related to experiencing greater minority stress (Mori et al., 2020), and also potential hesitations to seek help from fear of being stigmatized by the therapist for their gender identity (Calton et al., 2016). As a result, there is an imperative to include transgender people and their experiences related to self-stigma in future research to better understand the clinical implications and develop effective treatments and to eradicate the erasure of trans men from men and masculinity research.

Race/Ethnicity

Most of this work on self-stigma has examined samples that were predominantly White. Recently, efforts have expanded this work, with the largest number of these studies supporting similar links between self-stigma and attitudes and intentions to seek services across different US racial/ethnic groups (De Luna & Kawabata, 2020; Freitas-Murrell & Swift, 2015; Shannon et al., 2022; Soheilian & Inman, 2009). However, some differences have been noted. For example, Asian students were found to have greater self-stigma than other racial/ethnic students (Cheng et al., 2013; Sigal & Plunkett, 2023). The link between self-stigma and help-seeking decisions has also been found to be the strongest for Asian individuals (Phillips et al., 2022; Saykeo & Lawrence, 2018). One possible reason is individuals who adhere to Asian cultural values might perceive emotional self-disclosure to authority figures (i.e., mental health professionals) as less comfortable than individuals who adhere to Western cultural values that value more emotional suppression and self-control (Kim & Zane, 2016).

In turn, results tend to show that self-stigma is the least predictive of attitudes and intentions to seek services for African Americans (Saykeo & Lawrence, 2018). Lannin et al. (2020) found that Black students reported lower self-stigma and clicked on the link to receive online mental health information at a higher rate than White students. One proposed explanation is based on a positive racial/ethnic identity being associated with less self-stigma for Black individuals but not for other racial/ethnic groups (Cheng et al., 2013). Overall, future work is needed to further examine the potential benefits of racial/ethnic identity and other cultural identity factors in protecting against the effects of self-stigma. Specifically, work is needed to examine culturally relevant factors (e.g., racial-ethnic identity, enculturation, loss of face) as moderators (De Luna & Kawabata, 2020; Ma et al., 2021).

Age

Studies directly examining age differences have found that self-stigma may explain why older adults and younger individuals are less likely to seek mental health services than middle-aged adults (Murphy & Mackenzie, 2023). For example, a study examining adolescents found that self-stigma was negatively related to attitudes and intent to seek help (Shechtman et al., 2018). Another study with middle school students also found that self-stigma was linked to willingness to seek help (Chen et al., 2014). Interestingly, Mackenzie et al. (2019a) did not find that older individuals had more total self-stigma, but that age moderates the links between self-stigma and help seeking, with older individuals being the most sensitive to the effects of self-stigma. As such, it may be possible that different age cohorts are exposed to different external influences—such as social norms, social scripts, and social models—that affect the internalization and expression of public stigma.

Global/Region

While much of the research on self-stigma has occurred in the United States, there is a growing body of work from around the world (Koutra et al., 2023; Shechtman et al., 2018; Topkaya et al., 2017; Vogel et al., 2017). Studies have also been done with international individuals residing in other countries (e.g., Lee et al., 2014; Ma et al., 2021). Studies tend to show universal importance of self-stigma around the world (Tomczyk et al., 2020). Interestingly, samples from Asian countries tend to show higher mean levels of self-stigma compared with US samples (Yamawaki & Green, 2020). However, North American and European countries tend to exhibit stronger links between self-stigma and outcomes compared with many other countries (Lannin & Bible, 2022; Vogel et al., 2013a). These variations may be the result of country-specific factors that affect individuals' sense of self. For example, the extant research has largely examined the impact of self-stigma from an individualistic approach ("I will be perceived as crazy") rather than from a collectivistic perspective ("my family will be viewed negatively"). Given the importance of collectivist values in many parts of the world, concerns about how seeking help would affect the family/significant others could be uniquely salient in decisions to seek treatment (Topkaya et al., 2017). As such, future work could directly examine the relevant contributions of a collectivistic self-stigma within countries with varying levels of independent and collectivistic values to further enhance our understanding.

Intersectionality

Though minoritized groups may be at greater risk of mental health concerns due to experiencing stigmatization and discrimination (Meyer, 2003), these effects may be enhanced for those who have multiple stigmatized identities (Vidales, 2022). As such, it may be beneficial to examine self-stigma from the lens of intersectionality—which reflects the manner in which multiple social systems and/or individual identities such as gender, race, ethnicity, and age may intersect to produce and sustain complex inequalities (Crenshaw, 1989).Holding multiple minoritized identities while experiencing a mental health issue can lead to a double stigma that further exacerbates difficulties associated with seeking mental health services (Gary, 2005). Research aimed at understanding how intersecting identities influence the experience and consequences of self-stigma is still in its nascent stages (Oexle & Corrigan, 2018).

One salient example involves the intersection of race and gender. Previous work, as noted already, has linked gender with self-stigma of seeking help, such that men experience the effects of self-stigma to a greater degree and are less likely to admit mental health needs than women (Heath et al., 2017a). This finding points to differences in societal gendered expectations, where traditional masculine norms maintain that admitting to a mental health need is a weakness (Berger et al., 2013). However, this research has largely assumed that all men experience masculinity in similar ways. This is not the case. Coleman-Kirumba et al. (2023) note that Black men's experience of masculinity intersects across their identities because Black men develop their sense of masculinity within larger sociopolitical environments that devalue them (Wade & Rochlen, 2013). As a result, Black men experience aspects of their masculine identity, not just as part of their overall sense of being a man (e.g., having certain responsibilities) but also in terms of their sense of being a Black man (e.g., having certain experiences with racism and discrimination; Coleman-Kirumba et al., 2023). Consistent with this notion, Coleman-Kirumba et al. (2023) found that Black men's endorsement of traditional, Black, and intersecting notions of masculinity all independently predicted public stigma, which then predicted self-stigma.

Other identities may also intersect. For example, Vogel et al. (2011) also found that the link between masculinity and stigma present only for straight men, with no significant relationship between masculinity and attitudes among gay men. Moreover, Lytle et al. (2018) found that gay men were less likely to seek help than lesbians and bisexual men. However, more research is needed on self-stigma within the context of other intersectional identities. The majority of research in this area has focused on intersecting identities for men. This is an important limitation as research has found a link between the experience of intersectional discrimination by sexually diverse women of color and higher levels of self-stigma of seeking help (Cerezo & O'Shaughnessy, 2021). Vidales (2022) also discusses how "lesbian, gay, bisexual, transgender, and queer (LGBTQ+) populations are unique in that they historically have been stigmatized both by the psychology profession (e.g., having one's identity being pathologized by the American Psychiatric Association), as well as the larger society" (p. 241). They also note that work in this area needs to expand beyond monosexuality (i.e., focusing on gay men and lesbian women) to include asexual individuals and bisexual individuals. Similarly, as previously noted, the transgender/gender nonconforming community has been largely ignored by mental health researchers and often included only as an extension of sexuality research leading to limited knowledge of their experiences of stigma. Yet transgender people of color are at the greatest risk of being the subject of anti-LGBTQ+ stigma and discrimination (Whitfield et al., 2014). As such, there is great need for additional awareness of transgender issues around self-stigma. Overall, it may be important to consider the identities and ecological systems in which a person is embedded to better understand their experience of stigma. Each system may influence the individual directly as well as indirectly through other systems. The overall impact of intersectional identities may have complex relations with self-stigma, and future quantitative and qualitative research is needed to better understand these complexities.

Measuring Self-Stigma of Seeking Help

To allow for the exploration of the self-stigma of seeking help, Vogel et al. (2006) developed the Self-Stigma of Seeking Help Scale (SSOSH). Based on Corrigan's (2004) discussion of self-stigma, the SSOSH assesses concerns about the loss in self-esteem a person would feel if they decided to seek help from a psychologist or other mental health professional. The SSOSH has been cited over 1,700 times (Google Scholar, July 2023) and has been administered in countries worldwide (Vogel et al., 2013a, 2017). Respondents rate 10 items such as, "I would feel inadequate if I went to a therapist for help" (Vogel et al., 2006, p. 328) on a 5-point Likert-type scale ranging from 1 = *strongly disagree* to 5 = *strongly agree* (see Table 9.1 for full scale items). Five items are reverse-scored so that higher scores correspond to higher self-stigma.

The SSOSH scores typically reflect a unidimensional construct in US samples. Exploratory factor analyses among college students (Vogel et al., 2006) and community adults (Brenner et al., 2021) and confirmatory factor analyses among college students (Vogel et al., 2006) support a one-factor structure. In addition, SSOSH scores have demonstrated a univariate construct with internal consistency among community ($\alpha = 0.92$) samples and college ($\alpha = 0.90$) samples (Tucker et al., 2013), as well as two-month test–retest reliability (0.72) among college students (Vogel et al., 2006). A meta-analytic estimate of Cronbach's alpha ($k = 129$) for the SOSSH found high internal consistency ($\alpha = 0.84$, 95% CI = [0.83, 0.85]; Lannin & Bible, 2022). The Hedge's Q test also indicated that internal consistency is likely heterogeneous across samples and that variations reflected actual differences in population parameters across studies.

Cross-culturally, the SSOSH is also supported as a unidimensional construct, with minor exceptions consistent with the challenges among translated measures (Wong et al., 2003). Vogel et al. (2013a, 2017)

Table 9.1 Items from the SSOSH-10

SSOSH-10
1. I would feel inadequate if I went to a therapist for psychological help
2. My self-confidence would NOT be threatened if I sought professional help
3. Seeking psychological help would make me feel less intelligent
4. My self-esteem would increase if I talked to a therapist
5. My view of myself would not change just because I made the choice to see a therapist
6. It would make me feel inferior to ask a therapist for help
7. I would feel okay about myself if I made the choice to seek professional help
8. If I went to a therapist, I would be less satisfied with myself
9. My self-confidence would remain the same if I sought professional help for a problem I could not solve
10. I would feel worse about myself if I could not solve my own problems

Participants are presented with, "Directions: People at times find that they face problems that they consider seeking help for. This can bring up reactions about what seeking help would mean. Please use the 5-point scale to rate the degree to which each item describes how you might react in this situation."
Participants rate items on the following scale: 1 = *strongly disagree*; 2 = *disagree*; 3 = *agree/disagree equally*; 4 = *agree*; 5 = *strongly agree*.
Note. Vogel et al. (2006).

found psychometric support for the original 10-item single-factor SSOSH across countries. For example, Vogel et al. (2013a) used a confirmatory factor analysis framework to conduct measurement invariance analysis and latent mean comparisons of the SSOSH across six countries: England, Greece, Israel, Taiwan, Turkey, and the United States. Results suggested that the SSOSH has a similar univariate structure across countries and is sufficiently invariant across countries to be used to explore cultural differences in the way that self-stigma relates to help-seeking behavior. Any differences tended to comprise reverse-coded items that seemed to have more difficulty in the translation process. This aligns with previous literature that detailing problems in obtaining cross-cultural measurement equivalence with reverse-worded items (Wong et al., 2003).

Consistent with this, the single-factor model garnered full support in samples from Columbia (Larrahondo et al., 2021), Greece (Efstathiou et al., 2019), and Germany (Apolinário-Hagen et al., 2016; Zhou et al., 2019). However, some studies in Turkey (Kaya et al., 2015; Sezer & Kezer, 2013; Topkaya, 2021) suggested a two-factor model, and one study with Chinese samples Zhou et al., 2019) did not find a good fit to the one-factor model. In each of the studies, the reverse-coded items tended to be the reason for lower fit or comprised a large part of the second factor. To examine this lower fit, Vogel et al. (2017) in a study examining the SSOSH across 10 countries removed the five reverse-worded items for the SSOSH and reexamined the measurement invariance. The remaining five items of the self-stigma yielded good overall model fit. The five items on each scale loaded significantly in each country and region. Furthermore, for each scale, the ΔCFI between the multiple group models where item loadings were allowed to freely estimate and the model where the item loadings were fixed were both within the proposed cutoff of <0.01. Therefore, they used the five-items versions of the measures in their analyzes. This is consistent with research in US samples finding that three reverse-scored items provided the least information and that reverse-scored items can be removed without meaningfully affecting the validity of the SSOSH (Brenner et al., 2021). As such, researchers should consider examining the factor structure of the SSOSH in their sample to decide whether the full or a briefer version better fits their data.

Briefer versions of the SSOSH have shown some validity. Brenner et al. (2021) used item response theory (IRT) to develop a screener (SSOSH-3) and brief versions (SSOSH-7) of the SSOSH. Results supported removal of three reverse-scored items to create the SSOSH-7, as they provided the least amount of information among community adults and college students in the United States. The SSOSH-3 consisted of the three most useful items and did not include any reverse-scored items. The SSOSH-7 and SSOSH-3 were both highly correlated with the original 10-item SSOSH and demonstrated significant correlations with help-seeking constructs and in similar magnitude to the original SSOSH.

Importantly, more work on the validity of the SSOSH across diverse samples is needed. Few studies have examined the measurement invariance of the SSOSH across diverse groups within countries. As one exception, Vidales et al. (2022) recently examined the measurement invariance and latent mean differences of the three versions of the SSOSH (10, 7, and 3 items) across demographic profiles of men. Results revealed strong invariance for the three scales across all demographic groups based on their race/ethnic group, sexuality, and age cohort. This suggests that a range of groups of men understand the scale in the same way, and thus the scale can be used to compare their scores.

Despite evidence that self-stigma of seeking psychological help is a construct that can be assessed across numerous cultures, measurement is not without its challenges. Cultural factors and individual differences may influence the way that people interpret the construct and complete scale items. Comparing self-stigma across cultures may require adaptation of the measurement and may also need to account for intervening variables that influence the nature of the construct. For example, self-stigma may be a more proximal variable for individuals in cultures that value individualism, but less salient for individuals in cultures that value collectivism. Indeed, the way that self-stigma is understood and measured not only affects the way that it is assessed but also has implications for the nature of the interventions that might be effective in mitigating its effects.

Interventions

A growing body of research has taken on the challenge of reducing stigma, though most interventions focus on reducing the self-stigma of *mental illness* rather than *seeking help*. Given the impact of the self-stigma of seeking help on people's decisions to seek out treatment, interventions to mitigate this stigma are needed. However, effective interventions are difficult to design and implement given that they need to reach an audience that is, almost by definition, avoidant of psychological intervention in the first place. Despite this, researchers examining help-seeking self-stigma interventions have identified several promising avenues: (a) providing psychoeducation and normative messaging; (b) building resilience against self-stigmatizing beliefs; and (c) decreasing avoidance of perceived self-stigma.

Psychoeducation and Normative Messaging

Most interventions designed to mitigate help-seeking self-stigma have focused on reducing stigmatized beliefs through psychoeducation and messages designed to normalize the process of seeking help. For example, Cornish et al. (2019) developed an intervention targeting military personnel that used an educational brochure and video to reframe help seeking as a courageous act. Results of the study indicated that the intervention led to a larger decrease in self-stigma relative to a control group (Cornish et al., 2019). In another study, Hammer and Vogel (2010) asked men to read a brochure about how men experience depression and the benefits of seeking psychological help and found that, compared with a control group, men reported lower levels of help-seeking self-stigma. Stanley et al. (2018) also attempted to directly change stigmatized beliefs through providing feedback about the accuracy of self-stigmatizing statements believed to be true or false by participants. This intervention yielded a reduction in self-stigma levels but did not significantly differ from a control group that was given psychoeducational information. Future efforts might also use established health education techniques including (a) providing an explanation for the symptoms a person is experiencing (Schreiber & Hartrick, 2002); (b) providing information that problems are not their fault and are reversible (Rosen et al., 2000), and (c) showing that symptoms improve through treatment (Mann & Himelein, 2004).

Interventions prioritizing direct (or indirect) contact with those who have previously sought help may also be effective in reducing stigma through normalizing the behavior. For example, in the Cornish et al. (2019) study, the intervention included testimonials from former service personnel who had previously sought therapy. Recently, Keum and Ogrodniczuk (2023) also had participants watch a video of a man who had sought help. Importantly, the video appeared to disrupt the link between self-stigma and help-seeking attitudes. Gronholm and Thornicroft (2022) noted that these types of help-seeking self-disclosures from celebrities may further reduce self-stigma as it normalizes the behavior from someone many can connect to. There is evidence that social media influencers are starting to talk about mental health more often; however, only a small percentage of posts appear to directly address specific mental health difficulties (Pretorius et al., 2022), and further research is needed to understand the best messenger and formats to deliver these types of messages.

Building Resilience

Other research has begun to examine ways to build resilience against negative self-stigmatizing beliefs so that they do not result in negative outcomes. One area that has shown some potential is self-compassion (Heath, 2022). Self-compassion is a nonjudgmental and accepting approach toward the self in which an individual treats themselves with kindness and care in the face of challenges or perceived inadequacies (Neff, 2003). Self-compassion has been connected to a reduced likelihood of experiencing shame (Johnson & O'Brien, 2013). Several cross-sectional studies have found that higher self-compassion helps to mitigate (reduce) the internalization of help-seeking stigma (Heath et al., 2018), particularly for men (Booth et al., 2019; Heath et al., 2017a). However, more research is needed to examine these effects experimentally.

Decreasing Avoidance

Researchers have noted that interventions designed to directly combat self-stigmatizing beliefs often show mixed results due to possible rebound effects where the very act of thinking about seeking help elicits the very fears (self-stigma) that the intervention was trying to diminish (Cornish et al., 2019). For example, distressed students instructed to view a psychoeducational brochure and contemplate personal reasons to seek therapy (or not) reported higher self-stigma and were less willing to receive personalized results from a distress screening tool than their noncontemplative peers (Lannin et al., 2019). Similarly, higher initial self-stigma of seeking help can lead to spending less time reading a brochure designed to decrease self-stigma (Cornish et al., 2019). As such, interventions designed to reach those who are avoidant of psychological intervention may need to be able to reduce this initial unwillingness for individuals to even engage with the intervention. Self-affirmation, or reflecting on aspects of the self that are viewed positively, appears to be one approach that could help mitigate this (Lannin et al., 2022; Seidman, 2022). Specifically, self-affirmations can increase sources of self-worth, which increases ones' resistance to threatening information to other aspects of the self (Sherman, 2013). Consistent with this, Lannin et al. (2013) found that participants in a self-affirmed intervention, compared with a control intervention, reported lower levels of self-stigma associated with seeking help. Subsequently, Lannin et al. (2017) found that participants who engaged in self-affirmation task reported less of a threat response to mental health information and improved beliefs about seeking help relative to a no-affirmation control group (Lannin et al., 2017). Future work is needed to further understand how self-affirmation tasks can be embedded in other self-stigma reduction interventions to enhance their effects for those most likely to not engage with the intervention (i.e., have stronger initial self-stigma).

Implications

Building on the aforementioned work, it is important to develop and test interventions that are practical and scalable. Because many help avoiders may not be in contact with providers, it may be useful for efforts to occur in nontraditional environments such as physicians' offices or nonclinical environments. Medical practitioners, for example, are an important referral source as most clients seek help for psychological distress from their primary care physician first rather than a psychologist (Druss et al., 2008). Unsurprisingly, medical intake forms increasingly include mental health screens for depression or anxiety (Mitchell, 2019), and now with the development of the three-item SSOSH-3

(Brenner et al., 2021) it could also be possible to include an ultra-brief assessment of self-stigma, which would allow medical practitioners to make referrals easier for mental health services. This could also lead to basic trainings with medical providers regarding how to discuss seeking help with distressed patients with high self-stigma.

Overall Critique

Although the extant literature indicates that self-stigma is a robust barrier to seeking psychological help, the research is not without limitations. Importantly, there is a need for future research to continue to examine the effects of self-stigma in global populations as well as in subpopulations that are not WEIRD (i.e., Western, educated, industrialized, rich, and democratic). Furthermore, people of color (Maura & de Mamani, 2017), sexual minorities, transgender and gender nonconforming individuals (Borgogna et al., 2019), and people from other marginalized communities experience mental health disparities. As such, a more comprehensive understanding of self-stigma of seeking help within these communities is needed. Of particular importance is the need to examine intersecting identities and how these influence experiences and consequences of self-stigma (Oexle & Corrigan, 2018). Culturally relevant factors (e.g., racial/ethnic identity, enculturation, loss of face) are often salient moderators of mental health outcomes (De Luna & Kawabata, 2020; Ma et al., 2021), suggesting this may also be an important area for future research.

Another key limitation of the literature is that most studies have utilized self-reported attitudes and intentions to seek help as proxies for help-seeking behavior. One way to address this would be through studies that examine help-seeking behavior over time (see Fox et al., 2018; Seidman et al., 2019b). With the development of shorter self-stigma measures, there is an increased ability to conduct this work in applied settings, as it removes some of the limited time and patient fatigue barriers (Brenner et al., 2021). If longitudinal examination is not possible, researchers and clinicians should consider other help-seeking–related behaviors, for example, decisions to seek information about counseling by clicking on a link (Lannin et al., 2016), time spent reading a treatment brochure (Cornish et al., 2019), or willingness to receive results from a mental health screening measure (Brenner et al., 2019).

The literature has also almost exclusively utilized self-reported assessments of self-stigma (for exceptions see Freitag et al., 2019; Rüsch et al., 2010). Although an individual is often the best expert regarding their experiences of self-stigma, this may not always be the case. Some experiences of self-stigma may be outside of conscious awareness. There is evidence that both explicit and implicit self-stigma may independently predict variance in mental health–related outcome variables (Rüsch et al., 2010), but to date no studies have examined the effects of implicit self-stigma on decisions to seek help.

As noted already, an important direction in self-stigma research is understanding the impact of self-stigma on the therapy process itself. The effects of self-stigma may be present not only when people are contemplating the possibility of seeking help but also when they are receiving it. Specifically, self-stigma inhibits comfort in self-disclosing to a counselor (Seidman et al., 2019a), is related to the development of a working alliance (Seidman et al., 2023), deters treatment adherence, and contributes to early therapy dropout (Wade et al., 2011). These effects may be most noticeable for clients experiencing heightened psychological distress (Seidman et al., 2022), leading to a period in which clients are simultaneously most likely to need help yet least likely to feel allied with their therapist. As such, research is needed to better understand the complex ways that distress and stigma may interact to predict help-seeking outcomes. It may also be important for therapists to consider fluctuations in self-stigma and distress when developing and maintaining the working alliance.

Conclusion

People often experience heightened self-stigma—feeling shame because they believe that negative labels and stereotypes apply to them—associated with seeking help for mental health concerns. Self-stigma presents a two-pronged challenge that impedes recovery. First, self-stigma of seeking help harms peoples' self-esteem, which means that people feel demoralized and worthless for needing help. Second, people often want to avoid mental health services to forestall having negative labels associated with and applied to their identity. As such, the extant scientific literature provides strong evidence that self-stigma of seeking help is a serious barrier to attaining and maintaining optimal mental health and well-being. A number of factors moderate the antecedents and consequences of self-stigma, and research is ongoing to examine the nuances between cultures, groups, and individuals. Theory-based intervention development and testing are burgeoning, and there is reason to be hopeful. However, much more work is needed, and future research is urged to continue these efforts—especially for groups that have been marginalized, hold multiple marginalized identities, and continue to experience inequitable access to mental health treatment.

References

Addis, M. E., & Mahalik, J. R. (2003). Men, masculinity, and the contexts of help seeking. *American Psychologist, 58*, 5–14. https://doi.org/10.1037/0003-066X.58.1.5

Angermeyer, M. C., & Dietrich, S. (2006). Public beliefs about and attitudes towards people with mental illness: A review of population studies. *Acta Psychiatrica Scandinavica, 113*, 163–179. https://doi.org/10.1111/j.1600-0447.2005.00699.x

Apolinário-Hagen, J., Trachsel, D. A., Anhorn, A., Holsten, B., Werner, V., & Krebs, S. (2016). Exploring individual differences in online and face-to-face help-seeking intentions in case of impending mental health problems: The role of adult attachment, perceived social support, psychological distress and self-stigma. *Journal of Health and Social Sciences, 1*, 223–240. https://doi.org/10.19204/2016/xplr24

Avery, A. M., Hellman, R. E., & Sudderth, L. K. (2001). Satisfaction with mental health services among sexual minorities with major mental illness. *American Journal of Public Health, 91*, 990–991. https://doi.org/10.2105/ajph.91.6.990

Berger, J. L., Addis, M. E., Green, J. D., Mackowiak, C., & Goldberg, V. (2013). Men's reactions to mental health labels, forms of help-seeking, and sources of help-seeking advice. *Psychology of Men & Masculinity, 14*, 433–443. https://doi.org/10.1037/a0030175

Booth, N. R., McDermott, R. C., Cheng, H. L., & Borgogna, N. C. (2019). Masculine gender role stress and self-stigma of seeking help: The moderating roles of self-compassion and self-coldness. *Journal of Counseling Psychology, 66*, 755–762. https://doi.org/10.1037/cou0000350

Borgogna, N. C., McDermott, R. C., Aita, S. L., & Kridel, M. M. (2019). Anxiety and depression across gender and sexual minorities: Implications for transgender, gender nonconforming, pansexual, demisexual, asexual, queer, and questioning individuals. *Psychology of Sexual Orientation and Gender Diversity, 6*, 54–63. https://doi.org/10.1037/sgd0000306

Brenner, R. E., Colvin, K. F., Hammer, J. H., & Vogel, D. L. (2021). Using item response theory to develop revised (SSOSH-7) and ultra-brief (SSOSH-3) self-stigma of seeking help scales. *Assessment, 28*, 1488–1499. https://doi.org/10.1177/1073191120958496

Brenner, R.E., Hammer, J. H., Vogel, D. L., Bitman-Heinrichs, R. L., Heath, P. J., & Wade, N. G. (2019, August). *Extending the theoretical understanding of mental illness and help-seeking self-stigmas*. American Psychological Association, Chicago, IL.

Calton, J. M., Cattaneo, L. B., & Gebhard, K. T. (2016). Barriers to help seeking for lesbian, gay, bisexual, transgender, and queer survivors of intimate partner violence. *Trauma, Violence & Abuse, 17*(5), 585–600. https://doi.org/10.1177/1524838015585318

Cerezo, A., & O'Shaughnessy, T. (2021). Psychological distress, alcohol misuse and stigma to seek psychological help in a community sample of sexual diverse women of color. *Journal of LGBTQ Issues in Counseling, 15*, 59–76. https://doi.org/10.1080/15538605.2021.1868374

Chan, K. K. S., Tsui, J. K. C., & Tang, A. T. Y. (2023). Longitudinal impact of self-compassion and psychological flexibility on mental illness recovery: The mediating roles of self-stigma and mental health service engagement. *Mindfulness, 14*, 1125–1134. https://doi.org/10.1007/s12671-023-02127-2

Chen, H., Fang, X., Liu, C., Hu, W., Lan, J., & Deng, L. (2014). Associations among the number of mental health problems, stigma, and seeking help from psychological services: A path analysis model among Chinese adolescents. *Children and Youth Services Review, 44*, 356–362. https://doi.org/10.1016/j.childyouth.2014.07.003

Cheng, H.-L., Kwan, K.-L. K., & Sevig, T. (2013). Racial and ethnic minority college students' stigma associated with seeking psychological help: Examining psychocultural correlates. *Journal of Counseling Psychology, 60*, 98–111. https://doi.org/10.1037/a0031169

Clement, S., Schauman, O., Graham, T., Maggioni, F., Evans-Lacko, S., Bezborodovs, N., Morgan, C., Rüsch, N., Brown, J. S. L., & Thornicroft, G. (2015). What is the impact of mental health-related stigma on help-seeking?

A systematic review of quantitative and qualitative studies. *Psychological Medicine*, *45*, 11–27. https://doi.org/10.1017/S0033291714000129

Coleman-Kirumba, L. M., Cornish, M. A., Horton, A. J., & Alvarez, J. C. (2023). Experiences of black men: Forms of masculinity and effects on psychological help-seeking variables. *Journal of Black Psychology*, *49*, 32–57. https://doi.org/10.1177/00957984221098122

Cornish, M., Brenner, R., Vogel, D., & Wade, N. (2019). Evaluation of an online help seeking stigma-reduction intervention for military personnel. *Stigma and Health*, *4*, 480–486. https://doi.org/10.1037/sah0000167

Corrigan, P. W. (1998). The impact of stigma on severe mental illness. *Cognitive and Behavioral Practice*, *5*, 201–222. https://doi.org/10.1016/S1077-7229(98)80006-0

Corrigan, P. W. (2004). How stigma interferes with mental health care. *American Psychologist*, *59*, 614–625. https://doi.org/10.1037/0003-066X.59.7.614

Crabb, R., & Hunsley, J. (2006). Utilization of mental health care services among older adults with depression. *Journal of Clinical Psychology*, *62*, 299–312. https://doi.org/10.1002/jclp.20231

Crenshaw, K. (1989). Demarginalizing the intersection of race and sex: A black feminist critique of antidiscrimination doctrine, feminist theory and antiracist politics. *University of Chicago Legal Forum*, *140*, 139–167. https://doi.org/10.3917/drs1.108.0465

De Luna, M. J. F., & Kawabata, Y. (2020). The role of enculturation on the help-seeking attitudes among Filipino Americans in Guam. *International Perspectives in Psychology*, *9*, 84–95. https://doi.org/10.1037/ipp0000127

Druss, B. G., Marcus, S. C., Campbell, J., Cuffel, B., Harnett, J., Ingoglia, C., & Mauer, B. (2008). Medical services for clients in community mental health centers: Results from a national survey. *Psychiatric Services*, *59*, 917–920. https://doi.org/10.1176/appi.ps.59.8.917

Efstathiou, G., Kouvaraki, E., Ploubidis, G., & Kalantzi-Azizi, A. (2019). Self-stigma, public-stigma and attitudes towards professional psychological help: Psychometric properties of the Greek version of three relevant questionnaires. *International Journal for the Advancement of Counselling*, *41*, 175–186. https://doi.org/10.1007/s10447-018-9364-9

Fox, A. B., Smith, B. N., & Vogt, D. (2018). How and when does mental illness stigma impact treatment seeking? Longitudinal examination of relationships between anticipated and internalized stigma, symptom severity, and mental health service use. *Psychiatry Research*, *268*, 15–20. https://doi.org/10.1016/j.psychres.2018.06.036

Freitag, S., Stolzenburg, S., Schomerus, G., & Schmidt, S. (2019). Brief implicit association tests of stigmatizing attitudes, awareness of mental distress and label-avoidance: A study in people with depressive symptoms. *Community Mental Health Journal*, *55*, 507–518. https://doi.org/10.1007/s10597-019-00372-1

Freitas-Murrell, B., & Swift, J. K. (2015). Predicting attitudes toward seeking professional psychological help among Alaska natives. *American Indian and Alaska Native Mental Health Research*, *22*, 21–35. https://doi.org/10.5820/aian.2203.2015.21

Gary, F. A. (2005). Stigma: Barrier to mental health care among ethnic minorities. *Issues in Mental Health Nursing*, *26*, 979–999. https://doi.org/10.1080/01612840500280638

Griffiths, S., Mond, J. M., Li, Z., Gunatilake, S., Murray, S. B., Sheffield, J., & Touyz, S. (2015). Self-stigma of seeking treatment and being male predict an increased likelihood of having an undiagnosed eating disorder. *The International Journal of Eating Disorders*, *48*(6), 775–778. https://doi.org/10.1002/eat.22413

Gronholm, P. C., & Thornicroft, G. (2022). Impact of celebrity disclosure on mental health-related stigma. *Epidemiology and Psychiatric Sciences*, *31*, e62. https://doi.org/10.1017/S2045796022000488

Hammer, J. H., & Vogel, D. L. (2010). Men's help seeking for depression: The efficacy of a male-sensitive brochure about counseling. *The Counseling Psychologist*, *38*, 296–313. https://doi.org/10.1177/0011000009351937

Hammer, J. H., & Vogel, D. L. (2017). Development of the help-seeker stereotype scale. *Stigma and Health*, *2*, 121–136. https://doi.org/10.1037/sah0000048

Heath, P. J. (2022). Mindfulness and self-compassion interventions for stigma. In D. L. Vogel & N. G. Wade (Eds.), *The Cambridge handbook of stigma and mental health* (pp. 449–465). Cambridge University Press. https://doi.org/10.1017/9781108920995.026

Heath, P. J., Brenner, R. E., Lannin, D. G., & Vogel, D. L. (2018). Self-compassion moderates the relationship of public and anticipated self-stigma of seeking help. *Stigma and Health*, *3*, 65–68. https://doi.org/10.1037/sah0000072

Heath, P. J., Brenner, R. E., Vogel, D. L., Lannin, D. G., & Strass, H. A. (2017a). Masculinity and barriers to seeking counseling: The buffering role of self-compassion. *Journal of Counseling Psychology*, *64*, 94–103. https://doi.org/10.1037/cou0000185

Heath, P. J., Seidman, A. J., Vogel, D. L., Cornish, M. A., & Wade, N. G. (2017b). Help-seeking stigma among men in the military: The interaction of restrictive emotionality and distress. *Psychology of Men & Masculinity*, *18*, 193–197. https://doi.org/10.1037/men0000111

Jennings, K., Goguen, K., Britt, T. W., Jeffirs, S., Wilkes, J. R., III, Brady, A., Pittman, R., & DiMuzio, D. (2017). The role of personality traits and barriers to mental health treatment seeking among college students. *Psychological Services*, *14*, 513–523. https://doi.org/10.1037/ser0000157

Johnson, E. A., & O'Brien, K. A. (2013). Self-compassion soothes the savage ego-threat system: Effects on negative affect, shame, rumination, and depressive symptoms. *Journal of Social and Clinical Psychology*, *32*, 939–963. https://doi.org/10.1521/jscp.2013.32.9.939

Kaya, C., Tansey, T., Chan, F., Bezyak, J., Melekoğlu, M. A., Çakıroğlu, O., & Köse, S. (2015). Dimensionality of the Turkish version of the self-stigma of seeking help scale: Results from exploratory and confirmatory factor analyses. *International Journal for the Advancement of Counselling*, *37*, 105–116. https://doi.org/10.1007/s10447-014-9230-3

Keum, B. T., & Ogrodniczuk, J. S. (2023). The role of first-person depression storytelling online video on men's self-stigma of seeking help, traditional masculinity ideology, and psychological help-seeking attitudes. *The Journal of Men's Studies*, *31*, 241–260. https://doi.org/10.1177/10608265221108511

Kim, J. E., & Zane, N. (2016). Help-seeking intentions among Asian American and White American students in psychological distress: Application of the health belief model. *Cultural Diversity & Ethnic Minority Psychology*, *22*, 311–321. https://doi.org/10.1037/cdp0000056

Koutra, K., Pantelaiou, V., & Mavroeides, G. (2023). Why don't young people seek help for mental illness? A cross-sectional study in Greece. *Youth*, *3*, 157–169. https://doi.org/10.3390/youth3010011

Lannin, D. G., & Bible, J. (2022). Self-stigma of seeking help: A meta-analysis. In D. L. Vogel & N. G. Wade (Eds.), *The Cambridge handbook of stigma and mental health* (pp. 111–142). Cambridge University Press. https://doi.org/10.1017/9781108920995.009

Lannin, D. G., Guyll, M., Vogel, D. L., & Madon, S. (2013). Reducing the stigma associated with seeking psychotherapy through self-affirmation. *Journal of Counseling Psychology*, *60*(4), 508–519. https://doi.org/10.1037/a0033789

Lannin, D. G., Ludwikowski, W. M., Heath, P. J., Vogel, D. L., Wolf, L. J., & Wicker, I. M. (2020). How are personal values linked to help-seeking stigma? *The Counseling Psychologist*, *48*, 249–276. https://doi.org/10.1177/0011000019884815

Lannin, D. G., Tucker, J. R., Streyffeler, L., Harder, S., Ripley, B., & Vogel, D. L. (2019). How medical Students' compassionate values influence help-seeking barriers. *Teaching and Learning in Medicine*, *31*(2), 170–177. https://doi.org/10.1080/10401334.2018.1522259

Lannin, D. G., Vogel, D. L., Brenner, R. E., Abraham, W. T., & Heath, P. J. (2016). Does self-stigma reduce the probability of seeking mental health information? *Journal of Counseling Psychology*, *63*, 351–358. https://doi.org/10.1037/cou0000108

Lannin, D. G., Vogel, D. L., Brenner, R. E., & Tucker, J. R. (2015). Predicting self-esteem and intentions to seek counseling: The internalized stigma model. *The Counseling Psychologist*, *43*, 64–93. https://doi.org/10.1177/0011000014541550

Lannin, D. G., Vogel, D. L., & Heath, P. J. (2017). Can reflecting on personal values online increase positive beliefs about counseling? *Journal of Counseling Psychology*, *64*, 261–268. https://doi.org/10.1037/cou0000201

Lannin, D. G., Vogel, D. L., & Heath, P. J. (2022). Reducing help-seeking stigma through self-affirmation. In W. Goodfriend & A. Nordstrom (Eds.), *Innovative stigma and discrimination reduction programs across the world* (pp. 53–64). Routledge/Taylor & Francis. https://doi.org/10.1037/a0033789

Larrahondo, B. F., García Valencia, J., Rangel Martínez-Villalba, A. M., Zapata Ospina, J. P., & Aguirre-Acevedo, D. C. (2021). Validation of the self stigma of seeking help (SSOSH) scale in a population of Colombian medical students. *Revista Colombiana de Psiquiatría*, *50*, 82–91. https://doi.org/10.1016/j.rcpeng.2020.01.002

Lee, E. J., Ditchman, N., Fong, M. W., Piper, L., & Feigon, M. (2014). Mental health service seeking among Korean international students in the United States: A path analysis. *Journal of Community Psychology*, *42*, 639–655. https://doi.org/10.1002/jcop.21643

Levant, R. F., Stefanov, D. G., Rankin, T. J., Halter, M. J., Mellinger, C., & Williams, C. (2013). Moderated path analysis of the relationships between masculinity and men's attitudes toward seeking psychological help. *Journal of Counseling Psychology*, *60*, 392–406. https://doi.org/10.1037/a0033014

Link, B. G., Cullen, F. T., Struening, E., Shrout, P. E., & Dohrenwend, B. P. (1989). A modified labeling theory approach to mental disorders: An empirical assessment. *American Sociological Review*, *54*, 400–423. https://doi.org/10.2307/2095613

Lytle, M. C., Blosnich, J. R., De Luca, S. M., & Brownson, C. (2018). Association of religiosity with sexual minority suicide ideation and attempt. *American Journal of Preventive Medicine*, *54*, 644–651. https://doi.org/10.1016/j.amepre.2018.01.019

Ma, S., Zhu, Y., & Bresnahan, M. (2021). Chinese international students' face concerns, self-stigma, linguistic factors, and help-seeking intentions for mental health. *Health Communication*, *37*, 1–9. https://doi.org/10.1080/10410236.2021.1910167

Mackenzie, C. S., Heath, P. J., Vogel, D. L., & Chekay, R. (2019a). Age differences in public stigma, self-stigma, and attitudes toward seeking help: A moderated mediation model. *Journal of Clinical Psychology*, *75*, 2259–2272. https://doi.org/10.1002/jclp.22845

Mackenzie, C. S., Visperas, A., Ogrodniczuk, J. S., Oliffe, J. L., & Nurmi, M. A. (2019b). Age and sex differences in self-stigma and public stigma concerning depression and suicide in men. *Stigma and Health*, *4*, 233–241. https://doi.org/10.1037/sah0000138

Mann, C. E., & Himelein, M. J. (2004). Factors associated with stigmatization of persons with mental illness. *Psychiatric Services, 55*, 185–187. https://doi.org/10.1176/appi.ps.55.2.185

Maura, J., & de Mamani, A. W. (2017). Mental health disparities, treatment engagement, and attrition among racial/ethnic minorities with severe mental illness: A review. *Journal of Clinical Psychology in Medical Settings, 24*, 187–210. https://doi.org/10.1007/s10880-017-9510-2

Mejia-Lancheros, C., Lachaud, J., Woodhall-Melnik, J., O'Campo, P., Hwang, S. W., & Stergiopoulos, V. (2021). Longitudinal interrelationships of mental health discrimination and stigma with housing and well-being outcomes in adults with mental illness and recent experience of homelessness. *Social Science & Medicine, 268*, 113463. https://doi.org/10.1016/j.socscimed.2020.113463

Meyer, I. H. (2003). Prejudice, social stress, and mental health in lesbian, gay, and bisexual populations: Conceptual issues and research evidence. *Psychological Bulletin, 129*, 674–697. https://doi.org/10.1037/0033-2909.129.5.674

Mitchell, A. J. (2019). Screening for psychosocial distress and psychiatric disorders in medicine: From concepts to evidence. In L. Grassi, M. B. Riba, & T. Wise (Eds.), *Person centered approach to recovery in medicine* (pp. 57–78). Springer. https://doi.org/10.1007/978-3-319-74736-1_4

Mori, D. L., Sloan, C. A., Flynn, H. W., & Burgess, C. (2020). Transgender Health. *The Wiley Encyclopedia of Health Psychology*, 219–227. https://doi.org/10.1002/9781119057840.ch205

Murphy, D. J., & Mackenzie, C. S. (2023). Experiential avoidance moderates the degree to which internalized stigma affects older adults' attitudes and intentions to seek mental health services. In *Stigma and health*. Advance online publication. https://doi.org/10.1037/sah0000444

Neff, K. (2003). Self-compassion: An alternative conceptualization of a healthy attitude toward oneself. *Self and Identity, 2*, 85–101. https://doi.org/10.1080/15298860309032

Oexle, N., & Corrigan, P. W. (2018). Understanding mental illness stigma toward persons with multiple stigmatized conditions: Implications of intersectionality theory. *Psychiatric Services, 69*, 587–589. https://doi.org/10.1176/appi.ps.201700312

Owen, J., Thomas, L., & Rodolfa, E. (2013). Stigma for seeking therapy: Self-stigma, social stigma, and therapeutic processes. *The Counseling Psychologist, 41*, 857–880. https://doi.org/10.1177/0011000012459365

Parcesepe, A. M., & Cabassa, L. J. (2013). Public stigma of mental illness in the United States: A systematic literature review. *Administration and Policy in Mental Health and Mental Health Services Research, 40*, 384–399. https://doi.org/10.1007/s10488-012-0430-z

Pescosolido, B. A., Halpern-Manners, A., Luo, L., & Perry, B. (2021). Trends in public stigma of mental illness in the US, 1996–2018. *JAMA Network Open, 4*, e2140202. https://doi.org/10.1001/jamanetworkopen.2021.40202

Phillips, M. S., Steelesmith, D. L., Brock, G., Benedict, J., Muñoz, J., & Fontanella, C. A. (2022). Mental health service utilization among medical students with a perceived need for care. *Academic Psychiatry, 46*, 223–227. https://doi.org/10.1007/s40596-021-01584-y

Pretorius, C., McCashin, D., & Coyle, D. (2022). Mental health professionals as influencers on TikTok and Instagram: What role do they play in mental health literacy and help-seeking? *Internet Interventions, 30*. Article 100591. https://doi.org/10.1016/j.invent.2022.100591

Richter, D., Wall, A., Bruen, A., & Whittington, R. (2019). Is the global prevalence rate of adult mental illness increasing? Systematic review and meta-analysis. *Acta Psychiatrica Scandinavica, 140*, 393–407. https://doi.org/10.1111/acps.13083

Rosen, A., Walter, G., Casey, D., & Hocking, B. (2000). Combating psychiatric stigma: An overview of contemporary initiatives. *Australasian Psychiatry, 8*, 19–26. https://doi.org/10.1046/j.1440-1665.2000.00239.x

Rüsch, N., Corrigan, P. W., Todd, A. R., & Bodenhausen, G. V. (2010). Implicit self-stigma in people with mental illness. *The Journal of Nervous and Mental Disease, 198*, 150–153. https://doi.org/10.1097/NMD.0b013e3181cc43b5

Santomauro, D. F., Mantilla Herrera, A. M., Shadid, J., Zheng, P., Ashbaugh, C., Pigott, D. M., Abbafati, C., Adolph, C., Amlag, J. O., Aravkin, A. Y., Bang-Jensen, B. L., Bertolacci, G. J., Bloom, S. S., Castellano, R., Castro, E., Chakrabarti, S., Chattopadhyay, J., Cogen, R. M., Collins, J. K., … Penberthy, L. (2021). Global prevalence and burden of depressive and anxiety disorders in 204 countries and territories in 2020 due to the COVID-19 pandemic. *The Lancet, 398*(10312), 1700–1712. https://doi.org/10.1016/S0140-6736(21)02143-7

Saykeo, S. P., & Lawrence, E. (2018). Factors that affect help-seeking: Examining racial differences between Whites, Asians, and African Americans. *Modern Psychological Studies, 24*(1), 8.

Schnyder, N., Panczak, R., Groth, N., & Schultze-Lutter, F. (2017). Association between mental health-related stigma and active help-seeking: Systematic review and meta-analysis. *The British Journal of Psychiatry, 210*, 261–268. https://doi.org/10.1192/bjp.bp.116.189464

Schreiber, R., & Hartrick, G. (2002). Keeping it together: How women use the biomedical explanatory model to manage the stigma of depression. *Issues in Mental Health Nursing, 23*, 91–105. https://doi.org/10.1080/016128402753542749

Seidman, A. J. (2022). Self-affirmation interventions to reduce mental health stigma. In D. L. Vogel & N. G. Wade (Eds.), *The Cambridge handbook of stigma and mental health* (pp. 429–448). Cambridge University Press. https://doi.org/10.1017/9781108920995.025

Seidman, A. J., Lannin, D. G., Heath, P. J., & Vogel, D. L. (2019a). Setting the stage: The effect of affirming personal values before psychotherapy intake screenings on perceptions of self-stigma and self-disclosure. *Stigma and Health, 4*, 256–259. https://doi.org/10.1037/sah0000140

Seidman, A. J., Vogel, D. L., & Lannin, D. G. (2023). Examining between-and within-person effects of the self-stigma of seeking psychological help on the therapeutic working alliance: The moderating role of psychological distress. *Psychotherapy, 60*, 206–211. https://doi.org/10.1037/pst0000482

Seidman, A. J., Wade, N. G., & Geller, J. (2022). The effects of group counseling and self-affirmation on stigma and group relationship development: A replication and extension. *Journal of Counseling Psychology, 69*, 701–710. https://doi.org/10.1037/cou0000614

Seidman, A. J., Wade, N. G., Vogel, D. L., & Armistead-Jehle, P. (2019b). The impact of stigma on behavioral health care utilization among active duty service members. *Military Psychology, 31*, 11–17. https://doi.org/10.1080/08995605.2018.1522927

Sezer, S., & Kezer, F. (2013). The reliability and validity of self stigma of seeking help scale (SSOSH) in a Turkish sample. *Dusunen Adam: Journal of Psychiatry & Neurological Sciences, 26*, 148–156. https://doi.org/10.5350/DAJPN2013260204

Shannon, J., Seward, D. X., Liu, Y., & Luke, M. (2022). Stigma, help-seeking, and counseling with African American male college students. *Journal of Counseling & Development, 100*, 421–432. https://doi.org/10.1002/jmcd.12275

Shechtman, Z., Vogel, D. L., Strass, H. A., & Heath, P. J. (2018). Stigma in help-seeking: The case of adolescents. *British Journal of Guidance & Counselling, 46*, 104–119. https://doi.org/10.1080/03069885.2016.1255717

Sherman, D. K. (2013). Self-affirmation: Understanding the effects. *Social and Personality Psychology Compass, 7*(11), 834–845. https://doi.org/10.1111/spc3.12072

Sibicky, M., & Dovidio, J. (1986). Stigma of psychological therapy: Stereotypes, interpersonal reactions, and the self-fulfilling prophecy. *Journal of Counseling Psychology, 33*, 148–154. https://doi.org/10.1037/0022-0167.33.2.148

Sigal, M., & Plunkett, S. W. (2023). Gender and ethnic differences in University students' attitudes about mental health services. *Journal of College Student Psychotherapy*, 1–18. https://doi.org/10.1080/87568225.2023.2179286

Soheilian, S. S., & Inman, A. G. (2009). Middle eastern Americans: The effects of stigma on attitudes toward counseling. *Journal of Muslim Mental Health, 4*, 139–158. https://doi.org/10.1080/15564900903245766

Stanley, I., Hom, M., & Joiner, T. (2018). Modifying mental health help-seeking stigma among undergraduates with untreated psychiatric disorders: A pilot randomized trial of a novel cognitive bias modification intervention. *Behaviour Research and Therapy, 103*, 33–42. https://doi.org/10.1016/j.brat.2018.01.008

Sun, S., Hoyt, W. T., Brockberg, D., Lam, J., & Tiwari, D. (2016). Acculturation and enculturation as predictors of psychological help-seeking attitudes (HSAs) among racial and ethnic minorities: A meta-analytic investigation. *Journal of Counseling Psychology, 63*, 617–632. https://doi.org/10.1037/cou0000172

Terlizzi, E. P., & Norris, T. (2021) Mental health treatment among adults: United States, 2020. *National Center for Health Statistics Data Brief.* https://www.cdc.gov/nchs/products/databriefs/db419.htm

Tomczyk, S., Schmidt, S., Muehlan, H., Stolzenburg, S., & Schomerus, G. (2020). A prospective study on structural and attitudinal barriers to professional help-seeking for currently untreated mental health problems in the community. *The Journal of Behavioral Health Services & Research, 47*, 54–69. https://doi.org/10.1007/s11414-019-09662-8

Topkaya, N. (2021). Predictors of attitudes toward seeking professional psychological help among Turkish college students. *Children and Youth Services Review, 120*, 105782. https://doi.org/10.1016/j.childyouth.2020.105782

Topkaya, N., Vogel, D. L., & Brenner, R. E. (2017). Examination of the stigmas toward help seeking among Turkish college students. *Journal of Counseling & Development, 95*, 213–225. http://dx.doi.org/10.1002/jcad.12133

Tucker, J. R., Hammer, J. H., Vogel, D. L., Bitman, R. L., Wade, N. G., & Maier, E. J. (2013). Disentangling self-stigma: Are mental illness and help-seeking self-stigmas different? *Journal of Counseling Psychology, 60*, 520–531. https://doi.org/10.1037/a0033555

Vidales, C. A. (2022). *Mental health stigma among LGBTQ+ populations.* In D. L. Vogel & N. Wade (Eds.), *The Cambridge handbook of stigma and mental health* (pp. 241–262). Cambridge University Press and Assessment. https://doi.org/10.1017/9781108920995

Vidales, C. A., Vogel, D. L., & Levant, R. F. (2022). The self-stigma of seeking help (SSOSH) scale: Measurement invariance across men from different backgrounds. *Measurement and Evaluation in Counseling and Development*, 1–15. https://doi.org/10.1080/07481756.2022.2160356

Vogel, D. L., Armstrong, P. I., Tsai, P. C., Wade, N. G., Hammer, J. H., Efstathiou, G., Holtham, E., Kouvaraki, E., Liao, H. Y., Shechtman, Z., & Topkaya, N. (2013a). Cross-cultural validity of the self-stigma of seeking help (SSOSH) scale: Examination across six nations. *Journal of Counseling Psychology, 60*, 303–310. https://doi.org/10.1037/a0032055

Vogel, D. L., Bitman, R. L., Hammer, J. H., & Wade, N. G. (2013b). Is stigma internalized? The longitudinal impact of public stigma on self-stigma. *Journal of Counseling Psychology, 60*, 311–316. https://doi.org/10.1037/a0031889

Vogel, D. L., Heimerdinger-Edwards, S. R., Hammer, J. H., & Hubbard, A. (2011). "Boys don't cry": Examination of the links between endorsement of masculine norms, self-stigma, and help-seeking attitudes for men from diverse backgrounds. *Journal of Counseling Psychology*, *58*, 368–382. https://doi.org/10.1037/a0023688

Vogel, D. L., Strass, H. A., Heath, P. J., Al-Darmaki, F. R., Armstrong, P. I., Baptista, M. N., Brenner, R. E., Gonçalves, M., Lannin, D. G., Liao, H.-Y., Mackenzie, C. S., Mak, W. W. S., Rubin, M., Topkaya, N., Wade, N. G., Wang, Y.-F., & Zlati, A. (2017). Stigma of seeking psychological services: Examining college students across ten countries/regions. *The Counseling Psychologist*, *45*, 170–192. https://doi.org/10.1177/0011000016671411

Vogel, D. L., Wade, N. G., & Ascheman, P. (2009). Measuring perceptions of stigmatization by others for seeking psychological help: Reliability and validity of a new stigma scale with college students. *Journal of Counseling Psychology*, *56*, 301–308. https://doi.org/10.1037/a0014903

Vogel, D. L., Wade, N. G., & Haake, S. (2006). Measuring the self-stigma associated with seeking psychological help. *Journal of Counseling Psychology*, *53*, 325–337. https://doi.org/10.1037/0022-0167.53.3.325

Wade, J. C., & Rochlen, A. B. (2013). Introduction: Masculinity, identity, and the health and well-being of African American men. *Psychology of Men & Masculinity*, *14*, 1. https://doi.org/10.1037/a0029612

Wade, N. G., Post, B. C., Cornish, M. A., Vogel, D. L., & Tucker, J. R. (2011). Predictors of the change in self-stigma following a single session of group counseling. *Journal of Counseling Psychology*, *58*, 170–182. https://doi.org/10.1037/a0022630

Wang, P. S., Berglund, P. A., Olfson, M., & Kessler, R. C. (2004). Delays in initial treatment contact after first onset of a mental disorder. *Health Services Research*, *39*, 393–416. https://doi.org/10.1111/j.1475-6773.2004.00234.x

Whaley, A. L., & Dubose, J. (2018). Intersectionality of ethnicity/race and gender in the phenomenology of African American college students' presenting problems: A profile analysis using nonmetric multidimensional scaling. *International Journal for the Advancement of Counselling*, *40*, 279–297. https://doi.org/10.1007/s10447-018-9326-2

Whitfield, D. L., Walls, N. E., Langenderfer-Magruder, L., & Clark, B. (2014). Queer is the new black? Not so much: Racial disparities in anti-LGBTQ discrimination. *Journal of Gay & Lesbian Social Services*, *26*, 426–440. https://doi.org/10.1080/10538720.2014.955556

Wong, N., Rindfleisch, A., & Burroughs, J. E. (2003). Do reverse-worded items confound measures in cross-cultural consumer research? The case of the material values scale. *Journal of Consumer Research*, *30*, 72–91. https://doi.org/10.1086/374697

World Health Organization. (2022). *World mental health report: transforming mental health for all.* World Health Organization. https://www.who.int/publications/i/item/9789240049338

Yamawaki, N., & Green, J. (2020). Stigma and self-efficacy as predictors of intention to seek help among American and Japanese college students. *International Journal of Psychology and Counselling*, *12*, 63–72. https://doi.org/10.5897/IJPC2020.0614

Yu, B. C., Chio, F. H., Chan, K. K., Mak, W. W., Zhang, G., Vogel, D., & Lai, M. H. (2023). Associations between public and self-stigma of help-seeking with help-seeking attitudes and intention: A meta-analytic structural equation modeling approach. *Journal of Counseling Psychology*, *70*, 90–102. https://doi.org/10.1037/cou0000637

Yu, B. C. L., Chio, F. H. N., Mak, W. W. S., Corrigan, P. W., & Chan, K. K. Y. (2021). Internalization process of stigma of people with mental illness across cultures: A meta-analytic structural equation modeling approach. *Clinical Psychology Review*, *87*, 102029. https://doi.org/10.1016/j.cpr.2021.102029

Zhou, Y., Lemmer, G., Xu, J., & Rief, W. (2019). Cross-cultural measurement invariance of scales assessing stigma and attitude to seeking professional psychological help. *Frontiers in Psychology*, *10*, 1249. https://doi.org/10.3389/fpsyg.2019.01249

10

Advancing the Measurement of Mental Illness Stigma: Considerations of Time, Structural Stigma, and Intersectionality

Annie B. Fox[1], Xueli Qiu[2], Mohammad Mousavi[3], and Valerie A. Earnshaw[3]

[1] MGH Institute of Health Professions
[2] Johns Hopkins University
[3] University of Delaware

Mental health communication and stigma are inherently linked, as stigma is both experienced and communicated via language, behaviors, and structural or institutional forces. Mental health communication campaigns are often designed to reduce stigma and increase help-seeking behaviors. Yet, despite many national and international stigma reduction campaigns over the past two decades (Borschmann et al., 2014; Evans-Lacko et al., 2014; Jorm et al., 2005), mental illness (MI) stigma continues to be a significant barrier to help seeking. Stigma is fundamentally a social process whereby certain attributes, characteristics, and/or identities become devalued and discredited (Goffman, 1963; Link & Phelan, 2001). MI stigma impacts individuals across the course of MI (i.e., from symptom onset to remission), and along every step of the mental health treatment continuum (Pence et al., 2012), from self-identification of symptoms as a potential MI, to completing a course of treatment. Understanding how MI stigma impacts people at these different stages continues to be a priority for public health researchers (Earnshaw et al., 2022b). Further, a better understanding of the multiple and complex ways MI stigma impacts individuals is necessary to developing mental health communication campaigns that reduce or eliminate stigma. But none of this can be accomplished without strong, psychometrically sound MI stigma measures that capture the ways stigma is experienced among individuals and embodied in structures that shape and influence people's lives.

While early conceptions characterized stigma as a "deeply discrediting" mark (Goffman, 1963, p. 3) and focused on the characteristics of stigma (e.g., Jones et al., 1984), stigma researchers now embrace the multidimensional nature of stigma, recognizing the different cognitive, affective, and behavioral ways people communicate and experience stigma (Corrigan et al., 2010; Fox et al., 2018). As our understanding of MI stigma has expanded, so too have the number and breadth of MI stigma measures (Fox et al., 2018). However, important gaps remain. For example, we need more research to determine whether the psychometric properties of our measures vary across developmental stages. Further, the measurement of structural MI stigma lags behind measurement advances in other areas of stigma research, including HIV/AIDS (Ferguson et al., 2022), sexual orientation (Pachankis et al., 2021), and race/ethnicity (Groos et al., 2018). For example, research focused on the experiences of lesbian, gay, bisexual, and transgender individuals has measured structural stigma in a number of ways, including hate crime statistics within geographic areas (e.g., Duncan et al., 2014); composite variables of state laws, policies, and/or attitudes (e.g., Hatzenbuehler et al., 2014; Pachankis

The Handbook of Mental Health Communication, First Edition.
Edited by Marco C. Yzer and Jason T. Siegel.

et al., 2014); and indicators of school climate like antibullying policies and the presence of Gay-Straight Alliances (Saewyc et al., 2014). Finally, measures are still needed to sufficiently address the intersection of stigmatized statuses, including MI with race, ethnicity, sexual/gender identities, and other stigmatized health conditions (e.g., weight, chronic illness, HIV/AIDs). These three areas—time, structural stigma, and intersectionality—are key to advancing the measurement of MI stigma and will therefore be the focus of this review.

The foundation of good measurement is clear and concise operational definitions. In order to advance MI stigma measurement, we first need to understand how stigma mechanisms have been defined and how they have been measured. Thus, the first section of this chapter briefly reviews definitions of MI stigma, summarizes existing measures, and describes current trends in MI stigma measurement. The sections that follow identify and describe three important areas of development that we argue will be key to advancing MI stigma measurement: time, structural stigma, and intersectional perspectives. Because our focus is on advancing the measurement of MI stigma, principles of good measurement, recommendations for specific stigma measures, and treatment-related stigma are beyond the scope of this chapter. Readers interested in such topics are directed to Brohan et al. (2022), Fox et al. (2018), and Brenner et al. (2022) for reviews of the literature in each of these areas.

Defining and Measuring Mental Illness Stigma

We cannot advance MI stigma measurement without consensus around defining and operationalizing MI stigma. Stigma is fundamentally a social process that occurs when "elements of labeling, stereotyping, separating, status loss, and discrimination co-occur in a power situation that allows the components of stigma to unfold" (Link & Phelan, 2001, p. 382). Because stigma is a social process, it is manifested at the interpersonal, intrapersonal, and structural levels. The majority of MI stigma research has focused on interpersonal and intrapersonal experiences of stigma. This distinction is sometimes referred to as public versus self-stigma (Corrigan et al., 2010) and reflects experiences of stigma based on whether an individual is perpetrating stigma (interpersonal) or is the target of stigmatization (intrapersonal) (Fox et al., 2018).

The mental illness stigma framework (MISF; Fox et al., 2018) identifies four distinct stigma mechanisms at the interpersonal level: ***stereotypes*** (negative beliefs about people with MI), ***prejudice*** (emotional reactions to people with MI), ***discrimination*** (negative behaviors directed toward people with MI), and ***perceived stigma*** (perceptions/awareness of stigma within the community/public). Stereotypes, prejudice, and discrimination represent the cognitive, affective, and behavioral components of stigma. While these stigma mechanisms can be measured in all people regardless of MI status, there are other stigma mechanisms that are specific to the experience of MI. At the intrapersonal level, the MISF describes three stigma mechanisms individuals who are the target of stigmatization may experience: ***anticipated stigma*** (concern about being the target of discrimination), ***enacted stigma*** (experienced discrimination), or ***internalized stigma*** (applying negative stereotypes of MI to the self).

When measuring MI stigma, researchers have at their disposal several excellent, well-validated measures, and there is at least one psychometrically valid measure for each stigma mechanism described in the MISF. Researchers interested in selecting well-validated measures should consult one of several reviews that identify and describe the overall quality and psychometric characteristics of existing measures, several of which use the Consensus-based Standards for the Selection of Health Measurement Instruments (COSMIN) checklist (Terwee et al., 2007) to guide their measurement evaluation. These reviews include Fox et al. (2018), Wei et al. (2018), and Brohan et al. (2022).

MI Stigma Measures 2015–2023

Examining recent developments in MI stigma measurement can tell us what researchers in the field are prioritizing and give clues to where the field might be headed. Although a comprehensive review is beyond the scope of this chapter, we performed a basic literature search for MI stigma measures published between 2015 and 2023 using PsycINFO, PubMed, and Google Scholar and identified 64 articles. Interestingly, more than half (*n* = 36) of the articles we identified involved a cross-cultural validation of an existing stigma measure or the development of a stigma measure for use in a specific cultural context. Further, nearly half of the 36 articles (*n* = 16) validated a measure of internalized stigma. The Internalized Stigma of Mental Illness Scale (ISMI; Ritsher et al., 2003) is one of the most cited measures of stigma since its publication (Google Scholar = 1800 citations as of July 2023). The ISMI was the subject of five additional validations involving either a short form (ISMI-9, ISMI-10) or adaptation to a specific MI (e.g., schizophrenia) or population (e.g., adolescents). Although not definitive, these findings suggest that both internalized stigma and the cross-cultural measurement of stigma have become priorities. This may be evidence of a shift in focus away from public stigma (stereotypes, prejudice, discrimination), which dominated MI stigma research for decades, to prioritizing the experience of stigma among individuals experiencing an MI, and in particular, how MI is experienced across different cultures.

Our search also identified 19 new measures, several of which address intriguing areas for future stigma measurement, including microaggressions, associative stigma, and stigma resistance. Ezell et al. (2018) developed the Daily Indignities of MI scale (DIMI) to measure the microaggressions experienced by people with MI. Such a measure addresses an important gap in MI stigma measurement, as most measures of experienced stigma focus on experiences of macrolevel aggressions (e.g., losing a job). Associative stigma (sometimes referred to as courtesy, affiliate, or familial stigma) is the stigma experienced by friends, family members, or health care professionals who are related to, live with, support, or treat individuals experiencing a mental health problem (Mak & Cheung, 2008; Verhaeghe & Bracke, 2012). Morris et al. (2018) developed the Self-Stigma in Relatives of People with Mental Illness Scale (SSRMI), which measures the extent to which first-degree relatives have internalized stigma associated with a family member who is experiencing a MI. Affiliate stigma has also been a focus of measurement among researchers studying stigma in Asian cultures (e.g., Chang et al., 2019) where stigma by association may be more prevalent due to cultural beliefs that situate the cause of MI not only in an individual but also in their family (Yang & Pearson, 2002).

Finally, stigma resistance has been conceptualized as resisting the process of internalizing the negative stereotypes of MI (Ritsher & Phelan, 2004). In fact, the ISMI contains a stigma resistance subscale; however, it is often found to be unreliable (Boyd et al., 2014) and therefore omitted from the published papers of researchers using the ISMI (Firmin et al., 2017). Firmin et al. (2017) developed a new psychometrically validated measure of stigma resistance that captures multiple ways people may resist stigma. The scale contains five subscales: (a) self–other differentiation (ability to separate stigmatizing attitudes of others versus those of the self); (b) personal identity (ability to find meaning in life outside mental illness); (c) personal cognitions (cognitive strategies used to challenge stigmatizing beliefs); (d) peer stigma resistance (desire to help others resist stigma); and (e) public stigma resistance (ways people publicly resist stigma). Furthering our understanding of stigma resistance may be especially useful for intervention development and clinical treatment. For example, scores on the different stigma resistance subscales may be used to determine appropriate targets for intervention, that is, individuals low in personal cognitions may benefit from learning cognitive strategies or techniques to deal with stigmatizing thoughts or beliefs (Firmin et al., 2017). Further, Firmin et al. found that stigma resistance was strongly correlated with self-efficacy, positive aspects of mental illness, recovery attitudes, and quality of life. Thus, targeting stigma resistance in interventions may be particularly beneficial to individuals experiencing MI.

The MI stigma literature has historically been plagued by an overabundance of unvalidated, often redundant, measures of stigma. But our brief review of new MI stigma measures suggests the field is moving in important new directions that capture the nuances of how people with MI (as well as their families and health care providers) experience, or resist, MI stigma. Further, the trend of cross-culturally validating measures is evidence that researchers not only are acknowledging the importance of cultural differences in how people experience stigma but also trying to make sure that we have the measurement tools to accurately reflect those experiences.

Incorporating Time into MI Stigma Research

Recent scholarship has highlighted the time-varying nature of stigma (Earnshaw et al., 2022b). As a dynamic social process, structural MI stigma has increased and decreased throughout history alongside changing conceptualizations of MI. Moreover, individuals may have different experiences of MI stigma at different developmental stages, and the impact of MI stigma may change over the life course. Finally, symptoms of MI may change over time as people develop, receive treatment, and transition into remission, further shaping experiences of MI stigma. Although longitudinal research on MI stigma is still sorely lacking (Livingston & Boyd, 2010), some emerging findings point to the importance of considering time when measuring MI stigma.

What Has Been Done?

At the societal level, evidence suggests that the extent to which MI is stigmatized within societies evolves. Researchers have documented decreases (Gagné et al., 2023), increases (Phelan et al., 2000), and lack of changes (Schomerus et al., 2012) in MI stigma over the past century. Importantly, findings suggest that stigma associated with different mental illnesses appears to change at different rates. For example, Schomerus et al. (2022) found that stigma associated with schizophrenia worsened whereas stigma associated with depression slightly improved in Germany from 1990 to 2020. To date, much of this research has been conducted by including MI stigma-related constructs such as social distance (Gagné et al., 2023; Schomerus et al., 2022) and stereotypes (Phelan et al., 2000) in repeated cross-sectional studies.

At the individual level, evidence suggests that MI stigma changes over the life course. A systematic review found that MI stigma exists among children, and several studies show that stigma increases with age over the course of childhood and adolescence as youth become more aware of their own and others' mental health problems (Kaushik et al., 2016). Until recently, much research with children and adolescents had been conducted with scales developed for adults. In the past several years, MI scales have been developed and tested for children and adolescents specifically (McKeague et al., 2015). Evidence suggests that levels of MI stigma may continue to evolve in adulthood, with some work suggesting that internalized stigma is higher among middle-aged than older-aged adults (Mackenzie et al., 2019; West et al., 2011). Yet, underscoring the complexity of associations between MI stigma and health across the lifespan, research suggests that older adults may be the most vulnerable to MI stigma as older adults appear to have the strongest associations between internalized MI stigma and worse attitudes toward help seeking (Mackenzie et al., 2019). Studies comparing MI stigma among adults often use the same scales for participants of different ages (Mackenzie et al., 2019; West et al., 2011). More work is needed to determine the extent to which these scales generalize to participants of different ages. For example, sources of stigma and social contexts in which stigma manifests may shift over time; therefore, scales that have been developed for one age group may or may not adequately capture stigma among another age group (Earnshaw et al., 2022b).

Also at the individual level, experiences and impacts of stigma may change as MI symptoms develop, are treated, and transition into remission. Some work suggests that MI stigma may be higher around the time of diagnosis (Grover et al., 2017). Suggesting an intersection between age and status course or MI stage, findings indicate that MI diagnoses at younger ages are associated with greater MI stigma (Grover et al., 2017; Kaushik et al., 2016). Studies additionally emphasize that MI stigma persists during treatment and remission (Link et al., 1997). However, few studies measure MI stigma across symptom development, treatment, and remission; therefore, it is difficult to determine the extent to which experiences of stigma change over these periods.

What Is Next?

To date, little research has explored the extent to which the nature of MI stigma changes across historical contexts, developmental stages, and MI stages (Earnshaw et al., 2022b). Yet it is possible that stereotypes surrounding and prejudice toward people with MI change across historical contexts and that the ways individuals with MI experience and anticipate stigma from others change over the life course and alongside the development, treatment, and remission of MI symptoms. The question of whether the nature of MI stigma changes holds profound implications for measurement validity: If researchers use measures that are attuned to the previous decade, life stage, or MI stage, they may underestimate the extent to which participants are experiencing MI stigma. Indeed, researchers have critiqued the use of MI stigma measures that were developed for adults with child populations (McKeague et al., 2015). Measures developed for adults may miss important experiences (e.g., bullying) or sources (e.g., teachers) of stigma more commonly experienced among children, potentially underestimating the degree to which children experience stigma. Exploratory, qualitative research may help to elucidate whether experiences of stigma change across time and inform measurement efforts. Moreover, it may be important to reestablish the validity of MI stigma measures when working in new historical contexts, developmental stages, or MI stages.

Measurement Issues to Consider

Researchers may feel a tension between using established MI stigma measures versus time-specific MI stigma measures. The use of established MI measures enables comparison of findings between studies and can be critical for accurate syntheses of bodies of research (e.g., meta-analyses) (Siddaway et al., 2019). Funding bodies such as the National Institutes of Health in the United States may additionally encourage the use of common measures to facilitate cross-study analyses. Yet established, popular measures may not be the most accurate way to measure MI stigma at a particular historical context, developmental stage, or MI stage. When choosing MI stigma measures, we recommend that researchers carefully consider and weigh the importance of comparing their findings with those of other studies versus measuring time-specific aspects of MI stigma. There may be studies wherein it is most important to compare findings across studies, and therefore the use of established, popular measures is preferable. There may be other studies wherein it is most important to measure MI stigma in the most accurate and valid way possible, and therefore the use of time-specific measures is preferable. If researchers choose to use time-specific measures, we encourage them to carefully develop and validate their measures to avoid contributing to the proliferation of unvalidated MI stigma measures (Fox et al., 2018).

Measuring Structural MI Stigma

Structural stigma refers to the "societal-level conditions, cultural norms, and institutional practices that constrain the opportunities, resources, and well-being for stigmatized populations" (Hatzenbuehler & Link, 2014, p. 2). Structural stigma affects people with MI across the entire range of life domains, including education, housing, health care, parenting, travel, employment, privacy, technology, media, engagement with the criminal justice system, and participation in civic duties (Livingston, 2020). Importantly, structural stigma plays a pivotal role in the mental health treatment cascade. There is widespread consensus that eliminating structural stigma is a priority for improving mental health outcomes, and there have been continuous calls for measuring and integrating structural stigma into mental health stigma research. However, for researchers to be able to incorporate structural stigma into their research, we need to have both strong operationalizations and corresponding measurement tools available that can be feasibly implemented.

What Has Been Done?

Similar to the measurement of individual-level experiences of stigma, self-report data has been used to capture structural stigma. Researchers have aggregated stigma scores within specific geographic areas as an estimate of stigma within those areas and then examined relationships between community-level stigma and individual-level outcomes. For example, individuals living in countries with lower stigmatizing attitudes and higher rates of help seeking reported experiencing less self-stigma and discrimination

(Evans-Lacko et al., 2012), and individuals who live in countries with more stigmatizing beliefs encountered more barriers to seeking treatment (Bracke et al., 2019). Self-report measures have also been used to measure the attitudes and behaviors of health care providers, which can often reflect the larger culture of an institution (Henderson et al., 2014). Although studies measuring provider attitudes may capture interpersonal stigma, they can also be categorized as structural stigma when those attitudes are not isolated to just a few individuals but rather reflect the larger organizational culture (Livingston, 2013).

Given its complexity, measuring structural stigma often requires different methodological approaches (Hatzenbuehler, 2014). For example, structural MI stigma is sometimes measured with content coding, as many manifestations of structural stigma may be evident in the text of laws, bills, or print media (e.g., Corrigan et al., 2005b). Corrigan et al. (2005b) examined all the mental health-related bills that were introduced in 2002 in all 50 states of the United States; bills were coded as either expanding or contracting the liberty, discrimination, and/or privacy of people with MI. In another study, Corrigan et al. (2005a) examined newspaper articles for evidence of structural stigma, finding that 39% of MI-related articles focused on dangerousness and violence.

There are many other potential data sources for collecting and measuring structural stigma, including governments, hospital systems, insurance companies, health care providers, and people with lived experiences (Livingston, 2021). The health care and insurance systems are arguably the most important sources of structural stigma for people with MI (Pugh et al., 2015). Indicators of structural stigma include access to and quality of mental health care (Livingston, 2020; Misra et al., 2021), resource distribution (Ricciardelli et al., 2020; Schomerus et al., 2011), compulsory treatment, funding allocations (Corrigan et al., 2004; Liese et al., 2019), methods of teaching mental health care in medical school curricula (Sukhera et al., 2022; Thomas et al., 2013), and the language used to describe patients with mental health conditions (Healy et al., 2022; Weiner et al., 2023). Geographically tied data regarding insurance coverage rates, reimbursement rates for mental health providers, the size of the mental health workforce, mortality and comorbidity rates, wait times for mental health services, and number of mental health referrals can also serve as indicators of structural stigma.

An excellent source for more information regarding measuring structural stigma for mental health and substance use is the work of the Mental Health Commission of Canada, which in 2019 launched a multiyear program for addressing structural stigma for people with MI or substance use disorders. Its work includes an excellent review of structural stigma assessment with an emphasis on the health care system (Livingston, 2021), a framework for action (Knaak et al., 2020), and the beginning development of an audit tool for structural stigma that will include a range of structural stigma measures (Ungar & Moothathamby, 2020).

What Is Next?

Given there are so many sources of data for capturing structural stigma and that stigma may change over time, we need ways to quickly collect and aggregate data so that they can be analyzed in the context of individual experiences and outcomes. Luckily, technology has advanced in ways that can now facilitate the collection and analysis of structural-level data. Web-scraping technology, artificial intelligence linked to analysis software (e.g., R, Python), and techniques like sentiment analysis all allow for quickly culling, coding, and analyzing qualitative data (text) on websites, newspapers, and social media. Further, these technologies may be leveraged for collecting quantitative data from websites that regularly publish indicators of structural stigma. The more efficient we can be in measuring structural stigma, the better able we will be to address structural stigma through intervention in real time.

One potential technological and quantitative tool that may be leveraged as a measure of structural stigma is Google Trends (GT; https://trends.google.com), a publicly available tool that provides both real-time and historical estimates of search word (or phrase) volume across Google products (e.g., Google Search Engine, YouTube). The use of GT data as a tool for measuring MI stigma is nascent. However, a small number of studies in the broader stigma literature suggest that GT has the potential to provide useful geographic, longitudinal, and population-level data regarding MI stigma.

For example, GT search volume for the full spelling of the term *N-word* is associated with Black mortality attributed to heart disease and cancer (Chae et al., 2015); preterm birth and low birth rate among Black women in the United States (Chae et al., 2018); and increased depression among Black people (Isoya & Yamada, 2021). Applying a similar analysis to MI-related GT search data has the potential to better inform our understanding of the connection between structural stigma and outcomes for people with MI.

Measurement Issues to Consider

It is possible to become easily overwhelmed by the number of potential sources of structural-level stigma data. Thus, it will be important for researchers to think carefully about what structural indicators fit their research questions and connect those to their operational definition of structural stigma. From both a measurement and methodological perspective, structural stigma research may benefit from consideration and testing of latent variable models that allow for multiple indicators of structural stigma, as single indicator measures may not fully capture the complexity of structural stigma. The development of a structural MI stigma index that includes a range of indicators across the different life domains may be particularly useful.

The measurement of individual-level stigma has evolved over the years to better capture the multitude of ways people experience stigma. The measurement of structural stigma will also need to undergo a similar process. Livingston (2021) argues that the assessment of structural stigma for people with MI must be multimodal, collecting data from a range of quantitative and qualitative sources; it should be participatory and intersectional, capturing the lived experiences of people with MI who may also experience stigma related to other aspects of their identities; and it should be cross-level and longitudinal, as structural stigma may be experienced at multiple levels of a particular system or organization and may change over time.

Measuring Intersectional MI Stigma

Scholars have paid increasing attention to the role of intersectionality in stigma processes over the past two decades. Intersectional stigma emerges when individual forms of stigma intersect to create unique and sometimes new stigmatizing experiences and conditions (Berger, 2004). Although often overlooked in intersectional stigma scholarship, intersectionality frameworks emphasize that all forms of oppression (including stigma) are multilevel in nature and encourage action-oriented scholarship that aims to dismantle these systems (Logie et al., 2021).

Recent scholarship has demonstrated that accounting for intersectionality can yield important insights into the experiences and outcomes of stigma. For example, in their review of cultural aspects of MI stigma, Misra et al. (2021) found that Asian, Black, and Latinx Americans experience MI stigma in unique ways. These include specific experiences of structural stigma (e.g., service barriers due to immigration and historical racism), affiliative stigma (e.g., among family members), public stigma (e.g., rooted in specific cultural beliefs), and internalized stigma (e.g., failing to fulfill lineage obligations). In their systematic review and meta-analysis, Eylem et al. (2020) found that racial minorities report slightly more stereotypes, prejudice, and discrimination toward people with MI than racial majorities. Based on their scoping review, McKenzie et al. (2022) found that gender norms characterizing men as strong, self-reliant, and healthy may exacerbate internalized stigma among men.

What Has Been Done?

Researchers have arguably struggled with how to best operationalize intersectional stigma. To date, researchers have primarily focused on how to account for the multidimensional aspect of intersectionality, or the ways multiple forms of stigma shape experiences and outcomes of stigma at the individual level (Earnshaw et al., 2022a). Many researchers address intersectionality via analytic approaches.

In these approaches, researchers may use one MI stigma scale for all participants in their study and then consider intersectionality within their analyses. Popular analytic approaches are to compare mean levels of MI stigma across groups with different social statuses or explore whether social statuses moderate associations between stigma with outcomes.

Although less popular than analytic approaches to intersectional stigma, there are at least three common approaches to incorporating intersectionality into the measurement of MI stigma (Earnshaw et al., 2022a). First, parallel measures use separate items (i.e., unique scales or subscales) to independently measure stigma experienced with MI and other unique social statuses. For example, in their research on associations between stigma and HIV risk among women with MI, Collins et al. (2008) included separate measures of enacted MI stigma and enacted racial/ethnic stigma. Second, intercategorical measures are designed to capture experiences of stigma across a range of social statuses. The Everyday Discrimination Scale, which asks people to indicate the frequency with which they have experienced enacted stigma and their attributions for these experiences, is perhaps the most widely used example of this type of measure (Williams et al., 1997) and has been applied to MI stigma research (Gabbidon et al., 2014). The Intersectional Discrimination Index is another example that does not include attributions for experiences of stigma, instead asking people to indicate experiences that occurred "because of who you are" (Scheim & Bauer, 2019). Third, group-specific measures are tailored to the unique experiences of individuals at the intersection of specific social statuses. For example, ***Preguntas con Cartas*** was developed to measure stigma toward people with MI among Latinos in faith-based settings (Caplan, 2016).

What Is Next?

Critics have argued that the field's current focus on developing approaches to operationalize the multidimensional aspects of intersectional stigma overlooks key elements of intersectionality frameworks (Bowleg, 2021; Earnshaw et al., 2022a). Beyond calling attention to the multidimensional aspect of stigma, intersectionality calls on researchers to attend to the ways in which stigma is a multilevel and multidirectional construct as well as engage in action-oriented scholarship to dismantle systems of oppression that lead to and maintain stigma. Researchers can attend to the multilevel nature of intersectional MI stigma by measuring stigma at multiple social–ecological levels (Earnshaw et al., 2022a). Structural-level measures can be incorporated alongside individual- and interpersonal-level measures of stigma.

Researchers can further attend to the multidirectional nature of intersectional MI stigma by considering the ways stigma at one social–ecological level impacts stigma at other social–ecological levels longitudinally (Earnshaw et al., 2022a). Finally, researchers can engage in action-oriented scholarship by partnering with communities at all stages of their work (Corrigan, 2020; Corrigan & Oppenheim, 2023; Earnshaw et al., 2022a). From a measurement perspective, researchers can additionally incorporate empowerment-based factors (e.g., resilience, activism) alongside measures of intersectional stigma to avoid scholarship that takes a deficits-only approach (Logie et al., 2021).

Measurement Issues to Consider

Researchers may grapple with several measurement-related issues as they study MI stigma through the lens of intersectionality. Researchers continue to debate the importance of measuring participants' attributions for experiences of stigma. This debate has at least two layers. First, researchers disagree about the extent to which participants are able to attribute experiences of stigma to specific social statuses (e.g., MI versus race). Some qualitative research suggests that it can be difficult for participants to determine the causes of experiences of stigma, such as whether experiences were due to race, sexual orientation, or gender (Bowleg, 2012). The use of intercategorial measures that do not require participants to make attributions for experiences of stigma and group-specific measures enable participants to report on experiences of discrimination without having to identify attributions for those experiences. In contrast, the stereotype content model (Fiske et al., 2002) suggests that people experience unique forms of stigma associated with specific social statuses and therefore may be able to attribute experiences of stigma to specific social statuses. The use of parallel and intercategorial measures that require participants to make attributions for experiences of stigma assumes that individuals are able to ascribe their experiences to specific social statuses.

Second, researchers may disagree about the extent to which attributions for stigma matter in terms of health outcomes. Some researchers emphasize the frequency of experiences of stigma rather than attributions for stigma. For example, the Intersectional Discrimination Index measures the frequency with which participants experience stigma and the extent to which they anticipate stigma but not their attributions for these experiences (Scheim & Bauer, 2019). Other researchers emphasize attributions for discrimination alongside frequency. For example, Russell and colleagues found that the magnitude of the association between stigma-based bullying with substance use and school-related outcomes differed depending on attributions for bullying (Russell et al., 2012). More research is needed to determine whether attributing stigma to MI versus other stigmatized statuses matters in terms of health outcomes.

The Future of Mental Illness Stigma Measurement

The measurement of MI stigma has evolved significantly over the past several decades, in line with our evolving understanding of the complexity of MI stigma. Importantly, we have begun to accumulate an excellent set of tools for capturing the complex ways in which people experience stigma. Recent years have seen an increase in cross-cultural validations of existing measures, as well as the development of culture-specific measures. We have also seen an expansion of stigma measurement to include those who love, support, or treat people with MI as well as how people do (or do not) resist stigma. By expanding measurement efforts in these directions, researchers may better capture the broad scope of the impact of MI stigma and more successfully integrate strengths-based perspectives into MI stigma research (Logie et al., 2021).

Yet critical work still needs to be done to develop and validate MI stigma measures that capture the complex and varied ways people experience stigma. As such, it is vitally important researchers think carefully about whether the measures they plan to use are sufficient to capture the experiences of individuals who are affected by MI stigma, and work to fill in the gaps. We have argued that there are three primary areas of development needed to further advance the measurement of MI stigma: time, structural stigma, and intersectionality. These three areas for growth are inherently linked by an underlying acknowledgment of MI stigma as a multilevel and evolving social process. Researchers, organizations, and governments engaged in stigma reduction efforts via interventions, campaigns, and policy changes need to be able to accurately and comprehensively measure MI stigma to gauge the effectiveness of their efforts. Stigma campaigns that target individual-level attitudes but do not measure or address structural factors may be missing a key mechanism for reducing stigma. Interventions designed to improve help seeking among people with MI may fail without consideration of how MI stigma may change over the course of illness, and stigma reduction efforts that only focus on MI without consideration for intersectional statuses may miss important opportunities for dismantling systems of oppression. Ultimately, strong measures are needed to support efforts to dismantle MI stigma and improve the well-being of people with MI.

References

Berger, M. T. (2004). *Workable sisterhood: The political journey of stigmatized women with HIV/AIDS*. Princeton University Press.

Borschmann, R., Greenberg, N., Jones, N., & Henderson, R. C. (2014). Campaigns to reduce mental illness stigma in Europe: A scoping review. *Die Psychiatrie*, *11*(1), 43–50. https://doi.org/10.1055/s-0038-1670735

Bowleg, L. (2012). "Once you've blended the cake, you can't take the parts back to the main ingredients": Black gay and bisexual men's descriptions and experiences of intersectionality. *Sex Roles*, *68*(11–12), 754–767. https://doi.org/10.1007/s11199-012-0152-4

Bowleg, L. (2021). Evolving intersectionality within public health: From analysis to action. *American Journal of Public Health*, *111*(1), 88–90. https://doi.org/10.2105/AJPH.2020.306031

Boyd, J. E., Adler, E. P., Otilingam, P. G., & Peters, T. (2014). Internalized stigma of mental illness (ISMI) scale: A multinational review. *Comprehensive Psychiatry*, *55*(1), 221–231. https://doi.org/10.1016/j.comppsych.2013.06.005

Bracke, P., Delaruelle, K., & Verhaeghe, M. (2019). Dominant cultural and personal stigma beliefs and the utilization of mental health services: A cross-national comparison. *Frontiers in Sociology*, *4*, 40. https://doi.org/10.3389/fsoc.2019.00040

Brenner, R. E., Egli, M. R., & Hammer, J. H. (2022). Disentangling mental illness and help-seeking stigmas. In D. L. Vogel & N. Wade (Eds.), *Cambridge handbook of stigma and mental health* (pp. 31–51). Cambridge University Press. https://doi.org/10.1017/9781108920995.004

Brohan, E., Milenova, M., Bakolis, I., Evans-Lacko, S., Kohrt, B. A., & Thornicroft, G. (2022). Measurement of mental illness stigma and discrimination. In D. L. Vogel & N. Wade (Eds.), *Cambridge handbook of stigma and mental health* (pp. 52–72). Cambridge University Press. https://doi.org/10.1017/9781108920995.005

Caplan, S. (2016). A pilot study of a novel method of measuring stigma about depression developed for Latinos in the faith-based setting. *Community Mental Health Journal*, *52*(6), 701–709. https://doi.org/10.1007/s10597-016-0005-7

Chae, D. H., Clouston, S., Hatzenbuehler, M. L., Kramer, M. R., Cooper, H. L. F., Wilson, S. M., Stephens-Davidowitz, S. I., Gold, R. S., & Link, B. G. (2015). Association between an internet-based measure of area racism and black mortality. *PLoS One*, *10*(4), e0122963. https://doi.org/10.1371/journal.pone.0122963

Chae, D. H., Clouston, S., Martz, C. D., Hatzenbuehler, M. L., Cooper, H. L. F., Turpin, R., Stephens-Davidowitz, S., & Kramer, M. R. (2018). Area racism and birth outcomes among Blacks in the United States. *Social Science & Medicine*, *199*, 49–55. https://doi.org/10.1016/j.socscimed.2017.04.019

Chang, C. C., Su, J. A., Chang, K. C., Lin, C. Y., Koschorke, M., Rüsch, N., & Thornicroft, G. (2019). Development of the family stigma stress scale (FSSS) for detecting stigma stress in caregivers of people with mental illness. *Evaluation & the Health Professions*, *42*(2), 148–168. https://doi.org/10.1177/0163278717745658

Collins, P. Y., Elkington, K. S., von Unger, H., Sweetland, A., Wright, E. R., & Zybert, P. A. (2008). Relationship of stigma to HIV risk among women with mental illness. *The American Journal of Orthopsychiatry*, *78*(4), 498–506. https://doi.org/10.1037/a0014581

Corrigan, P. W. (2020). Community-based participatory research (CBPR), stigma, and health. *Stigma and Health*, *5*(2), 123–124. https://doi.org/10.1037/sah0000175

Corrigan, P. W., Larson, J. E., & Kuwabara, S. A. (2010). Social psychology of the stigma of mental illness: Public and self-stigma models. In J. E. Maddux (Ed.), *Social psychological foundations of clinical psychology* (Vol. 555, pp. 51–68). The Guilford Press.

Corrigan, P. W., & Oppenheim, M. (2023). The power of community-based participatory research (CBPR). *Psychiatric Rehabilitation Journal*, *47*(1), 2–8. https://doi.org/10.1037/prj0000568

Corrigan, P. W., Watson, A. C., Gracia, G., Slopen, N., Rasinski, K., & Hall, L. L. (2005a). Newspaper stories as measures of structural stigma. *Psychiatric Services*, *56*(5), 551–556. https://doi.org/10.1176/appi.ps.56.5.551

Corrigan, P. W., Watson, A. C., Heyrman, M. L., Warpinski, A., Gracia, G., Slopen, N., & Hall, L. L. (2005b). Structural stigma in state legislation. *Psychiatric Services*, *56*(5), 557–563. https://doi.org/10.1176/appi.ps.56.5.557

Corrigan, P. W., Watson, A. C., Warpinski, A. C., & Gracia, G. (2004). Stigmatizing attitudes about mental illness and allocation of resources to mental health services. *Community Mental Health Journal*, *40*(4), 297–307. https://doi.org/10.1023/b:comh.0000035226.19939.76

Duncan, D. T., Hatzenbuehler, M. L., & Johnson, R. M. (2014). Neighborhood-level LGBT hate crimes and current illicit drug use among sexual minority youth. *Drug and Alcohol Dependence*, *135*, 65–70. https://doi.org/10.1016/j.drugalcdep.2013.11.001

Earnshaw, V. A., Rendina, J. H., Bauer, G. R., Bonett, S., Bowleg, L., Carter, J., English, D., Friedman, M. R., Hatzenbuehler, M. L., Johnson, M. O., McCree, D. H., Neilands, T. B., Quinn, K. G., Robles, G., Scheim, A. I., Smith, J. C., Smith, L. R., Sprague, L., Taggart, T., ... Kerrigan, D. L. (2022a). Methods in HIV-related intersectional stigma research: Core elements and opportunities. *American Journal of Public Health*, *112*(S4), S413–S419. https://doi.org/10.2105/AJPH.2021.306710

Earnshaw, V. A., Watson, R. J., Eaton, L. A., Brousseau, N. M., Laurenceau, J.-P., & Fox, A. B. (2022b). Integrating time into stigma and health research. *Nature Reviews Psychology*, *1*(4), 236–247. https://doi.org/10.1038/s44159-022-00034-2

Evans-Lacko, S., Brohan, E., Mojtabai, R., & Thornicroft, G. (2012). Association between public views of mental illness and self-stigma among individuals with mental illness in 14 European countries. *Psychological Medicine*, *42*(8), 1741–1752. https://doi.org/10.1017/S0033291711002558

Evans-Lacko, S., Corker, E., Williams, P., Henderson, C., & Thornicroft, G. (2014). Effect of the time to change anti-stigma campaign on trends in mental-illness-related public stigma among the English population in 2003–13: An analysis of survey data. *The Lancet Psychiatry*, *1*(2), 121–128. https://doi.org/10.1016/S2215-0366(14)70243-3

Eylem, O., de Wit, L., van Straten, A., Steubl, L., Melissourgaki, Z., Danışman, G. T., de Vries, R., Kerkhof, A. J. F. M., Bhui, K., & Cuijpers, P. (2020). Stigma for common mental disorders in racial minorities and majorities a systematic review and meta-analysis. *BMC Public Health*, *20*(1), 879. https://doi.org/10.1186/s12889-020-08964-3

Ezell, J. M., Choi, C.-W. J., Wall, M. M., & Link, B. G. (2018). Measuring recurring stigma in the lives of individuals with mental illness. *Community Mental Health Journal*, *54*(1), 27–32. https://doi.org/10.1007/s10597-017-0156-1

Ferguson, L., Gruskin, S., Bolshakova, M., Yagyu, S., Fu, N., Cabrera, N., Rozelle, M., Kasoka, K., Oraro-Lawrence, T., Stackpool-Moore, L., Motala, A., & Hempel, S. (2022). Frameworks and measures for HIV-related internalized stigma, stigma and discrimination in healthcare and in laws and policies: A systematic review. *Journal of the International AIDS Society*, *25*(S1), e25915. https://doi.org/10.1002/jia2.25915

Firmin, R. L., Lysaker, P. H., McGrew, J. H., Minor, K. S., Luther, L., & Salyers, M. P. (2017). The stigma resistance scale: A multi-sample validation of a new instrument to assess mental illness stigma resistance. *Psychiatry Research*, *258*, 37–43. https://doi.org/10.1016/j.psychres.2017.09.063

Fiske, S. T., Cuddy, A. J. C., Glick, P., & Xu, J. (2002). A model of (often mixed) stereotype content: Competence and warmth respectively follow from perceived status and competition. *Journal of Personality and Social Psychology*, *82*(6), 878–902. https://doi.org/10.1037/0022-3514.82.6.878

Fox, A. B., Earnshaw, V. A., Taverna, E. C., & Vogt, D. (2018). Conceptualizing and measuring mental illness stigma: The mental illness stigma framework and critical review of measures. *Stigma and Health*, *3*(4), 348–376. https://doi.org/10.1037/sah0000104

Gabbidon, J., Farrelly, S., Hatch, S. L., Henderson, C., Williams, P., Bhugra, D., Dockery, L., Lassman, F., Thornicroft, G., & Clement, S. (2014). Discrimination attributed to mental illness or race-ethnicity by users of community psychiatric services. *Psychiatric Services*, *65*(11), 1360–1366. https://doi.org/10.1176/appi.ps.201300302

Gagné, T., Henderson, C., & McMunn, A. (2023). Is the self-reporting of mental health problems sensitive to public stigma towards mental illness? A comparison of time trends across English regions (2009–19). *Social Psychiatry and Psychiatric Epidemiology*, *58*(4), 671–680. https://doi.org/10.1007/s00127-022-02388-7

Goffman, E. (1963). *Stigma: Notes on the management of spoiled identity*. Simon and Schuster.

Groos, M., Wallace, M., Hardeman, R., & Theall, K. P. (2018). Measuring inequity: A systematic review of methods used to quantify structural racism. *Journal of Health Disparities Research and Practice*, *11*(2), 13. https://digitalscholarship.unlv.edu/jhdrp/vol11/iss2/13

Grover, S., Avasthi, A., Singh, A., Dan, A., Neogi, R., Kaur, D., Lakdawala, B., Rozatkar, A. R., Nebhinani, N., Patra, S., Sivashankar, P., Subramanyam, A. A., Tripathi, A., Gania, A. M., Singh, G. P., & Behere, P. (2017). Stigma experienced by patients with severe mental disorders: A nationwide multicentric study from India. *Psychiatry Research*, *257*, 550–558. https://doi.org/10.1016/j.psychres.2017.08.027

Hatzenbuehler, M. L. (2014). Structural stigma and the health of lesbian, gay, and bisexual populations. *Current Directions in Psychological Science*, *23*(2), 127–132. https://doi.org/10.1177/0963721414523775

Hatzenbuehler, M. L., Jun, H. J., Corliss, H. L., & Austin, S. B. (2014). Structural stigma and cigarette smoking in a prospective cohort study of sexual minority and heterosexual youth. *Annals of Behavioral Medicine*, *47*(1), 48–56. https://doi.org/10.1007/s12160-013-9548-9

Hatzenbuehler, M. L., & Link, B. G. (2014). Introduction to the special issue on structural stigma and health. *Social Science & Medicine*, *103*, 1–6. https://doi.org/10.1016/j.socscimed.2013.12.017

Healy, M., Richard, A., & Kidia, K. (2022). How to reduce stigma and bias in clinical communication: A narrative review. *Journal of General Internal Medicine*, *37*(10), 2533–2540. https://doi.org/10.1007/s11606-022-07609-y

Henderson, C., Noblett, J., Parke, H., Clement, S., Caffrey, A., Gale-Grant, O., Schulze, B., Druss, B., & Thornicroft, G. (2014). Mental health-related stigma in health care and mental health-care settings. *The Lancet*, *1*(6), 467–482. https://doi.org/10.1016/S2215-0366(14)00023-6

Isoya, H., & Yamada, H. (2021). Hidden internet-based measure of discrimination and mental health of Black people. *Social Science & Medicine*, *273*, 113776. https://doi.org/10.1016/j.socscimed.2021.113776

Jones, E. E., Farina, A., Hastorf, A. H., Markus, H., Miller, D. T., & Scott, R. A. (1984). *Social stigma: The psychology of marked relationships. Freeman*. https://doi.org/10.1146/annurev.psych.56.091103.070137

Jorm, A. F., Christensen, H., & Griffiths, K. M. (2005). The impact of *Beyondblue*: The national depression initiative on the Australian public's recognition of depression and beliefs about treatments. *The Australian and New Zealand Journal of Psychiatry*, *39*(4), 248–254. https://doi.org/10.1080/j.1440-1614.2005.01561.x

Kaushik, A., Kostaki, E., & Kyriakopoulos, M. (2016). The stigma of mental illness in children and adolescents: A systematic review. *Psychiatry Research*, *243*, 469–494. https://doi.org/10.1016/j.psychres.2016.04.042

Knaak, S., Livingston, J., Stuart, H., & Ungar, T. (2020). *Combating mental illness-and substance use-related structural stigma in health care*. Mental Health Commission of Canada. https://mentalhealthcommission.ca/wp-content/uploads/2021/09/Combating-Mental-Illness-and-Substance-Use-Related-Structural-Stigma-in-Health-Care.pdf

Liese, B. H., Gribble, R. S. F., & Wickremsinhe, M. N. (2019). International funding for mental health: A review of the last decade. *International Health*, *11*(5), 361–369. https://doi.org/10.1093/inthealth/ihz040

Link, B. G., & Phelan, J. C. (2001). Conceptualizing stigma. *Annual Review of Sociology*, *27*(1), 363–385. https://doi.org/10.1146/annurev.soc.27.1.363

Link, B. G., Struening, E. L., Rahav, M., Phelan, J. C., & Nuttbrock, L. (1997). On stigma and its consequences: Evidence from a longitudinal study of men with dual diagnoses of mental illness and substance abuse. *Journal of Health and Social Behavior*, *38*(2), 177–190. http://www.jstor.org/stable/2955424

Livingston, J. D. (2013). *Mental illness-related structural stigma*. Mental Health Commission of Canada. https://commissionsantementale.ca/wp-content/uploads/drupal/MHCC_OpeningMinds_MentalIllness-Related SructuralStigmaReport_ENG_0_0.pdf

Livingston, J. D. (2020). *Structural stigma in health-care contexts for people with mental health and substance use issues*. Mental Health Commission of Canada. https://www.mentalhealthcommission.ca/wp-content/uploads/drupal/2020-07/structural_stigma_in_healthcare_eng.pdf

Livingston, J. D. (2021). *A framework for assessing structural stigma in health-care contexts for people with mental health and substance use issues*. Mental Health Commission of Canada. https://mentalhealthcommission.ca/wp-content/uploads/2021/09/Structural_Stigma_Assessment_Report_eng.pdf

Livingston, J. D., & Boyd, J. E. (2010). Correlates and consequences of internalized stigma for people living with mental illness: A systematic review and meta-analysis. *Social Science & Medicine*, *71*(12), 2150–2161. https://doi.org/10.1016/j.socscimed.2010.09.030

Logie, C. H., Earnshaw, V., Nyblade, L., Turan, J., Stangl, A., Poteat, T., Nelson, L., & Baral, S. (2021). A scoping review of the integration of empowerment-based perspectives in quantitative intersectional stigma research. *Global Public Health*, *17*(8), 1451–1466. https://doi.org/10.1080/17441692.2021.1934061

Mackenzie, C. S., Heath, P. J., & Vogel, D. L. (2019). Age differences in public stigma, self-stigma, and attitudes toward seeking help: A moderated mediation model. *Journal of Clinical Psychology*, *75*(12), 2073–2292. https://onlinelibrary.wiley.com/doi/abs/10.1002/jclp.22845

Mak, W. W. S., & Cheung, R. Y. M. (2008). Affiliate stigma among caregivers of people with intellectual disability or mental illness. *Journal of Applied Research in Intellectual Disabilities*, *21*(6), 532–545. https://doi.org/10.1111/j.1468-3148.2008.00426.x

McKeague, L., Hennessy, E., O'Driscoll, C., & Heary, C. (2015). Peer mental health stigmatization scale: Psychometric properties of a questionnaire for children and adolescents. *Child and Adolescent Mental Health*, *20*(3), 163–170. https://doi.org/10.1111/camh.12088

McKenzie, S. K., Oliffe, J. L., Black, A., & Collings, S. (2022). Men's experiences of mental illness stigma across the lifespan: A scoping review. *American Journal of Men's Health*, *16*(1). https://doi.org/10.1177/15579883221074789

Misra, S., Jackson, V. W., Chong, J., Choe, K., Tay, C., Wong, J., & Yang, L. H. (2021). Systematic review of cultural aspects of stigma and mental illness among racial and ethnic minority groups in the United States: Implications for interventions. *American Journal of Community Psychology*, *68*(3–4), 486–512. https://doi.org/10.1002/ajcp.12516

Morris, E., Hippman, C., Murray, G., Michalak, E. E., Boyd, J. E., Livingston, J., Inglis, A., Carrion, P., & Austin, J. (2018). Self-stigma in relatives of people with mental illness scale: Development and validation. *The British Journal of Psychiatry*, *212*(3), 169–174. https://doi.org/10.1192/bjp.2017.23

Pachankis, J. E., Hatzenbuehler, M. L., Bränström, R., Schmidt, A. J., Berg, R. C., Jonas, K., Pitoňák, M., Baros, S., & Weatherburn, P. (2021). Structural stigma and sexual minority men's depression and suicidality: A multilevel examination of mechanisms and mobility across 48 countries. *Journal of Abnormal Psychology*, *130*(7), 713–726. https://doi.org/10.1037/abn0000693

Pachankis, J. E., Hatzenbuehler, M. L., & Starks, T. J. (2014). The influence of structural stigma and rejection sensitivity on young sexual minority men's daily tobacco and alcohol use. *Social Science & Medicine*, *103*, 67–75. https://doi.org/10.1016/j.socscimed.2013.10.005

Pence, B. W., O'Donnell, J. K., & Gaynes, B. N. (2012). The depression treatment cascade in primary care: A public health perspective. *Current Psychiatry Reports*, *14*(4), 328–335. https://doi.org/10.1007/s11920-012-0274-y

Phelan, J. C., Link, B. G., Stueve, A., & Pescosolido, B. A. (2000). Public conceptions of mental illness in 1950 and 1996: What is mental illness and is it to be feared? *Journal of Health and Social Behavior*, *41*(2), 188–207. https://doi.org/10.2307/2676305

Pugh, T., Hatzenbuehler, M., & Link, B. (2015). *Structural stigma and mental illness*. Commissioned paper for Committee on the Science of Changing Behavioral Health Social Norms, Mailman School of Public, Columbia University (August 2015). https://sites.nationalacademies.org/cs/groups/dbassesite/documents/webpage/dbasse_170045.pdf

Ricciardelli, R., Carleton, R. N., Mooney, T., & Cramm, H. (2020). "Playing the system": Structural factors potentiating mental health stigma, challenging awareness, and creating barriers to care for Canadian public safety personnel. *Health*, *24*(3), 259–278. https://doi.org/10.1177/1363459318800167

Ritsher, J. B., Otilingam, P. G., & Grajales, M. (2003). Internalized stigma of mental illness: Psychometric properties of a new measure. *Psychiatry Research*, *121*(1), 31–49. https://doi.org/10.1016/j.psychres.2003.08.008

Ritsher, J. B., & Phelan, J. C. (2004). Internalized stigma predicts erosion of morale among psychiatric outpatients. *Psychiatry Research, 129*(3), 257–265.

Russell, S. T., Sinclair, K. O., Poteat, V. P., & Koenig, B. W. (2012). Adolescent health and harassment based on discriminatory bias. *American Journal of Public Health, 102*(3), 493–495. https://doi.org/10.2105/AJPH.2011.300430

Saewyc, E. M., Konishi, C., Rose, H. A., & Homma, Y. (2014). School-based strategies to reduce suicidal ideation, suicide attempts, and discrimination among sexual minority and heterosexual adolescents in Western Canada. *International Journal of Child, Youth & Family Studies, 5*(1), 89–112. https://doi.org/10.18357/ijcyfs.saewyce.512014

Scheim, A. I., & Bauer, G. R. (2019). The intersectional discrimination index: Development and validation of measures of self-reported enacted and anticipated discrimination for intercategorical analysis. *Social Science & Medicine, 226*, 225–235. https://doi.org/10.1016/j.socscimed.2018.12.016

Schomerus, G., Lucht, M., Holzinger, A., Matschinger, H., Carta, M. G., & Angermeyer, M. C. (2011). The stigma of alcohol dependence compared with other mental disorders: A review of population studies. *Alcohol and Alcoholism, 46*(2), 105–112. https://doi.org/10.1093/alcalc/agq089

Schomerus, G., Schindler, S., Sander, C., Baumann, E., & Angermeyer, M. C. (2022). Changes in mental illness stigma over 30 years - improvement, persistence, or deterioration? *European Psychiatry, 65*(1), e78. https://doi.org/10.1192/j.eurpsy.2022.2337

Schomerus, G., Schwahn, C., Holzinger, A., Corrigan, P. W., Grabe, H. J., Carta, M. G., & Angermeyer, M. C. (2012). Evolution of public attitudes about mental illness: A systematic review and meta-analysis. *Acta Psychiatrica Scandinavica, 125*(6), 440–452. https://doi.org/10.1111/j.1600-0447.2012.01826.x

Siddaway, A. P., Wood, A. M., & Hedges, L. V. (2019). How to do a systematic review: A best practice guide for conducting and reporting narrative reviews, meta-analyses, and meta-syntheses. *Annual Review of Psychology, 70*, 747–770. https://doi.org/10.1146/annurev-psych-010418-102803

Sukhera, J., Knaak, S., Ungar, T., & Rehman, M. (2022). Dismantling structural stigma related to mental health and substance use: An educational framework. *Academic Medicine, 97*(2), 175–181. https://doi.org/10.1097/ACM.0000000000004451

Terwee, C. B., Bot, S. D. M., de Boer, M. R., van der Windt, D. A. W. M., Knol, D. L., Dekker, J., Bouter, L. M., & de Vet, H. C. W. (2007). Quality criteria were proposed for measurement properties of health status questionnaires. *Journal of Clinical Epidemiology, 60*(1), 34–42. https://doi.org/10.1016/j.jclinepi.2006.03.012

Thomas, S., Pai, N., Dawes, K., Wilson, C., & Williams, V. (2013). Updating medical school psychiatry curricula to meet projected mental health needs. *Australasian Psychiatry, 21*(6), 578–582. https://doi.org/10.1177/1039856213500092

Ungar, T., & Moothathamby, N. (2020). *Structural stigma in health care for mental health and substance use.* Mental Health Commission of Canada. https://www.mentalhealthcommission.ca/wp-content/uploads/drupal/2020-07/structural_stigma_in_health_care_for_mental_health_and_substance_use_eng.pdf

Verhaeghe, M., & Bracke, P. (2012). Associative stigma among mental health professionals: Implications for professional and service user well-being. *Journal of Health and Social Behavior, 53*(1), 17–32. https://doi.org/10.1177/0022146512439453

Wei, Y., McGrath, P., Hayden, J., & Kutcher, S. (2018). The quality of mental health literacy measurement tools evaluating the stigma of mental illness: A systematic review. *Epidemiology and Psychiatric Sciences, 27*(5), 433–462. https://doi.org/10.1017/S2045796017000178

Weiner, S. G., Lo, Y.-C., Carroll, A. D., Zhou, L., Ngo, A., Hathaway, D. B., Rodriguez, C. P., & Wakeman, S. E. (2023). The incidence and disparities in use of stigmatizing language in clinical notes for patients with substance use disorder. *Journal of Addiction Medicine, 17*(4), 424–430. https://doi.org/10.1097/ADM.0000000000001145

West, M. L., Yanos, P. T., Smith, S. M., Roe, D., & Lysaker, P. H. (2011). Prevalence of internalized stigma among persons with severe mental illness. *Stigma Research and Action, 1*(1), 3–10. https://doi.org/10.5463/sra.v1i1.9

Williams, D. R., Yu, Y., Jackson, J. S., & Anderson, N. B. (1997). Racial differences in physical and mental health socioeconomic status, stress and discrimination. *Journal of Health Psychology, 2*, 335–351. https://doi.org/10.1177/135910539700200305

Yang, L., & Pearson, V. (2002). Understanding families in their own context: Schizophrenia and structural family therapy in Beijing. *Journal of Family Therapy, 24*(3), 233–257. https://doi.org/10.1111/1467-6427.00214

11

Refining the Concept of Mental Health Literacy: Criteria for Determining What the Public Needs to Know

Anthony F. Jorm
University of Melbourne

Together with some colleagues, I introduced the term *mental health literacy* in Australia in 1997. We defined it as "knowledge and beliefs about mental disorders which aid their recognition, management or prevention" (Jorm et al., 1997, p. 182). We elaborated on the concept by stating that "mental health literacy includes the ability to recognize specific disorders; knowing how to seek mental health information; knowledge of risk factors and causes, of self-treatments, and of professional help available; and attitudes that promote recognition and help-seeking" (p. 182).

The aim of introducing the term was simply to draw attention to a neglected area. At that time, there was considerable interest in Australia in educating health professionals, such as general practitioners, about how to recognize and better manage mental disorders, but educating the public was not seen as a priority. Members of the public were seen as passive recipients of the actions taken by health professionals for their benefit rather than as active participants in influencing their own mental health. By creating a concept that captured the need for education to empower members of the public to take action to improve mental health, we hoped to increase the national focus on this area.

Subsequently, I expanded on the concept by highlighting the stark contrast between public awareness of physical and mental health actions. While people generally know how to take action on prevention, early intervention and treatment of physical diseases, they are often ignorant about preventing mental disorders, delay or avoid seeking treatment, and are unsure how to help others with mental health problems (Jorm, 2012). I proposed that mental health literacy has many components, including:

> (a) Knowledge of how to prevent mental disorders, (b) recognition of when a disorder is developing, (c) knowledge of help-seeking options and treatments available, (d) knowledge of effective self-help strategies for milder problems, and (e) first aid skills to support others who are developing a mental disorder or are in a mental health crisis. (Jorm, 2012, p. 231)

More recently, I have expressed concern that, while the concept of mental health literacy has been very influential, much of the research on the topic has not led to any practical benefit (Jorm, 2020). This is because research has generally focused on measuring mental health literacy, surveying mental health literacy in various populations, and examining its association with other variables, such as help-seeking intentions and stigma. There has been much less work on changing behavior or improving mental health. I pointed out that the original definition of mental health literacy included a link to action: "....which aid their recognition, management and prevention" (Jorm et al., 1997, p. 182).

The Handbook of Mental Health Communication, First Edition.
Edited by Marco C. Yzer and Jason T. Siegel.

Later, I made this link more explicit (Jorm, 2012, p. 231): "It is important to note that mental health literacy is not simply a matter of having knowledge…. Rather it is knowledge that is linked to the possibility of action to benefit one's own mental health or that of others." This definition implies a causal link from mental health literacy to mental health action to better mental health. To put more emphasis on the importance of behavior change, I proposed a new complementary concept of *mental health action*, which I defined as "action that individuals or groups take to benefit their own mental health or that of others" (Jorm, 2020, p. 1).

These conceptualizations of mental health literacy and action do not take account of any specific requirements for particular stages of the lifespan or social roles. Recognizing that adults who interact with children may need specific knowledge to benefit child mental health, Hart et al. (2023, p. 339) have proposed the concept of *mental health literacy for supporting children,* which they defined as "adults' knowledge and beliefs that support action to prevent or manage mental health problems in children." Hart et al. (2023, p. 339) see mental health literacy for supporting children as involving the:

1 ability to recognize when a child is developing a mental health problem (e.g., not coping, experiencing increasing distress, or difficulty functioning as expected)
2 knowledge and attitudes about (a) how to seek and engage critically with information about child mental health, (b) risk factors and causes of mental health problems in children, and (c) sources of formal and informal help for both the child and caregivers
3 ability to communicate about child mental health and supportive strategies with (a) the child in a developmentally appropriate manner; and (b) other adults who care for or are responsible for the child

This developmentally aligned concept is quite compatible with earlier definitions of mental health literacy and mental health action by Jorm et al. (1997) and Jorm (2020).

Alternative Conceptualizations of Mental Health Literacy

Since the original definition was proposed, others have proposed alternative definitions or extensions of the concept. The most influential alternative definition, as judged by citations, is from Kutcher and colleagues (Kutcher et al., 2015, 2016). Influenced by evolving definitions of health literacy more generally and focusing on the needs of young people, they defined mental health literacy as:

> understanding of how to obtain and maintain positive mental health; understanding mental disorders and their treatments; decreasing stigma related to mental disorders; and, enhancing help-seeking efficacy (knowing when and how to seek help and developing competencies designed to improve one's mental health care and self-management capabilities). (Kutcher et al., 2016, p. 155)

Essentially, Kutcher et al. (2015, 2016) have broadened the original concept to include an understanding of positive mental health (aka well-being), help-seeking efficacy, and reduction of stigma. On the other hand, they have removed knowledge of how to assist others who have mental health problems.

Other authors have proposed definitions of mental health literacy that have emphasized positive mental health, although these definitions have been much less influential than the alternative offered by Kutcher and colleagues. Kusan (2013, p.14) argued that the original definition of Jorm et al. (1997) was overly narrow and based on "the dominant biomedical orientation of the mental health field" (p. 1). He defined mental health literacy as "the self-generated and acquired knowledge with which people negotiate their mental health" (p. 1). He saw this broader definition as including concepts from positive psychology, including resilience, salutogenesis, and mindfulness.

Bjørnsen and colleagues (2017a, 2017b) also emphasized the importance of young people knowing about what contributes to positive mental health. Their concept of *positive mental health literacy* elaborated the first component of Kutcher et al.'s (2015, 2016) definition (i.e., understanding of how to obtain and maintain positive mental health). This positive mental health literacy involved knowing about the importance of factors such as handling stressful situations in a good manner, believing in yourself, having good sleep routines, making decisions based on your own will, setting limits for your actions, feeling that you belong to a community, mastering your own negative thoughts, setting limits for what is OK for you, feeling valuable regardless of your own accomplishments, and experiencing school mastery.

How Broad Should the Concept of Mental Health Literacy Be?

Spiker and Hammer (2018) have questioned the expansion of the concept of mental health literacy beyond mental health knowledge. They gave three reasons for concern about the expansion: (a) It is important to have a consistent definition of mental health literacy to allow comparison across studies; (b) if mental health literacy is defined too broadly, it loses its meaningfulness, as it incorporates features of other constructs; and (c) a broader definition results in a proliferation of constructs that overlap with existing constructs. They state that "the inclusion of attitudes, stigma, positive mental health and help-seeking efficacy in [mental health literacy's] content domain simply repackages these well-established constructs into a broader construct with a new name...which can create confusion among researchers" (p. 239).

To overcome this problem, Spiker and Hammer (2018) argued that mental health literacy needs to be reconceptualized as a multiconstruct theory, which specifies the interrelationships among constructs such as mental health knowledge, stigma, attitudes, positive mental health, and help-seeking efficacy. They did not themselves propose such a theory but stated:

> To further MHL as a theory, researchers must (i) agree upon what forms of mental health knowledge should be incorporated into the mental health knowledge construct and (ii) be explicit about the interrelationships among the various constructs invoked by the theory. (Spiker & Hammer, 2018, p. 241)

I agree with Spiker and Hammer's (2018) concerns. The concepts of stigma and positive mental health are themselves multidimensional and have their own complex literatures on measurement and approaches to intervention. Rather than a broadening of the concept of mental health literacy, I believe we need a tighter specification of what should be incorporated into the concept. As a first step in this direction, in the current chapter, I present a proposal for how researchers should determine what knowledge should be incorporated into the construct.

Proposed Criteria for Determining What the Public Needs to Know

The original definition of mental health literacy and the subsequent definition of mental health action imply a causal link from knowledge to action to better mental health. Based on these causal links, I propose the following criteria for determining what members of the public need to know:

1 *The knowledge is relevant.* The knowledge concerns mental health problems that are relevant to the person's stage of life (e.g. adolescent, adult), their social roles (e.g., parent, work supervisor, carer), and their culture (e.g., the problem is prevalent in the culture). In the area of prevention, for example, it is relevant for parents of adolescents to know what actions they can take to reduce their children's risk of misusing substances. An example of relevant knowledge in the area of mental health first aid is for an adult to know what to do if someone in their social network is suicidal. In the area of professional help seeking, it is relevant for a person with symptoms that impair their functioning to know about evidence-based options for professional help in their community.
2 *The knowledge underpins action.* The knowledge can be translated into specific actions that an individual can feasibly take to improve their own mental health or that of others. This criterion would exclude, for example, many types of psychiatric textbook knowledge that are unlikely to inform

action, such as findings on prevalence, diagnostic methods, genetics, neurochemistry, or brain imaging. If applied to the examples given for criterion 1, the knowledge would need to specify particular parenting strategies that can be used to reduce adolescents' risk of misusing substances, specific first aid actions that a member of the public should take to reduce a person's risk of suicide, and the particular types of evidence-based help a person with symptoms should seek.

3 *The action benefits mental health.* There is evidence that the action is associated with better mental health outcomes. Ideally, the evidence would indicate that any association is likely to be causal, with longitudinal or experimental evidence more convincing than cross-sectional associations. In the previous examples, this criterion would entail showing that specific parenting strategies prevent substance misuse in adolescents, that suicide first aid strategies reduce the risk of suicidal actions, and that seeking evidence-based professional help reduces symptoms.

Considered in terms of the links from knowledge to action to mental health, criterion 2 covers the knowledge–action link, while criterion 3 covers the action–mental health link.

Some Case Studies Fulfilling the Criteria

To illustrate how the criteria might be used in practice, this chapter presents two case studies in which methods consistent with the criteria have been used to determine what the public needs to know about some specific components of mental health literacy.

Parenting Strategies for Prevention of Depression and Anxiety

The first example concerns what parents of adolescents should know about parenting strategies that can reduce their children's risk of developing depression and anxiety symptoms, which is a type of universal prevention. There is evidence that a range of modifiable parenting factors increase the risk for depression or anxiety in adolescents, including less warmth, more interparental conflict, overinvolvement, aversiveness, and less autonomy granting and monitoring (Yap et al., 2014a). However, the research showing the association of these factors with increased risk does not provide detailed advice on what parents should actually do, for example, what specific behaviors should a parent engage in to show warmth or provide monitoring. To provide this detail, Yap et al. (2014b) carried out a Delphi expert consensus study. A literature search identified 402 recommendations for parenting strategies, which were rated by a panel of international experts for their preventive importance. To help their judgments, the experts were provided with a systematic review of the risk and protection factor evidence on parenting. The experts endorsed 190 of the parenting strategies, which were categorized under 11 headings:

1. You can reduce your child's risk of depression and anxiety problems
2. Establish and maintain a good relationship with your teenager
3. Be involved and support increasing autonomy
4. Establish family rules and consequences
5. Minimize conflict in the home
6. Encourage supportive relationships
7. Help your teenager deal with problems
8. Encourage good health habits
9. Help your teenager to deal with anxiety
10. Encourage professional help seeking when needed
11. Do not blame yourself.

A range of interventions was then developed to increase parents' use of the strategies, with varying degrees of intensity of intervention used to produce change (Yap et al., 2017a). The simplest level of intervention was a set of parenting guidelines that could be downloaded from the Internet (Yap et al. 2017b). In an evaluation of these guidelines, parents who downloaded them were asked one month later about the impact of reading them. Most parents reported that the guidelines were useful and that they had tried to make positive changes in their parenting.

The next level of intervention involved providing parents with tailored feedback on their parenting. The Parenting to Reduce Adolescent Depression and Anxiety Scale (PRADAS) was developed to measure a parent's concordance with the practices recommended in the guidelines (Cardamone-Breen, et al., 2017). Most parents of adolescents were found to have considerable room for improvement in their parenting. As expected, parents who had higher concordance had fewer depression and anxiety symptoms in their child (Cardamone-Breen et al., 2017). The PRADAS was then used for tailoring an online intervention called Partners in Parenting to improve preventive parenting (Yap et al., 2017). After completing the PRADAS, a parent was given a personalized feedback report on what they were doing well and on areas where they could improve. Recommendations were made for a series of online interactive modules in areas of parenting where improvements could be made. Parents then received links to the modules on a weekly basis and prompts to complete them. Parents could either complete the modules independently or also receive additional phone support from a coach who discussed the content with them.

A randomized trial has compared Partners in Parenting with a control condition in which parents received web-based fact sheets on adolescent development and well-being. Immediately after intervention, the Partners in Parenting intervention was found to produce an improvement in self-reporting parenting behaviors, consistent with what was taught in the modules (Yap et al., 2018). A 12-month follow-up showed that these gains in parenting persisted and that parents who received Partners in Parenting also reported a greater reduction in their child's depressive symptoms (Yap et al., 2019). A mediation analysis showed that the reduction in depressive symptoms was mediated by the improvements in parenting.

This series of studies meets the three criteria for identifying what parents of adolescents need to know about reducing their child's risk of depression and anxiety. First, the knowledge is relevant, as demonstrated by the expert consensus from the Delphi study and parents' assessment that the guidelines provided useful information. Second, the knowledge underpins action, as shown by the improvement in parenting when parents downloaded the guidelines or received the Partners in Parenting intervention. Finally, the action benefits mental health, as shown by the correlation of parents' PRADAS scores with better mental health in their adolescent child and by the mediation analysis linking improvements in parenting behavior after completing Partners in Parenting with perceived reduction in their child's depressive symptoms.

Self-Help Strategies for Sub-Threshold Depression

The second example concerns what people with sub-threshold depressive symptoms should know about informal self-help strategies to prevent progression to a depressive disorder, which is a type of indicated prevention. Informal self-help strategies are those used by people to deal with mental health problems without professional guidance. Surveys of the public show that members of the public rate informal self-help strategies as likely to be helpful for mental health problems and that they commonly use them (Jorm, 2012). I have previously included knowledge of effective self-help strategies for milder problems as one of the components of mental health literacy.

To find out which self-help strategies might be helpful for sub-threshold depression, Morgan and Jorm (2009) carried out a literature search to identify 282 potential self-help strategies. They carried out a Delphi expert consensus study with both professional and depression consumer experts to find out which of these strategies were most likely to be helpful as well as feasible to carry out. Panelists were provided with a systematic review of available trials of self-help interventions to assist their judgments (Morgan & Jorm, 2008). Fourteen strategies were identified as both likely to be helpful and feasible. The endorsed strategies were generally lifestyle changes (e.g., "Engage in exercise or physical activity") or psychosocial activities (e.g., "Talk over problems or feelings with someone who is supportive and caring").

Morgan et al. (2012) created a questionnaire about the use of the 14 strategies and their perceived helpfulness, which was administered to a sample of people with sub-threshold depression symptoms. The strategies were rated on a four-point scale for frequency of use over the previous month. Where a strategy had been used, it was also rated for perceived helpfulness on a 4-point scale. The strategies varied considerably in how frequently they were used and how helpful they were perceived to be. However, there was only a small association ($r = 0.21$) between the mean ratings of frequency of use and the mean ratings of helpfulness. This indicated that the most helpful strategies were not necessarily the ones most frequently used and that there was considerable potential to increase the use of the more helpful strategies.

Morgan et al. (2013) carried out a randomized controlled trial of an online intervention to promote the use of the 14 strategies to people with sub-threshold depressive symptoms. Participants were sent emails twice weekly over six weeks, with the experimental group receiving messages promoting the self-help strategies and the control group given general information about depression. The intervention led to an increase in reported use of self-help strategies and also a reduction in depressive symptoms. A mediation analysis showed that the effect of the email intervention on depressive symptoms was mediated by the increased use of the strategies.

This series of studies meets the three criteria for identifying what people with sub-threshold depressive symptoms need to know about self-help. First, the knowledge is relevant, as demonstrated by the expert consensus from the Delphi study. Second, the knowledge underpins action, as shown by the increase in the use of the recommended strategies when they were promoted via regular emails. Finally, the action benefits mental health, as shown by the mediation analysis linking the use of the strategies to improvement in depressive symptoms.

Evaluation of Commonly Used Mental Health Literacy Measures Against the Criteria

The three proposed criteria for what the public needs to know about mental health can be used to assess the content of existing mental health literacy measures. A systematic review by Wei et al. (2016) identified 16 mental health knowledge scales, which they evaluated for measurement properties. Most of these scales have had limited use and were not rated highly by Wei et al. (2016) for measurement properties. By far the most cited of these measures (as indicated by Google Scholar) are the Mental Health Knowledge Schedule (MAKS; Evans-Lacko et al., 2010) and the Mental Health Literacy Scale (MHLS; O'Connor and Casey, 2015). The MHLS was also the most highly rated scale by Wei et al. (2016). For these reasons, these two scales are reviewed here.

Mental Health Knowledge Schedule

The MAKS was developed by Evans-Lacko et al. (2010) as a measure of the knowledge component of stigma. Items were developed based on a literature review of types of knowledge that might influence subsequent mental health-related attitudes and behaviors and by advice on content coverage from an international panel of experts. The MAKS consists of 12 items covering knowledge of professional help, treatments and recovery, and various mental health problems. The authors stated that the content of the scale was intentionally heterogeneous and was not designed to be unidimensional. The original MAKS development study examined the feasibility of completing the scale in a reasonable time, looked for floor and ceiling effects, and assessed test–retest reliability. However, it provided little evidence relevant to the three criteria proposed above. Arguably, the content of the scale fulfills criterion 1 (relevance) for adults, as all adults are at risk of developing a mental health problem and will have contact with others who have mental health problems, so the sort of knowledge covered by the MAKS will be of personal relevance to them.

Subsequent research on the MAKS from Waldmann et al. (2020) provides evidence relevant to criterion 2 (underpins action) and criterion 3 (benefits mental health). These authors carried out a cross-sectional survey of unemployed persons with mental health problems in Germany. In addition to the MAKS, participants were assessed for help-seeking behaviors and mental health. Higher MAKS scores were associated with greater help seeking from health professionals and from family and friends, while help seeking from professionals (but not from family and friends) was associated with fewer symptoms of mental ill health. While these associations are consistent with criteria 2 and 3, the data were cross-sectional, so the causal link from knowledge to action to better mental health is only weakly supported. Longitudinal data on these associations would strengthen the credibility of the MAKS as a measure of mental health literacy which informs professional help-seeking actions.

Mental Health Literacy Scale

The MHLS was developed by O'Connor and Casey (2015) using Jorm et al.'s (1997) definition of mental health literacy as a guiding framework. It consists of 35 items covering the ability to recognize disorders, knowledge of how to seek mental health information, knowledge of risk factors and causes, knowledge of self-treatments, knowledge of professional help available, and attitudes that promote recognition and appropriate help seeking. The items were generated using the consensus advice of a clinical panel and pilot testing of a larger pool of items to remove those with poorer psychometric properties. Supporting the validity of the scale, the authors found that people who would be expected to have greater mental health literacy (mental health professionals and individuals who had had a mental illness) had higher scores on the scale.

The content of the MHLS satisfies criterion 1 (relevance) for adults, as all the items are relevant to action on adult mental health. However, the evidence for satisfying Criterion 2 (underpins action) and Criterion 3 (benefits mental health) is weak. O'Connor and Casey (2015) reported that the MHLS had a positive correlation with intentions to seek help for a mental health problem as measured by the General Help-Seeking Questionnaire, but provided no data on whether MHLS scores were associated with actual help seeking. A number of subsequent cross-sectional studies have also found an association between the MHLS and help-seeking intentions (Almanasef, 2021; Gorczynski et al., 2017; Moss et al., 2022), but other studies have not found a significant association (Gorczynski et al., 2020a, 2020b). Again, no data were reported on help-seeking actions. A number of these studies also reported on the correlation of the MHLS with psychological distress, with some finding a small negative correlation (Gorczynski et al., 2017; Moss et al., 2022) and others finding no significant association (O'Connor & Casey, 2015; Gorczynski et al., 2020a, 2020b).

Conclusion and Future Directions

Various definitions of mental health literacy have been proposed, leading to potential confusion about the concept and blurring its boundaries with other related concepts. Progress in mental health literacy research has also been hampered by a strong focus on knowledge with a relative neglect of putting this knowledge into action to benefit mental health. To clarify what mental health knowledge should be promoted to the public, three criteria are proposed here: the knowledge is relevant, the knowledge underpins action, and the action benefits mental health. These criteria define a subset of knowledge that has strong evidence of mental health benefits. The original definition of mental health literacy can be modified to incorporate both the concept of mental health action and the proposed criteria. Putting these together, we could say that mental health literacy is knowledge about mental health problems that underpins action that can benefit mental health. This definition involves a tightening of the concept, in contrast to proposals that others have put to broaden it.

This modified conceptualization of mental health literacy has clear implications for developing measures. To develop measures meeting all three criteria is a major task and will necessarily proceed in stages. Fulfilling criterion 1 (relevance) is comparatively straightforward and can be done during scale construction. Providing evidence for criterion 2 (underpins action) and criterion 3 (benefits mental health) is more demanding and will necessitate a program of research involving longitudinal and experimental evidence. The two case studies presented herein involved the development of measures that are quite specific in the knowledge and actions they assess. However, it would be possible to also develop broader multicomponent measures of mental health literacy that meet the proposed criteria.

The two most popular generic mental health literacy scales, the MAKS and the MHLS, only partially meet the criteria at present. Future work is needed to determine whether higher scores on these measures are associated with benefits to mental health.

As well as more clearly specifying that types of knowledge should be subsumed under mental health literacy, the modified definition links the concept more closely to intervention. When setting goals for improving mental health literacy, there needs to be an explicit program logic in which mental health literacy leads to action to improve mental health, which in turn leads to better mental health. Evaluations of interventions to improve mental health literacy then need to be based on this program logic.

The concept of mental health literacy was originally introduced to draw attention to the need for education to empower members of the public to take action to improve mental health. By more clearly specifying what types of knowledge are covered by the concept and making explicit the link to action for improving mental health, the hope is that this chapter will further advance this goal.

References

Almanasef, M. (2021). Mental health literacy and help-seeking behaviours among undergraduate pharmacy students in Abha, Saudi Arabia. *Risk Management and Healthcare Policy*, *14*, 1281–1286. https://doi.org/10.2147/rmhp.s289211

Bjørnsen, H. N., Eilertsen, M. B., Ringdal, R., Espnes, G. A., & Moksnes, U. K. (2017a). Positive mental health literacy: Development and validation of a measure among Norwegian adolescents. *BMC Public Health*, *17*(1). https://doi.org/10.1186/s12889-017-4733-6

Bjørnsen, H. N., Espnes, G. A., Eilertsen, M.-E. B., Ringdal, R., & Moksnes, U. K. (2017b). The relationship between positive mental health literacy and mental well-being among adolescents: Implications for school health services. *Journal of School Nursing*, *35*(2), 107–116. https://doi.org/10.1177/1059840517732125

Cardamone-Breen, M. C., Jorm, A. F., Lawrence, K. A., Mackinnon, A. J., & Yap, M. B. H. (2017). The parenting to reduce adolescent depression and anxiety scale: Assessing parental concordance with parenting guidelines for the prevention of adolescent depression and anxiety disorders. *PeerJ*, *5*, e3825. Portico. https://doi.org/10.7717/peerj.3825

Evans-Lacko, S., Little, K., Meltzer, H., Rose, D., Rhydderch, D., Henderson, C., & Thornicroft, G. (2010). Development and psychometric properties of the mental health knowledge schedule. *The Canadian Journal of Psychiatry*, *55*(7), 440–448. https://doi.org/10.1177/070674371005500707

Gorczynski, P., Gibson, K., Clarke, N., Mensah, T., & Summers, R. (2020a). Examining mental health literacy, help-seeking behaviours, distress, and wellbeing in UK coaches. *European Physical Education Review*, *26*(3), 713–726. https://doi.org/10.1177/1356336x19887772

Gorczynski, P., Sims-Schouten, W., Hill, D., & Wilson, J. C. (2017). Examining mental health literacy, help seeking behaviours, and mental health outcomes in UK university students. *The Journal of Mental Health Training, Education and Practice*, *12*(2), 111–120. https://doi.org/10.1108/jmhtep-05-2016-0027

Gorczynski, P., Sims-Schouten, W., & Wilson, C. (2020b). Evaluating mental health literacy and help-seeking behaviours in UK university students: A country wide study. *Journal of Public Mental Health*, *19*(4), 311–319. https://doi.org/10.1108/jpmh-10-2019-0086

Hart, L. M., Morgan, A. J., Tully, L., & Jorm, A. F. (2023). Mental health literacy for supporting children: The need for a new field of research and intervention. *World Psychiatry*, *22*(2), 338–339. https://doi.org/10.1002/wps.21099

Jorm, A. (2020). We need to move from 'mental health literacy' to 'mental health action'. *Mental Health & Prevention*, *18*, 200179. https://doi.org/10.1016/j.mhp.2020.200179

Jorm, A. F. (2012). Mental health literacy: Empowering the community to take action for better mental health. *American Psychologist*, *67*(3), 231–243. https://doi.org/10.1037/a0025957

Jorm, A. F., Korten, A. E., Jacomb, P. A., Christensen, H., Rodgers, B., & Pollitt, P. (1997). Mental health literacy: A survey of the public's ability to recognise mental disorders and their beliefs about the effectiveness of treatment. *Medical Journal of Australia*, *166*(4), 182–186. https://doi.org/10.5694/j.1326-5377.1997.tb140071.x

Kusan, S. (2013). Dialectics of mind, body, and place: Groundwork for a theory of mental health literacy. *SAGE Open*, *3*(4), 215824401351213. https://doi.org/10.1177/2158244013512131

Kutcher, S., Bagnell, A., & Wei, Y. (2015). Mental health literacy in secondary schools: A Canadian approach. *Child and Adolescent Psychiatric Clinics of North America*, *24*(2), 233–244. https://doi.org/10.1016/j.chc.2014.11.007

Kutcher, S., Wei, Y., & Coniglio, C. (2016). Mental health literacy: Past, present, and future. *Canadian Journal of Psychiatry*, *61*(3), 154–158. https://doi.org/10.1177/0706743715616609

Morgan, A. J., & Jorm, A. F. (2008). Self-help interventions for depressive disorders and depressive symptoms: A systematic review. *Annals of General Psychiatry*, *7*(1). https://doi.org/10.1186/1744-859x-7-13

Morgan, A. J., & Jorm, A. F. (2009). Self-help strategies that are helpful for sub-threshold depression: A Delphi consensus study. *Journal of Affective Disorders, 115*(1–2), 196–200. https://doi.org/10.1016/j.jad.2008.08.004

Morgan, A. J., Jorm, A. F., & Mackinnon, A. J. (2012). Usage and reported helpfulness of self-help strategies by adults with sub-threshold depression. *Journal of Affective Disorders, 136*(3), 393–397. https://doi.org/10.1016/j.jad.2011.11.015

Morgan, A. J., Mackinnon, A. J., & Jorm, A. F. (2013). Behavior change through automated e-mails: Mediation analysis of self-help strategy use for depressive symptoms. *Behaviour Research and Therapy, 51*(2), 57–62. https://doi.org/10.1016/j.brat.2012.11.002

Moss, R. A., Gorczynski, P., Sims-Schouten, W., Heard-Laureote, K., & Creaton, J. (2022). Mental health and wellbeing of postgraduate researchers: Exploring the relationship between mental health literacy, help-seeking behaviour, psychological distress, and wellbeing. *Higher Education Research & Development, 41*(4), 1168–1183. https://doi.org/10.1080/07294360.2021.1906210

O'Connor, M., & Casey, L. (2015). The mental health literacy scale (MHLS): A new scale-based measure of mental health literacy. *Psychiatry Research, 229*(1–2), 511–516. https://doi.org/10.1016/j.psychres.2015.05.064

Spiker, D. A., & Hammer, J. H. (2018). Mental health literacy as theory: Current challenges and future directions. *Journal of Mental Health, 28*(3), 238–242. https://doi.org/10.1080/09638237.2018.1437613

Waldmann, T., Staiger, T., Oexle, N., & Rüsch, N. (2020). Mental health literacy and help-seeking among unemployed people with mental health problems. *Journal of Mental Health, 29*(3), 270–276. https://doi.org/10.1080/09638237.2019.1581342

Wei, Y., McGrath, P. J., Hayden, J., & Kutcher, S. (2016). Measurement properties of tools measuring mental health knowledge: A systematic review. *BMC Psychiatry, 16*(1). https://doi.org/10.1186/s12888-016-1012-5

Yap, M. B. H., Cardamone-Breen, M. C., Rapee, R. M., Lawrence, K. A., Mackinnon, A. J., Mahtani, S., & Jorm, A. F. (2019). Medium-term effects of a tailored web-based parenting intervention to reduce adolescent risk of depression and anxiety: 12-month findings from a randomized controlled trial. *Journal of Medical Internet Research, 21*(8), e13628. https://doi.org/10.2196/13628

Yap, M. B. H., Lawrence, K. A., Rapee, R. M., Cardamone-Breen, M. C., Green, J., & Jorm, A. F. (2017a). Partners in Parenting: A multi-level web-based approach to support parents in prevention and early intervention for adolescent depression and anxiety. *JMIR Mental Health, 4*(4), e59. https://doi.org/10.2196/mental.8492

Yap, M. B. H., Mahtani, S., Rapee, R. M., Nicolas, C., Lawrence, K. A., Mackinnon, A., & Jorm, A. F. (2018). A tailored web-based intervention to improve parenting risk and protective factors for adolescent depression and anxiety problems: Postintervention findings from a randomized controlled trial. *Journal of Medical Internet Research, 20*(1), e17. https://doi.org/10.2196/jmir.9139

Yap, M. B. H., Martin, P. D., & Jorm, A. F. (2017b). Online parenting guidelines to prevent adolescent depression and anxiety: Evaluating user characteristics and usefulness. *Early Intervention in Psychiatry, 12*(5), 951–958. Portico. https://doi.org/10.1111/eip.12503

Yap, M. B. H., Pilkington, P. D., Ryan, S. M., & Jorm, A. F. (2014a). Parental factors associated with depression and anxiety in young people: A systematic review and meta-analysis. *Journal of Affective Disorders, 156*, 8–23. https://doi.org/10.1016/j.jad.2013.11.007

Yap, M. B. H., Pilkington, P. D., Ryan, S. M., Kelly, C. M., & Jorm, A. F. (2014b). Parenting strategies for reducing the risk of adolescent depression and anxiety disorders: A Delphi consensus study. *Journal of Affective Disorders, 156*, 67–75. https://doi.org/10.1016/j.jad.2013.11.017

Part III

Digital Media and Mental Health

12

Cracking the Code of Gaming Disorder: Effective Communication for Parents, Children, and Policymakers

Kylie Woodman and René Weber
University of California Santa Barbara

In an ever-evolving digital society, the issue of excessive media use, especially in the context of gaming, often sparks debates on whether it constitutes a disorder or mental illness. While deep engagement with activities like gaming, violin playing, or dancing can be immersive, what sets apart a healthy passion from a behavioral addiction remains a complex puzzle. Understanding the distinctions between healthy and pathological, excessive behaviors requires a clear conceptualization of what a disorder—here gaming disorder—looks like, what unique aspects of video gaming separate it from other behaviors, and how it is measured. Through unraveling the intricacies of a gaming disorder, also called gaming addiction,[1] we can chart a path toward clear communication and meaningful interventions to support individuals facing the challenges of a gaming disorder.

To illustrate the fine line between behaviors that are perceived as healthy or pathological, let us take the example of two young adolescents. One 13-year-old girl named Malenia plays the violin, and a 13-year-old boy named Godrick plays video games. Each adolescent spends every day after school exclusively engaging in their activity: Malenia trying to perfect each note and stroke of her bow, and Godrick attempting to land the perfect combos and strategically dodge all the attacks of a difficult boss in his game. Both adolescents are comparable in their high skill level obtained compared with other gamers/violin players. Engaging in these activities after school every day for many hours is enough time that it will take away from diversified activities that could be more enriching such as going outside, hanging out with friends, or delving into schoolwork. Both Malenia and Godrick are often unable to reduce their playing behaviors despite their attempts to do so. Godrick's and Malenia's prioritization of playing over other essential activities in their life leads to a neglect of schoolwork, social interactions, and even physical health (e.g., sedentary behaviors or minimal sleep). Further, their excessive playing leads to adverse consequences, such as declining academic performance and a battle of negative emotions when they cannot play. However, only Godrick is referred to a mental health professional and is diagnosed with gaming disorder (diagnostic code 6C51; World Health Organization, 2023). In contrast, while the behavioral patterns are similar, Malenia is diagnosed neither with violin playing disorder, which does not formally exist, nor with any other behavioral disorder. Malenia is labeled a passionate violinist, while Godrick is labeled an addicted gamer. But what crucially distinguishes Malenia's passion from Godrick's addiction?

The Handbook of Mental Health Communication, First Edition.
Edited by Marco C. Yzer and Jason T. Siegel.

What Classifies a Behavior as an Addiction?

The line between normal, healthy behaviors and a behavioral disorder is not always clear-cut and can vary based on cultural, societal, and individual factors. *Behavioral addictions* are excessive behaviors that persevere despite knowledge of adverse consequences leading to suffering (Alavi et al., 2012; Grant et al., 2010). Dissecting this definition provides meaningful insights into the difference between passion-driven behavior and dysfunction.

First, what is considered excessive behavior? Excessive is dependent on the societal and cultural norms around a specific behavior. A normal behavior is typically within a range of expected actions or responses to various situations and is perceived to be within an individual's conscious control; these behaviors are usually not extreme in their expression or frequency (Punzi, 2016). In comparison, excessive behavior is characterized by significantly more intense, severe, or frequent behaviors than what is considered typical; these behaviors are often enacted beyond one's better judgment and in a context where control is perceived as needed (Punzi, 2016). For example, Malenia's violin playing could be viewed by her family and herself as an expected and typical behavior for an aspiring violinist in which she has control and choice over her behaviors. Thus, her behaviors are viewed as functional and even rewarded by family and society. However, for Godrick, the amount of video game playing is seen as excessive by both himself and his family. Because his increased video game playing is likely perceived as a less desirable behavior, there is a higher expectation for control over his behavior, and the increased amount of gaming is more likely to be labeled as dysfunctional, ignored, and punished. Normal behaviors are consistent with the individual, societal, and cultural expectations of the behavior; are met with recognition and rewards; and thus do not require behavioral control. Pathological, excessive behaviors exhibit patterns of actions that deviate from these norms, are considered maladaptive for both the individual and those around them, and thus require behavioral control.

Second, what is considered a negative impact of excessive behaviors? The definition of negative impact is based on the assumption that normal behaviors do not significantly impair a person's ability to carry out daily activities, maintain relationships, or perform their responsibilities. In contrast, a disorder often interferes with a person's ability to function effectively in various areas of life, such as work, school, relationships, or self-care (Robbins & Clark, 2015). While experiencing occasional stress or discomfort is a normal part of life, a behavioral disorder involves significant distress or impairment caused by excessive behaviors. This distress is often a key factor in seeking professional help.

An individual's distressing experience from excessive behaviors can be partially explained by the *dualistic model of passion* outlined by Vallerand (2016). The dualistic model of passion examines how behaviors are either synchronized or unsynchronized from an individual's identity and self-esteem. For individuals with a *harmonious passion*, a behavior promotes well-being and happiness and becomes part of the self in an integrated and positive way. In contrast, an *obsessive passion*, like that of Godrick's video game playing, is internalized in a way that one's self-esteem will directly be dependent on the possibility of engaging in the activity. Obsessive passions are often driven by the relief of negative feelings promoting a rigid and compulsive involvement that goes beyond free will. For an individual with an obsessive passion, their actions do not align with their identity and often result in feelings of distress after the behaviors (Billieux et al., 2015; Vallerand, 2016).

Based on these conceptualizations of a behavioral addiction, it can be concluded that what separates a normal, healthy behavior from a pathological, disordered behavior or an addiction is the deviation of personal and societal expectations for behaviors that causes distress to themselves or others. With this definition, any behavior could be eligible to be diagnosed as an addiction. Nonetheless, very few behaviors have warranted specific diagnostic labels and criteria—one of which is gaming disorder.

What Is Gaming Disorder Anyway?

A gaming disorder is defined as a behavioral addiction characterized by impaired control over gaming behaviors, the prioritization of gaming over all other interests, and the continued escalation of gaming use despite negative consequences persisting for at least 12 months. A meta-analysis by Stevens et al.

(2021) determined that the worldwide prevalence rate of gaming disorder is between 2% and 3% of the general population. For youth aged 8–18, the prevalence increases to about 8% (Gao et al., 2022; Gentile, 2009), with the most common group to receive a diagnosis are 16-year-old males (APA, 2013).

Conceptualizing Gaming Disorders

Many terms have been used to describe problematic gaming throughout the years, including *gaming addiction, problematic gaming, gaming disorder*, and *Internet gaming disorder*. Since the term *video game addiction* first appeared in Soper and Miller (1983), researchers have used various terms, definitions, and criteria to describe the same phenomena of problematic gaming behaviors. Before its formalization as a diagnosis, the American Psychological Association (APA) recognized Internet gaming disorder (IGD) as a diagnosis under consideration in the *Diagnostic and Statistical Manual*, 5th edition (DSM-5) in 2013. Gaming disorder was only recently recognized as a diagnosable behavioral addiction in the World Health Organization's (WHO) International Classification of Diseases-11 (ICD-11) in 2018. Over the past 35 years, research on gaming disorder has been spread across various labels, definitions, and methodologies to understand the phenomenon. Only recently is the terminology converging around gaming disorder and adopting the criteria outlined by the DSM-5 and the ICD-11.

DSM-5: Internet Gaming Disorder

The DSM-5's IGD criteria are similar to that of gaming disorder but are based on the diagnostic criteria for substance addiction—using almost identical language. The criteria include (a) preoccupation or obsession with gaming, (b) development of withdrawal symptoms, (c) developed tolerance (e.g., increasing dosage/playing is needed over time), (d) the unsuccessful ability to reduce playing or quit, (e) loss of interest in activities other than gaming, (f) continuing to game despite problems (i.e., conflicts with family over gaming or emotion regulation issues due to dependency), (g) deception of use, (h) escape of negative feelings, and (i) developing functional impairment outside of gaming (i.e., failing classes or losing a job). The DSM-5 defines IGD as a condition warranting further research consideration. To be diagnosed with IGD, an individual must exhibit at least five of the eight symptoms within a year, which, for instance, would allow for an IGD diagnosis without gaming related conflicts, deception, and functional impairments. In addition, individuals have to be diagnosed by a professional to rule out any other overlapping comorbidities that may better address the symptoms experienced.

ICD-11: Gaming Disorder

WHO was the first to officially recognize gaming disorder (GD) as a diagnosable mental health concern (WHO, 2023). The ICD-11 defines gaming disorder as a mental health condition characterized by (a) impaired control over gaming, (b) increasing gaming priority over other activities to the extent that it takes precedence in daily life, and (c) continuing gaming despite negative consequences. These behavioral patterns must be present for at least 12 months and cause significant distress to the individual or others close to them to be diagnosed with gaming disorder. Consequently, GD diagnosis requires the experience of negative consequences (conflict) and functional impairments.

DSM-5 Versus ICD-11

Both DSM-5 and ICD-11 define criteria aimed at identifying and diagnosing problematic gaming behavior. Despite having a common focus, there are notable differences in their criteria and approaches. One of the significant distinctions is the general framing of the disorders. The DSM-5 frames IGD as identical to substance abuse (e.g., alcohol addiction or cocaine addiction)—using equivalent language and diagnostic criteria, whereas the ICD-11 frames gaming disorder as an impulse-control disorder (e.g., binge eating disorder, gambling disorder; Király & Demetrovics, 2017). The final differentiators are the criteria, such as DSM-5's inclusion of deception and using gaming to escape negative feelings or the ICD-11's emphasis on functional impairment in various life domains. Although these formalized definitions and criteria have standardized the discussion around gaming disorder, more research is needed to best categorize gaming disorder.

Risk Factors for Developing a Gaming Disorder

The development of gaming disorder is significantly influenced by individual risk factors, and researchers have identified several key predictors in this context. Several models have emerged as guides to explain how gaming disorder develops, such as the interaction of person–affect–cognition–execution model (I-PACE; Brand et al., 2019) and Richard et al.'s (2022) model of developmental risk factors of gaming disorder. These models all emphasize the role of predisposing factors and cognitive mechanisms contributing to gaming disorder.

Predisposing Factors

Predisposing factors for gaming disorder include impulsivity, mental health comorbidities, sex, and environmental stressors. These factors collectively contribute to an individual's vulnerability to developing addictive behaviors such as gaming disorder.

Impulsivity

Of all the individual risk factors, impulsivity stands out as a consistent predictor of gaming disorder. Impulsivity refers to the inability to consider alternative solutions, acting on immediate urges without assessing consequences, and a lack of self-control when presented with rewards and punishments. Highly impulsive individuals are more susceptible to the instant rewards and reinforcement provided by video games, which can result in a cycle of excessive gaming and compulsive behavior (as defined in Şalvarlı & Griffiths, 2022). Impulsive individuals have quicker response times, which could be a strategic advantage in gaming; however, the information concerning the decisions may not be fully integrated—resulting in a less-than-optimal outcome (Wang et al., 2017). A systematic review by Şalvarlı and Griffiths (2022) highlighted the relationship between impulsivity and gaming disorder, noting that the consistent findings are associated with deficits in executive control. This suggests that impulsivity may be a behavioral indication of cognitive dysfunction, specifically reduced activity in executive control centers of the brain (e.g., the medial prefrontal cortex) during decisions related to video gaming. The dysfunction of the executive control centers of the brain impairs a person's ability to assess the magnitude of rewards, process postponed rewards, and delay gratification (Wang et al., 2017). By identifying individuals with high impulsivity early on, interventions can be implemented to improve executive functioning before it manifests into an addiction.

Internalizing Comorbidities

Comorbidities, also known as the coexistence of multiple health disorders, are common in mental health conditions. Internalizing is a broad term to classify internal mental struggles such as depression, anxiety, attention issues, and emotion dysregulation (Ehrenreich & Underwood, 2016). Internalizing issues are deeply intertwined with gaming disorder to the extent that the DSM-5 and ICD-11 provide specific instructions to clinicians to examine for comorbidities before determining a final diagnosis and treatment plan. Common comorbid psychopathologies found that of individuals with IGD, 92% had anxiety, 89% depression, 85% attention deficit hyperactivity disorder (ADHD), and 75% a social phobia or other emotion-processing difficulties (González-Bueso et al., 2018; Richard et al., 2022).

It is unclear if there is a causal relationship between gaming disorder and other disorders, for example, if anxiety leads individuals to develop a gaming disorder or if excessively playing video games leads to heightened anxiety. Some studies have run statistical tests (e.g., cross-lagged panel analyses) to try and better understand the causal directions and found that increased depression and anxiety symptoms predicted IGD one year later. However, IGD scores did not predict anxiety scores a year later (Teng et al., 2021). This supports the *compensatory hypothesis* indicating that individuals engage with excessive media to alleviate negative moods and psychosocial problems (Kardefelt-Winther, 2014; Krossbakken et al., 2018). Conversely, a longitudinal study by Gentile et al. (2011) found that anxiety and depression increased due to pathological gaming. It is likely that internalizing psychopathy and the development of gaming disorders define a complex, mutually reinforcing relationship where cause and effect over time are difficult to separate. Nevertheless, incorporating internalizing psychopathy as a risk factor in the study of gaming disorder, and vice versa, incorporating gaming disorder as a risk factor for internalizing psychopathy not only sheds light on the complex interplay between mental struggles and excessive gaming behavior but also underscores the importance of thorough assessment and treatment considerations in addressing gaming disorder.

Sex

Sex is another prominent correlate with gaming disorder, albeit a less understood factor, in the development of gaming disorders. Currently, males are reported to not only play more video games but have a four times higher diagnosis rate of gaming disorders compared with females (Bagot et al., 2022; Lopez-Fernandez et al., 2019). Since the COVID-19 pandemic, more females have begun to play video games, yet this did not result in an increase in gaming addiction scores (Han et al., 2022; Nagata et al., 2022). A study by Dong et al. (2018) identified that gaming elicited more craving-related activations in the brain (e.g., thalamus) for males than females. These results provide a neurological basis for why males may be more vulnerable than females in developing gaming disorder. Once again emphasizing that gaming disorder is multifaceted and more than just time spent playing video games.

Most research on gaming disorder has been on male-dominated populations, which contributes to a lack of understanding of potentially different manifestations of female gaming addictions (Lopez-Fernandez et al., 2019). For example, a study by Lopez-Fernandez et al. (2016) found that women's gaming disorders often manifest with other dysfunctional behaviors, such as excessive social media use (Bagot et al., 2022). A common sex difference in behavioral addictions is that females tend to develop them later in life and develop symptoms more quickly compared with males—a phenomenon known as telescoping (Zakiniaeiz et al., 2017). Although little research has been conducted on telescoping with gaming disorder (King & Potenza, 2020), it may prompt different adjustments to the diagnostic criteria of having symptoms present for at least 12 months. Finally, females diagnosed with IGD tend to have longer play times, heightened competitiveness, higher depression scores, and negative mood compared with males with gaming disorder (Dong & Potenza, 2022; Lopez-Fernandez et al., 2019). These differences may indicate that female manifestations of gaming disorder symptoms are more similar to an emotion regulation disorder, whereas in males gaming disorder symptomatic aligns closer with dysfunction in impulse control.

Environmental Factors

Adverse environmental factors that induce stress not only have the potential to prompt individuals to turn to gaming as a means of escape or coping but also can serve as triggers for gaming cravings. Early life experiences, such as negative early life events and family conflict (Bonnaire & Phan, 2017; Bussone et al., 2020), are additional biopsychological factors that may heighten susceptibility to gaming disorder. Familial environment, especially family conflict, plays a role in shaping children's and adolescents' gaming use, as a potential coping mechanism, and catalyzes the emergence of a gaming disorder (Bussone et al., 2020). The interplay between vulnerability to stress and maladaptive coping strategies can lead individuals to resort to gaming use as a means of mood regulation (Schneider et al., 2018). Gaming offers relief from negative emotions that can be brought on by early life experiences, family conflict, or other environmental stressors.

Cognitive Mechanisms of Gaming Disorder

Gaming disorder models such as those previously ones mentioned integrate concepts from neurobiological theories, such as the incentive-sensitization theory (Robinson & Berridge, 2008), and the competing neurobehavioral decision system theory (CNDS; Bickel et al., 2014). Theories such as CNDS propose a cognitive dual system: the impulsive reward-driven system (system 1) and the executive control system (system 2). The progression toward addictive behaviors involves an increasing imbalance between the two systems. For example, a teenager with a gaming addiction would have a prominent system 1, and when presented with a game, system 1 will automatically decide to engage in the behavior before system 2 can have input, limiting the teen's decision options to the more impulsive decision. The dual-system framework of CNDS connects how gamers with poor inhibition (weaker system 2) are more likely to experience the rewarding features of video games and take advantage of their reward processing system in system 1. While the hyperactivity in system 1 is related to limbic structures in human brains (e.g., amygdala, ventral striatum), the hypoactivity in system 2 is related to prefrontal-striatal circuits (Volkow et al., 2013). The insula in particular plays a mediating role in this process, and dopamine and serotonergic projections, as well as glutamate and GABA systems, are implicated (Naaijen et al., 2015). Both internal and external stimuli can be conditioned within an addiction process, leading to the triggering of affective and cognitive processes that influence gaming behavior. External (i.e., family conflict, a game with reward schedules conducive to addictive behavior) and internal triggers (i.e., depression, anxiety, or stress) in the early stages prompt gaming behavior, while the high rewards from gaming strengthen associations between responses, decisions, and gaming (Brand et al., 2019). As gaming disorder progresses, cue reactivity, craving, and diminished inhibitory control lead to habitual behaviors. Reduced executive functions and inhibitory control also play a significant role in addictive behaviors, affecting decision-making, reward balance, and shifting brain circuits.

The cognitive and neurobiological underpinnings of gaming disorder emphasize the role of heightened reward processing, impaired decision-making, and weakened cognitive control in the gaming addiction process and offer insights into how individuals with gaming disorder may process messages differently.

Why Are Video Games Addictive?

Video games possess unique characteristics that contribute to their addictive potential compared to other media and activities. Although the term video games encompass many genres, styles, and modes of engagement, they can be defined as digital or virtual environments programmed with rewards and punishments which engage players through immediate feedback to reach a desired outcome (based on the definitions by Salen & Zimmerman, 2003; Tavinor, 2008). The challenges and engagement offered by video games, coupled with engaging content and competitive aspects like leaderboards, sustain player interest through novel rewards. There are many approaches to understanding the appeal of video games, but among the leading theories are the motivational model of video game engagement with its inherent self determination perspective and traditional operant conditioning.

Self-Determination Motivations

The motivation model of video game engagement (Przybylski et al., 2010; Ryan et al., 2006), based on self-determination theory (SDT; Ryan & Deci, 2017), highlights the significance of intrinsic motivations in gaming. SDT focuses on three basic psychological needs that motivate individuals toward psychological well-being. The three psychological needs are competence (possessing adequate knowledge), relatedness (feeling a sense of belonging), and autonomy (perceiving ownership of one's decisions). The motivation model of video game Engagement suggests that playing video games can satisfy those psychological needs, and the more video games satisfy the needs, the more enjoyment players receive. For example, players satisfy the need for competence through gaming contexts, which allow for opportunities to acquire and master various skills; they experience relatedness through various opportunities for social interaction in multiplayer contexts. Gamers receive autonomy through, for instance, customization options and general control over the video game and its virtual worlds. The overall impact of any gaming activity on well-being is determined by the person's experience of need satisfaction, particularly with respect to autonomy, competence, and relatedness. The fact that video games seem to be so effective in satisfying these important basic needs of all individuals seems to be an important reason for their addictive potential.

Operant Conditioning

One primary factor contributing to the addictiveness of gaming is a complex, adaptive reward and punishment system, which provides immediate feedback for easy learning and quick development of an addiction compared with other behaviors. Humans' reward systems are best explained by the theory of operant conditioning in behavioral psychology (Akpan, 2020; Skinner, 1965). Rewards are stimuli that provide positive reinforcement, increasing the likelihood of a behavior in the future, while punishments provide negative reinforcement and decrease the probability of a behavior occurring (Lutz & Widmer, 2014). Video games primarily use rewards such as in-game currency, novel stimuli, power buffs, or social acknowledgment through scoreboards; these are considered secondary rewards, which create intrinsic motivation and stable reward value independent of physiological states (Lutz & Widmer, 2014). In video games, rewards are processed within the context of other rewards and punishments, creating reward patterns. These patterns can be influenced by the four fundamental reward schedules: fixed interval, variable interval, fixed ratio, and variable ratio reward schedule.

Fixed ratio rewards are consistent rewards that occur after a behavior is executed a certain number of times. In video games, this could be the act of collecting 30 tokens and then turning them in to complete a quest. *Fixed interval rewards* are similar, but rather than dependent on a behavior that occurs, the reward is delivered after a consistent interval in time. A common example would be weapon spawn points in first-person shooter games, where a new weapon appears in a specific location after a fixed amount of time. *Variable interval rewards* are delivered at an unknown interval of time after the behavior. For example, in some game types, as a player moves through the environment, they will encounter a power-up at random intervals to reinforce their progress. *Variable ratio rewards* are considered one of the most addictive reward patterns, where rewards are given at a random number of times a behavior is executed. Loot boxes are examples of variable ratio rewards; players will repeatedly engage with a game mechanism in hopes of getting a large reward but, more often, not getting the reward. In the foundational Skinner's experiments, mice ravenously and compulsively pressed a reward lever during variable ratio conditions. In a study by Nagle et al. (2014) comparing the variable ratio to fixed ratio reward patterns in video games, players with variable ratio reward patterns played longer, reported more enjoyment in the game, and a strong desire to continue playing. Another addictive feature of variable rewards is the result of a partial reinforcement effect that results in the learned behaviors that are resistant to extinction, or unlearning of the behavior compared with consistent reinforcement.

For years, video game companies have used human psychology theories such as SDT and operant conditioning as ways to teach players gaming mechanics and skills to achieve the goals established by the game, but these theories have also been used to increase play time and engagement of gamers—creating many addictive features within video games.

Message Processing for Individuals with Gaming Disorder

Understanding how individuals with gaming disorder respond to messages compared to those without this disorder is a complex issue. While direct literature on this topic is limited, we can draw insights from related research and similar disorders to provide speculative guidance on crafting effective messages for individuals with gaming disorder.

Gaming Messages

One of the most direct studies to message processing and gaming disorder was conducted by Chau et al. (2019). Their team created the Wise IT-use (WIT) program to address issues related to IGD and risky online behaviors. The program used gamified features to effectively reduce symptoms of IGD and the proportion of students at risk of the disorder—mitigating withdrawal and mood disturbances when not gaming. This provides some indication that individuals with gaming disorder will be receptive to health messages when conveyed in a gamified setting.

Similar studies on in-game advertising have shown that even advertisements which are embedded in game play can influence gamers' attitudes and behaviors (Cianfrone et al., 2008; Hussain et al., 2022). In-game advertisements offer unique opportunities to encourage positive health behaviors and general mass communication within the gaming community, as they can have implicit effects on memories and behaviors. Further, virtual communities within the gaming community can be effective in disseminating information, particularly when known community influencers are involved (Goodman et al., 2018).

It may be counterintuitive to think that individuals will be able to effectively process advertisements while playing intensive video games. However, for an individual with ADHD or with executive dysfunction like problematic gamers, there seem to be a larger capacity to process multiple streams of information. In a research study conducted by Fisher and Keene (2017), the investigators examined the ability to process messages by individuals with ADHD within a secondary task reaction time (STRT) paradigm. Both individuals with ADHD and without had similar message recall of short advertisements; however, individuals with ADHD had quicker STRTs indicating that ADHD individuals were able to maintain recall while allocating additional available resources for attending to a simultaneous secondary task. For individuals with gaming disorder, which is both comorbid with ADHD and displays similar executive dysfunctions, it is likely that sufficient cognitive resources are available to simultaneously process gaming disorder messages and game demands. Based on Fisher and Keen's findings it may even be the case that individuals with ADHD and gaming disorder would become bored with just seeing a message, and may respond more positively with additional demands present like a gamified task or opportunities to explore novel game features.

Executive Dysfunction

A shared indicator of gaming disorder, ADHD, depression, and anxiety is executive dysfunction, which is often conceptualized as a cognitive imbalance of reflective and reflexive brain systems in neuroimaging studies (see above). Given this dysfunction and underlying neurological imbalance a few (dual process) models from the persuasion and consumer behavior literature may offer clues how this imbalance may impact message processing. For instance, the elaboration likelihood model (ELM) in persuasion argues that the ability and motivation to process messages predicts whether individuals process messages through a central route involving critical thinking, deliberation, and conscious decision-making, or through a peripheral route, which is more intuitive and automatic. Individuals with gaming disorder may be more likely to take the peripheral route when processing messages due to poor executive functioning. An exception to this would be for topics that are particularly salient and motivating for them—such as gaming related information. Research on gaming disorders indicates that individuals are more reactive to gaming related cues and often act more impulsively toward those cues. People with gaming disorder may exhibit a memory bias toward gaming-related content—leading to better recall of messages because their minds are more attuned to such content and it triggers a craving response (Van Holst et al., 2012). To what extent this higher motivation to process game-related messages leads to effective processing of antigaming messages and not to severe counterarguing is an open question (see Weber et al., 2015).

Effectively Communicating Gaming Disorder

With a better understanding of gaming disorder, we now turn to the question of how gaming disorder can be effectively communicated to parents, their children, and policymakers.

Parents and Children

Parents often find themselves juggling various responsibilities, including their children's well-being, daily routines, career expectations, and more. When faced with concerns about their child's frequent video game playing, it can be tempting to use gaming as a scapegoat and react with panic. However, it is essential to approach the issue with an informed and balanced perspective and avoid placing undue blame solely on gaming or the child. We suggest parents use a mediation approach to video games, which includes understanding and discussion.

Understanding

Developing gaming literacy for parents begins with an active investigation to acquire the skills and information needed to understand video games. A default preventive measure for gaming disorders may be to simply limit all screen time, including that of video games. However, video games are complex and can be very enriching to a child's development (e.g., cooperation and problem-solving skills; Adachi & Willoughby, 2013; peer group building—especially for shy individuals; Kowert et al., 2014). Parents can acquire general game rating information from the Entertainment Software Rating Board (esrb.org) as a start. However, one of the best ways to understand video games is simply to play them. Co-playing between a parent and child allows parents to learn more about the game, learn about their child's gaming behavior, and increase family bonds and communication (Wang et al., 2017). Understanding the content, mechanics, and potential effects of video games can help parents make informed decisions and engage in meaningful conversations with their children. Learning about video games does not mean advocating for unlimited screen time, but rather it enables parents to have informed discussions and establish healthy boundaries.

Parents should also learn about behavioral addictions and disorders (as provided in this chapter) and keep in mind that any mental disorder, including gaming disorder, is complex and rarely results from a single cause. Because comorbidities, or co-existing disorders, are common with gaming disorders, recognizing this complexity can help parents avoid seeking simplistic monocausal explanations for their child's gaming behaviors and instead approach the situation with openness and understanding. In cases in which parents favor rather simple explanations seemingly providing quick answers to their child's (and the family's) problems, it can help that instead of solely focusing on a checklist of symptoms, parents may benefit from learning more about the research domain criteria approach (RDoC). This approach, introduced by the National Institute of Mental Health (NIMH), emphasizes that mental health is simultaneously influenced by broad domains such as the environment in which individuals grow up, developmental stage (i.e., toddler vs. teenager), genetic predispositions, and neurobiological systems and that all these domains interact in their contribution to behavior and mental disorders. Explaining gaming disorder in the context of RDoC can help parents comprehend that mental disorders have multiple causes and consequences and are likely not well explained by a specific and rigid set of symptoms.

By adopting a comprehensive approach that includes understanding video games, understanding behavioral disorders, acknowledging comorbidities, and considering the broader context of mental health through the RDoC perspective, parents can have more productive and empathetic conversations about gaming disorders with their children and make well-informed decisions to support their well-being.

Communication

When parents are communicating with their children about gaming disorders and gaming behaviors, effective communication strategies can foster understanding, empathy, and a supportive environment. Honesty and empathy are foundational to successful communication. Parents should be well-informed about gaming disorders, drawing from the knowledge gained in the previous sections, to provide accurate information to the child. Conversations should be approached with honesty and openness, explaining that gaming disorder is a real condition without dramatizing or using fear as a communication tool.

Parents can normalize feelings and disorder experiences by emphasizing that gaming disorders can be as disabling as other disorders and that mental disorders, in general, are relatively common, especially during the teenage years. Parents can reassure their children that disorders are not permanent or fixed; they can come and go, and seeking help is a positive step toward managing them. The use of simple language, avoiding technical terms, and utilizing examples and metaphors aids understanding. Employing humor while being sensitive to the seriousness of the disorder can also be an effective communication tool. Parents should clearly communicate the actions they are willing to take, such as seeking professional help, and let their children know that they are on their side and supportive, regardless of any disorder. During conversations about help seeking, expressing love and care provides a sense of security during this conversation.

Parents can encourage ongoing communication by creating a safe and nonjudgmental environment. Parents should invite their children to share their feelings and thoughts openly, and parents should be prepared to be attentive listeners, avoid punitive behaviors, or use access to gaming as a reward or punishment during the conversation, as this can be threatening and cause a child to shut down or become defensive.

It is advisable that parents engage in conflict with openness, avoiding aggression. If aggressive feelings arise, they should be discussed openly and honestly. Parents should share their own feelings and fears and work together to define boundaries and address the negative consequences of excessive gaming. It is wise to avoid assigning blame or inducing guilt, as this approach can be counterproductive and hinder productive dialogue.

By employing these effective communication strategies, parents can create a supportive and understanding environment for discussing gaming disorders and gaming behaviors with their children. Open communication and empathy can foster trust and facilitate the journey toward seeking appropriate help and support for managing gaming-related challenges.

Policymakers and Public Health Officials

Policymakers and public health officials play a critical role in addressing gaming disorder. Like parent–child communication, the first step is being informed about gaming disorder. To effectively address gaming disorder, officials should consider the complex interplay of psychological and neurobiological factors that contribute to excessive gaming.

Drawing on communication principles, policymakers and health officials can develop targeted communication campaigns to raise awareness about gaming disorder, potential consequences, and support. Message framing should be carefully considered, emphasizing both the negative outcomes of excessive gaming and the benefits of balanced gaming to influence attitudes and behaviors related to gaming habits. Recent studies have examined how to craft effective health messages to individuals with gaming disorder, such as a study with Chinese adolescents, which found that structuring messages in a narrative format led to higher acceptance of gaming disorder as a serious condition compared to information fact sheets (Ren & Shen, 2022). Although this method was effective for that population, targeted prevention approaches should consider age and culture to most effectively persuade their audience.

To address the emergence of increased video gaming and gaming disorder, officials should consider prosocial preventive measures that promote healthier gaming habits. Many policies have already arisen out of concerns over gaming disorder; however, some are more effective than others. First, restrictive limits (e.g., shutdown policy and parental controls) are a common preventive measure for gaming time; while controlling time can be a useful step (Davies & Blake, 2016; Király et al., 2018), it does not address the core dysfunction of a gaming disorder. Second, implementing structural changes to games, such as including warning messages and decreasing addictive reward schedules (like that of loot boxes and variable reward ratios), can also be an effective step in addressing the addictive potential of games (Király et al., 2018). Moreover, warning labels on video games, particularly concerning features like loot boxes, may not effectively inform consumer decisions for those with gaming disorder. Garrett et al. (2023) found that individuals with gaming disorder perceive potential harm differently, and existing warning labels do not align closely with their perceived risks, leading to potential misunderstandings. Third, adjusting support infrastructure to better address factors impacting the psychological and motivational levels of gamers through either prevention campaigns or the funding of counseling services specifically tailored to gaming disorders (Dau et al., 2015; Király et al., 2018). Individually these measures are not fully effective, but in combination, they may work to significantly decrease gaming disorder prevalence. Thus, going forward, officials should consider an integrative preventative policy approach utilizing mild restrictions, structural gaming changes, and structural support for individuals with a gaming disorder.

Conclusion

In an ever-evolving digital society, the issue of excessive media use, particularly gaming, has sparked debates on whether it constitutes a disorder or mental illness. Understanding the distinctions between healthy and pathological behaviors requires a clear conceptualization of what a disorder looks like, what unique aspects of video gaming separate it from other behaviors, and how it is measured. Through unraveling the intricacies of gaming disorder, we can chart a path toward clear communication and meaningful interventions to support individuals facing its challenges.

As we move forward in the digital age, the complexities of gaming disorder will continue to evolve, requiring ongoing research and collaboration among various stakeholders to effectively address this emerging mental health challenge. With a balanced understanding of gaming and its impact on individuals, we can foster a supportive environment and develop targeted interventions to help individuals and communities navigate the challenges of excessive gaming while promoting overall well-being.

Note

1 This chapter uses the terms ***pathological, excessive gaming, gaming disorder, gaming addiction,*** and ***video game addiction*** interchangeably.

References

Adachi, P. J. C., & Willoughby, T. (2013). Do video games promote positive youth development? *Journal of Adolescent Research, 28*(2), 155–165. https://doi.org/10.1177/0743558412464522

Akpan, B. (2020). Classical and operant conditioning—Ivan Pavlov; Burrhus Skinner. In B. Akpan & T. J. Kennedy (Eds.), *Science education in theory and practice: An introductory guide to learning theory* (pp. 71–84). Springer International Publishing. https://doi.org/10.1007/978-3-030-43620-9_6

Alavi, S. S., Ferdosi, M., Jannatifard, F., Eslami, M., Alaghemandan, H., & Setare, M. (2012). Behavioral addiction versus substance addiction: Correspondence of psychiatric and psychological views. *International Journal of Preventive Medicine, 3*(4), 290–294. https://www.ncbi.nlm.nih.gov/pmc/articles/PMC3354400

American Psychiatric Association. (2013). *Diagnostic and statistical manual of mental disorders* (5th ed.). https://doi.org/10.1176/appi.books.9780890425596

Bagot, K., Tomko, R., Marshall, A. T., Hermann, J., Cummins, K., Ksinan, A., Kakalis, M., Breslin, F., Lisdahl, K., Mason, M., Redhead, J., Squeglia, L., Thompson, W., Wade, T., Tapert, S., Fuemmeler, B., & Baker, F. (2022). Youth screen use in the ABCD® study. *Developmental Cognitive Neuroscience, 57*, 101150. https://doi.org/10.1016/j.dcn.2022.101150

Bickel, W. K., Moody, L., Quisenberry, A. J., Ramey, C. T., & Sheffer, C. E. (2014). A competing neurobehavioral decision systems model of SES-related health and behavioral disparities. *Preventive Medicine, 68*, 37–43. https://doi.org/10.1016/j.ypmed.2014.06.032

Billieux, J., Schimmenti, A., Khazaal, Y., Maurage, P., & Heeren, A. (2015). Are we over pathologizing everyday life? A tenable blueprint for behavioral addiction research. *Journal of Behavioral Addictions, 4*(3), 119–123. https://doi.org/10.1556/2006.4.2015.009

Bonnaire, C., & Phan, O. (2017). Relationships between parental attitudes, family functioning and internet gaming disorder in adolescents attending school. *Psychiatry Research, 255*, 104–110. https://doi.org/10.1016/j.psychres.2017.05.030

Brand, M., Wegmann, E., Stark, R., Müller, A., Wölfling, K., Robbins, T. W., & Potenza, M. N. (2019). The interaction of person-affect-cognition-execution (I-PACE) model for addictive behaviors: Update, generalization to addictive behaviors beyond internet-use disorders, and specification of the process character of addictive behaviors. *Neuroscience & Biobehavioral Reviews, 104*, 1–10. https://doi.org/10.1016/j.neubiorev.2019.06.032

Bussone, S., Trentini, C., Tambelli, R., & Carola, V. (2020). Early-life interpersonal and affective risk factors for pathological gaming. *Frontiers in Psychiatry, 11*, 547450. https://doi.org/10.3389/fpsyt.2020.00423

Chau, C., Tsui, Y. Y., & Cheng, C. (2019). Gamification for internet gaming disorder prevention: Evaluation of a wise IT-use (WIT) program for Hong Kong primary students. *Frontiers in Psychology, 10*, 489688. https://doi.org/10.3389/fpsyg.2019.02468

Cianfrone, B. A., Trail, G. T., Zhang, J. J., & Lutz, R. J. (2008). Effectiveness of in-game advertisements in sport video games: An experimental inquiry on current gamers. *International Journal of Sport Communication*, *1*(2), 195–218. https://doi.org/10.1123/ijsc.1.2.195

Dau, W., Hoffmann, J. D. G., & Banger, M. (2015). Therapeutic interventions in the treatment of problematic internet use—Experiences from Germany. In C. Montag & M. Reuter (Eds.), *Internet addiction: Neuroscientific approaches and therapeutical interventions* (pp. 183–217). Springer International Publishing. https://doi.org/10.1007/978-3-319-07242-5_12

Davies, B., & Blake, E. (2016). Evaluating existing strategies to limit video game playing time. *IEEE Computer Graphics and Applications*, *36*(2), 47–57. https://doi.org/10.1109/MCG.2016.25

Dong, G., Wang, L., Du, X., & Potenza, M. N. (2018). Gender-related differences in neural responses to gaming cues before and after gaming: Implications for gender-specific vulnerabilities to internet gaming disorder. *Social Cognitive and Affective Neuroscience*, *13*(11), 1203–1214. https://doi.org/10.1093/scan/nsy084

Dong, G.-H., & Potenza, M. N. (2022). Considering gender differences in the study and treatment of internet gaming disorder. *Journal of Psychiatric Research*, *153*, 25–29. https://doi.org/10.1016/j.jpsychires.2022.06.057

Ehrenreich, S. E., & Underwood, M. K. (2016). Adolescents' internalizing symptoms as predictors of the content of their Facebook communication and responses received from peers. *Translational Issues in Psychological Science*, *2*(3), 227–237. https://doi.org/10.1037/tps0000077

Fisher, J. T., & Keene, J. R. (2017). *Examining cognitive load and recall for educational multimedia messages in ADHD and high media multitasking populations* [Conference presentation]. The 67th annual meeting of the International Communication Association. San Diego, CA, USA.

Gao, Y. X., Wang, J. Y., & Dong, G. H. (2022). The prevalence and possible risk factors of internet gaming disorder among adolescents and young adults: Systematic reviews and meta-analyses. *Journal of Psychiatric Research*, *154*, 35–43. https://doi.org/10.1016/j.jpsychires.2022.06.049

Garrett, E. P., Drummond, A., Lowe-Calverley, E., & Sauer, J. D. (2023). Current loot box warnings are ineffective for informing consumers. *Computers in Human Behavior*, *139*, 107534. https://doi.org/10.1016/j.chb.2022.107534

Gentile, D. (2009). Pathological video-game use among youth ages 8 to 18: A national study. *Psychological Science*, *20*(5), 594–602. https://doi.org/10.1111/j.1467-9280.2009.02340.x

Gentile, D. A., Choo, H., Liau, A., Sim, T., Li, D., Fung, D., & Khoo, A. (2011). Pathological video game use among youths: A two-year longitudinal study. *Pediatrics*, *127*(2), e319–e329. https://doi.org/10.1542/peds.2010-1353

González-Bueso, V., Santamaría, J. J., Fernández, D., Merino, L., Montero, E., & Ribas, J. (2018). Association between internet gaming disorder or pathological video-game use and comorbid psychopathology: A comprehensive review. *International Journal of Environmental Research and Public Health*, *15*(4), 668. https://doi.org/10.3390/ijerph15040668

Goodman, W., McFerran, E., Purves, R., Redpath, I., & Beeken, R. J. (2018). The untapped potential of the gaming community: Narrative review. *JMIR Serious Games*, *6*(3), e10161. https://doi.org/10.2469/faj.v27.n2.12

Grant, J. E., Potenza, M. N., Weinstein, A., & Gorelick, D. A. (2010). Introduction to behavioral addictions. *The American Journal of Drug and Alcohol Abuse*, *36*(5), 233–241. https://doi.org/10.3109/00952990.2010.491884

Han, T. S., Cho, H., Sung, D., & Park, M.-H. (2022). A systematic review of the impact of COVID-19 on the game addiction of children and adolescents. *Frontiers in Psychiatry*, *13*, 976601. https://doi.org/10.3389/fpsyt.2022.976601

Hussain, M., Islam, T., & Rehman, S. U. (2022). What you see is what you get: Assessing in-game advertising effectiveness. *Journal of Research in Interactive Marketing*, *17*(4), 527–543. https://doi.org/10.1108/JRIM-03-2022-0087

Kardefelt-Winther, D. (2014). A conceptual and methodological critique of internet addiction research: Towards a model of compensatory internet use. *Computers in Human Behavior*, *31*, 351–354. https://doi.org/10.1016/j.chb.2013.10.059

King, D. L., & Potenza, M. N. (2020). Gaming disorder among female adolescents: A hidden problem? *Journal of Adolescent Health*, *66*(6), 650–652. https://doi.org/10.1016/j.jadohealth.2020.03.011

Király, O., & Demetrovics, Z. (2017). Inclusion of gaming disorder in ICD has more advantages than disadvantages. *Journal of Behavioral Addictions*, *6*(3), 280–284. https://doi.org/10.1556/2006.6.2017.046

Király, O., Griffiths, M. D., King, D. L., Lee, H.-K., Lee, S.-Y., Bányai, F., Zsila, Á., Takacs, Z. K., & Demetrovics, Z. (2018). Policy responses to problematic video game use: A systematic review of current measures and future possibilities. *Journal of Behavioral Addictions*, *7*(3), 503–517. https://doi.org/10.1556/2006.6.2017.050

Kowert, R., Domahidi, E., & Quandt, T. (2014). The relationship between online video game involvement and gaming-related friendships among emotionally sensitive individuals. *Cyberpsychology, Behavior and Social Networking*, *17*(7), 447–453. https://doi.org/10.1089/cyber.2013.0656

Krossbakken, E., Pallesen, S., Mentzoni, R. A., King, D. L., Molde, H., Finserås, T. R., & Torsheim, T. (2018). A cross-lagged study of developmental trajectories of video game engagement, addiction, and mental health. *Frontiers in Psychology*, *9*, 412655. https://doi.org/10.3389/fpsyg.2018.02239

Lopez-Fernandez, O., González-Bueso, V., Montero, E., Santamaría, J. J., & Merino, L. (2016). Validation in clinical population of the problematic internet entertainment use scale for adults (PIEUSAd). *Cuadernos de Medicina Psicosomática y Psiquiatría de Enlace, 117*, 61–71. https://irep.ntu.ac.uk/id/eprint/32654

Lopez-Fernandez, O., Williams, A. J., Griffiths, M. D., & Kuss, D. J. (2019). Female gaming, gaming addiction, and the role of women within gaming culture: A narrative literature review. *Frontiers in Psychiatry, 10*, 449322. https://doi.org/10.3389/fpsyt.2019.00454

Lutz, K., & Widmer, M. (2014). What can the monetary incentive delay task tell us about the neural processing of reward and punishment? *Neuroscience and Neuroeconomics, 3*, 33–45. https://doi.org/10.2147/NAN.S38864

Naaijen, J., Lythgoe, D. J., Amiri, H., Buitelaar, J. K., & Glennon, J. C. (2015). Fronto-striatal glutamatergic compounds in compulsive and impulsive syndromes: A review of magnetic resonance spectroscopy studies. *Neuroscience & Biobehavioral Reviews, 52*, 74–88. https://doi.org/10.1016/j.neubiorev.2015.02.009

Nagata, J. M., Cortez, C. A., Cattle, C. J., Ganson, K. T., Iyer, P., Bibbins-Domingo, K., & Baker, F. C. (2022). Screen time use among US adolescents during the COVID-19 pandemic: Findings from the adolescent brain cognitive development (ABCD) study. *JAMA Pediatrics, 176*(1), 94–96. https://doi.org/10.1001/jamapediatrics.2021.4334

Nagle, A., Wolf, P., Riener, R., & Novak, D. (2014). The use of player-centered positive reinforcement to schedule in-game rewards increases enjoyment and performance in a serious game. *International Journal of Serious Games, 1*(4), 35–47. https://doi.org/10.17083/ijsg.v1i4.47

Przybylski, A. K., Rigby, C. S., & Ryan, R. M. (2010). A motivational model of video game engagement. *Review of General Psychology, 14*(2), 154–166. https://doi.org/10.1037/a0019440

Punzi, E. H. (2016). Excessive behaviors in clinical practice—A state of the art article. *International Journal of Qualitative Studies on Health and Well-Being, 11*, 30055. https://doi.org/10.3402/qhw.v11.30055

Ren, Y., & Shen, F. (2022). Effects of narratives and behavioral involvement on adolescents' attitudes toward gaming disorder. *Health Communication, 37*(6), 657–667. https://doi.org/10.1080/10410236.2020.1862397

Richard, J., Temcheff, C., Fletcher, É., Lemieux, A., Derevensky, J., & Déry, M. (2022). An empirical investigation of the externalizing and internalizing pathways to disordered gaming behavior: A longitudinal study across childhood and adolescence. *Computers in Human Behavior, 128*, 107096. https://doi.org/10.1016/j.chb.2021.107096

Robbins, T., & Clark, L. (2015). Behavioral addictions. *Current Opinion in Neurobiology, 30*, 66–72. https://doi.org/10.1016/j.conb.2014.09.005

Robinson, T. E., & Berridge, K. C. (2008). The incentive sensitization theory of addiction: Some current issues. *Philosophical Transactions of the Royal Society B: Biological Sciences, 363*(1507), 3137–3146. https://doi.org/10.1098/rstb.2008.0093

Ryan, R. M., & Deci, E. L. (2017). *Self-determination theory: Basic psychological needs in motivation, development, and wellness.* Guilford Publications.

Ryan, R. M., Rigby, C. S., & Przybylski, A. (2006). The motivational pull of video games: A self-determination theory approach. *Motivation and Emotion, 30*(4), 344–360. https://doi.org/10.1007/s11031-006-9051-8

Salen, K., & Zimmerman, E. (2003). *Rules of play: Game design fundamentals.* The MIT Press.

Şalvarlı, Ş. İ., & Griffiths, M. D. (2022). The association between internet gaming disorder and impulsivity: A systematic review of literature. *International Journal of Mental Health and Addiction, 20*(1), 92–118. https://doi.org/10.1007/s11469-019-00126-w

Schneider, L. A., King, D. L., & Delfabbro, P. H. (2018). Maladaptive coping styles in adolescents with internet gaming disorder symptoms. *International Journal of Mental Health and Addiction, 16*(4), 905–916. https://doi.org/10.1007/s11469-017-9756-9

Skinner, B. F. (1965). *Science and human behavior.* Simon and Schuster.

Soper, W. B., & Miller, M. J. (1983). Junk-time junkies: An emerging addiction among students. *The School Counselor, 31*(1), 40–43. https://www.jstor.org/stable/23900931

Stevens, M. W., Dorstyn, D., Delfabbro, P. H., & King, D. L. (2021). Global prevalence of gaming disorder: A systematic review and meta-analysis. *Australian & New Zealand Journal of Psychiatry, 55*(6), 553–568. https://doi.org/10.1177/0004867420962851

Tavinor, G. (2008). Definition of videogames. *Contemporary Aesthetics (Journal Archive), 6*(1), 16. http://hdl.handle.net/2027/spo.7523862.0006.016

Teng, Z., Pontes, H. M., Nie, Q., Griffiths, M. D., & Guo, C. (2021). Depression and anxiety symptoms associated with internet gaming disorder before and during the COVID-19 pandemic: A longitudinal study. *Journal of Behavioral Addictions, 10*(1), 169–180. https://doi.org/10.1556/2006.2021.00016

Vallerand, R. J. (2016). The dualistic model of passion: Theory, research, and implications for the field of education. In W. C. Liu, J. C. K. Wang, & R. M. Ryan (Eds.), *Building autonomous learners: Perspectives from research and practice using self-determination theory* (pp. 31–58). Springer. https://doi.org/10.1007/978-981-287-630-0_3

Van Holst, R. J., Lemmens, J. S., Valkenburg, P. M., Peter, J., Veltman, D. J., & Goudriaan, A. E. (2012). Attentional bias and disinhibition toward gaming cues are related to problem gaming in male adolescents. *The Journal of Adolescent Health, 50*(6), 541–546. https://doi.org/10.1016/j.jadohealth.2011.07.006

Volkow, N. D., Wang, G.-J., Tomasi, D., & Baler, R. D. (2013). Unbalanced neuronal circuits in addiction. *Current Opinion in Neurobiology*, *23*(4), 639–648. https://doi.org/10.1016/j.conb.2013.01.002

Wang, Y., Hu, Y., Xu, J., Zhou, H., Lin, X., Du, X., & Dong, G. (2017). Dysfunctional prefrontal function is associated with impulsivity in people with internet gaming disorder during a delay discounting task. *Frontiers in Psychiatry*, *8*, 302647. https://doi.org/10.3389/fpsyt.2017.00287

Weber, R., Huskey, R., Mangus, J. M., Westcott-Baker, A., & Turner, B. (2015). Neural predictors of message effectiveness during counterarguing in antidrug campaigns. *Communication Monographs*, *82*(1), 4–30. https://doi.org/10.1080/03637751.2014.971414

World Health Organization. (2023). *6C51 gaming disorder*. In *International statistical classification of diseases and related health problems* (11th ed.). https://icd.who.int/browse11/l-m/en#/http://id.who.int/icd/entity/1448597234

Zakiniaeiz, Y., Cosgrove, K. P., Mazure, C. M., & Potenza, M. N. (2017). Does telescoping exist in male and female gamblers? Does it matter? *Frontiers in Psychology*, *8*, 283447. https://doi.org/10.3389/fpsyg.2017.01510

13

Chatbots for Mental Health: A Network-Oriented Modeling Perspective

Gert-Jan de Bruijn[1], Fakhra Jabeen[2], and Tibor Bosse[2]

[1] University of Antwerp

[2] Radboud University

Mental health issues are a global public health problem. Particularly depression and anxiety are key causes of the global burden of disease. In the 2019 systematic scientific assessment on the global burden of over 350 diseases and injuries in over 200 countries on years of life lost, years lived with disability, and disability-adjusted life-years, depression ranked no. 13 in all age categories, just below HIV/AIDS and tuberculosis (Collaborators et al., 2020). Depression and anxiety ranked no. 4 and no. 6, respectively, in the age category 10–24 years, and no. 6 and no. 15 in the age category 25–49 years. Prevalence estimates have also painted a worrisome picture, with pooled prevalence estimates of 14.9% and 19.1% reported for depression and anxiety in children, adolescents, and young adults, respectively (Barker et al., 2020). Moreover, studies have also reported that prevalence rates of subthreshold anxiety—symptoms that are too few and/or too short-term to reach the standardized diagnostic threshold in the *Diagnostic and Statistical Manual of Mental Disorders* (DSM)—are nearly double those of anxiety disorders, which, if left untreated, will lead to even higher prevalence estimates in the next decade. Finally, the economic burden of depression and anxiety is enormous: In 2018, the economic burden of major depressive disorder was nearly 330 billion USD, up by over a third since 2010 (236 billion USD, 37.9%) (Greenberg et al., 2021). These numbers indicate a strong need to provide not only adequate treatment to those suffering from depression and/or anxiety but also effective preventive tools for those with subclinical symptoms of anxiety and depression. Unfortunately, these increasing trends have not been paralleled by increases in the availability of relevant health care services that can provide adequate care, treatment, and prevention to those in need of mental health support.

In general, two strands of treatment and prevention of depression and anxiety exist: pharmaceutical and nonpharmaceutical. For pharmaceutical treatments, antidepressant medications such as selective serotonin reuptake inhibitors have proven effective for treatment and relapse prevention in depression (Arıkan et al., 2023), whereas benzodiazepine has proven effective for anxiety treatment (Stimpfl et al., 2023). For nonpharmaceutical treatments, evidence points to cognitive behavior therapy (CBT), including such elements as behavioral activation and cognitive restructuring, as an effective method to reduce anxiety and/or depressive symptoms (Chen et al., 2022; Oud et al., 2019). Nevertheless, those in need of mental health care treatment and prevention oftentimes do not get the treatment they need. First, increasing demand for mental health care services has led to long waiting lists for those in need of care. Second, mental health help seeking is suboptimal: recent numbers indicate that some two-thirds of adolescents and (young) adults who suffer from anxiety disorders have not sought formal mental health care help, and those who do report only minimum contact with psychotherapists (Niermann et al., 2021). Moreover, interventions that seek to improve mental health help-seeking

The Handbook of Mental Health Communication, First Edition.
Edited by Marco C. Yzer and Jason T. Siegel.

behaviors are generally effective only in the short-term and only in (older) adults, but they are not effective in children and adolescents (Xu et al., 2018).

Digital Solutions for Mental Health

To cope with the increasing demand for mental health care services, interventions based on digital technology are often put forward as a promising solution. Indeed, in recent years, several digital tools have been developed to enhance mental health care. Some of these tools are based on conversational technology, or chatbots (e.g., Abd-alrazaq et al., 2019; Vaidyam et al., 2019). The following section presents the state of the art in (a) general digital tools and (b) chatbot technology for mental health.

Digital Tools and Mental Health

Earlier digital tools—such as mobile apps and telehealth technologies—have been used as supplements or alternatives to regular mental health care because they may reduce the barriers people experience in mental health help seeking. Among these, popular mobile apps for mental health are arguably to most used in everyday life. However, content analysis of popular mobile apps for anxiety and depression have also demonstrated that effective treatment elements are generally not included in these apps (Wasil et al., 2019, 2020). For instance, Wasil et al. (2019) reviewed 27 mobile health apps for depression and anxiety and found that—for the 16 included depression apps—various evidence-based treatment protocols, such as problem-solving, behavioral contracting, and communication skills, were completely absent from these apps, while other evidence-based treatment protocols, such as goal setting, relaxation, and self-monitoring, were absent in over 60% of these apps. Similar results were found for the 17 anxiety-related apps, where evidence-based treatments such as problem-solving and modeling were absent for these apps, while exposure, cognitive restructuring, and self-monitoring were absent in over 75% of the apps. In a follow-up study of these findings, Wasil et al. (2020) also reported that the two apps that accounted for 90% of the total number of monthly users and 96% of the total number of daily mental health app users contained a maximum of five (out of a possible 20) effective treatment elements.

Digital tools have also been used in purposeful treatment interventions for depression and anxiety. Nevertheless, meta-analyses on the effects of these digital interventions as treatment solutions have provided mixed results. For instance, in a systematic review and meta-analysis on the effects of e-health depression and anxiety interventions for children and adolescents with long-term conditions, the effects of five e-health intervention studies were summarized and resulted in a nonsignificant pooled standardized mean difference of −0.06 and − 0.07 for depression and anxiety symptoms: Nonsignificant differences were found regardless of follow-up duration (immediate follow-up or three- to six-month follow-up) or comparison group (care-as-usual or attention placebo or any comparator) (Thabrew et al., 2018). A more recent meta-analysis on digital interventions for the treatment of depression (Moshe et al., 2021) summarized 88 studies—of which the majority were Internet or computer based—and found an overall modest effect-sized difference for digital interventions versus all control conditions. In line with an earlier meta-analysis (Richards & Richardson, 2012), this effect was particularly strong when the digital intervention included a human support component, such as email follow-up or progress feedback. However, given the paucity of evidence, no clear conclusions could be drawn for children and adolescent target groups, and—when compared with face-to-face interventions—these digital interventions were not more effective in reducing depression or depressive symptoms.

The fact that digital interventions become more effective when a human support component is added indicates that adding technologies with human-like capabilities would benefit mental health care. Nowadays, the increasing computational capabilities of computers combined with advances in artificial intelligence and computational linguistic techniques have led to the development of chatbots—text-based conversational systems—that can not only understand humanlike text input but also generate humanlike text in conversations. The next section first briefly describes what chatbots are, followed by an overview of the evidence base on the effectiveness of these chatbots for depression and anxiety.

Chatbots and Mental Health

Chatbot is an umbrella term used for a wide range of (embodied and nonembodied) conversational agents that are capable of interacting with users through conversational interfaces (Vaidyam et al., 2019). The main goal is to simulate real-time conversations by "…exploiting natural language technologies to engage users in text-based information-seeking, and task-oriented dialogs" (Mott et al., 2004, p. 2). Researchers and practitioners in various areas of the health care sector have started to apply chatbot technology to create effective solutions in terms of usability and efficacy. This is because this type of technology can help alleviate pressure on health care systems in terms of time, cost, and availability (Abd-alrazaq et al., 2019). Chatbots are not only accessible 24/7 but also can have an almost unlimited number of conversations simultaneously. Additionally, chatbots are able to converse in a nonstigmatizing way, thereby overcoming the stigma associated with regular mental health care help seeking.

Research indicates that chatbot technology holds the potential to promote well-being and behavior management (Abd-alrazaq et al., 2019; Fitzpatrick et al., 2017; He et al., 2023; Inkster et al., 2018). ELIZA, the very first chatbot reported in the literature, was created to simulate a psychotherapist based on simple *scripts* (Weizenbaum, 1983). Since then, the capabilities of chatbots have improved significantly (Abd-alrazaq et al., 2019; Fitzpatrick et al., 2017; Inkster et al., 2018). By leveraging various methods from artificial intelligence (AI) and machine learning (ML), chatbots can efficiently comprehend input from users and respond accordingly using different modalities (e.g., text or audio). Moreover, chatbots can be of different levels of sophistication, depending on the extent to which they use these AI techniques. On one end of the spectrum, *rule-based* or decision tree-based chatbots use a predefined sequence or flow to communicate with users to achieve their goal (e.g., customer care or reservations bots) (Abd-alrazaq et al., 2019). In contrast, *AI-based* chatbots use advanced AI-based techniques to understand and track conversations and generate responses in a flexible manner (Zhu et al., 2022). As chatbots are able to deduce not only the topics humans talk about but also the related sentiments (Krahmer et al., 2022), they have the potential to build a certain *rapport* with the user, which can be beneficial in enhancing the mental health of the individual (Devaram, 2020; Inkster et al., 2018; Zhang et al., 2022).

Indeed, chatbots might use psychological or behavioral techniques to enhance psychological and mental health. For instance, *Woebot* uses CBT to improve mental health and support users to overcome depression (Fitzpatrick et al., 2017; He et al., 2023). Similarly, *Wysa* uses a decision support system and behavioral therapy to support people who are facing anxiety and depression (Inkster et al., 2018). Other examples where chatbots are used to promote different aspects of well-being include a fitness-related bot in which dialogues are analyzed to motivate and track the user's progress (Kocielnik et al., 2018), a nutrition chatbot in which conversations are analyzed for food tracking (Graf et al., 2015), a meditation chatbot that uses sensors and breathing rate to develop the conversational experience (Shamekhi & Bickmore, 2015), or a virtual coach to provide mindfulness training through conversation analysis (Hudlicka, 2016). Research shows that users had positive experiences with chatbots regarding diagnostic quality, therapeutic efficacy, and acceptability (Vaidyam et al., 2020). Focusing on clinical samples, Lim et al. (2022) reviewed chatbots, including embodied chatbots and chatbots using different combinations of gestures and written and spoken responses, to deliver CBT and/or problem-solving therapy (PST) to adults with (sub)clinical depression and/or anxiety. Their meta-analytical findings showed that chatbot-delivered therapy—relative to human-supervised care-as-usual or waitlist control conditions was significantly more effective in reducing depressive symptoms (Hedges' $g = 0.54$, $p < 0.001$).

To improve the quality of human–chatbot interaction, the usage of *tailored* responses is a promising direction. For example, Graf et al. (2015) incorporated users' personal preferences to create a personalized interaction with a chatbot to record their intake by using motivational strategies like suggestion, self-monitoring, comparison, and competition. Currently, large language models (LLMs) such as GPT-3 and Bloom are widely used and can have the potential to further improve human–chatbot interaction because of their ability to generate highly human-like text at runtime. These models are trained based on massive datasets using deep learning. Deep learning is one of the latest AI techniques, which processes information based on artificial neural networks consisting of multiple layers, loosely inspired by the human brain. Thanks to their almost human-level performance, chatbots based on LLMs can be used for a wide variety of applications; for instance, for practicing counseling skills through role play (Maurya, 2023). However, as LLMs are trained using diverse datasets and are generative by nature, it is hard to fully control their output. This may have serious implications, such as misleading information or biased output, that can impact the mental health of users. Hence, developers should always keep an eye on whether they truly fulfill their purpose (Assayed et al., 2023).

Some design methodologies have been considered to improve chatbot technology so that it can fulfill end users' goals and desires. For instance, in co-creation researchers codeveloped a chatbot by considering input from multiple stakeholders (like health care practitioners and psychotherapists), which provides promising results (Grové, 2021) in terms of personalized care, or using an agile method to improve the outcomes based on users' feedback. Different parameters were also considered to estimate the usability of a chatbot, for example, ease of use, responsiveness, reliability, understandability, trustworthiness, or enjoyability (Abd-alrazaq et al., 2019). Most studies concluded that chatbots are trustworthy and easy to talk to (Abd-alrazaq et al., 2020), yet some studies point to limitations in terms of understanding user intent, providing a reliable response (Chow et al., 2023), or a lack of creativity (Babulak, 2023). Overall, research indicates that chatbots that effectively use personalization (Zhu et al., 2022), and adaptive features are still in their infancy (He et al., 2023).

With respect to the effectiveness of mental health chatbots, to date, several pilot studies and controlled trials have been conducted. For instance, Goonesekera and Donkin (2022) developed a chatbot named Otis that incorporated CBT techniques such as psychoeducation, exposure, and cognitive restructuring and tested its acceptability and effectiveness on anxiety reduction in 29 (young) adults recruited via convenience sampling. On average, these participants engaged for nearly 10 days with Otis, after which they reported significantly lower scores on general anxiety and significantly higher scores on personal well-being and quality of life.

In summary, there is some evidence that chatbots can act as an effective and efficient solution for mental health care, even though the quality of the trials tends to be low and the positive short-term effects do not translate into long-term positive effects. One thing current chatbot-based trials tend to have in common is that their theoretical backdrop is derived from traditional psychological and psychiatric models, which assume that depressive and/or anxiety symptoms (e.g., lack of sleep) arise from a common overarching cause (i.e. depression). However, in the past two decades, advances have been made in theory development that regard a mental health disorder—including depression and anxiety—not as a latent construct but rather as a *network* of interacting symptoms. The next sections explain how this network-oriented perspective can be used to develop chatbots that have the ability to reason about the (mental) state of individuals.

A Network-Oriented Modeling Approach

This section first briefly describes the network-oriented approach from a psychological perspective and then how the network-oriented paradigm can be addressed from a computational perspective. Subsequently, it discusses how the combination of these two perspectives can be used to develop and apply network-based mental health chatbots.

Psychological Perspective

From a traditional common cause perspective, a mental health disorder is regarded as a latent higher-order construct that is the root cause of the symptoms of that disorder. In other words, symptoms that are reported by an individual are being caused by the mental health disorder. For instance, if an individual reports depressed mood, fatigue, hopelessness, and sleep problems, the traditional perspective postulates that an overarching property (e.g., depression) is causing these symptoms. It also assumes that there is no relevant interaction between these symptoms. Treatment based on this traditional perspective focuses solely on reducing these symptoms, and effective treatment is assumed to have occurred if mean scores of these symptoms have changed in the healthier direction. In contrast, the network perspective of mental health postulates that a mental health condition can be modeled as a ***network*** that consists of ***interacting symptoms*** in an individual. In this approach, nodes (symptoms) and edges (connections between symptoms) allow for identifying (how and when) which symptoms get activated and/or provide feedback loops to other symptoms (McElroy et al., 2018). This perspective also focuses on so-called bridge symptoms, which are pathways that can connect different disorders. Treatment based on this network perspective specifies a focus not on changing mean scores of symptoms but rather on identifying and modifying symptoms that are key for the connectivity between symptoms in the network (Borsboom, 2017).

Since its inception almost two decades ago, substantial research has focused on identifying the network structures of depression and anxiety. For instance, Rouquette et al. (2018) used data from the Quebec Longitudinal Study of Kindergarten Children to estimate Gaussian graphical models (GGM)—a network structure estimation model—to identify how behavioral and emotional symptoms are related to depression and anxiety in adolescence and early adulthood. Their results demonstrated that irritability, solidarity, blaming others, feeling not liked, and often crying were distinctive symptoms in the network; moreover, their results showed that not being liked and irritability at a younger age were positive predictors of an anxiety diagnosis at an early adult age. In a study on the elderly, Yang et al. (2022) used GGM to estimate the network structure of anxiety and depression to understand how comorbidity arises and/or is maintained. They found that particularly irritability and concentration difficulties were bridge symptoms linking depression and anxiety.

The evidence from network structures has also been implemented in depression and anxiety interventions. As stated, these network-based treatment interventions diverge from traditional treatment interventions in focusing more explicitly on outcomes that are related to the dynamics and interconnectivity of symptoms rather than on mean scores of symptoms. Arguably because of the relative novelty of the network theory of mental health, only a handful of interventions have been implemented to date (McElroy et al., 2018). For instance, a study of over 8,000 8-to-18-year olds obtained from 81 child and adolescent mental health services in the United Kingdom found that the connectivity of the network was associated with treatment response, such that those who respond to early treatment have less densely connected symptom networks. In another study, a randomized controlled trial design was used to compare the network structure of those allocated to the treatment condition (i.e. mindfulness-based cognitive therapy, or MCBT) with those allocated to a waiting-list control condition (Snippe et al., 2017). Using data from the mind-Maastricht trial, Snippe et al. (2017) not only found that those receiving MCBT had not only reduced depressive symptoms but also marginal changes in the network structure compared with those in the control conditions. Specifically, those who received MCBT had a stronger negative association between feeling down and cheerfulness after MCBT treatment.

Computational Perspective

As explained in the previous section, a modern perspective on mental health conceptualizes mental health conditions as a network of interacting symptoms which can be related to presence of (positive) feelings as well as psychological wellbeing (Peter et al., 2011). Interestingly, the psychological perspective has considerable overlap with recent computational modeling approaches in AI, in particular the idea of ***network-oriented modeling*** (Kuipers, 1984; Treur, 2020). Here, we briefly explain what computational modeling is and how it can be used to study any complex phenomenon.

Modeling is a well-established concept, serving as a versatile tool capable of representing growth or decay of any phenomenon by reflecting changes over time. For example, in archeology ***spatial analysis*** utilizes data models for population distributions to analyze growth patterns of different infrastructure networks, like roads or utilities (McCoy & Ladefoged, 2009). Similarly, ***predictive modeling*** relies on statistical models based on extracted features to study different trends in data. The data collected are related to a certain domain (e.g., epidemiology or health care), which are analyzed over time for prediction and to improve decision-making (Kuhn & Johnson, 2013). Many researchers use ***computational models*** to study dynamics of various complex processes. An example can be how humans interact with other individuals in a crowd or how or what factors can influence an ecosystem. Such processes may involve multiple components or factors interacting together to exhibit an emergent phenomenon, which can also be modeled and analyzed. Some widely used modeling techniques include agent-based modeling (ABM), complex networks, and temporal-causal modeling.

- ABM is a technique that allows researchers to study the dynamics of complex systems. An ABM consists of (large) numbers of individuals represented as computational agents, which are simulated to understand the behavior of a whole system in certain circumstances or scenarios. The behaviors of the individual agents are typically formalized in a specific format, for instance, using logical expressions, mathematical equations, or decision rules (micro level). Hence, the researcher has the flexibility to analyze the resulting emergent behaviors of an entire system (macro level) by running simulations in an artificial environment.
- *Complex networks* have some similarities with ABM in the sense that they also have the goal to study the behavior of complex systems computationally. However, they treat the individual units not as agents but rather as nodes in the network. For example, these individual units may represent neurons, components, or cities, which interact together to exhibit an entire complex system. Complex networks typically represent the system as graph structures where different components interact with each other in meaningful ways.
- *Temporal–causal modeling* is another mathematical and computational approach used to study the dynamics of various complex processes (varying from transportation systems to social networks, psychological or biological phenomena, and more), by representing them as a causal network of multiple (sub)systems or components. The main difference with the aforementioned modeling techniques is that it uses an explicit notion of time to describe the components' interaction. As a consequence, temporal–causal models can be used to simulate the dynamics of a system, enabling modelers to have insights into various real-time behaviors, addressing questions like why, when, what, or how. For example, how the occurrence of an event (or intervention) is responsible for a (behavioral) change, and how this change can have certain consequences (Kuipers, 1984; Treur, 2020).

The approach we present in this chapter, *network-oriented modeling* (Kuipers, 1984; Treur, 2020), is inspired by all of these approaches. The main underlying idea is that any complex system in nature can be modeled computationally as a network of interacting components or factors (represented formally as numerical variables). More specifically, a causal relationship between an event and its consequences can be represented by two or more variables (or nodes) connected through a weighted directional arrow (Treur, 2020). The causal relationships between these factors can be modeled using mathematical formulae (e.g., difference equations), which can be used to simulate their behavior over time.

To illustrate this, consider a combination of factors (from the literature) that have been found to influence stress. For instance, Jiang et al. (2016) mention the *use of music to reduce stress.* Such a relationship can be formally represented by two variables connected via a directional arrow, i.e., music → stress (or $W \rightarrow Z$, where W = music and Z = stress). Similarly, the finding that a *mindfulness-based intervention could reduce stress* (Ireland et al., 2017) can be represented as mindfulness-based intervention → stress (or $X \rightarrow Z$, where X = mindfulness-based intervention and Z = stress). Moreover, a person might be under *unusual stress,* caused by a *large number of stressful life events* (LaRocca, 1984) represented by $Y \rightarrow Z$, where Y = stressful life event and Z = stress. Taken together, these causal–temporal relationships can be represented graphically as shown in Figure 13.1, where music and meditation reduce stress (dotted arrows), while stressful life event (like chronic illness) increases stress (solid arrow).

The impact of each of the incoming states varies as per the strength of a connection. To illustrate it further, consider the impact of the mindfulness intervention in the example: *Higher levels* of mindfulness can significantly reduce stress (Dehghan et al., 2020). This effect can be represented by an *increased connection strength* for the connection from state mindfulness to stress (higher values of $\omega_{\text{mindfulness,stress}}$). This impact can be calculated over time, so when mindfulness is higher (at time

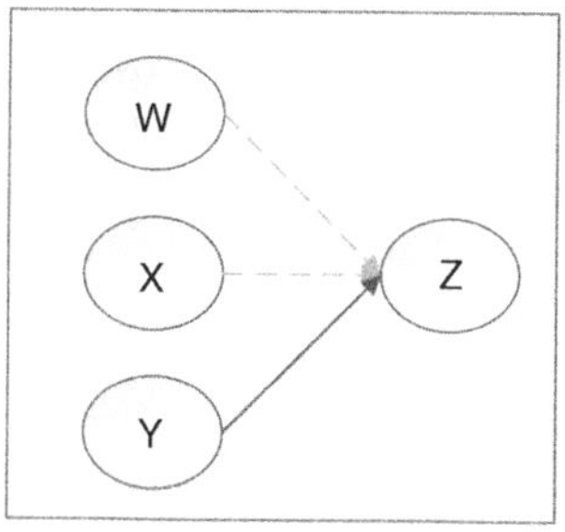

Figure 13.1 Example visualization of a causal–temporal relationship of different factors influencing stress.

point t), it will reduce stress. In a formal notation, impact of an incoming *state variable* at a time point t can be computed as

$$\textbf{impact}_{X,Y}(t) = \omega_{X,Y}\, X(t)$$

After adding the relevant details to a designed model (for details see Treur, 2020), the impact of all relevant variables on stress (i.e., music, mindfulness intervention, ...) is aggregated to estimate the total impact. This network-oriented approach enables researchers to study the dynamics of the entire system by running simulations and applying mathematical verification (Treur, 2020). Some efforts demonstrate that (part of) these models can also be validated against empirical data (Jabeen, 2018; Jabeen et al., 2020). However, collecting appropriate data that can be directly mapped to the variables used in the models has always been challenging (Igelström et al., 2022).

In contrast to other modeling techniques, such as inferential (e.g., regression models, Bayes models) or predictive modeling (e.g., neural networks, support vector machines), network-oriented models do not rely solely on data analytics to estimate their outcomes. Instead, they enable researchers to observe the causal–temporal associations among variables (through simulations), facilitating a deeper understanding of underlying complex phenomena. Also, they are able to explain various behaviors using different simulation experiments. Moreover, they have the potential to complement other computational methods while reflecting their causality (Igelström et al., 2022; Jabeen, 2018; Jabeen et al., 2020). The next section explains how network-oriented models of mental health may be applied in practice, for instance, to run what if simulations that allow the researcher to predict the hypothetical effect of a certain intervention for an individual. The next section discuss how this approach could be implemented within mental health chatbots, allowing the chatbot itself to reason about the mental state of its user.

Using Network-Oriented Models in Practice

In the digital solutions for mental health section, we discussed that chatbots can be valuable for improving one's mental health by using different intervention strategies (e.g., behavioral therapies, emotion regulation). Next, in the network-oriented modeling approach section, we explained how network-oriented modeling can be applied to study the dynamics of any complex phenomenon, including mental health. This section puts forward an approach to combine these two developments to come up with chatbots that can reason about the mental health of individual users. This approach is taken in the *What's BOThering You* project,[1] a research collaboration between several universities in the Netherlands and Flanders funded by Netherlands Organization Health Research and Development ZonMw.

The underlying idea of our approach is that a network-oriented model of mental health is developed, which will be incorporated as a dedicated module within a mental health chatbot. The chatbot conversations would be inspired by the designed models and will help to collect information regarding the (causal) components/factors. Once the data are collected (via conversations), the models can help estimate the user's mental health. These models can also be used to study the influence of possible interventions, thus allowing the chatbot to provide insights regarding the effects of (hypothetical) interventions. As a result, the chatbot is endowed with the ability to predict what will happen in the hypothetical case that a certain node in the network is changed (in other words, what will happen if a certain intervention is applied). By using the network-oriented model, the chatbot will then be capable of deriving the consequences of this hypothetical intervention for the individual's mental health. And if these consequences match the desired pattern and outcome, it may decide to actually apply this intervention. Such decisions may be implemented either through simple decision rules (e.g., "If the hypothetical intervention is predicted to result in >10% increase in overall mental health, then apply it") or they may be the outcome of a machine learning component, which has been trained on historical data.

Moreover, to be able to reason and interact about the mental health of a user, the chatbot should have information about their current state and its related factors. A simple example can be estimating an emotion (positive/negative affect) in relation with certain feedback in a certain context. It is to be noted that such observations also require data that can be mapped to the variables used in a network-oriented model. In the literature, different techniques are used to collect these kinds of data. For example, some studies use one-time data via surveys (Andrews et al., 2006), while others use data over time (e.g., longitudinal: Lemyre et al., 2023; Schindler et al., 2021), or ecological momentary assessment (EMA) (Asselbergs et al., 2016). Interview-based methods are also used to estimate the mental health of students (Andrews et al., 2006). Different studies also used machine learning techniques (e.g., natural language processing or deep learning; Zhang et al., 2022) or conversational analysis (Weizenbaum, 1983) to enhance the conversational and prediction capabilities of a chatbot. This is usually done by enriching knowledge corpora or learning from conversations (Abd-alrazaq et al., 2020; Assayed et al., 2023; Babulak, 2023). These techniques can help in understanding users' messages and predicting the relevant factors based on a semantic analysis of the text.

As soon as the chatbot has collected relevant data, this can be combined with certain reasoning techniques (i.e., network models) to predict the future development of a model. For instance, network models can be used to identify most relevant or interacting nodes (i.e., symptoms). So along with EMA data, complex structural patterns can be analyzed and predicted (Heshmati et al., 2022). Also, causality can be studied through observational data, which can be helpful to reason about and predict variations in behaviors over time (Igelström et al., 2022; Jabeen, 2018; Jabeen et al., 2020). Yet, it is to be noted that, for these types of models, data collection (for latent variables) can be challenging (Igelström et al., 2022). Thus, available data can also be analyzed by considering fewer variables to understand the essence of models (Igelström et al., 2022; Jabeen et al., 2020). Such an analysis can be helpful in understanding the context of a conversation. An example can be to understand a pattern during a conversation (e.g., absence of purpose in life); the chatbot can predict its consequences (by network models) and can intervene to regulate and improve the individual's mental health (e.g., by giving an optimistic response like, "You may think of doing yoga; this might help you focus on your life more").

In all, different prediction techniques are being used to complement conversational technologies to foster mental health and well-being (Abd-alrazaq et al., 2019). However, the combination of network-oriented modeling and chatbots opens new possibilities that, to our knowledge, have not been applied before. Integrating network-oriented modeling techniques into chatbot development has the potential to enhance user–chatbot interactions for several reasons. First, the models are designed in a scenario-based manner and thus can reflect different (causal) phenomenon or illnesses (Borsboom, 2017; Treur, 2020). Second, these models can be constructed by considering inter- and intrapersonal relations of an individual (or their network), which can help researchers to understand and predict the possible outcomes. Third, these approaches are supported by data, and with the advancement in data analytics, the possible outcomes can be estimated more accurately. Fourth, these models can help identify which symptoms or factors need to be regulated to avoid any undesired state. Fifth, mental health is a complex phenomenon that is multidimensional and varies over time. That is, it includes (the absence of) not merely psychological complaints (e.g., stress, low mood, concentration difficulties) but also wellness components (e.g., positive emotions, attitude, social interactions) of an individual, which may vary over time. This can conveniently be captured by network-oriented models.

Although the proposed methodology may have several benefits to provide better health solutions, its possible limitations have to be kept in mind during the design of a chatbot. For instance, like other AI-based techniques, causal models can answer only the specific research questions for which they have been developed (Treur, 2020). In other words, their output is deterministic by nature, so they can reflect only the modeled behavior. So, although they can explain the user interaction and behavioral development, the designed chatbot can sometimes act more like a rule-based chatbot. Also, the network models are typically based on a set of assumptions that are sometimes difficult to validate based on the literature. Therefore, if underlying assumptions are not validated before using a chatbot, this may negatively influence its performance. Moreover, these models are validated based on certain data, which may vary with different settings or environments and thus can introduce bias (Igelström et al., 2022). Despite these potential limitations of network-oriented models, we believe they can inspire conversational designers to enhance the effectiveness of mental health chatbots by using network models. This approach can help them in better understanding and explaining human behaviors and to design chatbots to interact with users in a more personalized manner.

Note

1 https://www.ru.nl/en/research/research-projects/whats-bothering-you

References

Abd-alrazaq, A. A., Alajlani, M., Alalwan, A. A., Bewick, B. M., Gardner, P., & Househ, M. (2019). An overview of the features of chatbots in mental health: A scoping review. *International Journal of Medical Informatics*, *132*, 103978. https://doi.org/10.1016/j.ijmedinf.2019.103978

Abd-Alrazaq, A. A., Rababeh, A., Alajlani, M., Bewick, B. M., & Househ, M. (2020). Effectiveness and safety of using chatbots to improve mental health: Systematic review and meta-analysis. *Journal of Medical Internet Research*, *22*(7), e16021. https://doi.org/10.2196/16021

Andrews, B., Hejdenberg, J., & Wilding, J. (2006). Student anxiety and depression: Comparison of questionnaire and interview assessments. *Journal of Affective Disorders*, *95*(1), 29–34. https://doi.org/10.1016/j.jad.2006.05.003

Arıkan, M. K., Ilhan, R., Pogarell, O., & Metin, B. (2023). When to stop medication in unipolar depression: A systematic review and a meta-analysis of randomized controlled trials. *Journal of Affective Disorders*, *325*, 7–13. https://doi.org/10.1016/j.jad.2023.01.024

Assayed, S. K., Alkhatib, M., & Shaalan, K. (2023). *A generative AI chatbot in high school advising: A qualitative analysis of domain-specific chatbot and chatgpt*. Research Square. https://doi.org/10.21203/rs.3.rs-3710923/v1

Asselbergs, J., Ruwaard, J., Ejdys, M., Schrader, N., Sijbrandij, M., & Riper, H. (2016). Mobile phone-based unobtrusive ecological momentary assessment of day-to-day mood: An explorative study. *Journal of Medical Internet Research*, *18*(3), e72. https://doi.org/10.2196/jmir.5505

Babulak, E. (2023). Introductory chapter: Journey to AI driven chatbots. In *Chatbots—The AI-driven front-line services for customers*. IntechOpen. https://doi.org/10.5772/intechopen.112461

Barker, M. M., Bland, M., & Fraser, L. K. (2020). Anxiety and depression prevalence in children, adolescents, and young adults with life-limiting conditions—Reply. *JAMA Pediatrics*, *174*(2), 208–209. https://doi.org/10.1001/jamapediatrics.2019.4809

Borsboom, D. (2017). A network theory of mental disorders. *World Psychiatry*, *16*(1), 5–13. https://doi.org/10.1002/wps.20375

Chen, G. J., Kunik, M. E., Marti, C. N., & Choi, N. G. (2022). Cost-effectiveness of tele-delivered behavioral activation by lay counselors for homebound older adults with depression. *BMC Psychiatry*, *22*(1), 648. https://doi.org/10.1186/s12888-022-04272-9

Chow, J. C. L., Sanders, L., & Li, K. (2023). Impact of ChatGPT on medical chatbots as a disruptive technology. *Frontiers in Artificial Intelligence*, *6*, 1166014. https://doi.org/10.3389/frai.2023.1166014

Dehghan, M., Jazinizade, M., Malakoutikhah, A., Madadimahani, A., Iranmanesh, M. H., Oghabian, S., Mohammadshahi, F., Janfaza, F., & Zakeri, M. A. (2020). Stress and quality of life of patients with cancer: The mediating role of mindfulness. *Journal of Oncology*, *2020*, 1–10. https://doi.org/10.1155/2020/3289521

Devaram, S. (2020). *Empathic Chatbot: Emotional intelligence for empathic chatbot: Emotional intelligence for mental health well-being*. ArXiv. https://doi.org/10.48550/ARXIV.2012.09130

Fitzpatrick, K. K., Darcy, A., & Vierhile, M. (2017). Delivering cognitive behavior therapy to young adults with symptoms of depression and anxiety using a fully automated conversational agent (Woebot): A randomized controlled trial. *JMIR Mental Health*, *4*(2), e19. https://doi.org/10.2196/mental.7785

GBD 2019 Risk Factors Collaborators. (2020). Global burden of 87 risk factors in 204 countries and territories, 1990–2019: A systematic analysis for the global burden of disease study 2019. *The Lancet*, *396*(10258), 1223–1249. https://doi.org/10.1016/S0140-6736(20)30752-2

Goonesekera, Y., & Donkin, L. (2022). A cognitive behavioral therapy chatbot (Otis) for health anxiety management: Mixed methods pilot study. *JMIR Formative Research*, *6*(10), e37877. https://doi.org/10.2196/37877

Graf, B., Krüger, M., Müller, F., Ruhland, A., & Zech, A. (2015, November). Nombot: Simplify food tracking. *Proceedings of the 14th International Conference on Mobile and Ubiquitous Multimedia*. https://doi.org/10.1145/2836041.2841208

Greenberg, P. E., Fournier, A. A., Sisitsky, T., Simes, M., Berman, R., Koenigsberg, S. H., & Kessler, R. C. (2021). The economic burden of adults with major depressive disorder in the United States (2010 and 2018). *PharmacoEconomics*, *39*(6), 653–665. https://doi.org/10.1007/s40273-021-01019-4

Grové, C. (2021). Co-developing a mental health and wellbeing chatbot with and for young people. *Frontiers in Psychiatry*, *11*, 606041. https://doi.org/10.3389/fpsyt.2020.606041

He, Y., Yang, L., Qian, C., Li, T., Su, Z., Zhang, Q., & Hou, X. (2023). Conversational agent interventions for mental health problems: Systematic review and meta-analysis of randomized controlled trials. *Journal of Medical Internet Research*, *25*, e43862. https://doi.org/10.2196/43862

Heshmati, S., Oravecz, Z., Brick, T. R., & Roeser, R. W. (2022). Assessing psychological well-being in early adulthood: Empirical evidence for the structure of daily well-being via network analysis. *Applied Developmental Science*, *26*(2), 207–225. https://doi.org/10.1080/10888691.2020.1766356

Hudlicka, E. (2016). Enhancing mindfulness-based cognitive therapy with a virtual mindfulness coach. In M. M. Maheu, K. P. Drude, & S. D. Wright (Eds.), *Career paths in telemental health* (pp. 171–182). Springer. https://doi.org/10.1007/978-3-319-23736-7_16

Igelström, E., Craig, P., Lewsey, J., Lynch, J., Pearce, A., & Katikireddi, S. V. (2022). Causal inference and effect estimation using observational data. *Journal of Epidemiology and Community Health*, *76*(11), 960–966. https://doi.org/10.1136/jech-2022-219267

Inkster, B., Sarda, S., & Subramanian, V. (2018). An empathy-driven, conversational artificial intelligence agent (Wysa) for digital mental well-being: Real-world data evaluation mixed-methods study. *JMIR mHealth and uHealth*, *6*(11), e12106. https://doi.org/10.2196/12106

Ireland, M., Spencer, L., O'Connor, A., Clough, B., & Gill, K. (2017). A randomized controlled trial of mindfulness to reduce stress and burnout among intern medical practitioners. *Medical Teacher*, *39*(4), 409–414. https://doi.org/10.1080/0142159X.2017.1294749

Jabeen, F. (2018). How happy you are: A computational study of social impact on self-esteem. In S. Staab, O. Koltsova, & D. Ignatov (Eds.), *Lecture notes in computer science* (pp. 108–117). Springer. https://doi.org/10.1007/978-3-030-01159-8_10

Jabeen, F., Gerritsen, C., & Treur, J. (2020). Narcissism and fame: A complex network model for the adaptive interaction of digital narcissism and online popularity. *Applied network. Science*, *5*(1). https://doi.org/10.1007/s41109-020-00319-6

Jiang, J., Rickson, D., & Jiang, C. (2016). The mechanism of music for reducing psychological stress: Music preference as a mediator. *The Arts in Psychotherapy*, *48*, 62–68. https://doi.org/10.1016/j.aip.2016.02.002

Kocielnik, R., Xiao, L., Avrahami, D., & Hsieh, G. (2018). Reflection companion: A conversational system for engaging users in reflection on physical activity. *Proceedings of the ACM on Interactive, Mobile, Wearable and Ubiquitous Technologies*, *2*(2), 1–26. https://doi.org/10.1145/3214273

Krahmer, E., Bosse, T., & de Bruijn, G. (2022). Chatbots and health. In E. Ho, C. Bylund, & J. Van Weert (Eds.), *The international encyclopedia of health communication* (pp. 1–9). John Wiley & Sons. https://doi.org/10.1002/9781119678816.iehc0724

Kuhn, M., & Johnson, K. (2013). *Applied predictive modeling*. Springer New York. https://doi.org/10.1007/978-1-4614-6849-3

Kuipers, B. (1984). Commonsense reasoning about causality: Deriving behavior from structure. *Artificial Intelligence*, *24*(1), 169–203. https://doi.org/10.1016/0004-3702(84)90039-0

LaRocca, N. G. (1984). Psychosocial factors in multiple sclerosis and the role of stress. *Annals of the New York Academy of Sciences*, *436*, 435–442. https://doi.org/10.1111/j.1749-6632.1984.tb14816

Lemyre, A., Palmer-Cooper, E., & Messina, J. P. (2023). Wellbeing among university students during the COVID-19 pandemic: A systematic review of longitudinal studies. *Public Health*, *222*, 125–133. https://doi.org/10.1016/j.puhe.2023.07.001

Lim, S. M., Shiau, C. W. C., Cheng, L. J., & Lau, Y. (2022). Chatbot-delivered psychotherapy for adults with depressive and anxiety symptoms: A systematic review and meta-regression. *Behavior Therapy*, *53*(2), 334–347. https://doi.org/10.1016/j.beth.2021.09.007

Maurya, R. K. (2023). *Using AI based chatbot chatGPT for practicing counseling skills through role-play. PsyArXiv.* https://doi.org/10.31234/osf.io/s47jb

McCoy, M. D., & Ladefoged, T. N. (2009). New developments in the use of spatial technology in archaeology. *Journal of Archaeological Research, 17*(3), 263–295. https://doi.org/10.1007/s10814-009-9030-1

McElroy, E., Shevlin, M., Murphy, J., & McBride, O. (2018). Co-occurring internalizing and externalizing psychopathology in childhood and adolescence: A network approach. *European Child Adolescent Psychiatry, 27*(11), 1449–1457. https://doi.org/10.1007/s00787-018-1128-x

Moshe, I., Terhorst, Y., Philippi, P., Domhardt, M., Cuijpers, P., Cristea, I., Pulkki-Råback, L., Baumeister, H., & Sander, L. B. (2021). Digital interventions for the treatment of depression: A meta-analytic review. *Psychological Bulletin, 147*(8), 749–786. https://doi.org/10.1037/bul0000334

Mott, B., Lester, J., & Branting, K. (2004). Conversational agents. In M. Singh (Ed.), *The practical handbook of internet computing.* Chapman & Hall/CRC. https://doi.org/10.1201/9780203507223.ch10

Niermann, H. C., Voss, C., Pieper, L., Venz, J., Ollmann, T. M., & Beesdo-Baum, K. (2021). Anxiety disorders among adolescents and young adults: Prevalence and mental health care service utilization in a regional epidemiological study in Germany. *Journal of Anxiety Disorders, 83*, 102453. https://doi.org/10.1016/j.janxdis.2021.102453

Oud, M., de Winter, L., Vermeulen-Smit, E., Bodden, D., Nauta, M., Stone, L., van den Heuvel, M., Taher, R. A., de Graaf, I., Kendall, T., Engels, R., & Stikkelbroek, Y. (2019). Effectiveness of CBT for children and adolescents with depression: A systematic review and meta-regression analysis. *European Psychiatry, 57*, 33–45. https://doi.org/10.1016/j.eurpsy.2018.12.008

Peter, T., Roberts, L. W., & Dengate, J. (2011). Flourishing in life: An empirical test of the dual continua model of mental health and mental illness among Canadian university students. *International Journal of Mental Health Promotion, 13*(1), 13–22. https://doi.org/10.1080/14623730.2011.9715646

Richards, D., & Richardson, T. (2012). Computer-based psychological treatments for depression: A systematic review and meta-analysis. *Clinical Psychology Review, 32*(4), 329–342. https://doi.org/10.1016/j.cpr.2012.02.004

Rouquette, A., Pingault, J.-B., Fried, E. I., Orri, M., Falissard, B., Kossakowski, J. J., Vitaro, F., Tremblay, R., Cote, S. M., & Borsboom, D. (2018). Emotional and behavioral symptom network structure in elementary school girls and association with anxiety disorders and depression in adolescence and early adulthood: A network analysis. *JAMA Psychiatry, 75*(11), 1173–1181. https://doi.org/10.1001/jamapsychiatry.2018.2119

Schindler, A. K., Polujanski, S., & Rotthoff, T. (2021). A longitudinal investigation of mental health, perceived learning environment and burdens in a cohort of first-year German medical students' before and during the COVID-19 "new normal.". *BMC Medical Education, 21*(1), 413. https://doi.org/10.1186/s12909-021-02798-2

Shamekhi, A., & Bickmore, T. (2015). Breathe with me: A virtual meditation coach. In W.-P. Brinkman, J. Broekens, & D. Heylen (Eds.), *Intelligent virtual agents* (pp. 279–282). Springer. http://dx.doi.org/10.1007/978-3-319-21996-7_29

Snippe, E., Viechtbauer, W., Geschwind, N., Klippel, A., de Jonge, P., & Wichers, M. (2017). The impact of treatments for depression on the dynamic network structure of mental states: Two randomized controlled trials. *Scientific Reports, 7*(1), 1–10. https://doi.org/10.1038/srep46523

Stimpfl, J. N., Mills, J. A., & Strawn, J. R. (2023). Pharmacologic predictors of benzodiazepine response trajectory in anxiety disorders: A Bayesian hierarchical modeling meta-analysis. *CNS Spectrums, 28*(1), 53–60. https://doi.org/10.1017/S1092852921000870

Thabrew, H., Stasiak, K., Hetrick, S. E., Wong, S., Huss, J. H., & Merry, S. N. (2018). E-health interventions for anxiety and depression in children and adolescents with long-term physical conditions. *Cochrane Database of Systematic Reviews, 8.* https://doi.org/10.1002/14651858.CD012489.pub2

Treur, J. (2020). *Network-oriented modeling for adaptive networks: Designing higher-order adaptive biological, mental and social network models.* Springer. https://doi.org/10.1007/978-3-030-31445-3

Vaidyam, A. N., Linggonegoro, D., & Torous, J. (2020). Changes to the psychiatric chatbot landscape: A systematic review of conversational agents in serious mental illness. *The Canadian Journal of Psychiatry, 66*(4), 339–348. https://doi.org/10.1177/0706743720966429

Vaidyam, A. N., Wisniewski, H., Halamka, J. D., Kashavan, M. S., & Torous, J. B. (2019). Chatbots and conversational agents in mental health: A review of the psychiatric landscape. *The Canadian Journal of Psychiatry, 64*(7), 456–464. https://doi.org/10.1177/0706743719828977

Wasil, A. R., Gillespie, S., Patel, R., Petre, A., Venturo-Conerly, K. E., Shingleton, R. M., ... DeRubeis, R. J. (2020). Reassessing evidence-based content in popular smartphone apps for depression and anxiety: Developing and applying user-adjusted analyses. *Journal of Consulting and Clinical Psychology, 88*(11), 983–993. https://doi.org/10.1037/ccp0000604

Wasil, A. R., Venturo-Conerly, K. E., Shingleton, R. M., & Weisz, J. R. (2019). A review of popular smartphone apps for depression and anxiety: Assessing the inclusion of evidence-based content. *Behaviour Research and Therapy, 123*, 103498. https://doi.org/10.1016/j.brat.2019.103498

Weizenbaum, J. (1983). ELIZA — A computer program for the study of natural language communication between man and machine. *Communications of the ACM, 26*(1), 23–28. https://doi.org/10.1145/357980.357991

Xu, Z., Huang, F., Koesters, M., Staiger, T., Becker, T., Thornicroft, G., & Ruesch, N. (2018). Effectiveness of interventions to promote help-seeking for mental health problems: Systematic review and meta-analysis. *Psychological Medicine*, *48*(16), 2658–2667. https://doi.org/10.1017/S0033291718001265

Yang, T., Guo, Z., Cao, X., Zhu, X., Zhou, Q., Li, X., Wang, H., Wang, X., Wu, L., Wu, S., & Liu, X. (2022). Network analysis of anxiety and depression in the functionally impaired elderly. *Frontiers in Public Health*, *10*, 1067646. https://doi.org/10.3389/fpubh.2022.1067646

Zhang, T., Schoene, A. M., Ji, S., & Ananiadou, S. (2022). Natural language processing applied to mental illness detection: A narrative review. *npj Digital Medicine*, *5*(1), 46. https://doi.org/10.1038/s41746-022-00589-7

Zhu, Y., Wang, R., & Pu, C. (2022). "I am chatbot, your virtual mental health adviser." What drives citizens' satisfaction and continuance intention toward mental health chatbots during the COVID-19 pandemic? An empirical study in China. *DIGITAL HEALTH*, *8*, 205520762210900. https://doi.org/10.1177/20552076221090031

14

mHealth for Mental Health: Expanding the Reach of Care

Nancy Lau[1,2], Lola Kola[3,4,5], Xin Zhao[1,2], Seth Asafo[6,7], Dzifa Attah[6], and Dror Ben-Zeev[1,4]

[1] Department of Psychiatry and Behavioral Sciences, University of Washington School of Medicine
[2] Center for Child Health, Behavior and Development, Seattle Children's Research Institute
[3] WHO Collaborating Centre for Research and Training in Mental Health, Neurosciences and Drug and Alcohol Abuse
[4] BRiTE Center, University of Washington
[5] Centre for Global Mental Health, David Goldberg Centre, Institute of Psychiatry, Psychology and Neuroscience, King's College London
[6] Department of Psychiatry, University of Ghana Medical School
[7] Department of Psychology, Accra College of Medicine

Mental health disorders are leading contributors to the global burden of disease and disability. The majority of people with mental health problems worldwide do not have access to high-quality mental health care. The COVID-19 pandemic has further exacerbated the mental health crisis with increasing incidence of new onset of mental health disorders and worsening of symptoms for those with preexisting mental health conditions (Moreno et al., 2020; Mukhtar, 2020). Mental health disorders cost the global economy $2.5 trillion USD annually in health care and lost productivity in 2010; annual cost is projected to increase to $6 trillion USD by 2030 (Campion et al., 2022). Common barriers to mental health services include limited human resources, geographic constraints, mental health stigma, and cost of services (Wainberg et al., 2017).

Technological advances have allowed us to begin to overcome traditional barriers to accessing in-person mental health services. The demands for mental health services cannot be met with in-person mental health services alone due to limited provider availability disproportionate to need and treatment cost (Aboujaoude et al., 2020). Smartphones have become ubiquitous across all aspects of work and life domains irrespective of gender, race and ethnicity, and socioeconomic status (Aboujaoude et al., 2020). The total number of smartphone users is 6.92 billion, with 86% of the world's population owning a smartphone (Turner, 2023). There are over 350,000 health care apps available for public download, and more than 90,000 apps were added in 2020 (IQVIA Institute for Human Data Science, 2021). Mobile health (mHealth) utilizes mobile phones and other handheld devices to deliver

The Handbook of Mental Health Communication, First Edition.
Edited by Marco C. Yzer and Jason T. Siegel.

mental health resources as users go about their daily lives (Price et al., 2014). The implementation of mHealth-based care delivery has the potential to reduce health disparities; for example, 73% of families living below the poverty line have one or more smartphones and digital interventions have been proposed as a feasible means of disseminating health programs in homeless populations (Rhoades et al., 2017). mHealth interventions demonstrate advantages in self-pacing, anonymity, reduced human resources and infrastructure requirements, and cost-effectiveness (Ebert et al., 2015; Ybarra & Eaton, 2005). The use of mHealth interventions has the potential to overcome disparities in access to evidence-based mental health care, improve patient education and involvement in treatment, and enhance the adoption and uptake of evidence-based practices (Price et al., 2014).

mHealth for mental health is a relatively nascent field. The COVID-19 pandemic has further accelerated the use and uptake of mHealth interventions for mental health, with more than 10,000 publicly available mHealth apps focused on self-management of mental health symptoms. mHealth interventions cover a wide array of functions/features such as symptom monitoring, psychoeducation, e-connecting to providers, facilitation of psychotherapy-assigned homework, journaling, cognitive and/or behavioral skills practice, and gamification. There is some evidence that mHealth interventions for mental health may be associated with moderate effect sizes for anxiety and depression, similar to the treatment benefits of in-person interventions (Firth et al., 2017a, 2017b). Other systematic reviews have shown mixed findings with generally low study quality, diminished treatment effect sizes with active comparison conditions, and no long-term efficacy studies (Goldberg et al., 2022; Marcolino et al., 2018). Additionally, a recent review of 1,000+ publicly available stress management and wellness apps showed that <1% had peer-reviewed publications in support of their efficacy (Lau et al., 2020).

The World Health Organization (WHO) has promoted initiatives for the adoption of mHealth mental health services (Grist et al., 2017). Research has shown that traditionally underserved populations who have limited access to or decline in-person mental health services are less reluctant to use digital and mHealth interventions (Price et al., 2014). However, whereas the implementation of mHealth has the potential to expand the reach of care to high-needs and underserved populations across the lifespan, the popularity of mHealth applications far outpaces that of the evidence in support of their use. mHealth tools, although promising in clinical and scientific potential, exist in a rapidly accelerating and unregulated space (Marzano et al., 2015). Here, we summarize the state of the science, discuss clinical implications, and future research directions. We focus our review on three major public health priorities that warrant attention from health care, industry, and research communities: supporting mental health gaps for children and young people (CYP), people living with serious mental illness (SMI), and those who reside in low- and middle-income countries (LMIC).

Children and Young People

The prevalence of mental health disorders in CYP continues to rise, with a global prevalence rate of 13.4% (Polanczyk et al., 2015). Approximately one-fourth of CYP have experienced a mental health disorder in the past year, and approximately one-third across their lifetimes (Merikangas et al., 2022). Less than half of CYP with mental health needs receive treatment (Merikangas et al., 2022). These mental health symptoms negatively impact critical stages of development, cause significant distress, disrupt social relationships, impair academic and occupational functioning, and are associated with poor health-related quality of life. Research has shown that a majority of adults with mental health disorders experience symptom onset in childhood and adolescence (Kessler et al., 2007). Symptoms often persist across the lifespan into adulthood if left untreated and increase the risk of developing comorbid mental health disorders. This highlights the importance of early intervention (Weisz et al., 2013).

mHealth interventions may be particularly appealing to CYP who are digital natives accustomed to interacting on smartphones and the Internet (Granger et al., 2016). The Internet and smartphones have shaped how CYP learn, create, and maintain social relationships; spend their free time; and engage with the world (The Lancet Child & Adolescent Health, 2018). A developmental science framework suggests that meeting CYP where they are necessitates the use of technology and a paradigm shift in treatment norms (Giovanelli et al., 2020). In the United States, 95% of teens have access to a smartphone (Vogels et al., 2022). The Internet serves as a primary means of mental health–related information-seeking and communication platform for CYP (Gulliver et al., 2010). Research has shown strong acceptability of digital interventions among CYP and that digital interventions provide a sense of autonomy (Venturo-Conerly et al., 2022). Motivating mechanisms for technology use include entertainment, information seeking, reinforcement, mastery, and self-efficacy (Giovanelli et al., 2020).

Anxiety and depression are among the most common mental health problems in CYP. A recent meta-analysis reported that global prevalence rates of clinically elevated anxiety and depressive symptoms in CYP are 20.5% and 25.2%, respectively (Racine et al., 2021). From 2016 to 2020, there has been a significant increase in CYP's anxiety disorder diagnoses (from 7.1% to 9.2%) and depression diagnoses (from 3.1% to 4%; Lebrun-Harris et al., 2022). A majority of mHealth interventions for CYP developed and tested in research settings target anxiety symptoms, depression symptoms, or both and incorporate strategies from in-person cognitive behavior therapy (CBT). CBT is the gold standard evidence-based psychotherapy for anxiety and depression with comparable treatment effects to that of psychiatric medications (David et al., 2018). Core treatment components are psychoeducation, cognitive restructuring, problem-solving, and behavioral techniques. At-home skills practice is a significant predictor of treatment response in CYP-focused anxiety and depression interventions, which can be facilitated by mHealth (Cummings et al., 2014).

A systematic review found that about half of commercially available apps for CYP with anxiety incorporated at least one evidence-based therapeutic ingredient, and about one-fourth contained more than one evidence-based therapeutic ingredient (Bry et al., 2018). The most frequently included therapeutic ingredient was exposure and cognitive restructuring, found in one-fifth of anxiety apps (Bry et al., 2018). Exposure is a key ingredient in CBT for anxiety disorders, in which anxious individuals are systematically exposed to feared stimuli to facilitate habituation and fear extinction (Kendall et al., 2005).

As for depression, many commercially available apps are not based on evidence-based therapeutic ingredients (or do not specify their use of evidence-based content; Cliffe et al., 2021). The relatively few apps that are informed by evidence-based treatments incorporate CBT, dialectical behavior therapy (DBT), interpersonal psychotherapy (IPT), and acceptance and commitment therapy (ACT; Cliffe et al., 2021). Most commercially available mental health apps are not supported by research (Neary & Schueller, 2018). Formats range from mHealth apps to texting services.

In research settings, mHealth interventions targeting CYP with anxiety and depression have established usability and feasibility. These are typically not available for public download. SmartCAT (Smartphone-enhanced Child Anxiety Treatment) is an example of an mHealth app that provides opportunities for reviewing CBT skills, exposure coaching in real time, and asynchronous communication between therapists and patients (Pramana et al., 2014). Therapists can utilize a therapist portal to exchange secure text messages or audiovisual files with patients, monitor adherence to treatment plans, track patient's anxiety ratings, and assign reward points. Patients and therapists have found SmartCAT to be acceptable, feasible, and understandable (Pramana et al., 2014). In the few available research trials of mHealth depression interventions, treatment effects were similar to those of active controls (Garrido et al., 2019). For example, in a double-blind randomized controlled trial (RCT), a CBT-based mHealth tool (MEMO) targeting depression prevention using text messages, videos, and animations yielded similar outcomes on depressive symptoms compared with the placebo group, although more from the active treatment group endorsed that the intervention was helpful (Whittaker et al., 2017). Additionally, many mHealth interventions were initially developed and tested in the adult population and then adapted for CYP. For example, the app-based platform IntelliCare was initially developed for adults and adapted for younger populations, such as college students (Lattie et al., 2016). It includes a suite of CBT and positive psychology skills modules and targets symptoms of depression and anxiety.

mHealth interventions are highly appealing for CYP who grew up with the Internet and prefer online self-help. mHealth interventions for CYP have incorporated common evidence-based therapeutic content such as CBT and have demonstrated feasibility and acceptability in research settings. The majority of such interventions focus on improving anxiety and depression given their high symptom prevalence rates in CYP and incorporate opportunities to communicate with mental health providers asynchronously or in real time.

Limitations and Recommendations for Research

mHealth interventions for CYP do not match the attractiveness, engagement, and interactivity of digital media that CYP typically engage with (Scholten & Granic, 2019). Most research efforts have simply transferred intervention manual content to a digital platform. CYP, who value self-efficacy and a sense of control, perceive such interventions to be inflexible, impersonal, and unresponsive to their needs. The cognitive load of mHealth interventions may be too challenging for CYP (especially those who are younger), with lengthy treatment modules on cognitive skills (Scholten & Granic, 2019). CYP may not understand their need for or are unable to engage with mHealth interventions when experiencing acute symptoms (Aguirre Velasco et al., 2020). mHealth interventions for CYP commonly incorporate some form of therapist involvement, but the need for therapists compromises scalability and access (Liverpool et al., 2020; Scholten & Granic, 2019). Entirely self-guided mHealth interventions may work best for prevention and early intervention. A serious games approach to mHealth interventions may be particularly appealing to CYP (Scholten & Granic, 2019). Common gamification elements (e.g., challenges, points, badges, leader boards) may increase engagement and sustainability. Future research should encourage CYP involvement in the co-design, refinement, and implementation of mHealth interventions; incorporating CYP perspectives is a critical step toward creating an engaging and sustainable mHealth intervention. Finally, research should explore the additive value of caregiver involvement and caregiver-facing therapeutic content, especially for younger CYPs (Funnell et al., 2022).

People with Serious Mental Illness

Individuals with SMI, such as schizophrenia and bipolar disorder, experience significant functional impairments and stigmatization and have very limited access to traditional mental health services. SMI leads to major impairments in social, academic, and work domains. People with SMI experience social isolation, comorbid mental health conditions such as anxiety, depression, and substance use, cognitive impairments, and financial disability (John et al., 2015). In the United States alone, SMI affects approximately 14.1 million adults ages 18 and older, which represents 5.5% of the US adult population (Substance Abuse and Mental Health Services Administration, 2022). A significant majority of people living with SMI have unmet mental health needs that hinder their ability to live healthy and productive lives (Ben-Zeev & Atkins, 2017). People with SMI are subject to significant stigma, discrimination, and victimization (Subu et al., 2021). Persons living with SMI also experience an increased risk of physical health conditions, wrongful incarceration, unemployment (Chowdhury & Chakraborty, 2017), homelessness (Choi et al., 2022), and suicide (Melamed et al., 2020). This not only affects individuals but also has a significant socioeconomic impact (Ben-Zeev & Atkins, 2017) as SMI is one of the leading contributors to health care expenditures globally and places a significant burden on public sector funding (Rathod et al., 2017). Cognitive impairments, limited literacy, and severe and intrusive mental health symptoms present barriers to mental health services (Ben-Zeev & Atkins, 2017). Many individuals with SMI do not receive treatment regularly (Mojtabai et al., 2009) and a nominal percentage (<5%) received evidence-based care.

Past research has shown that mHealth interventions have the potential to mitigate this service gap. A meta-analysis of studies conducted across the globe showed that a majority of individuals with SMI own a smartphone and are interested in mHealth interventions for symptom management (Firth & Torous, 2015). Although smartphone ownership in individuals with SMI is lower than in the general population, most adults with SMI engage with digital resources and social media in a comparable manner to adults without SMI and are interested in using their devices to manage symptoms (Ben-Zeev et al., 2012). mHealth has shown promise in bridging gaps in the detection, diagnosis, and treatment of persons living with SMI (Carter et al., 2021). Members of the mental health community have shown great interest in the development and use of mobile apps that can be used in the treatment and management of SMIs (Fortuna et al., 2019). This suggests that mHealth interventions may provide a scalable solution for mental health care.

mHealth interventions for individuals with SMI vary greatly in terms of clinician involvement and clinical use (Buck & Ben-Zeev, 2019). Formats include automated texts and self-guided smartphone applications for medication adherence and skills practice in between sessions (Granholm et al., 2012), asynchronous communication with a clinician for symptom monitoring and relapse prevention (Španiel et al., 2012), and clinician-guided real-time intervention delivery through text messaging (Myin-Germeys et al., 2011). These are not intended to fully replace human-delivered treatment; instead, they were designed to support and augment clinician-delivered services. mHealth interventions have the potential to facilitate the implementation of the coordinated specialty care (CSC) model, which emphasizes that multidisciplinary team efforts are needed to address the complex needs and severe functional impairments of patients with SMI; mHealth interventions can streamline multidisciplinary communication and support care coordination (Ben-Zeev et al., 2019).

Ben-Zeev et al. (2021) conducted a fully remote RCT of CORE, a smartphone intervention designed to challenge dysfunctional thoughts that are common symptoms of SMI, self-stigmatizing attitudes, and maladaptive beliefs that influence care seeking and mental health status. The intervention utilizes brief daily game-like exercises to counteract maladaptive beliefs about the self, others, and the world. Findings showed that CORE is usable, acceptable, and effective in significantly improving psychiatric symptoms. Ben-Zeev et al. (2018) conducted another RCT to test the effectiveness of the FOCUS intervention, which included the FOCUS mobile app, clinician dashboard, and mHealth support specialists. FOCUS was designed to support self-assessment and symptom self-management. Compared to a clinic-based group intervention, patients assigned to FOCUS were more likely to start treatment and remain engaged; treatment satisfaction and clinical outcomes were comparable in both groups. Text messaging interventions facilitating asynchronous clinician–patient communications have been shown to improve medication adherence, socialization, and symptom management. A relapse prevention program called the Information Technology Aided Relapse Prevention Programme in Schizophrenia (ITAREPS) provides mobile phone-based telemedicine for weekly remote patient monitoring and disease management and has been shown to be effective in an RCT.

Ben-Zeev et al. (2021) leveraged partnership with healers in Ghana to co-design a prototype of an mHealth toolkit (M-Healer) to support the dissemination of evidence-based SMI information and mental health care in Western Africa. Prototype module content included a program introduction, brief mental health interventions, verbal deescalation strategies, guided relaxation exercises, and human rights training. Qualitative interview data with local healers revealed that this smartphone toolkit was user-friendly and the information presented was understandable; healers also made suggestions to further improve the content and usability of the toolkit.

mHealth interventions show major promise in the detection, diagnosis, and treatment of individuals with SMI. Advantages of utilizing mHealth interventions in place of or in addition to in-person care include reducing treatment dropout, improving treatment satisfaction, reducing relapse rates, and improvement in psychiatric symptoms. A diverse array of treatment modalities have been deployed successfully, including self-guided smartphone apps and clinician-guided text messaging interventions. In addition, Chandrashekar (2018) reviewed existing literature to analyze the efficacy of smartphone-based treatments on mobile apps as compared to traditional treatments for three psychological disorders with high 12-month global prevalence rates: depression, anxiety, and schizophrenia. Mobile apps were found to have high efficacy in delivering mental health interventions. Factors associated with the effectiveness of these apps included high patient engagement, simpler user interfaces, transdiagnostic capabilities, and self-monitoring features.

Limitations and Recommendations for Research

Few large RCTs have been conducted on mHealth interventions for adults with SMI. Well-validated larger-scale studies, including underrepresented populations, are needed to demonstrate the clinical efficacy and effectiveness of mHealth interventions for adults with SMI. Concerns, such as data security and patient privacy, app sustainability over time, and attrition pose challenges to the adoption and implementation of mHealth tools for SMI (Tomczyk et al., 2021). To understand the unique perspectives of individuals with SMI and improve adoption and engagement, future research should also encourage the involvement of diverse patients with lived experience and their family members, frontline clinicians, multidisciplinary care teams, and policymakers in the process of the co-design and implementation of mHealth interventions. This will help inform the development and implementation of multicomponent mental health reform strategies to improve care and reduce human rights violations for individuals with SMI across the globe.

Low- and Middle-Income Countries

Over 80% of the world's population living with mental illness reside in LMICs (Rathod et al., 2017). Systematic reviews and meta-analyses have reported high rates of anxiety, depression, and post-traumatic stress disorders ranging from 12% to 75% among different population groups in LMICs (Freeman, 2022; Kieling et al., 2011; Roddy Mitchell et al., 2023; Yatham et al., 2018). Some pervasive negative societal attitudes toward mental illness in LMICs reinforce stereotyped views, stigma, prejudice, and discrimination against people with mental illness (Thornicroft et al., 2016, 2022). Mental disorders have severe consequences on health and productivity, but mental health as a disease burden remains a relatively low priority in LMICs (The Lancet Global Health, 2020). There is a significant gap in care for mental health conditions within LMICs such that up to 90% of persons suffering from mental health conditions do not receive satisfactory mental health care and follow-up care (Carter et al., 2021; Fu et al., 2020; Rathod et al., 2017). Barriers to mental health care within LMICs include lack of awareness of available mental health services, shortages in human resource and infrastructure constraints (e.g., providers, medication, equipment, facilities), lack of context-appropriate mental health interventions, mental illness stigma, lack of mental health literacy, and use of nonevidence-based traditional practices to diagnose and treat mental illness (Wainberg et al., 2017). This is exacerbated by poverty, geopolitical issues, and other systemic issues. Many countries in LMICs are affected by armed conflict, natural disasters, and violence, which have a significant negative impact on mental health (Tol et al., 2011).

For those seeking care, treatment options are limited to nonexistent. The few trained mental health professionals are located in their countries' major cities. In some LMICs, alternative harmful local treatment practices may range from caging, seclusion, forced fasting, administration of herbal medicine, or physical abuse to dispel demonic spirits (Drew et al., 2011). Such vulnerable persons with SMI may then become further traumatized and socially isolated and experience exacerbating mental health symptoms.

mHealth Interventions in LMICs

The use of digital health to increase coverage in mental health care has come to the forefront of the WHO agenda (Cuijpers et al., 2022; World Health Organization Guidelines, 2019). For people who reside in LMICs with limited access to mental health care, mHealth interventions may prove especially promising with widespread access to mobile phones and the internet (Ben-Zeev & Atkins, 2017). Though progress has been slow compared with general health care and other areas of public health, there has been growing interest in mHealth for mental health interventions in LMICs over the past decade (Free et al., 2013). The rapid growth of personalized digital health in mental health education and treatment continues to offer new solutions to systems- and patient-level barriers to care (Jabeen et al., 2023; Naslund & Deng, 2021; Rathbone et al., 2017). Despite the opportunities for scale-up and service integration mHealth presents for clinical care in low-resource settings, research and testing in the general population remain limited (Anglada-Martinez et al., 2015; Farooq et al., 2020; Free et al., 2010, 2013; Ragul et al., 2022). However, several intuitive features of mHealth are appealing and appropriate for diverse populations in LMICs, namely, accessibility in day-to-day life outside of hospital settings, the potential to design personalized interventions tailored to individual needs, and the wide range of mHealth platforms that can be leveraged for health management purposes (Fedele et al., 2017; McCool et al., 2022). The mobile technologies landscape in LMICs and the increasing ownership of mobile phones can be leveraged as powerful platforms for the provision of mental health education and treatment of mental disorders (Aschbrenner et al., 2019; McCool et al., 2022; Odgers & Jensen, 2020).

Despite the potential of mHealth in LMICs, current literature presents limited information on clinical efficacy and has methodological limitations. Existing research has also largely focused on addressing mental health disorders in adult populations despite the high burden of mental disorders in the youth population in developing countries (Oldehinkel & Ormel, 2023). Naslund et al. (2017) in a narrative review of 49 studies from 20 LMICs reported on the feasibility, acceptability, and potential clinical effectiveness of online, text messaging, and telephone support of digital interventions in reducing symptoms of mental health disorders. The majority of studies were assessments of feasibility and acceptability and showed positive results. Over one-fourth of studies used digital technology to complement care delivery in clinical settings and to provide basic mental health education to health workers. Over one-fourth of studies used mobile phone text messaging, Internet-based interventions, and telehealth to provide psychosocial support. The few studies that focused on effectiveness showed significant improvements in mental health symptoms and medication adherence. Similarly, a recent review of digital mental health prevention and treatment showed evidence of feasibility and acceptability. Roughly half of the studies reported improvements in mental health symptoms (Carter et al., 2021). However, many of the studies were single-site pilot studies with small sample sizes and no active control conditions.

A major focus of mHealth interventions in LMICs has been on depression and anxiety (GBD 2019 Mental Disorders Collaborators, 2022). A recent systematic review and meta-analysis of 96 studies from LMICs reported moderate to high effectiveness of digital mental health interventions in reducing depression and anxiety symptoms (Kim et al., 2023). The studies included RCTs of a range of intervention formats including a mobile app, telephone, texting, and telehealth as a standalone or adjunctive treatment.

Cross-sectional studies from Brazil, Burundi, Jamaica, Nigeria, and South Africa have reported country-level interest in digital mental health among youths (Pavarini et al., 2023). High rates of receptiveness toward mHealth for behavioral health care and mental health education have been documented in China and Vietnam (Sit et al., 2021; Tran et al., 2018). In Nigeria and South Africa, the availability of free call bonuses, low-cost data bundles and other cost-saving measures from Internet providers and phone sharing increase the desirability of mHealth (Kola et al., 2021).

The overwhelming majority of individuals with mental health conditions live in LMICs and experience mental health stigma, low mental health literacy, and limited access to evidence-based mental health treatments. The use of digital mental health to bridge the clinical care divide in low-resource settings is an important priority for the WHO. Early research suggests that mHealth interventions are feasible and acceptable for individuals who reside in LMICs. Intervention formats have ranged from mobile apps to telehealth as a standalone or supplemental to in-person care. Pilot studies show evidence of improvements in mental health symptoms including anxiety and depression.

Limitations and Recommendations for Research

Advancing evidence-based mHealth interventions in LMICs would require moving beyond feasibility pilot studies that presently dominate mHealth literature in LMICs to efficacy and effectiveness testing in large-scale RCTs. Theory-grounded approaches are essential to the development of contextually relevant interventions and implementation strategies (Cho et al., 2018; Prestwich et al., 2014). Engaging local stakeholders in the design and implementation of mHealth interventions prioritizes local ownership for the successful uptake of mHealth interventions (Quanbeck, 2019). Interdisciplinary partnerships among researchers, clinicians, engineers, individuals with personal experience, policymakers, and other relevant parties are essential in the co-design and development of mHealth tools (Thornicroft et al., 2010).

Conclusion

In recent years, mHealth has catapulted to the forefront of digital solutions for mental health care inequities globally and in vulnerable populations and resource-constrained settings where the burden of mental health is the highest (Naslund et al., 2017). The COVID-19 pandemic has led to a technological health care revolution with $250 billion in health care spending projected to be digitally deployed in the United States alone (Bestsennyy et al., 2020). Mobile applications within mental health care may function to promote positive behavior change, increase treatment adherence, provide real-time mental health support, and enable symptom self-monitoring. The potential for mHealth to improve care quality and access to mental health services is growing along with the popularity of mHealth for mental health care worldwide (Ben-Zeev & Atkins, 2017). Here, we have described the potential for mHealth to bridge the care access gap in three vulnerable populations: CYP, those with SMI, and individuals who reside in LMICs. Portable low-cost technologies have the potential to revolutionize health care for these traditionally underserved populations with significant mental health needs.

Research on mHealth for mental health has demonstrated feasibility and acceptability, translating in-person treatment modalities such as CBT to the mHealth space. Efficacy testing is ongoing with promising early results. A plethora of mHealth interventions include synchronous or asynchronous communication with a trained mental health therapist. The role of health care providers and striking the right balance between self-guided and coached mHealth interventions and what works for whom warrants further exploration. A potential solution is a stepped care model whereby self-guided mHealth interventions serve as entry-level care and stepped-up adjunctive coaching is provided for higher-level, acute, and severe mental health concerns. In addition, the iterative co-design of mHealth interventions with end users is warranted in order to bolster continued engagement and sustainability with real-world in-the-moment interventions that provide instantaneous care at an individual's fingertips. Academic researchers who are interested in the development of mHealth interventions should prioritize technical and scientific knowledge, sensitivity to needs and contexts, the establishment of empirical evidence in support of their use, standardization of approaches, ethical, privacy, and safety considerations, and training needs of patients and clinicians. mHealth interventions have the potential to overcome the global mental health crisis, especially for vulnerable populations that have the greatest needs and are the hardest to reach.

References

Aboujaoude, E., Gega, L., Parish, M. B., & Hilty, D. M. (2020). Editorial: Digital interventions in mental health: Current status and future directions. *Frontiers in Psychiatry, 11*, 111. https://doi.org/10.3389/fpsyt.2020.00111

Aguirre Velasco, A., Cruz, I. S. S., Billings, J., Jimenez, M., & Rowe, S. (2020). What are the barriers, facilitators and interventions targeting help-seeking behaviours for common mental health problems in adolescents? A systematic review. *BMC Psychiatry, 20*(1), 293. https://doi.org/10.1186/s12888-020-02659-0

Anglada-Martinez, H., Riu-Viladoms, G., Martin-Conde, M., Rovira-Illamola, M., Sotoca-Momblona, J. M., & Codina-Jane, C. (2015). Does mHealth increase adherence to medication? Results of a systematic review. *International Journal of Clinical Practice, 69*(1), 9–32. https://doi.org/10.1111/ijcp.12582

Aschbrenner, K. A., Naslund, J. A., Tomlinson, E. F., Kinney, A., Pratt, S. I., & Brunette, M. F. (2019). Adolescents' use of digital technologies and preferences for mobile health coaching in public mental health settings. *Frontiers in Public Health, 7*, 178. https://doi.org/10.3389/fpubh.2019.00178

Ben-Zeev, D., & Atkins, D. C. (2017). Bringing digital mental health to where it is needed most. *Nature Human Behaviour, 1*(12), 849–851. https://doi.org/10.1038/s41562-017-0232-0

Ben-Zeev, D., Brian, R. M., Jonathan, G., Razzano, L., Pashka, N., Carpenter-Song, E., Drake, R. E., & Scherer, E. A. (2018). Mobile health (mHealth) versus clinic-based group intervention for people with serious mental illness: A randomized controlled trial. *Psychiatric Services, 69*(9), 978–985. https://doi.org/10.1176/appi.ps.201800063

Ben-Zeev, D., Buck, B., Kopelovich, S., & Meller, S. (2019). A technology-assisted life of recovery from psychosis. *NPJ Schizophrenia, 5*(1), 15. https://doi.org/10.1038/s41537-019-0083-y

Ben-Zeev, D., Chander, A., Tauscher, J., Buck, B., Nepal, S., Campbell, A., & Doron, G. (2021). A smartphone intervention for people with serious mental illness: Fully remote randomized controlled trial of CORE. *Journal of Medical Internet Research, 23*(11), 1–16. https://doi.org/10.2196/29201

Ben-Zeev, D., Drake, R. E., Corrigan, P. W., Rotondi, A. J., Nilsen, W., & Depp, C. (2012). Using contemporary technologies in the assessment and treatment of serious mental illness. *American Journal of Psychiatric Rehabilitation, 15*, 357–376. https://doi.org/10.1080/15487768.2012.733295

Bestsennyy, O., Gilbert, G., Harris, A., & Rost, J. (2020). *Telehealth: A quarter-trillion-dollar post-COVID-19 reality?* McKinsey & Company. https://www.mckinsey.com/industries/healthcare/our-insights/telehealth-a-quarter-trillion-dollar-post-covid-19-reality

Bry, L. J., Chou, T., Miguel, E., & Comer, J. S. (2018). Consumer smartphone apps marketed for child and adolescent anxiety: A systematic review and content analysis. *Behavior Therapy, 49*(2), 249–261. https://doi.org/10.1016/j.beth.2017.07.008

Buck, B., & Ben-Zeev, D. (2019). Using technology to advance early psychosis intervention. *Intervening Early in Psychosis: A Team Approach, 349.*

Campion, J., Javed, A., Lund, C., Sartorius, N., Saxena, S., Marmot, M., Allan, J., & Udomratn, P. (2022). Public mental health: Required actions to address implementation failure in the context of COVID-19. *The Lancet Psychiatry, 9*(2), 169–182. https://doi.org/10.1016/S2215-0366(21)00199-1

Carter, H., Araya, R., Anjur, K., Deng, D., & Naslund, J. A. (2021). The emergence of digital mental health in low-income and middle-income countries: A review of recent advances and implications for the treatment and prevention of mental disorders. *Journal of Psychiatric Research, 133*, 223–246. https://doi.org/10.1016/j.jpsychires.2020.12.016

Chandrashekar, P. (2018). Do mental health mobile apps work: Evidence and recommendations for designing high-efficacy mental health mobile apps. *mHealth, 4*, 6–6. https://doi.org/10.21037/mhealth.2018.03.02

Cho, Y.-M., Lee, S., Islam, S. M. S., & Kim, S.-Y. (2018). Theories applied to m-health interventions for behavior change in low- and middle-income countries: A systematic review. *Telemedicine Journal and E-Health: The Official Journal of the American Telemedicine Association, 24*(10), 727–741. https://doi.org/10.1089/tmj.2017.0249

Choi, K. R., Castillo, E. G., Seamans, M. J., Grotts, J. H., Rab, S., Kalofonos, I., Mead, M., Walker, I. J., & Starks, S. L. (2022). Mental health conservatorship among homeless people with serious mental illness. *Psychiatric Services, 73*(6), 613–619. https://doi.org/10.1176/appi.ps.202100254

Chowdhury, S., & Chakraborty, P. p. (2017). Universal health coverage—there is more to it than meets the eye. *Journal of Family Medicine and Primary Care, 6*(2), 169–170. https://doi.org/10.4103/jfmpc.jfmpc

Cliffe, B., Tingley, J., Greenhalgh, I., & Stallard, P. (2021). mHealth interventions for self-harm: Scoping review. *Journal of Medical Internet Research, 23*(4), e25140. https://doi.org/10.2196/25140

Cuijpers, P., Heim, E., Abi Ramia, J., Burchert, S., Carswell, K., Cornelisz, I., Knaevelsrud, C., Noun, P., van Klaveren, C., van't Hof, E., Zoghbi, E., van Ommeren, M., & El Chammay, R. (2022). Effects of a WHO-guided digital health intervention for depression in Syrian refugees in Lebanon: A randomized controlled trial. *PLoS Medicine, 19*(6), e1004025. https://doi.org/10.1371/journal.pmed.1004025

Cummings, C. M., Kazantzis, N., & Kendall, P. C. (2014). Facilitating homework and generalization of skills to the real world. In E. S. Sburlati, H. J. Lyneham, C. A. Schniering, & R. M. Rapee (Eds.), *Evidence-based CBT for anxiety and depression in children and adolescents* (pp. 141–155). John Wiley & Sons, Ltd. https://doi.org/10.1002/9781118500576.ch11

David, D., Cristea, I., & Hofmann, S. G. (2018). Why cognitive behavioral therapy is the current gold standard of psychotherapy. *Frontiers in Psychiatry, 9*. https://www.frontiersin.org/articles/10.3389/fpsyt.2018.00004

Drew, N., Funk, M., Tang, S., Lamichhane, J., Chávez, E., Katontoka, S., Pathare, S., Lewis, O., Gostin, L., & Saraceno, B. (2011). Human rights violations of people with mental and psychosocial disabilities: An unresolved global crisis. *Lancet, 378*(9803), 1664–1675. https://doi.org/10.1016/S0140-6736(11)61458-X

Ebert, D. D., Zarski, A.-C., Christensen, H., Stikkelbroek, Y., Cuijpers, P., Berking, M., & Riper, H. (2015). Internet and computer-based cognitive behavioral therapy for anxiety and depression in youth: A meta-analysis of randomized controlled outcome trials. *PLoS One, 10*(3), e0119895. https://doi.org/10.1371/journal.pone.0119895

Farooq Naeem, M., Omair Husain, M., & Ishrat Husain, A. J. (2020). Digital psychiatry in low- and middle-income countries post-COVID-19: Opportunities, challenges, and solutions. *Indian Journal of Psychiatry, 62*(supple3), s380–s382. https://doi.org/10.4103/psychiatry.IndianJPsychiatry

Fedele, D. A., Cushing, C. C., Fritz, A., Amaro, C. M., & Ortega, A. (2017). Mobile health interventions for improving health outcomes in youth: A meta-analysis. *JAMA Pediatrics, 171*(5), 461–469. https://doi.org/10.1001/jamapediatrics.2017.0042

Firth, J., & Torous, J. (2015). Smartphone apps for schizophrenia: A systematic review. *JMIR mHealth and uHealth, 3*(4), e4930. https://doi.org/10.2196/mhealth.4930

Firth, J., Torous, J., Nicholas, J., Carney, R., Pratap, A., Rosenbaum, S., & Sarris, J. (2017a). The efficacy of smartphone-based mental health interventions for depressive symptoms: A meta-analysis of randomized controlled trials. *World Psychiatry, 16*(3), 287–298. https://doi.org/10.1002/wps.20472

Firth, J., Torous, J., Nicholas, J., Carney, R., Rosenbaum, S., & Sarris, J. (2017b). Can smartphone mental health interventions reduce symptoms of anxiety? A meta-analysis of randomized controlled trials. *Journal of Affective Disorders, 218*, 15–22. http://dx.doi.org/10.1016/j.jad.2017.04.046

Fortuna, K., Barr, P., Goldstein, C., Walker, R., Brewer, L. P., Zagaria, A., & Bartels, S. (2019). Application of community-engaged research to inform the development and implementation of a peer-delivered mobile health intervention for adults with serious mental illness. *Journal of Participatory Medicine, 11*(1), 1–9. https://doi.org/10.2196/12380

Free, C., Phillips, G., Felix, L., Galli, L., Patel, V., & Edwards, P. (2010). The effectiveness of M-health technologies for improving health and health services: A systematic review protocol. *BMC Research Notes, 3*, 250. https://doi.org/10.1186/1756-0500-3-250

Free, C., Phillips, G., Watson, L., Galli, L., Felix, L., Edwards, P., Patel, V., & Haines, A. (2013). The effectiveness of mobile-health technologies to improve health care service delivery processes: A systematic review and meta-analysis. *PLoS Medicine, 10*(1), e1001363. https://doi.org/10.1371/journal.pmed.1001363

Freeman, M. (2022). Investing for population mental health in low and middle income countries-where and why? *International Journal of Mental Health Systems, 16*(1), 38. https://doi.org/10.1186/s13033-022-00547-6

Fu, Z., Burger, H., Arjadi, R., & Bockting, C. L. H. (2020). Effectiveness of digital psychological interventions for mental health problems in low-income and middle-income countries: A systematic review and meta-analysis. *The Lancet Psychiatry, 7*(10), 851–864. https://doi.org/10.1016/S2215-0366(20)30256-X

Funnell, E. L., Spadaro, B., Martin-Key, N., Metcalfe, T., & Bahn, S. (2022). mHealth solutions for mental health screening and diagnosis: A review of app user perspectives using sentiment and thematic analysis. *Frontiers in Psychiatry, 13*(April), 1–17. https://doi.org/10.3389/fpsyt.2022.857304

Garrido, S., Millington, C., Cheers, D., Boydell, K., Schubert, E., Meade, T., & Nguyen, Q. V. (2019). What works and what doesn't work? A systematic review of digital mental health interventions for depression and anxiety in young people. *Frontiers in Psychiatry, 10.* https://www.frontiersin.org/articles/10.3389/fpsyt.2019.00759

GBD 2019 Mental Disorders Collaborators. (2022). Global, regional, and national burden of 12 mental disorders in 204 countries and territories, 1990–2019: A systematic analysis for the global burden of disease study 2019. *The Lancet Psychiatry, 9*(2), 137–150. https://doi.org/10.1016/S2215-0366(21)00395-3

Giovanelli, A., Ozer, E. M., & Dahl, R. E. (2020). Leveraging technology to improve health in adolescence: A developmental science perspective. *Journal of Adolescent Health, 67*(2, Supplement), S7–S13. https://doi.org/10.1016/j.jadohealth.2020.02.020

Goldberg, S. B., Lam, S. U., Simonsson, O., Torous, J., & Sun, S. (2022). Mobile phone-based interventions for mental health: A systematic meta-review of 14 meta-analyses of randomized controlled trials. *PLOS Digital Health, 1*(1), e0000002. https://doi.org/10.1371/journal.pdig.0000002

Granger, D., Vandelanotte, C., Duncan, M. J., Alley, S., Schoeppe, S., Short, C., & Rebar, A. (2016). Is preference for mHealth intervention delivery platform associated with delivery platform familiarity? *BMC Public Health, 16*, 619. https://doi.org/10.1186/s12889-016-3316-2

Granholm, E., Ben-Zeev, D., Link, P. C., Bradshaw, K. R., & Holden, J. L. (2012). Mobile assessment and treatment for schizophrenia (MATS): A pilot trial of an interactive text-messaging intervention for medication adherence, socialization, and auditory hallucinations. *Schizophrenia Bulletin, 38*(3), 414–425. https://doi.org/10.1093/schbul/sbr155

Grist, R., Porter, J., & Stallard, P. (2017). Mental health mobile apps for preadolescents and adolescents: A systematic review. *Journal of Medical Internet Research, 19*(5), e7332. https://doi.org/10.2196/jmir.7332

Gulliver, A., Griffiths, K. M., & Christensen, H. (2010). Perceived barriers and facilitators to mental health help-seeking in young people: A systematic review. *BMC Psychiatry, 10*, 113. https://doi.org/10.1186/1471-244X-10-113

IQVIA Institute for Human Data Science. (2021). *Digital Health Trends 2021: Innovation, Evidence, Regulation, and Adoption* [Institute Report]. https://www.iqvia.com/insights/the-iqvia-institute/reports/digital-health-trends-2021

Jabeen, R., Salman, M. J., & Qazi, I. (2023). Evidence of mobile health integration into primary health care systems for better maternal mental health in LMICs during COVID-19 pandemic—Review. *JPMA. The Journal of the Pakistan Medical Association, 73*(1), 125–128. https://doi.org/10.47391/JPMA.5155

John, N., Lisa, M., Gregory, M., & Srephen, B. (2015). Emerging mHealth and eHealth intervention for serious mental illness. *Medical Image Analysis, 24*(5), 321–332. https://doi.org/10.3109/09638237.2015.1019054. Emerging

Kendall, P. C., Robin, J. A., Hedtke, K. A., Suveg, C., Flannery-Schroeder, E., & Gosch, E. (2005). Considering CBT with anxious youth? Think exposures. *Cognitive and Behavioral Practice, 12*(1), 136–148.

Kessler, R. C., Amminger, G. P., Aguilar-Gaxiola, S., Alonso, J., Lee, S., & Üstün, T. B. (2007). Age of onset of mental disorders: A review of recent literature. *Current Opinion in Psychiatry, 20*(4), 359–364. http://dx.doi.org/10.1097/YCO.0b013e32816ebc8c

Kieling, C., Baker-Henningham, H., Belfer, M., Conti, G., Ertem, I., Omigbodun, O., Rohde, L. A., Srinath, S., Ulkuer, N., & Rahman, A. (2011). Child and adolescent mental health worldwide: Evidence for action. *Lancet, 378*(9801), 1515–1525. https://doi.org/10.1016/S0140-6736(11)60827-1

Kim, J., Aryee, L. M. D., Bang, H., Prajogo, S., Choi, Y. K., Hoch, J. S., & Prado, E. L. (2023). Effectiveness of digital mental health tools to reduce depressive and anxiety symptoms in low- and middle-income countries: Systematic review and meta-analysis. *JMIR Mental Health, 10*(1), e43066. https://doi.org/10.2196/43066

Kola, L., Abiona, D., Adefolarin, A. O., & Ben-Zeev, D. (2021). Mobile phone use and acceptability for the delivery of mental health information among perinatal adolescents in Nigeria: Survey study. *JMIR Mental Health, 8*(1), e20314. https://doi.org/10.2196/20314

Lattie, E. G., Schueller, S. M., Sargent, E., Stiles-Shields, C., Tomasino, K. N., Corden, M. E., Begale, M., Karr, C. J., & Mohr, D. C. (2016). Uptake and usage of IntelliCare: A publicly available suite of mental health and well-being apps. *Internet Interventions, 4*(2), 152–158. https://doi.org/10.1016/j.invent.2016.06.003

Lau, N., O'Daffer, A., Colt, S., Yi-Frazier, J. P., Palermo, T. M., McCauley, E., & Rosenberg, A. R. (2020). Android and iPhone mobile apps for psychosocial wellness and stress management: Systematic search in app stores and literature review. *JMIR mHealth and uHealth, 8*(5), e17798. https://doi.org/10.2196/17798

Lebrun-Harris, L. A., Ghandour, R. M., Kogan, M. D., & Warren, M. D. (2022). Five-year trends in US children's health and well-being, 2016-2020. *JAMA Pediatrics, 176*(7), e220056. https://doi.org/10.1001/jamapediatrics.2022.0056

Liverpool, S., Mota, C. P., Sales, C. M. D., Čuš, A., Carletto, S., Hancheva, C., Sousa, S., Cerón, S. C., Moreno-Peral, P., Pietrabissa, G., Moltrecht, B., Ulberg, R., Ferreira, N., & Edbrooke-Childs, J. (2020). Engaging children and young people in digital mental health interventions: Systematic review of modes of delivery, facilitators, and barriers. *Journal of Medical Internet Research, 22*(6), e16317. https://doi.org/10.2196/16317

Marcolino, M. S., Oliveira, J. A. Q., D'Agostino, M., Ribeiro, A. L., Alkmim, M. B. M., & Novillo-Ortiz, D. (2018). The impact of mHealth interventions: Systematic review of systematic reviews. *JMIR mHealth and uHealth, 6*(1), e8873. https://doi.org/10.2196/mhealth.8873

Marzano, L., Bardill, A., Fields, B., Herd, K., Veale, D., Grey, N., & Moran, P. (2015). The application of mHealth to mental health: Opportunities and challenges. *The Lancet Psychiatry, 2*(10), 942–948. https://doi.org/10.1016/S2215-0366(15)00268-0

McCool, J., Dobson, R., Whittaker, R., & Paton, C. (2022). Mobile health (mHealth) in low- and middle-income countries. *Annual Review of Public Health, 43*, 525–539. https://doi.org/10.1146/annurev-publhealth-052620-093850

Melamed, O. C., Hahn, M. K., Agarwal, S. M., Taylor, V. H., Mulsant, B. H., & Selby, P. (2020). Physical health among people with serious mental illness in the face of COVID-19: Concerns and mitigation strategies. *General Hospital Psychiatry, 66*, 30–33. https://doi.org/10.1016/j.genhosppsych.2020.06.013

Merikangas, K. R., Nakamura, E. F., & Kessler, R. C. (2022). Epidemiology of mental disorders in children and adolescents. *Dialogues in Clinical Neuroscience, 11(1), 7-20.*

Mojtabai, R., Fochtmann, L., Chang, S.-W., Kotov, R., Craig, T. J., & Bromet, E. (2009). Unmet need for mental health care in schizophrenia: An overview of literature and new data from a first-admission study. *Schizophrenia Bulletin, 35*(4), 679–695. https://doi.org/10.1093/schbul/sbp045

Moreno, C., Wykes, T., Galderisi, S., Nordentoft, M., Crossley, N., Jones, N., Cannon, M., Correll, C. U., Byrne, L., Carr, S., Chen, E. Y. H., Gorwood, P., Johnson, S., Kärkkäinen, H., Krystal, J. H., Lee, J., Lieberman, J., López-Jaramillo, C., Männikkö, M., . . . Arango, C. (2020). How mental health care should change as a consequence of the COVID-19 pandemic. *The Lancet Psychiatry, 7*(9), 813–824. https://doi.org/10.1016/S2215-0366(20)30307-2

Mukhtar, S. (2020). Psychological health during the coronavirus disease 2019 pandemic outbreak. *International Journal of Social Psychiatry, 66*(5), 512–516. https://doi.org/10.1177/0020764020925835

Myin-Germeys, I., Birchwood, M., & Kwapil, T. (2011). From environment to therapy in psychosis: A real-world momentary assessment approach. *Schizophrenia Bulletin, 37*(2), 244–247. https://doi.org/10.1093/schbul/sbq164

Naslund, J. A., Aschbrenner, K. A., Araya, R., Marsch, L. A., Unützer, J., Patel, V., & Bartels, S. J. (2017). Digital technology for treating and preventing mental disorders in low-income and middle-income countries: A narrative review of the literature. *The Lancet Psychiatry, 4*(6), 486–500. https://doi.org/10.1016/S2215-0366(17)30096-2

Naslund, J. A., & Deng, D. (2021). Addressing mental health stigma in low-income and middle-income countries: A new frontier for digital mental health. *Ethics, Medicine, and Public Health, 19*, 100719. https://doi.org/10.1016/j.jemep.2021.100719

Neary, M., & Schueller, S. M. (2018). State of the field of mental health apps. *Cognitive and Behavioral Practice, 25*(4), 531–537. https://doi.org/10.1016/j.cbpra.2018.01.002

Odgers, C. L., & Jensen, M. R. (2020). Annual research review: Adolescent mental health in the digital age: Facts, fears, and future directions. *Journal of Child Psychology and Psychiatry, and Allied Disciplines, 61*(3), 336–348. https://doi.org/10.1111/jcpp.13190

Oldehinkel, A. J., & Ormel, J. (2023). Annual research review: Stability of psychopathology: Lessons learned from longitudinal population surveys. *Journal of Child Psychology and Psychiatry, 64*(4), 489–502. https://doi.org/10.1111/jcpp.13737

Pavarini, G., Booysen, C., Jain, T., Lai, J., Manku, K., Foster-Estwick, A., Gatera, G., Omari Juma, D., Karorero, D., Philip-Joe, K., Genevive Ukachukwu, C., Sartor, C., Zeitz, L., Farmer, M., & Singh, I. (2023). Agents of change for mental health: A survey of young people's aspirations for participation across five low- and middle-income countries. *Journal of Adolescent Health, 72*(1, Supplement), S96–S104. https://doi.org/10.1016/j.jadohealth.2021.10.037

Polanczyk, G. V., Salum, G. A., Sugaya, L. S., Caye, A., & Rohde, L. A. (2015). Annual research review: A meta-analysis of the worldwide prevalence of mental disorders in children and adolescents. *Journal of Child Psychology and Psychiatry, 56*(3), 345–365. http://dx.doi.org/10.1111/jcpp.12381

Pramana, G., Parmanto, B., Kendall, P. C., & Silk, J. S. (2014). The SmartCAT: An m-health platform for ecological momentary intervention in child anxiety treatment. *Telemedicine Journal and E-Health, 20*(5), 419–427. https://doi.org/10.1089/tmj.2013.0214

Prestwich, A., Sniehotta, F. F., Whittington, C., Dombrowski, S. U., Rogers, L., & Michie, S. (2014). Does theory influence the effectiveness of health behavior interventions? Meta-analysis. *Health Psychology : Official Journal of the Division of Health Psychology, American Psychological Association, 33*(5), 465–474. https://doi.org/10.1037/a0032853

Price, M., Yuen, E. K., Goetter, E. M., Herbert, J. D., Forman, E. M., Acierno, R., & Ruggiero, K. J. (2014). mHealth: A mechanism to deliver more accessible, more effective mental health care. *Clinical Psychology & Psychotherapy, 21*(5), 427–436. https://doi.org/10.1002/cpp.1855

Quanbeck, A. (2019). Using stakeholder values to promote implementation of an evidence-based mobile health intervention for addiction treatment in primary care settings. *JMIR mHealth and uHealth, 7*(6), e13301. https://doi.org/10.2196/13301

Racine, N., McArthur, B. A., Cooke, J. E., Eirich, R., Zhu, J., & Madigan, S. (2021). Global prevalence of depressive and anxiety symptoms in children and adolescents during COVID-19: A meta-analysis. *JAMA Pediatrics, 175*(11), 1142–1150. https://doi.org/10.1001/jamapediatrics.2021.2482

Ragul, G., Rohit Verma, K. S. D., & Chadda, R. K. (2022). Learning from telepsychiatry during COVID-19 pandemic in India: Boon for public mental health in low- & middle-income countries. *Indian Journal of Medical Research*, 197–199. https://doi.org/10.4103/ijmr.ijmr_1034_21

Rathbone, A. L., Clarry, L., & Prescott, J. (2017). Assessing the efficacy of mobile health apps using the basic principles of cognitive behavioral therapy: Systematic review. *Journal of Medical Internet Research, 19*(11), e399. https://doi.org/10.2196/jmir.8598

Rathod, S., Pinninti, N., Irfan, M., Gorczynski, P., Rathod, P., Gega, L., & Naeem, F. (2017). Mental health service provision in low- and middle-income countries. *Health Services Insights, 10.* https://doi.org/10.1177/1178632917694350

Rhoades, H., Wenzel, S. L., Rice, E., Winetrobe, H., & Henwood, B. (2017). No digital divide? Technology use among homeless adults. *Journal of Social Distress and Homeless, 26*(1), 73–77. https://doi.org/10.1080/10530789.2017.1305140

Roddy Mitchell, A., Gordon, H., Lindquist, A., Walker, S. P., Homer, C. S. E., Middleton, A., Cluver, C. A., Tong, S., & Hastie, R. (2023). Prevalence of perinatal depression in low- and middle-income countries: A systematic review and meta-analysis. *JAMA Psychiatry, 80*(5), 425–431. https://doi.org/10.1001/jamapsychiatry.2023.0069

Scholten, H., & Granic, I. (2019). Use of the principles of design thinking to address limitations of digital mental health interventions for youth: Viewpoint. *Journal of Medical Internet Research, 21*(1), e11528. https://doi.org/10.2196/11528

Sit, H. F., Hong, I. W., Burchert, S., Sou, E. K. L., Wong, M., Chen, W., Lam, A. I. F., & Hall, B. J. (2021). A feasibility study of the WHO digital mental health intervention step-by-step to address depression among Chinese young adults. *Frontiers in Psychiatry, 12*, 812667. https://doi.org/10.3389/fpsyt.2021.812667

Španiel, F., Hrdlička, J., Novák, T., Kožený, J., Höschl, C., Mohr, P., & Motlová, L. B. (2012). Effectiveness of the information technology-aided program of relapse prevention in schizophrenia (ITAREPS): A randomized, controlled, double-blind study. *Journal of Psychiatric Practice, 18*(4), 269–280. https://doi.org/10.1097/01.pra.000416017.45591.c1

Substance Abuse and Mental Health Services Administration. (2022). *Key substance use and mental health indicators in the United States: Results from the 2021 national survey on drug use and health.* HHS Publication No. PEP22-07-01-005; NSDUH Series H-57. Center for Behavioral Health Statistics and Quality, Substance Abuse and Mental Health Services Administration. https://www.samhsa.gov/data/report/2021-nsduh-annual-national-report

Subu, M. A., Wati, D. F., Netrida, N., Priscilla, V., Dias, J. M., Abraham, M. S., Slewa-Younan, S., & Al-Yateem, N. (2021). Types of stigma experienced by patients with mental illness and mental health nurses in Indonesia: A qualitative content analysis. *International Journal of Mental Health Systems, 15*(1), 1–12. https://doi.org/10.1186/s13033-021-00502-x

The Lancet Child & Adolescent Health. (2018). Growing up in a digital world: Benefits and risks. *The Lancet Child & Adolescent Health, 2*(2), 79. https://doi.org/10.1016/S2352-4642(18)30002-6

The Lancet Global Health. (2020). Mental health matters. *The Lancet. Global Health, 8*(11), e1352. https://doi.org/10.1016/S2214-109X(20)30432-0

Thornicroft, G., Alem, A., Antunes Dos Santos, R., Barley, E., Drake, R. E., Gregorio, G., Hanlon, C., Ito, H., Latimer, E., Law, A., Mari, J., McGeorge, P., Padmavati, R., Razzouk, D., Semrau, M., Setoya, Y., Thara, R., & Wondimagegn, D. (2010). WPA guidance on steps, obstacles and mistakes to avoid in the implementation of community mental health care. *World Psychiatry: Official Journal of the World Psychiatric Association (WPA), 9*(2), 67–77. https://doi.org/10.1002/j.2051-5545.2010.tb00276.x

Thornicroft, G., Mehta, N., Clement, S., Evans-Lacko, S., Doherty, M., Rose, D., Koschorke, M., Shidhaye, R., O'Reilly, C., & Henderson, C. (2016). Evidence for effective interventions to reduce mental-health-related stigma and discrimination. *The Lancet, 387*(10023), 1123–1132. https://doi.org/10.1016/S0140-6736(15)00298-6

Thornicroft, G., Sunkel, C., Alikhon Aliev, A., Baker, S., Brohan, E., El Chammay, R., Davies, K., Demissie, M., Duncan, J., Fekadu, W., Gronholm, P. C., Guerrero, Z., Gurung, D., Habtamu, K., Hanlon, C., Heim, E., Henderson, C., Hijazi, Z., Hoffman, C., . . . Winkler, P. (2022). The Lancet Commission on ending stigma and discrimination in mental health. *Lancet, 400*(10361), 1438–1480. https://doi.org/10.1016/S0140-6736(22)01470-2

Tol, W. A., Barbui, C., Galappatti, A., Silove, D., Betancourt, T. S., Souza, R., Golaz, A., & van Ommeren, M. (2011). Mental health and psychosocial support in humanitarian settings: Linking practice and research. *Lancet, 378*(9802), 1581–1591. https://doi.org/10.1016/S0140-6736(11)61094-5

Tomczyk, S., Barth, S., Schmidt, S., & Muehlan, H. (2021). Utilizing health behavior change and technology acceptance models to predict the adoption of COVID-19 contact tracing apps: Cross-sectional survey study. *Journal of Medical Internet Research, 23*(5), 1–19. https://doi.org/10.2196/25447

Tran, B. X., Zhang, M. W., Le, H. T., Nguyen, H. D., Nguyen, L. H., Nguyen, Q. L. T., Tran, T. D., Latkin, C. A., & Ho, R. C. (2018). What drives young Vietnamese to use mobile health innovations? Implications for health communication and behavioral interventions. *JMIR mHealth and uHealth, 6*(11), e194. https://doi.org/10.2196/mhealth.6490

Turner, A. (2023). How many people have smartphones worldwide (Jun 2023). Bank My Cell. https://www.bankmycell.com/blog/how-many-phones-are-in-the-world

Venturo-Conerly, K. E., Fitzpatrick, O. M., Horn, R. L., Ugueto, A. M., & Weisz, J. R. (2022). Effectiveness of youth psychotherapy delivered remotely: A meta-analysis. *American Psychologist, 77*, 71–84. https://doi.org/10.1037/amp0000816

Vogels, E. A., Gelles-Watnick, R., & Massarat, N. (2022). *Teens, Social Media and Technology 2022.* Pew Research Center. https://www.pewresearch.org/internet/2022/08/10/teens-social-media-and-technology-2022

Wainberg, M. L., Scorza, P., Shultz, J. M., Helpman, L., Mootz, J. J., Johnson, K. A., Neria, Y., Bradford, J.-M. E., Oquendo, M. A., & Arbuckle, M. R. (2017). Challenges and opportunities in global mental health: A research-to-practice perspective. *Current Psychiatry Reports, 19*(5), 28. https://doi.org/10.1007/s11920-017-0780-z

Weisz, J. R., Kuppens, S., Eckshtain, D., Ugueto, A. M., Hawley, K. M., & Jensen-Doss, A. (2013). Performance of evidence-based youth psychotherapies compared with usual clinical care: A multilevel meta-analysis. *JAMA Psychiatry, 70*(7), 750–761. https://doi.org/10.1001/jamapsychiatry.2013.1176

Whittaker, R., Stasiak, K., McDowell, H., Doherty, I., Shepherd, M., Chua, S., Dorey, E., Parag, V., Ameratunga, S., Rodgers, A., & Merry, S. (2017). MEMO: An mHealth intervention to prevent the onset of depression in adolescents: A double-blind, randomised, placebo-controlled trial. *Journal of Child Psychology and Psychiatry, and Allied Disciplines, 58*(9), 1014–1022. https://doi.org/10.1111/jcpp.12753

World Health Organization. (2019). WHO releases first guideline on digital health interventions. *WHO Newsletter. [Online] World Health Organization, April, 17.*

Yatham, S., Sivathasan, S., Yoon, R., da Silva, T. L., & Ravindran, A. V. (2018). Depression, anxiety, and post-traumatic stress disorder among youth in low and middle income countries: A review of prevalence and treatment interventions. *Asian Journal of Psychiatry, 38*, 78–91. https://doi.org/10.1016/j.ajp.2017.10.029

Ybarra, M. L., & Eaton, W. W. (2005). Internet-based mental health interventions. *Mental Health Services Research, 7*(2), 75–87. https://doi.org/10.1007/s11020-005-3779-8

15

Mental Health Apps and Privacy: Misunderstandings and Messaging

Jolynn Childers Dellinger
Duke Law School and Duke Science & Society

When we think about mental health and privacy in the United States, ideas we have about doctor–patient confidentiality or HIPAA—that law we all hear about every time we visit a doctor's office—may come to mind. In this digital era, however, instead of visiting providers in traditional offices, we may be using mobile apps or communicating with chatbots to seek mental health care. And HIPAA, the Health Insurance Portability and Accountability Act, does not apply to most mental health apps. Mental health data are sensitive and subject to misuse and abuse, but privacy protections for these data in our information economy are extremely limited. Communication and messaging designed to promote mental health should be informed by an understanding of the privacy implications of mental health apps—both the promise and the problems.

In an ideal world, these apps may promise a more privacy-oriented form of care—mental health care that people can access from the privacy of their homes or throughout the day on personal devices. People could forgo the trip to a doctor's office that may necessitate taking time off work or school and avoid having to explain why they need that time; they could access care expeditiously and on their own schedules. Although seeking mental health care should never entail embarrassment or shame, the stigma associated with seeking help in some communities or cultures may be a disincentive for some. For these individuals, the degree of privacy that apps appear to offer could be the difference between obtaining the help they need and forgoing that care. Some people could have difficulty revealing deeply personal, intimate information while sitting face to face with a relatively unknown healthcare professional, but they may be more comfortable texting with a provider they cannot physically see.[1] Still others may prefer to share sensitive information with a chatbot rather than a person. In an ideal world, individuals seeking care would be free to select the type of care delivery that best conforms to their needs, concerns, resources, and understandings of privacy.

But ours is not an ideal world. In our digital reality, the privacy promise of mental health apps is undermined by privacy problems. We live in an information economy in which many apps are advertised, arguably deceptively, as "free," powered not by consumer dollars but by user data and advertising. Companies thrive on the collection and monetization of data. And this pervasive collection and use of data are taking place in a virtually unregulated environment. And therein lies the privacy problem that inhibits the potential of the mental health app industry—in the real world, incredibly sensitive personal data is remarkably unprotected.

[1] See Surani et al. (2023) (young people preferred online to in person mental health services and felt more comfortable sharing their issues with the system rather than medical professionals).

The Handbook of Mental Health Communication, First Edition.
Edited by Marco C. Yzer and Jason T. Siegel.

Part I: Mental Health Apps and Personal Data

What Are Mental Health Apps?

Over 10,000 digital products and services[2] are available to help individuals obtain mental health care.[3] And recent reports indicate that the big tech companies—Apple, Google (now Alphabet), Meta, and Amazon are becoming more involved in the mental health space as well, a development that has significant implications for data collection and use.[4]

Some mental health apps are primarily intermediaries—digital platforms designed to connect people seeking care with licensed care providers who can provide therapy via messaging or live sessions using video or audio, for example, BetterHelp, Talkspace, and Ayana. These companies may charge monthly subscription fees[5] for user access to the service and providers, who are typically independent contractors. Some, like Talkspace, indicate that services are covered by some insurance plans.[6] Others, like BetterHelp, are not.[7] These intermediary apps may offer online communities for support and other resources for self-guided care in addition to virtual connections to therapists.

Another type of app offers care solely via text, connecting individuals with professionals or volunteers. Crisis Text Line, a nonprofit, offers support to those considering suicide or self-harm or dealing with anxiety, eating disorders, or depression (Crisis Text Line, 2024). Counslr is a service originally geared toward college students; it offers support but is not intended to be a substitute for therapy.

> "We are not a replacement for traditional therapy," COUNSLR CEO Joshua Liss said. "Meaning we don't diagnose, we don't treat [and] we don't prescribe medication. We are there to provide support, coping strategies, empathy, reflecting listening [and] the sharing of resources. . . . COUNSLR, the app, is like a best friend in your pocket who happens to be a licensed counselor."[8]

A subset of the texting apps offers "care"[9] via chatbots—nonhuman, interactive artificial intelligence (AI) products designed to help people with their problems, for example, Wysa and Woebot.

> "[A] chatbot is "a software program that interacts with users using natural language." Chatbots leverage algorithms to mimic a conversation "between a human user and a computer using natural language." This technology permits users to interact with computers in a way that is "natural" for them and is analogous to human conversation. (Stiefel, 2019, p. 337)

---

[2] See M-Health Index & Navigation Database (2024) (introductory video). See also Germain (2021) ("Type 'mental health' or a condition such as anxiety or depression into an app store search bar, and you can end up scrolling through endless screens of options.").

[3] This chapter focuses on direct-to-consumer mental health apps and websites. Technologies that doctors provide for their patients' use and telemedicine used by providers as a vehicle for the delivery of mental health services also raise privacy and security issues but are outside the scope of this chapter.

[4] Nosthoff et al. (2023) (describing Apple's Mindfulness app's State of Mind Feature, Alphabet's Fitbit LogMood feature and Amazon OneMedical's Mindset).

[5] BetterHelp Editorial Team, *How Much Does BetterHelp Online Therapy Cost?*, BetterHelp, https://www.betterhelp.com/advice/general/how-much-does-betterhelp-cost/# (May 31, 2024) (detailing subscription fees).

[6] Talkspace has entered into agreements with a number of insurers, including Optum of United Health, Aetna, and Cigna. Talkspace, Inc., *Annual Report, Transition Report* (Form 10-K) 45 (Mar. 8, 2023) ("Through our platform, we serve our business-to-business ('B2B') channel, comprised of . . . programs such as Aetna, Cigna, Premera, and Optum, who offer their employees and insured members access to the Company's platform while their employer is under an active contract with Talkspace"). On its website, Talkspace indicates its services may be covered by some insurance plans (Talkspace, n.d.-a).

[7] BetterHelp does not offer services covered by insurance. BetterHelp Editorial Team, *Will BetterHelp Therapy Take Insurance?*, BetterHelp, https://www.betterhelp.com/advice/general/does-betterhelp-take-insurance-what-to-know-about-paying-for-therapy/# (May 13, 2024) ("BetterHelp cannot submit claims to Medicare, Medicaid, or any health insurance plan. For this reason, it is not covered by insurance. . . . The therapists working as independent contractors through the platform cannot submit claims to insurance companies.").

[8] Stevens (2023). See also GlobeNewswire (2023) (reporting on use of Counslr in high school student populations).

[9] To the extent we imagine "care" to imply or be inclusive of empathy, compassion, feeling, sensitivity, concern, and relational capacity, the ability of AI to provide care raises ethical questions. AI resources may better be described as solutions, responses, or strategies. See generally, Kwan (2023) (describing ethics of care).

Yet another category includes wellness apps that purport to provide mental health support of some kind—providing journaling, symptom or mood tracking, guided meditations, chat rooms, relaxation exercises, cognitive behavioral therapy, activities and games, and other resources (e.g. Happify, PTSD Coach).

Many mental health apps are free. Others are free to download but offer a variety of in-app purchase or subscription options. And they are developed by a variety of entities: for profit companies, healthcare companies, nonprofit companies, academic institutions, and government.

These apps raise a number of issues: accessibility, efficacy, and privacy are all important topics deserving further study. Sometimes these issues are intertwined, and failure to provide adequate safeguards in one arena can compromise another. For example, Scott Stiefel has recognized the relationship between efficacy and privacy in his evaluation of chatbots: "The apps provide services akin to mental health professionals and involve users disclosing information they may consider sensitive. Because of this sensitivity, the efficacy of the apps is closely tied to the question of how the apps handle the privacy—or more aptly, confidentiality—of information provided by users" (Stiefel, 2019, p. 342). This chapter will focus on the privacy issues raised by these technologies.

What Kind of Data Do These Apps Collect?

Mental health apps often request personal information including name, contact information (email, phone number, and home address), age, race, nationality, gender, and sexual orientation (Surani et al., 2023). Users can complete questionnaires providing details about the problems they are experiencing in that moment, inclination to self-harm or suicide, symptoms, past traumas, diagnoses, or other aspects of medical history (Surani et al., 2023). They may convey concerns, worries, descriptions of anxiety and depression, coping mechanisms and strategies, and behavior patterns. They may provide a list of medications they are taking or information about drug and alcohol intake or substance abuse.

Apps also feature a variety of interactive mechanisms that facilitate the collection and analysis of user data. Text therapy apps collect text and chat transcripts. Apps offer journal or diary interfaces, mood assessments, and community chat functions, which provide opportunities for users to provide—and apps to collect—sensitive information. Apps may also access other user data generated on a phone including social network data, step count, sleep habits, and biometric data.

From a more technical perspective, apps may collect data using a device's camera and microphone, access contacts, and track and collect location data. Usage metadata can reveal how long a user is on an app, length of therapy sessions, when and how often messages are exchanged, approximate location, and how often and when an app is opened and used. Apps may collect unique IDs that are associated with individuals' smartphones. These IDs can be used to track users' activity across apps on their devices, and the data obtained can be combined with other datasets and used for targeted advertising.[10] In addition, some "mental health apps available on the market require permissions to access or alter the device's storage, read phone status, view Wi-Fi connections and others which are considered to be higher risk by guidelines for app developers."[11]

Importantly, the mere facts that a user downloads a mental health app or accesses content through the app are, in and of themselves, data related to health.[12] And this is the case regardless of whether a user actually creates an account, uses an app's features, or follows through with services.

---

[10] Apple's mobile IDs are referred to as Identifier for Advertisers (IDFA) and Google's are Advertising Identifiers (Ad IDs); each are 32-character IDs. Although these identifiers are pseudonymous in that they do not actually contain personal information, the data attached to these IDs can be matched to data in other databases to identify users. Because mobile IDs are connected to devices and people tend to carry their phones with them, mobile IDs can provide insight into locations people actually visit. Mobile IDs can also be connected to IP addresses. Notably, with the advent of iOS 14, Apple provided users the option to block mobile ID tracking across apps on their phones, and studies showed a substantial majority of users have asked apps not to track them when given the option. Balasubramanian (2022) (fewer than 20% of US users opt in to tracking).

[11] Parker et al. (2019) (identifying salient consumer issues related to privacy in the mental health app market to inform advocacy efforts to promoting consumer interests).

[12] These data points would not necessarily be ***accurate*** data about health, however. For example, I downloaded eight of these apps while writing this chapter. Inferences may be drawn about my mental health based on those actions, but they would not be accurate; the research context would not be evident from the raw data. But inaccurate data can also be harmful.

How Are Data About Mental Health Collected and Used?

Users intentionally provide personal information directly to apps by answering questions, texting, and participating in community chat groups and interactive activities. If people log in to mental health apps using Facebook or Google credentials, they may (perhaps unwittingly) associate their activity on a mental health app with their Facebook or Google accounts. This action may provide the app with additional information about the user and simultaneously provide Facebook or Google with information about the person's use of the mental health app. Not all disclosure is intentional. Users may be unaware, for example, of apps' collection of metadata and technical data from their devices.

Many apps solicit sensitive data from the outset of a user's experience. A 2017 study of 116 apps for depression noted that "[o]f the apps that did have a [privacy] policy, they were often only provided after users were asked for information, meaning the apps had collected data before alerting users how that data could be used" (O'Loughlin et al., 2019). Talkspace begins collecting personal information as soon as a user engages with the app. Among other things, the app asks the user to "tell us why you're looking for help today" and presents a number of choices including feeling anxious or panicky, relationship difficulty, traumatic experience, trouble sleeping, navigating addiction, depression, stress, or other. After answering several questions on successive screens, including an assessment of physical health, gender, birth date, and state in which the user spends the most time, the user has an opportunity to create an account. At that point, the app requests an email and phone number and, in smaller font, provides links to "Terms of Service" and a "Privacy Policy." The user can click the link to access the text of the policy or just select "I'll do this later" and go on to choose and pay for a plan. By contrast, as of the time of this writing, when I download and access BetterHelp, a pop-up immediately appears informing me about BetterHelp's privacy practices and providing links that would allow me to learn more. I have to click "okay" to acknowledge I have seen this message before I am able to continue with the app. Interfaces obscuring or delaying access to information about privacy while requesting completion of intake questionnaires create confusion and subvert users' ability to be informed about the app's practices.

Companies mine and use consumer data in a variety of ways: to improve their services and offerings, for research,[13] for advertising and marketing, to train algorithms, and for analytics. To use the data in these ways, apps often share, disclose, or sell it to third parties (Healey, 2023), including advertisers, analytics companies, data brokers, Meta and Google (e.g. Hunter & Merrill, 2022 re general health data; Tewari, 2022 re mental health data; Healey, 2023 re mental health data; Singer, 2023 re GoodRx; Marcelline, 2023 re Cerebral).[14]

Technologies used by developers may also disclose data. Software development kits (SDKs) are sets of tools that engineers use to build apps. They can include Application programming interfaces (APIs)—predefined pieces of code that allow two pieces of software to communicate with each other, provide a way for applications to access and share data, and enable the integration of an app with third-party services like social media platforms.[15] Facebook (now known as Meta), Google analytics, and Flurry analytics, among others, provide SDKs for developers' use. In a proceeding against FloHealth, the Federal Trade Commission (FTC) described the Flo app's use of SDKs from

> numerous third-party marketing and analytics firms . . . including Facebook, Flurry, Fabric, AppsFlyer, and Google. These SDKs gathered the unique advertising or device identifiers and Custom App Events of the millions of Flo App users. By including sensitive health information in the titles of the Custom App Events, [the app] conveyed the health information of millions of users to these third parties for years. This directly contradicted [Flo's] statements in its privacy policies that it would not divulge such information.[16]

---

[13] Research might pertain to health conditions and consumer needs but may also be conducted for marketing purposes. Some users may be willing to contribute to academic or medical research when they would decline to share data for advertising or marketing purposes; privacy policies often fail to provide adequate clarity.

[14] Consumer Reports found in its 2021 study that Sanity & Self and Wysa also sent data to Facebook, and Youper told Consumer Reports it was sharing with Facebook (Germain, 2021). See also Camacho et al. (2022) (explaining that a study of 578 mental health apps revealed that 44% shared data they collected with third parties).

[15] For more information on SDKs and APIs, see Yasar (2022).

[16] Complaint at 4, Flo Health, Inc., No. C-4747 (F.T.C. 2021).

Pixels are a tracking technology that can be hidden from sight and can track and send all sorts of personal data such as how a user interacts with a web page including specific items a user has purchased or information users have typed within a form while on the site. Businesses often want to use them to track consumer behavior (pageviews, clicks, interactions with ads) and target ads to users who may be more likely to engage or purchase something based on that prior online behavior.[17]

Users are largely unaware of the data transmission enabled by these technologies. Arguably, some engineers who use these prebuilt pieces of code also fail to recognize the ways the code permits data transfer. In July 2023, the US Department of Health and Human Services (HHS) Office for Civil Rights (OCR) and the FTC issued a joint letter drawing the attention of companies "to serious privacy and security risks related to the use of online tracking technologies that may be present on your website or mobile application (app) and impermissibly disclosing consumers' sensitive personal health information to third parties."[18]

Part II: The Legal Landscape

Why HIPAA Does Not Usually Protect Data Collected by Mental Health Apps

Intuitively, the data mental health apps collect and use feel like health data. And most people in the United States associate health data with HIPAA. But HIPAA's protections are far more limited than many people imagine,[19] and that law does not apply to most direct-to-consumer mental health apps and digital wellness products (Stiefel, 2019).[20] Designed to promote the portability and interoperability of patient records, HIPAA applies only to "covered entities" and "protected health information." Covered entities include health plans, health care clearinghouses, and providers[21] who transmit health information in electronic form in connection with a covered transaction, along with their "business associates."[22]

> In spite of [HIPAA's] broad definition of health care provider, a health care provider is not a covered entity unless and until the health care provider engages in an electronic transaction covered by the rule . . . *generally, the electronic submission of insurance claims causes a health care provider to become a covered entity*. (Stiefel, 2019, p. 355)

HIPAA limits covered entities' ability to disclose "protected health information" (PHI), which is a limited category of identifiable data related to health care.[23] When a covered entity violates HIPAA's

[17] Federal Trade Commission Office of Technology, *Lurking Beneath the Surface: Hidden Impacts of Pixel Tracking*, FTC(March 16, 2023), https://www.ftc.gov/policy/advocacy-research/tech-at-ftc/2023/03/lurking-beneath-surface-hidden-impacts-pixel-tracking; see *The Facebook Pixel*, Meta (February 5, 2021), https://www.facebook.com/government-nonprofits/blog/the-facebook-pixel; Fyler (2023) (describing the Meta pixel as "currently installed on around 30% of the world's most popular websites").

[18] Letter from Melanie Fontes Rainer, Dir., U.S. Dep't of Health & Hum. Servs. Off. of C.R. & Samuel Levine, Dir., FTC Bureau of Consumer Prot. (July 20, 2023) (on file with author).

[19] Some state laws may also provide additional protections for the confidentiality of health information. California recently passed a law to bring mental health apps within the scope of its Confidentiality of Medical Information Act. Jiang (n.d.) (describing AB 2089, effective Jan. 1, 2023).

[20] Mental health applications are software. Software can serve medical purposes and, in some cases, be considered a "medical device" within the purview of the Food and Drug Administration's (FDA's) regulatory authority. The FDA focuses on efficacy and safety and does not regulate privacy. See Stiefel, 2019 at 348.

[21] See 45 C.F.R. § 160.103 (2013) (defining all three terms).

[22] Business associates are people or companies that perform "certain functions or activities that involve the use or disclosure of protected health information on behalf of, or provides services to, a covered entity." *Business Associates*, U.S. Dep't of Health & Hum. Servs., https://www.hhs.gov/hipaa/for-professionals/privacy/guidance/business-associates/index.html (May 24, 2019). Those functions can include, among other things, data analysis, data aggregation, consulting, management and administrative services. 45 C.F.R. § 160.103. As of 2009, pursuant to the Health Information Technology for Economic and Clinical Health (HITECH) Act, Pub. L. No. 111–5, 123 Stat. 260 (2009), HHS could enforce HIPAA directly against business associates in addition to covered entities.

[23] 45 C.F.R. § 160.103.

Privacy Rule,[24] OCR can investigate complaints, conduct compliance reviews, take corrective actions, and impose civil monetary penalties. OCR can also refer potential violations of the criminal provisions of HIPAA to the Department of Justice (US Department of Health and Human Services, n.d.).

Apps that offer free texting services with volunteers, counselors, or chatbots do not engage in electronic transactions covered by the rule and are not covered entities under HIPAA.[25] Mental health apps that connect people seeking care with care providers but do not take insurance are also not covered by HIPAA (e.g. BetterHelp). Talkspace has relationships with a number of insurers and represents that it is covered by HIPAA.[26]

Notably, even where HIPAA does apply, deidentified data are not "protected health information." Some apps assert that they disclose only deidentified data. Talkspace told Consumer Reports that it uses "'de-identified' text chat logs for research and product development" (Germain, 2021). Apps may use data to improve their products to better serve the needs of users. Researchers and providers can use health data in ways designed to benefit patients, to find cures for disease, and deal with issues of public health. The ability to use deidentified data promotes these beneficial uses of data, and deidentification is meant to provide patients some degree of privacy protection. Privacy and data scholars have explained, however, that de-identification is becoming less and less protective in an era of big data. The proliferation of data increases the likelihood that data can be reidentified (Narayanan and Felten, 2014).[27]

In short, (a) HIPAA is not an all-encompassing protection of health data and (b) determining when HIPAA applies is often complicated and likely beyond the ability of a typical user. So, if HIPAA doesn't provide as much protection for health data as people imagine, how are the data collected by mental health apps protected?

The FTC: A Privacy Watchdog

The United States does not have a federal comprehensive privacy law.[28] Rather, Congress has approached data protection in a sector-specific way, regulating privacy in the context of education, credit reporting, children's privacy, finance, and patient data, among others. Since the 1990s and the emergence of the internet, Congress has looked to the FTC to protect privacy in the general commercial context through its enforcement of Section 5 of the Federal Trade Commission Act, a law pertaining to unfair and deceptive trade practices.[29]

Collecting data and making it available to advertisers is the business model that supports the provision of free services on the internet. Although people often do not pay dollars to use services, they provide tremendous amounts of data that companies can monetize. Accordingly, companies have an incentive to collect as much personal data as possible. Generally speaking, we rely on companies that

[24] 45 CFR §§ 160.101–160.105, 160.500–160.552 (2013); 45 C.F.R. § 164 (2013).

[25] ***Protecting the Privacy and Security of Your Health Information When Using Your Personal Cell Phone or Tablet***, U.S. Dep't of Health & Hum. Servs., https://www.hhs.gov/hipaa/for-professionals/privacy/guidance/cell-phone-hipaa/index.html (June 29, 2022) (providing HHS guidance explaining limited nature of HIPAA protections).

[26] (Talkspace, n.d.-b) (Talkspace privacy policy).

[27] See also Kaltwasser (2023) (studies of health data sets at Duke indicating "reidentification from deidentified data was possible between 86% and 100% of the time").

[28] In the past decade, numerous states have passed their own comprehensive privacy laws, including California, Colorado, Connecticut, Delaware, Florida, Indiana, Iowa, Kentucky, Maryland, Minnesota, Montana, Nebraska, New Hampshire, New Jersey, Oregon, Tennessee, Texas, Utah, and Virginia.

[29] Deceptive practices involve "a material representation, omission or practice that is likely to mislead a consumer acting reasonably in the circumstances. An act or practice is 'unfair' if it 'causes or is likely to cause substantial injury to consumers which is not reasonably avoidable by consumers themselves and not outweighed by countervailing benefits to consumers or to competition'." ***A Brief Overview of the Federal Trade Commission's Investigative, Law Enforcement, and Rulemaking Authority***, FTC, https://www.ftc.gov/about-ftc/mission/enforcement-authority (May 2021) (citing 15 U.S.C. § 45(n)). See also Chao et al. (2019) (discussing limitations of the FTC's unfair and deceptive practices authority).

collect and use consumer data to post privacy policies that describe how they collect, use, share, disclose, retain, and protect our data. It is up to us, as consumers, to read those policies and decide whether we want to use products and services on those terms. If we do not like the terms, we are free to choose a different product or service. In the event a company does not abide by the representations it has made in its privacy policy or engages in unfair conduct, the FTC may investigate or pursue an action against that company for deceptive or unfair practices. Notably, apps and services that fall outside the sector-specific laws (some of which require companies to have privacy policies), are not required by federal law to have a privacy policy at all. And numerous apps do not. In a study of 116 apps for depression conducted in October 2017, for example, only 49% had a privacy policy (O'Loughlin et al., 2019). In a 2020 study of 158 apps recommended by universities to student populations, 39% had no privacy policy (Melcher & Torous, 2020). An app without a privacy policy fails to inform consumers how their data will be used, compromising consumer agency and app accountability.[30]

Our system, heavily reliant on industry self-regulation, is referred to as a notice and choice approach to data protection. Unfortunately, this approach puts a substantial burden on consumers to protect their data, and it doesn't scale.[31] In reality, a vanishingly small subset of Americans actually reads privacy policies. The vast majority of us download apps, scroll right past the "your use of this app constitutes your agreement to our privacy policy" language, and start using the service. A 2014 Pew Research Center study showed that the majority of Americans believe that if a company has a privacy policy, that means the company is protecting the privacy of their data (Smith, 2014). That assumption could not be further from the truth. Our confusion about the degree to which our data are protected matters because our beliefs in this regard undoubtedly influence our propensity to disclose our information. Accordingly, the common perceptions that data disclosed to mental health apps will be protected because they are "health" data or that a company that has a privacy policy will protect user data may both lead people to share highly sensitive data with mental health apps.

Sometimes, mental health apps add to the confusion by displaying the HIPAA seal and representing that they are "HIPAA compliant." The Counslr app goes further, describing itself as "***truly*** HIPAA compliant."[32] Although a company can attempt to comply with HIPAA guidelines even when it is not a covered entity or business associate, a company does not bring itself within the jurisdiction of HHS by doing so. Recognizing that this representation can be confusing for consumers, the FTC's recent consent order with BetterHelp explicitly prohibits the app from misrepresenting "the extent to which [it] is a HIPAA-covered entity, and the extent that [its] privacy and information practices are in compliance with HIPAA requirements."[33] The FTC also raised misrepresentations about HIPAA compliance in its actions against GoodRx and Premom.

The FTC does its best to protect consumers' health data with the tools available. The agency has investigated a number of health care apps and services for allegedly misrepresenting their practices to consumers. Recent FTC actions also characterize as unfair the disclosure of sensitive health data to advertisers without informing users or obtaining affirmative consent.[34] And the FTC has begun pursuing unfairness claims against entities sharing user data with third parties through the use of SDKs and tracking technologies like pixels.[35]

[30] Chao et al. (2019) (discussing limitations of FTC's unfair and deceptive practices authority).

[31] Woodrow Hartzog, Professor of L. & Comput. Sci., Northeastern Univ. Sch. of L. & Khoury Coll. of Comput. Scis., Prepared Testimony and Statement for the Record, Hearing on Policy Principles for a Federal Data Privacy Framework in the United States 2 (Feb. 27, 2019).

[32] Counslr (2024) ("Compare the options. How we stand out from the rest"; Emphasis added).

[33] In re BetterHelp, Inc., Docket No. C-4796, File No. 2023169, at *7 (July 7, 2023).

[34] See, e.g., Complaint at 17, In re Flo Health, Inc., No. C-4747 (F.T.C. 2021); Complaint for Permanent Injunction, Civil Penalties, and Other Relief at 24–26, United States v. GoodRx Holdings, Inc., No. 23-cv-460 (N.D. Cal. 2023).

[35] For more information, see the following FTC matters: United States v. Easy Healthcare Corp., No. 1:23-cv-3107 (N.D. Ill. June 23, 2023); In re BetterHelp, Inc., Docket No. C-4796, File No. 2023169 (July 7, 2023); United States v. GoodRx Holdings, Inc., No. 23-cv-460 (N.D. Cal. 2023).

In addition to its Section 5 enforcement authority, the FTC enforces the Health Breach Notification Rule (HBNR),[36] which was designed to require entities that fall outside the scope of HIPAA to notify consumers in the event of a breach of unsecured personally identifiable health data in personal health records.[37] Since 2021, the FTC has begun interpreting this rule quite broadly,[38] characterizing developers of health apps as healthcare providers and construing the "sharing of covered information without an individual's authorization"[39] as a breach of security. The FTC characterized unauthorized disclosures in GoodRx and Premom as violations of the HBNR. In the spring of 2024, the agency finalized changes to the HBNR further clarifying its applicability to healthcare apps,[40] among other amendments, and the new rule took effect July 29, 2024.[41]

Although the FTC can investigate and bring an action against any company engaging in deceptive or unfair conduct or in violation of the HBNR, it is worthy of note that the FTC must proceed one case at a time. Moreover, there are only approximately 40 people in the agency charged with this privacy-protective work for the entire country, so resources are limited (Sherman, 2023).

Part III: Why Does All of This Matter?

The unauthorized or unanticipated disclosure of mental health data, in and of itself, violates an individual's privacy. Those data can be misused and abused and lead to further harm. Unauthorized disclosure of mental health data can lead to discrimination (jobs, schools), affect insurance coverage and the prices of retail products, and make people susceptible to scams and blackmail.[42] As the FTC has explained "even the disclosure of an individual's use of a health-related mobile application (e.g. an HIV management app, mental health app, or addiction recovery app) could, depending on the type of health app at issue, lead to a number of potential injuries, including embarrassment, social stigma, more expensive health insurance premiums, or even loss of employment."[43] This part of the chapter will discuss some of the risks and harms associated with the under-regulated use of mental health data.

Taking Advantage of Vulnerable People

People in need of mental health are a vulnerable population. Moreover, some mental health apps brand and advertise their services specifically to marginalized groups. BetterHelp, for example, has subdivisions targeting LGBTQ individuals, teens, and religious users: Pride Counseling, Teen Counseling, and Faithful Counseling, respectively. Ayana, an app designed to address the mental healthcare gap, is "focused on connecting marginalized communities, people of color, LGBTQ+, and disabled individuals to licensed therapists" (Raphael, 2019).

---

[36] Health Breach Notification Rule, 16 C.F.R. § 318 (2024).
[37] *Id.*
[38] U.S. Fed. Trade Comm'n, Statement of the Commission on Breaches by Health Apps and Other Connected Devices 2 (2021); see Kirk J. Nahra, Arianna Evers, & Ali A. Jessani, *FTC Proposes Changes To Clarify the Health Breach Notification Rule's Applicability to Health Apps and Other Evolving Technologies*, WilmerHale (June 8, 2023), https://www.wilmerhale.com/en/insights/blogs/wilmerhale-privacy-and-cybersecurity-law/20230608-ftc-proposes-changes-to-clarify-the-health-breach-notification-rule (discussing the proposed changes and noting the FTC's enforcement of the HBNR against GoodRx and Easy Healthcare's fertility-tracking app, PreMom, both of which involved unauthorized disclosure for advertising purposes).
[39] U.S. Fed. Trade Comm'n, *supra* note 38, at 2.
[40] *FTC Finalizes Changes to the Health Breach Notification Rule*, U.S. Fed. Trade Comm'n (Apr. 24, 2024), https://www.ftc.gov/news-events/news/press-releases/2024/04/ftc-finalizes-changes-health-breach-notification-rule.
[41] 16 C.F.R. § 318.
[42] Gooding and Kariotis (2022) (discussing harms from disclosure of mental health data).
[43] Health Breach Notification Rule 88 Fed. Reg. 37,819 (proposed June 9, 2023) (codified at 16 C.F.R. § 318).

Mental health apps have been touted for their ability to address the issue of mental healthcare deserts. Almost half of the people in the United States live in a place where it is difficult to obtain mental health care.[44] Members of Black (Vance, 2019), Brown (Duarte-Velez, 2023), and Native American communities (Mental Health America, n.d.) in the United States as well as people with fewer economic resources and those living in rural areas[45] have greater challenges obtaining care.[46] Unfortunately, however, privacy is also fundamentally less accessible to marginalized people; Black and Brown communities (Lai & Tanner, 2022), in particular, are more highly surveilled populations in the United States and have more interactions with the government that involve the collection and disclosure of personal data (Gellman & Adler-Bell, 2017).

Arguably, a heightened duty should exist when companies are dealing with people at risk. Even apps created with the best of intentions may fall short in the privacy area if developers do not understand the nature of the surveillance economy, the technologies they incorporate into their apps, and the lack of legal protection for data. But also, companies focused on the bottom line can take advantage of vulnerability and need by suggesting to users that apps are covered by HIPAA (when they are not) or that the privacy of their data will be protected (when it isn't). Featuring the HIPAA seal on an app not subject to HIPAA and making privacy policies difficult to find and hard to understand are ways companies can subvert users' ability to make informed decisions. The consequences of our failure to protect mental health data are likely to affect members of marginalized groups more substantially.

Targeted Advertising

Highly personalized microtargeted advertising is the lifeblood of the information economy. We use "free" apps and services and provide our data in return. When we shop online for a pair of sneakers at http://Nike.com, most of us are not surprised to see an ad for Nikes on the next site we visit. But analyzing and using people's sensitive health data to target ads to them (or to other individuals who have enough data points in common with them, i.e., "look alike audiences") raises substantially more complicated and arguably ethical issues. Sending a person struggling with an eating disorder ads for diuretics, for example, should not be permitted. Even following a person dealing with trauma or a mental health issue around the internet with constant reminders of her struggle is problematic.[47]

Data Broker Ecosystem

When health data make their way into the data broker ecosystem, they can become part of the profiles compiled, maintained, and sold on to other buyers. Data brokers sell mental health data (Harwell, 2023). A 2023 study from Duke University revealed that 10 of the brokers evaluated "advertised highly sensitive mental health data on Americans including data on those with depression, attention disorder, insomnia, anxiety, ADHD [attention deficit hyperactivity disorder], and bipolar disorder as well as data on ethnicity, age, gender, zip code, religion, children in the home, marital status, net worth, credit score, date of birth, and single parent status" (Kim, 2023, p. 4). In other words, there is a market for these data, and mental health apps and data brokers operate in an underregulated sphere that allows them to decide, on a company-by-company basis, how they want to use it. An app could elect to sell user data outright to data brokers. A company's practices in this regard should be set out in its privacy policy. When a company states that it will never sell identifiable data, a user should look for

---

[44] Haseltine (2023) ("Approximately 47 percent of the U.S. population [158 million people] live in a mental health workforce shortage area.").

[45] Livingston and Green (2022) ("Seventy-five percent of rural counties across the country have no mental health providers or fewer than 50 per 100,000 people.").

[46] Vasan and Le Melle (2021) and Carratala and Maxwell (2020) (noting some apps attempt to develop services addressing the needs of these communities.), Johnson (2020) and Raphael (2019) (discussing Ayana).

[47] See Paul (2017) (describing negative effects of receiving ads targeted at mental health).

representations about the use of "deidentified" data. Apps will often indicate that they do, in fact, sell, use, or otherwise monetize deidentified data, suggesting that data disconnected from its identifying characteristics, like names and contact information, cannot pose a risk to users. Many prominent scholars have explained, however, that big data and reidentification technologies substantially decrease the utility of deidentification as a privacy protective measure (Barocas & Nissenbaum, 2014; Narayanan & Felten, 2014). The data broker industry easily "link[s] mobile advertising IDs (MAIDs) collected by apps to a person's full name, physical address, and other personal identifiable information (PII)" (Cox, 2021).

Beyond Advertising, Implications for Content Provision

When health data are incorporated into profiles and shared with companies like Meta and Google or with data brokers, that information about a user may affect, not only advertising, but also content that a user sees in the future. Mozilla's Jen Caltrider has explained that "[p]olitical disinformation campaigns have targeted people whose profiles include specific characteristics related to mental health, such as depression."[48]

Perceptions That Discourage Care

Unsurprisingly, the lack of protection and the lack of clarity about the protection that does exist for mental health data in the United States concern many individuals. For some, there is stigma associated with seeking mental health care, and others are uncomfortable or embarrassed to be perceived as having such needs. For these people, the potential disclosure of their data or even the fact that they are using a mental health app, as well as the risk that their information may be used in ways they cannot anticipate, can be disincentives for seeking the care that they need. Even more unfortunately, communicating the facts that people need to know to make informed decisions about obtaining healthcare confidentially (i.e., the facts described in this chapter) will, in our current under-regulated environment, magnify that disincentive.

Notions of Informed Consent

Notions of informed consent developed in the latter half of the twentieth century have become a familiar principle of the modern medical experience (Bazzano et al., 2021). We want to ensure people fully understand what is happening when they undergo medical treatment or procedures and appreciate the risks. The notice and choice system we employ in the United States when it comes to data collection rests on a similar idea—that people should generally have the opportunity to understand how their data are going to be used before they download an app or use a website. In the case of mental health apps, these ideas overlap. Although many mental health apps claim they are not providing treatment or diagnoses, people certainly appear to be turning to these apps for help managing symptoms or developing coping strategies, to learn about concerning thoughts or behaviors, and to understand why they feel the way they do. All of these things sound a lot like treatment. In any event, whether using an app or accessing care in person, all people should have the right to understand how the very private, sensitive data they share in the process will be used and the risks that use may create.

Part IV: How to Communicate About Mental Health Apps

Although apps hold promise for privacy, our failure in the United States to adequately protect people's data creates privacy problems for users. The conundrum that this promise versus problems opposition creates for messaging is clear. We want to be able to broadly promote access to a full spectrum of care,

[48] Healey (2023) (paraphrasing Jen Caltrider, director of Mozilla's Privacy Not Included).

but we do not want to actively encourage people to share their very sensitive mental health information in environments that put them at risk. People who promote the use of digital mental health care have an ethical obligation to be aware of and appreciate the privacy risks that our approach to regulation in the United States has created and to communicate about mental health care possibilities in a manner that is informed by those risks.

The Message for Clinicians, Doctors, and Other Providers

Providers should be aware of the privacy implications of mental health apps and online services when they consider incorporating them into their practices or recommending them to patients or people seeking help. Providers associated with educational institutions—universities or high schools—should be especially aware of these concerns.[49]

Recent scholarship addresses the importance of evaluating and implementing apps in practice, noting privacy as a significant concern: "It is important to note that patients may assume that mHealth apps are adhering to the same privacy and security standards as health care entities, the same that they expect when interacting with their providers, but this may not be the case. Patient consent to use these apps should be informed and voluntary."[50] A variety of resources are available to help providers become more aware of privacy issues raised by mental health apps. Professional groups have made affirmative efforts to provide information about apps centering privacy as a concern. The American Counseling Association (ACA) explains that "[e]thics requires counselors to know about any technology one uses or recommends, including its privacy practices. Counselors should be aware of not just what companies say they do or don't do but also what they actually do with user information. Although many companies are transparent about what information they compile about and from their users (customers, patients, clients) and how they gather, use, store and sell that information, others are more vague or unclear" (American Counseling Association, n.d.). Highlighting the confusion around HIPAA compliance on its webpage devoted to this issue, the ACA provides additional informational and educational resources for providers.

The American Psychiatric Association (APA) has created an app evaluation model using a "hierarchical rating system and embedded rubric so that APA members, patients, and other providers, become familiar with important information that should be considered when picking an app," and privacy protection is one of the factors the model analyzes (American Psychiatric Association, n.d.). Using this APA model, the Digital Psychiatry Lab with the Beth Israel Deaconess Medical Center in Boston has created the M-Health Index and Navigation Database located at http://Mindapps.org (MINDApps), which contains evaluations of over 600 mental health apps available in app stores, each informed by 105 objective questions (Washington University School of Medicine, 2024). Although MINDapps does not endorse any of the evaluated apps, trained volunteers have analyzed the apps, and the database permits filtered searches. "Privacy & Security" is one of the primary categories, and the app condenses and highlights important terms from privacy policies pertaining to the collection, use and storage of user data, including deletion and opt-out options. Two of the factors are confusing: "Is PHI shared" and "Meets HIPAA." MINDApps appears to check the box for "Meets HIPAA" if an app ***claims*** to meet HIPAA or represents that it is "HIPAA-compliant"—a statement that does not provide actual protection for consumers and which can be affirmatively misleading as explained previously. "PHI" is also a HIPAA term meaning "Protected Health Information," but it appears MINDApps is using the term in a more colloquial sense to refer to "personal health information" entered into apps. Given the lack of clarity around HIPAA coverage, this use of the term PHI could further confuse users.

Overall, the database empowers consumers by providing them with information, but this approach has its limits for privacy protection. Including "privacy and security" as one of 12 filters and as 2 among over 100 factors a consumer might prioritize does not alleviate the burden on the consumer to

---

[49] Melcher and Torous (2020) (43% of 60 top schools studied in 2020 suggested a total of 218 apps to students; 39% had no privacy policy).

[50] King et al. (2023) (discussing steps clinicians should take when incorporating use of digital apps into their treatment of patients).

understand the digital environment, appreciate the risks and harms associated with our country's decision not to provide adequate protections for sensitive health data, and choose to limit their options accordingly. Still, some information is better than no information.

The Message for Developers, Companies, and Apps

Protect user privacy. Full stop. Use default settings, user interface options, and design to further the privacy interests of users, enable informed consent, and protect user data. Avoid the unconsented disclosure of personal data through the use of SDKs, APIs, and pixels. And provide fully encrypted communications.[51] Refuse to compromise patients' welfare in the pursuit of growth and engagement. The FTC has created an interactive tool to provide guidance "for anyone developing a mobile app that will access, collect, share, use, or maintain information related to an individual consumer's health, such as information related to diagnosis, treatment, fitness, wellness, or addiction."[52] Developers should also keep apprised of FTC enforcement actions that pertain to mental health apps and other health-related entities and use of health-related data because these actions provide insight into the agency's conception of best practices. Recent cases of interest involve BetterHelp, Flo Health, PreMom, GoodRx, Kochava, and X-Mode.

The Message for People in Need of Care

Researchers have demonstrated that consumers, including young adults, who want to use mental health apps care substantially about privacy and security.[53] As unfair as it is that the burden of protecting the privacy of mental health data in the commercial environment falls on individuals, consumers should be encouraged to become as informed as possible and to take steps to protect their privacy when using these apps and services. Some helpful ideas for users include:

- Read the privacy policy of the app to try to understand how the app will use and disclose your data. If an app does not have a privacy policy, absolutely do not use it.
- When creating accounts, use strong, unique passwords and multifactor authentication if available.
- Avoid logging in to mental health apps using other accounts like Facebook or Google.
- Be aware of default settings that make accounts or activity public and take care to set all profiles to private (which may take a bit of effort).
- Opt out of sharing data for market research and other nonessential purposes where possible.
- Be aware that community features, chat rooms, and texting with volunteers or bots provide far less privacy than 1:1 appointments with care providers who accept insurance, and restrict the sharing of sensitive data accordingly.
- Avoid using photos, use screen names as opposed to real names, turn off location sharing, and look for apps that encrypt communications.
- Take steps to delete your data and/or accounts when you are no longer using a service.

[51] Parker et al. (2019) (Offering specific recommendations for improved protection of user privacy "targeted at multiple stakeholders throughout the global mobile app ecosystem including government regulators, developers, and app stores); Iwaya et al. (2023).

[52] *Mobile Health App Interactive Tool*, U.S. Fed. Trade Comm'n (Dec. 2022), https://www.ftc.gov/business-guidance/resources/mobile-health-apps-interactive-tool.

[53] Kabacińska et al. (2022) (noting "well-grounded" security and privacy concerns expressed by young adults using mental health applications: privacy was in the top five criteria used to select mobile mental health apps ranked by the study participants, and security was one of the most salient themes that emerged from the qualitative analysis).

Before deciding on a service, people can consult recent reviews by consumer protection oriented entities, like Consumer Reports (Germain, 2021) and Mozilla (2023), which evaluate the privacy practices of mental health apps available in the Apple Store and Google Play. In its 2021 study, Consumer Reports' Digital Lab examined which companies received data from apps as they were being used, determined whether privacy settings were on or off by default, and analyzed whether the companies' privacy policies aligned with app behavior (Germain, 2021). Mozilla's "Privacy Not Included" team, led by Jen Caltrider, investigated and evaluated approximately 30 mental health apps in 2022 and 2023 (Caltrider et al., 2023). The team examined the data the apps were collecting, "what they told users they were doing with their personal information, whether users could change or delete the information collected, how solid their basic security practices were," and the developer's track records (Healey, 2023). Mozilla recommended two apps for their data handling practices: PTSD Coach, created by the US Department of Veterans' Affairs, and Wysa, a chatbot, but the vast majority of the apps reviewed earned a warning label. Mozilla provides fairly extensive reviews of each app and very specific information about why it has concerns about each product and recommends steps users can take to try to protect their data.[54] These reports are useful resources for both practitioners and consumers.

Ultimately, the burden of protecting privacy should be on apps offering mental health care, not on consumers. Apps collecting and using this sensitive data should owe a nonnegotiable duty of loyalty to their customers. Monetizing the health data of vulnerable individuals should be prohibited, and, at a minimum, heightened protections should be provided. But this is a job for Congress and for state legislatures. So the messaging about mental health apps should go beyond providers, developers, and consumers and reach all the way to Capitol Hill. Big tech is a powerful lobbying force; providers and people in the health care field can be a voice for people in need of mental health care—amplifying health policy concerns, the importance of privacy and confidentiality to the provision of mental health care, and the need for stronger regulation.

The Message for Congress and State Legislatures

Ideally, members of the mental health care community would act together to pressure Congress to take action to protect health data shared through digital platforms. Laws and regulations that can be enforced against bad actors will incentivize best practices. From a policy perspective, such protection would promote trust and encourage people to obtain the care they need. Protecting the privacy of mental health data will ultimately enable us to realize the promise of mental health apps. Consumers should also join this fight for greater data protection, but their voices will be stronger when supported by the healthcare industry.

In addition to enacting privacy protective legislation, members of Congress can conduct inquiries and investigate reported bad practices. In June 2022, for example, Senators Warren (D-MA), Booker (D-NJ), and Wyden (D-OR) sent letters of inquiry to BetterHelp and Talkspace asking them to clarify their privacy practices in response to reports about data mining and disclosure to third parties including data brokers, Meta, and Google.[55] These efforts increase transparency and contribute to popular understanding about what is happening with our data behind the scenes.

---

[54] Kabacińska et al. (2022) (suggesting concerns about privacy and security should inform the "development of a user-driven app-rating platform"). For user-driven ratings to be effective, users must be informed about the ways apps are using personal data and the risks that such uses pose.

[55] Letter from Elizabeth Warren, Sen., Cory A. Booker, Sen., Ron Wyden, Sen. to Alon Matas, Founder and President, BetterHelp (June 22, 2022) (on file with author); Press Release, Ron Wyden, US Sen. for Oregon, Wyden, Colleagues Call on Mental Health Apps to Provide Answers on Patient Data Privacy and Sharing Practice (June 24, 2022) (on file with author).

Conclusion

Making mental health care more accessible will benefit society. Mental health apps are a promising innovation that could enable more people to obtain care more privately, even from the comfort of their own homes. But at the moment, our regulatory approach is not designed to facilitate that eventuality. While we work toward that future, ideal world, approaching mental health apps with caution and with a clearer understanding of the privacy risks and potential harms they entail is paramount.

References

American Counseling Association. (n.d.). *Telehealth & emerging technology.* https://www.counseling.org/resources/topics/professional-counseling/technology-related/telehealth-apps

American Psychiatric Association. (n.d.). *The App Evaluation Model.* https://www.psychiatry.org/psychiatrists/practice/mental-health-apps/the-app-evaluation-model

Balasubramanian, M. (2022, May 2). *App tracking transparency opt-in rate—Monthly updates.* Flurry. https://www.flurry.com/blog/att-opt-in-rate-monthly-updates

Barocas, S., & Nissenbaum, H. (2014). Big data's end run around procedural privacy protections. *Communications of the ACM, 57*(11), 31–33. https://doi.org/10.1145/2668897

Bazzano, L. A., Durant, J., & Brantley, P. R. (2021). A modern history of informed consent and the role of key information. *Ochsner Journal, 21*(1), 81–85. https://doi.org/10.31486/toj.19.0105

Caltrider, J., Rykov, M., & MacDonald, Z. (2023, May 1). *Are mental health apps better or worse at privacy in 2023?* Mozilla. https://foundation.mozilla.org/en/privacynotincluded/articles/are-mental-health-apps-better-or-worse-at-privacy-in-2023

Camacho, E., Cohen, A., & Torous, J. (2022). Assessment of mental health services available through smartphone apps. *JAMA Network Open, 5*(12), e2248784. https://doi:10.1001/jamanetworkopen.2022.48784

Carratala, S., & Maxwell, C. (2020, May 7). *Health disparities by race and ethnicity.* Center for American Progress. https://www.americanprogress.org/article/health-disparities-race-ethnicity

Chao, B., Null, E., & Park, C. (2019, November 20). *Enforcing a new privacy law. Who should hold companies accountable?* New America. https://www.newamerica.org/oti/reports/enforcing-new-privacy-law

Counslr. (2024). *Untitled.* https://www.counslr.com

Cox, J. (2021, July 14). *Inside the industry that unmasks people at scale.* Vice. https://www.vice.com/en/article/epnmvz/industry-unmasks-at-scale-maid-to-pii

Crisis Text Line. (2024). *Untitled.* https://www.crisistextline.org

Duarte-Velez, Y. (2023, April 20). *Mental health and the Latinx/Hispanic community.* Lifespan. https://www.lifespan.org/lifespan-living/mental-health-and-latinxhispanic-community

Fyler, T. (2023, July 24). *Meta pixel at heart of data privacy cases—again.* TechHQ. https://techhq.com/2023/07/why-is-the-meta-pixel-at-heart-of-data-privacy-cases

Gellman, B., & Adler-Bell, S. (2017, December 21). *The disparate impact of surveillance.* The Century Foundation. https://tcf.org/content/report/disparate-impact-surveillance

Germain, T. (2021, March 2). *Mental health apps aren't all as private as you may think. Consumer Reports.* https://www.consumerreports.org/health/health-privacy/mental-health-apps-and-user-privacy-a7415198244

GlobeNewswire. (2023, October 25). *Counslr increases support in New York state, as need for mental health resources grows in high schools.* https://www.globenewswire.com/en/news-release/2023/10/25/2766234/0/en/Counslr-Increases-Support-in-New-York-State-As-Need-for-Mental-Health-Resources-Grows-in-High-Schools.html

Gooding, P., & Kariotis, T. (2022, November 15). *Mental health apps are not keeping your data safe. Scientific American.* https://www.scientificamerican.com/article/mental-health-apps-are-not-keeping-your-data-safe

Harwell, D. (2023, February 13). Now for sale: Data on your mental health. *Washington Post.* https://www.washingtonpost.com/technology/2023/02/13/mental-health-data-brokers

Haseltine, W. (2023, September 22). *Solving the mental health provider shortage. Psychology Today.* https://www.psychologytoday.com/us/blog/best-practices-in-health/202309/solving-the-mental-health-provider-shortage

Healey, J. (2023, May 2). Mental health apps may put your privacy at risk. Here's what to look for. *Los Angeles Times.* https://www.latimes.com/business/technology/story/2023-05-02/mental-health-apps-privacy-risk-what-to-look-for

Health Breach Notification Rule, 16 C.F.R. § 318. (2024). https://www.ecfr.gov/current/title-16/chapter-I/subchapter-C/part-318

Hunter, T., & Merrill, J. B. (2022, September 22). Health apps share your concerns with advertisers. HIPAA can't stop it. *Washington Post.* https://www.washingtonpost.com/technology/2022/09/22/health-apps-privacy

Iwaya, L. H., Babar, M. A., Rashid, A., & Wijayarathna, C. (2023). On the privacy of mental health apps: An empirical investigation and its implications for app development. *Empirical Software Engineering, 28*(1), 2. https://doi.org/10.1007/s10664-022-10236-0

Jiang, K. (n.d.). *California privacy legislation update: AB 2089, 984, 2677, and 2269*. California Lawyers Association. https://calawyers.org/privacy-law/california-privacy-legislation-update-ab-2089-984-2677-and-2269

Johnson, J. (2020, July 7). *These mental health apps are geared toward people of color. Forbes.* https://www.forbes.com/sites/forbestheculture/2020/07/07/these-mental-health-apps-are-geared-toward-people-of-color/?sh=7c8c0f0922e4

Kabacińska, K., McLeod, K., MacKenzie, A., Vu, K., Cianfrone, M., Tugwell, A., & Robillard, J. M. (2022). What criteria are young people using to select mobile mental health applications? A nominal group study. *Digital Health, 8*, 20552076221102775. https://doi.org/10.1177/20552076221102775

Kaltwasser, J. (2023, July 11). *"Deidentified" health data not so deidentified after all.* Managed Healthcare. https://www.managedhealthcareexecutive.com/view/-deidentified-health-data-not-so-deidentified-after-all

Kim, J. (2023, February 13). *Data brokers and the sale of Americans' mental health data.* Duke University Sanford School of Public Policy. https://techpolicy.sanford.duke.edu/wp-content/uploads/sites/4/2023/02/Kim-2023-Data-Brokers-and-the-Sale-of-Americans-Mental-Health-Data.pdf

King, D. R., Emerson, M. R., Tartaglia, J., Nanda, G., & Tatro, N. A. (2023). Methods for navigating the mobile mental health app landscape for clinical use. *Current Treatment Options in Psychiatry, 10*, 72–86. https://doi.org/10.1007/s40501-023-00288-4

Kwan, J. (2023, May 5). *Care ethics.* Santa Clara University. https://www.scu.edu/ethics/ethics-resources/ethical-decision-making/care-ethics/care-ethics.html

Lai, S., & Tanner, B. (2022, July 18). *Examining the intersection of data privacy and civil rights.* Brookings Institution. https://www.brookings.edu/articles/examining-the-intersection-of-data-privacy-and-civil-rights

Livingston, K., & Green, M. (2022, May 18). *America's mental health care deserts: Where is it hard to access care?* ABC News. https://abcnews.go.com/Health/americas-mental-health-care-deserts-hard-access-care/story?id=84301748

Marcelline, M. (2023, March 12). *Mental health startup shared patient data with Google, Facebook, Meta.* PCMag. https://www.pcmag.com/news/mental-health-startup-shared-patient-data-with-google-facebook-meta

Melcher, J., & Torous, J. (2020). Smartphone apps for college mental health: A concern for privacy and quality of current offerings. *Psychiatric Services, 71*(11), 1114–1119. https://doi.org/10.1176/appi.ps.202000098

Mental Health America. (n.d.). *Native and indigenous communities and mental health.* https://www.mhanational.org/issues/native-and-indigenous-communities-and-mental-health

M-Health Index & Navigation Database. (2024, May 10). *Welcome video.* https:/http://mindapps.org

Mozilla. (2023, May 2). *Shady mental health apps inch toward privacy and security improvements, but many still siphon personal data.* https://foundation.mozilla.org/en/blog/shady-mental-health-apps-inch-toward-privacy-and-security-improvements-but-many-still-siphon-personal-data

Narayanan, A., & Felten, E. W. (2014, July 9). *No silver bullet: De-identification still doesn't work.* Princeton University. https://www.cs.princeton.edu/~arvindn/publications/no-silver-bullet-de-identification.pdf

Nosthoff, A.-V., Maschewski, F., & Couldry, N. (2023, December 1). *Big Tech is exploiting the mental health crisis to monetize your data.* Jacobin. https://jacobin.com/2023/12/big-tech-mental-health-data-collection-colonization

O'Loughlin, K., Neary, M., Adkins, E. C., & Schueller, S. M. (2019). Reviewing the data security and privacy policies of mobile apps for depression. *Internet Interventions, 15*, 110–115. https://doi.org/10.1016/j.invent.2018.12.001

Parker, L., Halter, V., Karliychuk, T., & Grundy, Q. (2019). How private is your mental health app data? An empirical study of mental health app privacy policies and practices. *International Journal of Law and Psychiatry, 64*, 198–204. https://doi.org/10.1016/j.ijlp.2019.04.002

Paul, K. (2017, May 5). *When Facebook and Instagram think you're depressed.* Vice. https://www.vice.com/en/article/pg7d59/when-facebook-and-instagram-thinks-youre-depressed

Raphael, R. (2019, December 8). *This app matches marginalized communities to therapists who share their background.* FastCompany.https://www.fastcompany.com/90440201/this-app-matches-marginalized-communities-to-therapists-who-share-their-background

Sherman, J. (2023, July 14). *The key to protecting privacy is locked in an underfunded government agency.* Slate. https://slate.com/technology/2023/07/federal-trade-commission-funding-privacy.html

Singer, N. (2023, February 1). GoodRx leaked user health data to Facebook and Google, F.T.C. says. *New York Times.* https://www.nytimes.com/2023/02/01/business/goodrx-user-data-facebook-google.html

Smith, A. (2014, December 4). *Half of online Americans don't know what a privacy policy is.* Pew Research Center. https://www.pewresearch.org/short-reads/2014/12/04/half-of-americans-dont-know-what-a-privacy-policy-is

Stevens, S. (2023, December 17). *Text-based mental health app aims to help students.* Spectrum News 1. https://spectrumlocalnews.com/nys/central-ny/news/2023/12/16/text-based-mental-health-app-aims-to-help-students-

Stiefel, S. (2019). The chatbot will see you now: Protecting mental health confidentiality in software applications. *Science and Technology Law Review, 20*(2), 333–387. https://doi.org/10.7916/stlr.v20i2.4774

Surani, A., Bawaked, A., Wheeler, M., Kelsey, B., Roberts, N., Vincent, D., & Das, S. (2023, June). Security and privacy of digital mental health: An analysis of web services and mobile apps. In *Conference on Data and Applications Security and Privacy.* http://dx.doi.org/10.2139/ssrn.4469981

Talkspace. (n.d.-b) *Privacy policy.* Talkspace. https://www.talkspace.com/public/privacy-policy

Talkspace. (n.d.-a). *Online therapy covered by insurance.* Talkspace. https://www.talkspace.com/coverage/insurance

Tewari, S. (2022, September 28). *How to navigate mental health apps that may share your data.* American Civil Liberties Union. https://www.aclu.org/news/privacy-technology/how-to-navigate-mental-health-apps-that-may-share-your-data

US Department of Health and Human Services. (n.d.). *How OCR enforces the HIPAA privacy & security rules.* https://www.hhs.gov/hipaa/for-professionals/compliance-enforcement/examples/how-ocr-enforces-the-hipaa-privacy-and-security-rules/index.html

Vance, T. A. (2019, February 8). *Addressing mental health in the Black community.* Columbia University Irving Medical Center. https://www.columbiapsychiatry.org/news/addressing-mental-health-black-community

Vasan, A., & Le Melle, S. M. (2021, February 17). *Biden wants to fix racial inequality. Mental health access is an important place to start.* NBC News. https://www.nbcnews.com/think/opinion/biden-wants-fix-racial-inequality-mental-health-access-important-place-ncna1257376

Washington University School of Medicine. (2024). *Recommended apps & websites.* https://psychiatry.wustl.edu/wellness-resources/website-resources/

Yasar, K. (2022, October). *Software development kit (SDK).* TechTarget. https://www.techtarget.com/whatis/definition/software-developers-kit-SDK

Part IV

Special Populations, Mental Health Disparities, and Communication Inequalities

16

Considerations for Optimizing Mental Health Communication to Advance Mental Health Equity

Crystal L. Barksdale[1], Collene Lawhorn[2], Jennifer Alvidrez[3], and Kat Schwartz[3]

[1]National Institutes of Health, National Institute on Minority Health and Health Disparities
[2]National Institutes of Health, National Institute of Mental Health
[3]National Institutes of Health, Office of Disease Prevention

Mental health communication involves the study and practice of sharing information, raising awareness, and promoting dialogue to influence our understanding of mental health. Mental health communication can be an important tool for achieving health equity because, if implemented appropriately, it can help reduce stigma, ensure more equitable access to information and resources, improve mental health literacy, promote culturally and linguistically appropriate services, and drive advocacy and policy change.

Historically, mental health communication has been shaped by Western medicalized perspectives and a gross underappreciation for cultural diversity that contributed to longstanding disparities in mental health outcomes (Hsieh & Kramer, 2021). During the US Civil Rights era, a shift toward mental health advocacy, community-based care, and human rights for institutionalized individuals, families, and communities (Korr, 2020; Yohanna, 2013) contributed to the recognition of communication as a critical discipline for supporting mental health and well-being.

Although progress has been made, equity-focused mental health communication for culturally diverse populations has still not been fully integrated into mental healthcare services, and ongoing efforts should address mental health information access, culturally and linguistically appropriate resources, and inclusive dialogue that recognizes the diverse experiences of individuals and communities with mental health concerns.

Framing Mental Health and Mental Health Communication Among Culturally Diverse Populations

Although we want to avoid creating a narrative that reinforces stereotypes, there is an urgent need within the field of health communication broadly, and mental health communication more specifically, to use health communication theories and strategies to improve communication delivered to diverse populations. Improved communication can lead to better mental health outcomes, reduced mental health disparities,

The Handbook of Mental Health Communication, First Edition.
Edited by Marco C. Yzer and Jason T. Siegel.

and the achievement of mental health equity or providing all individuals with the same opportunity to experience mental wellness and effectively cope with mental illness by removing structural and social determinant barriers (Braveman et al., 2017; Schiavo, 2014; US Department of Health and Human Services, 2022). The groundbreaking Surgeon General report *Mental Health: Culture, Race, and Ethnicity* (US Department of Health and Human Services, 2001), released over 20 years ago, documented the existence of mental healthcare disparities for racially and ethnically diverse populations and established the knowledge base that contextualizes this pervasive public health problem. Unfortunately, mental health disparities, defined here as differences in health outcomes that adversely affect racially/ethnically minoritized individuals, populations of less privileged socioeconomic status (SES), underserved rural populations, and sexual and gender minoritized (SGM) individuals (Perez-Stable et al., 2021), have persisted or worsened in the last 2 decades despite our awareness of their existence, increased understanding of their causes, and efforts at reduction and mitigation. We use the term "minoritized" to use systems-centered language and in recognition that "minority" is a socially constructed term that acknowledges the active social processes in which systems disempower and place individuals into "minority" status (APA Presidential Task Force, 2023; Benitez, 2010; Sotto-Santiago, 2019). As mental health disparities have persisted, the achievement of mental health equity remains impossible.

A range of individual and population attributes are associated with mental health disparities, inequitable access to mental healthcare services, and increased marginalization. These include but are not limited to, race, ethnicity, nativity, age, gender identity, sexual orientation, geographic location, socioeconomic position/status, religion, language, and disability status (Alvidrez et al., 2019; Hsieh & Kramer, 2021). As these factors intersect to shape an individual's identity and all that this entails (i.e. socialization, interpersonal behavior, language, and communication preferences), it is also important to recognize how they intersect to influence other processes and experiences such as perceptions about and experiences with mental health and mental health care. Mental health disparities are often compounded at the intersection of multiple marginalized identities, yet research suggests that intersectional inequities are often overlooked, both in terms of the target of interventions and health communication approaches (APA Presidential Task Force, 2023; Collin & Blidge, 2020; Harrington et al., 2022). Thus, employing an intersectionality theoretical framework to mental health communications, which is necessary for understanding how individuals' multiple social identities or statuses (e.g. race, gender, sexual orientation, socioeconomic position/status) combine to form multiple interlocking systems of privilege and oppression (e.g. racism, sexism, heterosexism, classism; Bowleg, 2012), becomes essential to addressing mental health disparities and promoting equity. Acknowledging the existence of multiple social identities and considering the health information and communication needs of individuals with multiple marginalized identities is critical to understanding how mental health disparities arise, persist, and how best to intervene (Bowleg, 2012; Dhamoon, 2011; Harrington et al., 2022).

Landscape of Mental Health and Mental Healthcare Disparities

Disparities in mental health and mental health care are well documented and affect multiple diverse populations across the lifespan. For example, compared to White youth, Hispanic/Latino, and Asian youth are more likely to be diagnosed with mood disorders, whereas Black and Hispanic/Latino youth are more likely to be diagnosed with disruptive behavior disorders (Cummings et al., 2019; Huang et al., 2012; Merikangas et al., 2010). Among adults, findings from community-based studies suggest that racial and ethnic minoritized adults have a lower overall prevalence of mental disorders compared to White adults; however, once diagnosed, racial and ethnic minoritized adults are more likely to have more severe and persistent courses of disorders (Alvarez et al., 2019; Breslau et al., 2005; Williams et al., 2007). SGM individuals (e.g. those who identify as gay, lesbian, bisexual, or transgender) have consistently higher rates of depression, anxiety, and substance use compared to cisgender and heterosexual individuals (e.g. Henderson et al., 2022). Regarding geographic diversity, adults living in rural areas have a similar prevalence of most mental disorders compared to those living in urban areas (Breslau et al., 2014).

The death rate from suicide remains significantly higher among American Indian/Alaska Native populations from late adolescence through adulthood (Leavitt et al., 2018), and rates of suicide and suicidal thoughts and behaviors have been steadily increasing in recent years among Black and Asian youth (Bridge et al., 2018; Lindsey et al., 2019; Xiao & Lu, 2021). The death rate from suicide is also higher among those living in rural areas compared to those living in urban areas (Ivey-Stephenson et al., 2017), whereas the prevalence of suicidal thoughts and behaviors is higher among SGM individuals than among cisgender heterosexual individuals (Hottes et al., 2016; Raifman et al., 2020). Notably, differences across diverse populations in suicide and other mental health outcomes are driven by sociocultural and systemic factors, including bias in diagnosis (Fadus et al., 2020; Gara et al., 2019), cultural differences in identification and manifestation of symptoms (Marshall et al., 2009; Yang & Benson, 2016), and differential access to mental health care (US Department of Health and Human Services, 2001).

Mental healthcare disparities are especially problematic, as they not only jeopardize the achievement of mental health equity but also exacerbate existing disparities and disproportionalities in other health and social systems (e.g. in social services systems, carceral systems), and they increase the burden of illness on individuals, families, communities, and society. Historically, the mental healthcare system has not effectively addressed the needs of culturally diverse populations (President's New Freedom Commission on Mental Health, 2003), and often this is reflected in the lack of attention to the communication needs of diverse populations. As a result, communication about mental health is often not tailored to diverse populations.

Multilevel Approaches to Communicating About Mental Health Among Culturally Diverse Populations: How Health Professionals Communicate About Mental Health

This section addresses the considerations of health professionals who communicate directly with patients/clients/consumers about their mental health needs, diagnoses, prevention and treatment options, and how to maintain mental wellness. Individual-level approaches to mental health communication may rely on health professionals who are responsible for developing mental health promotion and prevention interventions, providing treatments, and monitoring and maintaining care of individuals across the continuum of mental health (i.e. those focused on mental wellness to those receiving prevention intervention programs and those receiving treatment and maintenance care; National Academies of Sciences, Engineering, and Medicine, 2019). Health professionals, including psychologists, psychiatrists and primary care physicians, social workers, psychiatric nurses, and other providers, often work within a larger healthcare system (organization) that has its own culture, with norms and practices that guide patient–provider interactions and communications about mental health (see the next section for a discussion of how organizations communicate about mental health). The culture of health care, and increasingly mental health care and the professionals who work within it, are shaped by a scientific, biomedical framework, which reinforces a specific, technical view of illness and patients' experiences of illness (Fancher, 2017; Hsieh & Kramer, 2021). The culture of mental health and the mental healthcare system and organizations therein, as well as professionals' own training and their personal sociocultural characteristics (i.e. racial/ethnic minoritized status, gender identity, sexual orientation, socioeconomic background, nativity, language preference, religious/spiritual background; Hsieh & Kramer, 2021; Lawrence et al., 2015; Ruben, 2016), are just a myriad of the inter- and intrapersonal cultural factors that shape how health professionals communicate about mental health with patients. Yet, these factors and their role in how professionals communicate may often go unnoticed given the tendency to default to culturally and professionally guided constructions of mental health and mental health care, which become manifested in the language and discussions (Van Beveren et al., 2023).

As society becomes increasingly diverse, mental healthcare practices will inevitability continue to evolve and blend with local preferences, cultural traditions, and strategies for mental prevention and wellness, which leads to, for example, community differences in preferences for and participation in care (Hsieh & Kramer, 2021). An important consideration at the individual level of communication is understanding what happens when the complex cultural milieu of the healthcare provider collides with the complex cultural milieu of the patient—a fusion, or a process of potential for adopting and modifying foreign ways into an already functional cultural system (Hsieh & Kramer, 2021). Thus, first and foremost, the interaction is not simply recognizing and identifying the cultural differences between the healthcare provider and the mental health client/patient but also appreciating that each is affected by multiple levels of influence that shape health/mental health behavior, outcomes, and communication (Hsieh & Kramer, 2021; Viswanath et al., 2021).

Intentional, Purposeful Content

The next consideration of health professionals' communication is the purpose and intent of the message content. For health professionals in the mental healthcare context, using patient-centered communication (PCC; Epstein & Street, 2007; Street, 2019) is a useful option for crafting an intentional and purposeful message. Through implementing the core concepts of PCC (i.e. eliciting patient perspectives, understanding the patient within their unique psychosocial and cultural context, and reaching a shared understanding of the patient's problems and treatments that are concordant with the patient's values; Epstein & Street, 2007), health professionals can help empower the patient and increase equitable participation in the communication process, as well as work toward achieving patient-centered care and other mental healthcare goals. Research suggests PCC indirectly affects health outcomes through factors such as adherence, patient self-efficacy, and patient satisfaction (e.g. Haskard-Zolnierek et al., 2021; Jiang, 2017; Schulz & Jiang, 2021). Enhanced PCC can also improve outcomes such as participation and continuation in treatment (White & Chanoff, 2011).

Beyond incorporating PCC core concepts, health professionals must integrate a cultural and structural approach in their communications to have an effective impact on mental health equity. This requires a sensitivity to the community's cultural norms as well as the patient's individual preferences (Hsieh & Kramer, 2021), while also understanding the influences of larger societal and structural factors on health communication behavior (Viswanath et al., 2021). A key component of this sensitivity is understanding who comprises the key group/intended audience of the intended message and (a) what are the priorities, needs, and preferences of that group related to mental health communication; (b) what are the geographic, economic, social, and psychological factors that shape the individual's behavior; and (c) what individual and community behaviors may shape perceptions of mental health (Schiavo, 2014). For example, if a health professional intends to talk with a young, Black woman about mental health screening and treatment, it would be helpful to know and consider that communication with health professionals about mental health treatment in the Black community has historically been limited due to concerns about stigma, mistrust, and historical trauma (e.g. Gaston et al., 2016; Taylor & Kuo, 2019). Among Black women, these conversations may be further complicated by the Superwoman Schema/strong Black woman archetype of being strong, resilient, and taking care of others while neglecting one's own health (e.g. Woods-Giscombe et al., 2016). This highlights the importance of crafting messaging through an intersectional lens to demonstrate an understanding of how multiple systems in which individuals operate affect mental health (Erving et al., 2021), which can maximize the impact of the message. Thus, health professionals should carefully consider how to employ PCC core concepts within culturally and linguistically appropriate frameworks when crafting their communications and messages to best inform mental health knowledge or behavior change among diverse populations.

Delivering Culturally and Linguistically Appropriate Communications

As with all health communication, communication about mental health must be culturally and linguistically appropriate, it must be provided in a language and communication style that meets the patient's preferences and needs, and it must be respectful of the patient's cultural norms and beliefs about mental health and mental health care. Attending to communication using a cultural lens will help address the underlying factors that perpetuate disparities, such as the therapeutic alliance, low mental health literacy, and the possibility of misdiagnosis (Kagawa-Singer & Kassim-Lakha, 2003; Magana, 2019; Tambling et al., 2021). To further ensure information is accurately exchanged between patient and provider, and to enhance understanding of patients' cultural norms and beliefs about mental health and mental health care, professionals may consider employing a cultural broker who can bridge any differences between the professional's and patient's cultural frame of reference (e.g. Barksdale et al., 2014; Park et al., 2011).

Multilevel Approaches to Communicating About Mental Health Among Culturally Diverse Populations: Organizations That Educate the Public About Mental Health

This section discusses considerations for organizations that educate, inform, and offer guidance to diverse populations about mental health. Examples of such organizations include healthcare organizations, insurers, mental health advocacy groups, professional societies, public health departments, and other governmental agencies, schools, and workplaces. Mental health information may be disseminated through a wide variety of formats and venues, including printed materials, online written materials, videos, or podcasts; as well as interactive formats such as classes, webinars, or social media chats or discussion forums. For this information to be beneficial, organizations must provide it in a way that is understandable, relevant, and respectful to its intended audiences.

Understandable Content

Mental health information, whether written or spoken, must be understandable and meaningful to the intended audience. This requires organizations to be familiar with their audiences regarding existing general and mental health literacy (Centers for Disease Control and Prevention, 2022). At a fundamental level, organizations must attend to factors that may affect comprehension of the material. Many online mental health resources are written well beyond the sixth-grade level recommended for public communications and may not be understandable by individuals with fewer years of formal education (Skierkowski et al., 2019).

If versions of materials are not already available in other languages besides English, appropriate translations should be developed that are understandable to a nonprofessional audience (Kiing et al., 2016). Translations should not be word-for-word literal translations but should appropriately reflect cultural constructs of mental health, idiomatic expressions, and shared positive and negative associations with certain words or phrases. For example, the meaning of the Spanish word *nervios* (literally translated as "nerves") varies across Spanish-speaking populations, and it can signify anything from somatic complaints to schizophrenia (Baer et al., 2003). Input from both mental health professionals and nonprofessional native speakers of the language who are familiar with the populations or communities of focus is therefore critical to producing understandable and meaningful translations (Acharya et al., 2017; Kiing et al., 2016).

Relevant Content

Whatever the specific content of mental health communication, it must resonate with the intended audience. It is important that materials or communications include representative images or personal narratives to signal their relevance or applicability to diverse populations. People are more likely to attend to and comprehend information if it is accompanied by images of people who look like them (Eisend et al., 2023; Good et al., 2010). This may be particularly important when organizations communicate about mental health to a racially and ethnically diverse audience, as there is a perception across groups that mental illness is more common in White populations (Boysen et al., 2023).

Using appropriate terms to refer to population groups is also critical to establish personal relevance or appeal of the information. Gender-neutral language (e.g. chairperson, spouse) can help increase relevance and acceptability of information for people who identify as gender nonbinary (Harris et al., 2017).

Umbrella terms that encompass multiple groups, such as Black, Indigenous, People of Color (BIPOC); Latinx; or Lesbian/Gay/Bisexual/Transgender/Queer and/or Questioning/Intersex/Asexual/Plus (LGBTQIA+), are not universally embraced and may be unlikely to be used for self-identification (Selvarajah et al., 2020). Referring explicitly to specific populations (e.g. gay and bisexual men instead of men who have sex with men) and providing more than a single identity label (Black or African American) may avoid confusion about who is being referred to and avoid alienating those who do not identify with certain umbrella or specific population terms.

Respectful Content

Mental health information that is either targeted (disseminated to specific populations) or tailored (developed for specific populations) may be particularly helpful to reach and engage diverse audiences (Schmid et al., 2008). However, the framing of this targeting or tailoring can influence whether the information is accepted or dismissed by the intended audience. For example, having a special segment or section of communication materials devoted to "special populations" may suggest that these groups are inferior or represent a deviation from normal (Sussman et al., 2020). Similarly, labeling an entire group as "at risk" or "vulnerable" based on population membership (e.g. that American Indian or Alaska Native youth are at risk of suicide) can imply that certain groups experience elevated rates of mental health problems because of inherent fragility or susceptibility that they have no control over and not because of societal oppression or disadvantage (Braveman & Parker Dominguez, 2021; Berchini, 2017). Taking disrespectful language a step further, the inappropriate use of the term "gender dysphoria" as a synonym for transgender status, rather than as a condition experienced by a subset of transgender individuals, implies that transgender identity is itself a mental illness (Ashley, 2021). It is also important for organizations to avoid using stigmatizing language that suggests people living in impoverished, oppressive, or abusive environments experience mental health problems solely because of poor or unhealthy "lifestyle choices" (Farrington-Douglas, 2022).

Multilevel Approaches to Communicating About Mental Health Among Culturally Diverse Populations: Mass Media Approaches to Communicating About Mental Health

This section discusses considerations for news organizations and media outlets regarding the coverage and portrayal of mental health among diverse populations. Media coverage and messages have the potential to increase awareness about mental health, reduce stigma, and encourage people to get help for mental health problems. Unfortunately, such coverage may also introduce and reinforce stigma and barriers to seeking help for certain populations.

Increasing Awareness

Media portrayals of individuals with mental health conditions often have little diversity and may create the impression that mental health problems are primarily experienced by cisgender, heterosexual White men or women (Boysen et al., 2023). Members of other population groups may not see themselves in such portrayals and therefore may not perceive the topic of mental health as relevant to them. Celebrities or public figures who are racial or ethnic minorities or SGM may play a particularly important role in increasing awareness of mental health issues and decreasing stigma in these populations (Calhoun & Gold, 2020).

Reducing Stigma

Although mental health stigma is ubiquitous, individuals from racial and ethnic minoritized groups often have more negative views toward mental illness (Eylem et al., 2020). Unfortunately, media coverage of race or ethnicity and mental illness may heighten stigma. An analysis of media coverage of mass shootings shows that shootings are more often attributed to mental illness for White and Latino individuals than for Black individuals and that Black and Latino individuals are portrayed less sympathetically than White shooters (Duxbury et al., 2018). Similarly, in an analysis of news articles about drug use (Lindsay & Vuolo, 2021), coverage of White individuals emphasized substance use as a medical issue requiring treatment, whereas coverage of Black individuals emphasized criminal behavior requiring punishment. More balanced coverage about mental illness among racially and ethnically minoritized individuals that highlights social and structural determinants of health and barriers to mental health care may promote more compassionate views by the public and increase support for decriminalizing substance use and mental illness (McGinty et al., 2018; Petty et al., 2017). However, more research is needed on the best ways to disentangle issues of mental health, SES, and race and ethnicity in health messages.

Encouraging Help-Seeking

Media organizations can play a key role in encouraging and normalizing mental health treatment for those who need it. Media coverage of celebrities and other public figures who have been open about receiving mental health treatment may be especially impactful for populations with low levels of help-seeking (Lutanco-Chua, 2022). However, even though such accounts may increase awareness and acceptance of mental health issues, they may not automatically lead to increased help-seeking because of the different life circumstances and treatment options between celebrities and the public. Particularly for individuals who live in rural or other underserved areas, have jobs with limited or no health insurance or sick leave, or cannot afford to pay for treatment out of pocket, it may not be possible to "take a mental health break," check themselves voluntarily into inpatient facilities, or receive psychotherapy. This may foster the impression that receiving mental health treatment is a luxury that is out of reach of most people (Sloat, 2022). More media coverage about when and how to access mental health care, including free resources or those covered by public and private health insurance, is needed to encourage more people to seek mental health care.

Another reason why the media message to simply "get help" may be problematic is that seeking help for mental health problems may be dangerous for some populations. Highly publicized examples of Black individuals in a mental health crisis being killed by police in the community or mental health facilities (Shadravan et al., 2021; Treisman, 2023) may instill fear in Black communities about asking for help. Reluctance to seek emergency assistance for a mental health crisis may increase the likelihood of eventual police involvement or delay appropriate mental health treatment (Kessell et al., 2009). Coverage of violent interactions can be accompanied by a discussion of alternatives to seek help that do not involve the police or advocating for programs that reduce violent encounters between police and individuals experiencing a mental health crisis (Shadravan et al., 2021). More generally, the media and others involved in mental health communication can play an important role in not just documenting mental health disparities but also heightening public awareness and support of policy changes to address those disparities (Holder & Treno, 1997).

Cross-Cutting Considerations for Optimizing Mental Health Communication for Culturally Diverse Populations Equity Considerations

Effective mental health communication should be guided by a health equity lens that emphasizes fairness, inclusivity, and justice. This requires it to be community centered, culturally appropriate, respectful, and relevant to the mental health needs of diverse populations. Effective mental health communication should also acknowledge and address mental health disparities and employ health equity messaging strategies that actively work to reduce them among populations that are disproportionately affected.

Accessibility

Communication equity ensures that mental health information is accessible to all individuals, regardless of their background, SES, or geographic location. When mental health information is available and easily accessible, it facilitates help-seeking within and across communities and facilitates conversations about mental health without significant barriers (Henderson et al., 2013). Mental health communication that is unclear, jargon filled, or does not incorporate a clear pathway of understanding for all, including those with mental health literacy challenges, limited English proficiency, and accessibility needs, can contribute to unjust healthcare systems and poor health outcomes (Gotlieb et al., 2022). As researchers have suggested, to ensure the delivery of easy-to-understand communications that are also culturally and linguistically appropriate, professionals, organizations, and the media should use open-ended questions to increase understanding of the audience's cultural context, use the active voice, and use plain language (i.e. language free of jargon; Aggarwal et al., 2016; Sedgwick et al., 2021).

Representation and Community Engagement

Mental health communication equity should also feature diverse representation (Stuart, 2016) at all levels that is culturally and contextually sensitive and respects the unique ways communities understand and address mental health issues. Health communication should strive to represent consumer needs and encourage active engagement in mental health care by using participatory approaches that convey a variety of perspectives, life experiences, and identities. Collaboration with and input from members of the intended audiences are critical ingredients for effective communication across these dimensions (Muvuka et al., 2020).

Inherent in using mental health communication as a tool to achieve mental health equity at any socioecological level is the role of the community. Community-engaged research approaches are widely recognized as instrumental in addressing health disparities; their use ensures that the communities and individuals served by the service sector and/or involved in the research enterprise are involved in the development, implementation, dissemination, and evaluation of the products of those partnerships. Similarly, mental health communication interventions, particularly those addressing culturally diverse populations and aiming to reduce disparities, should center on the community comprised of the intended individuals or audience(s) of the mental health communication. Communication-related community engagement includes defining who comprises the community, employing strategies to engage community members and/or gatekeepers of the community to understand the mental health issues and to develop messages to address those issues (and related stigma), engaging community members/gatekeepers to implement and disseminate the message, working with the community to evaluate and collect feedback about the message, and engaging community members/gatekeepers to develop and implement strategies to sustain the message to reduce disparities and achieve equity and other long term outcomes.

Message Framing to Promote Equity

Positive and strengths-based framing promotes mental health equity by highlighting the capabilities, resilience, and potential of diverse individuals from backgrounds and their communities (American Medical Association & Association of American Medical Colleges, 2021). By focusing on strengths and assets rather than deficits, mental health communication can challenge stereotypes and stigmatizing narratives that perpetuate inequities in marginalized and minoritized populations (Peinado et al., 2020). Positive message framing that highlights stories of recovery, personal growth, and success may inspire hope and promote the idea that mental health challenges can be overcome (Xie, 2013). Empowerment-oriented message framing does not absolve social and structural barriers that contribute to poor mental health outcomes for many communities but uses language that is co-created with communities and encourages individuals to take an active role in their mental health journey, seek support, and engage in self-care practices (Fagan et al., 2020; Krist et al., 2017).

Structural and Social Determinants

Equity in health communication involves recognizing and explicitly highlighting systemic structural inequities and the social determinants of mental health. By crafting messages that draw attention to social injustices, systemic barriers, and marginalized voices, communication can promote a more comprehensive understanding of the root causes of mental health inequities, encourage dialogue that leads to mental health policy changes (Viswanath, 2006), and embolden healthcare professionals, organizations, and media messengers to expand their roles as social change agents (Shim et al., 2018). Framing messages in a way that recognizes social determinants of mental health also serves to advance mental health equity by highlighting the impact of poverty, racism, discrimination, trauma, and access to resources (American Medical Association & Association of American Medical Colleges, 2021) and can help reduce stigma for marginalized and minoritized groups (Neff et al., 2017; Petty et al., 2017). However, an exclusive emphasis on larger, upstream social and structural determinants of mental health may suggest that mental health problems are inevitable and intractable. This may engender a sense of limited personal agency for members of marginalized and minoritized groups, which may in turn exacerbate mental health problems and deter help-seeking when necessary. It is therefore important to differentiate between social determinants of mental health, which are larger structural forces that are more difficult to modify on an individual level (e.g. neighborhood residential segregation), and social risks (e.g. a person's housing instability) or social needs (e.g. a person's need for housing assistance), which are more addressable through mental health treatment or other services (Alderwick & Gottlieb, 2019).

Interdisciplinary Collaboration

Communication scholars and practitioners with the cultural humility to address community mistrust can help forge partnerships and collaborations between mental health consumers, practitioners, and advocates—translating evidence-based research advancements into meaningful outcomes (Meffert et al., 2021). Teams that involve cross-disciplinary expertise, including but not limited to mental health researchers, communication scientists, public health professionals, care providers, and community members, can help foster a sense of ownership, informed decision-making, and empowerment for sustainable outcomes.

Evaluation and Impact Considerations

Evaluating the impact of mental health communication with diverse populations involves assessing multiple levels of efficacy. Evaluation metrics that address health communication exposure, impact, context, and predictors are important for assessing the effectiveness of mental health messages. Quality of information—including its meaningfulness, credibility, and utility for diverse communities—and factors such as geography, individual accessibility, affordability, availability of culturally and linguistically appropriate services and reduction in barriers to accessing mental health services and resources are critical for identifying areas for improvement and attention.

In mental health, determining thoughtful engagement includes employing measures that determine knowledge and awareness about mental health, changes in mental health literacy, and a greater understanding of mental illnesses and resources. It also involves determining the influence of messaging in shifting attitudes, beliefs, and behaviors about mental health in intended as well as unintended directions.

Social media tools provide a useful opportunity to gauge reach by assessing the number of views, shares, comments, subscribers, and likes in virtual spaces that may provide safe spaces for diverse voices. Partnerships with technology experts, social media platforms, and marketing experts that facilitate ethical data access could elucidate important trends in online health information seeking and areas for growth. Although the growing information ecosystem presents many opportunities to connect audiences that might not readily be connected, the spread of misinformation, disinformation, and exposure to poor-quality information also presents important challenges (Lawhorn et al., 2022).

Advancing Mental Health Communication for Diverse Populations: Implications for Mental Health Equity

Mental health communication is a vital tool to address mental health disparities and promote mental health equity. Through describing communication from an intersectional culturally framed, multilevel perspective, we have outlined several important factors for the field to consider in optimizing mental health communication approaches and strategies for culturally diverse populations and thus, ultimately, to work to achieve mental health equity.

Opportunities for Future Research

Although the field has progressed, several opportunities remain to advance the science of mental health communication and improve our understanding of how this tool may be used to achieve mental health equity for all. For example, more research is needed to understand the impact of different modalities and forms of mental health communication (e.g. verbal, nonverbal) on mental health and healthcare outcomes among diverse populations. Specifically, additional research is needed to develop evidence-based, culturally and linguistically appropriate communication strategies and interventions using accessible technology to reduce mental health stigma, improve mental health literacy, and help enhance access to appropriate mental health care for diverse populations. Addressing such factors and increasing the provision of relevant mental health information helps ensure that disparities in mental health are reduced (Kreps, 2019). In addition, as noted previously, there is much work that remains to appropriately integrate and implement an intersectional approach that will enhance our ability to address disparities more effectively.

Conclusion

In conclusion, the potential for mental health communication to promote positive health outcomes is unlikely to be fully realized if that communication is not equitably developed and implemented. The consequences of poor mental health communication are well described and dire for everyone, but especially for culturally diverse populations. An increased focus on equity in health and mental health communication has resulted in improved recognition of the importance of inclusivity, culturally and linguistically appropriate resources and information, and improved information access. Greater collaboration among health communication scholars, practitioners, and communities is needed to further optimize mental health communication for culturally diverse populations. We hope that the considerations presented herein encourage continued attention and discussion about the need for equity-focused mental health communication and the development and implementation of innovative mental health communication strategies to advance mental health equity.

Disclaimer

Drs. Barksdale, Lawhorn, and Alvidrez and Ms. Schwartz report no financial relationships with commercial interests. The views expressed in this article represent those of the authors and do not necessarily represent the views of NIH.

References

Acharya, B., Basnet, M., Rimal, P., Citrin, D., Hirachan, S., Swar, S., Thapa, P., Pandit, J., Pokharel, R., & Kohrt, B. (2017). Translating mental health diagnostic and symptom terminology to train health workers and engage patients in cross-cultural, non-English speaking populations. *International Journal of Mental Health Systems, 11*, 62. https://doi.org/10.1186/s13033-017-0170-2

Aggarwal, N. K., Pieh, M. C., Dixon, L., Guarnaccia, P., Alegria, M., & Lewis-Fernandez, R. (2016). Clinician descriptions of communication strategies to improve treatment engagement by racial/ethnic minorities in mental health series: A systematic review. *Patient Education and Counseling*, *99*(2), 198–209. https://doi.org/10.1016/j.pec.2015.09.002

Alderwick, H., & Gottlieb, L. M. (2019). Meanings and misunderstandings: A social determinants of health lexicon for health care systems. *Milbank Quarterly*, *97*(2), 407–419. https://doi.org/10.1111/1468-0009.12390

Alvarez, K., Fillbrunn, M., Green, J. G., Jackson, J. S., Kessler, R. C., McLaughlin, K. A., Sadikova, E., Sampson, N. A., & Alegria, M. (2019). Race/ethnicity, nativity, and lifetime risk of mental disorders in U.S. adults. *Social Psychiatry and Psychiatric Epidemiology*, *54*, 1–13. https://doi.org/10.1007/s00127-018-1644-5

Alvidrez, J., Castille, D., Laude-Sharp, M., Rosario, A., & Tabor, D. (2019). The National Institute on Minority Health and Health Disparities research framework. *American Journal of Public Health*, *109*(S1), S16–S20. https://doi.org/10.2105/AJPH.2018.304883

American Medical Association and Association of American Medical Colleges. (2021). *Advancing health equity: Guide on language, narrative and concepts*. https://www.ama-assn.org/system/files/ama-aamc-equity-guide.pdf

APA Presidential Task Force on Psychology and Health Equity. (2023). Report of the American Psychological Association presidential task force on psychology and health equity. *American Psychologist*, *78*, 259–267. https://doi.org/10.1037/amp0001125

Ashley, F. (2021). The misuse of gender dysphoria: Toward greater conceptual clarity in transgender health. *Perspectives on Psychological Science*, *16*(6), 1159–1164. https://doi.org/10.1177/1745691619872987

Baer, R. D., Weller, S. C., de Alba Garcia, J. G., Glazer, M., Trotter, R., Pachter, L., & Klein, R. E. (2003). A cross-cultural approach to the study of the folk illness *nervios*. *Culture, Medicine, and Psychiatry*, *27*(3), 315–337. https://doi.org/10.1023/a:1025351231862

Barksdale, C. L., Kenyon, J., Graves, D. L., & Jacobs, C. G. (2014). Addressing disparities in mental health agencies: Strategies to implement the national CLAS standards in mental health. *Psychological Services*, *11*(4), 369–376. https://doi.org/10.1037/a0035211

Benitez, M. (2010). Resituating culture centers within a social justice framework: Is there room for examining whiteness? In D. Patton (Ed.), *Culture centers in higher education: Perspectives on identity, theory, and practice* (pp. 119–134). Stylus.

Berchini, C. (2017, February 24). *Redefining "at-risk": New times call for new ground rules*. National Council of Teachers of English. https://ncte.org/blog/2017/02/redefining-risk-new-times-call-new-ground-rules

Bowleg, L. (2012). The problem with the phrase women and minorities: Intersectionality—An important theoretical framework for public health. *American Journal of Public Health*, *102*, 1267–1273. https://doi.org/10.2105/AJPH.2012.300750

Boysen, G. A., Axtell, E. L., Kishimoto, A. G., & Sampo, B. L. (2023). The racial stereotype about mental illness. *Journal of Social Psychology*, *163*(4), 501–514. https://doi.org/10.1080/00224545.2021.2023086

Braveman, P., Arkin, E., Orleans, T., Proctor, D., & Plough, A. (2017). *What is health equity? And what difference does a definition make?* Robert Wood Johnson Foundation.

Braveman, P., & Parker Dominguez, T. (2021). Abandon "race." Focus on racism [review]. *Frontiers in Public Health*, *9*, 689462. https://doi.org/10.3389/fpubh.2021.689462

Breslau, J., Kendler, K. S., Su, M., Gaxiola-Aguilar, S., & Kessler, R. C. (2005). Lifetime risk and persistence of psychiatric disorders across ethnic groups in the United States. *Psychological Medicine*, *35*(3), 317–327. https://doi.org/10.1017/S0033291704003514

Breslau, J., Marshall, G., Pincus, H., & Brown, R. (2014). Are mental disorders more common in urban than rural areas of the United States? *Journal of Psychiatric Research*, *56*, 50–55. https://doi.org/10.1016/j.jpsychires.2014.05.004

Bridge, J. A., Horowitz, L. M., Fontanella, C. A., Sheftall, A. H., Greenhouse, J., Kelleher, K. J., & Campo, J. V. (2018). Age-related racial disparity in suicide rates among US youths from 2001 through 2015. *JAMA Pediatrics*, *172*(7), 697–699. https://doi.org/10.1001/jamapediatrics.2018.0399

Calhoun, A. J., & Gold, J. A. (2020). "I feel like I know them": The positive effect of celebrity self-disclosure of mental illness. *Academic Psychiatry*, *44*(2), 237–241. https://doi.org/10.1007/s40596-020-01200-5

Centers for Disease Control and Prevention. (2022). *Health literacy: Understand your audience*. https://archive.cdc.gov/www_cdc_gov/healthliteracy/developmaterials/understandaudience/index.html

Collin, P., & Blidge, S. (2020). *Intersectionality*. Wiley.

Cummings, J. R., Ji, X., Lally, C., & Druss, B. G. (2019). Racial and ethnic difference in minimally adequate depression care among Medicaid-enrolled youth. *Journal of the American Academy of Child & Adolescent Psychiatry*, *58*(1), 128–138. https://doi.org/10.1016/j.jaac.2018.04.025

Dhamoon, R. K. (2011). Considerations on mainstreaming intersectionality. *Political Research Quarterly*, *64*(1), 230–243. https://doi.org/10.1177/1065912910379227

Duxbury, S. W., Frizzell, L. C., & Lindsay, S. L. (2018). Mental illness, the media, and the moral politics of mass violence: The role of race in mass shootings coverage. *Journal of Research in Crime and Delinquency*, *55*(6), 766–797. https://doi.org/10.1177/0022427818787225

Eisend, M., Muldrow, A. F., & Rosengren, S. (2023). Diversity and inclusion in advertising research. *International Journal of Advertising*, *42*(1), 52–59. https://doi.org/10.1080/02650487.2022.2122252

Epstein, R. M., & Street, R. L. (2007). *Patient-centered communication in cancer care: Promoting healing and reducing suffering*. National Cancer Institute.

Erving, C. L., Patterson, E. J., & Boone, J. (2021). Black women's mental health matters: Theoretical perspectives and future directions. *Sociology Compass, 15*(9), e12919. https://doi.org/10.1111/soc4.12919

Eylem, O., de Wit, L., van Straten, A., Steubl, L., Melissourgaki, Z., Danışman, G. T., de Vries, R., Kerkhof, A. J. F. M., Bhui, K., & Cuijpers, P. (2020). Stigma for common mental disorders in racial minorities and majorities a systematic review and meta-analysis. *BMC Public Health, 20*(1), 879. https://doi.org/10.1186/s12889-020-08964-3

Fadus, M. C., Ginsburg, K. R., Sobowale, K., Halliday-Boykins, C. A., Bryant, B. E., Gray, K. M., & Squeglia, L. M. (2020). Unconscious bias and the diagnosis of disruptive behavior disorders and ADHD in African American and Hispanic youth. *Academic Psychiatry, 44*, 95–102. https://doi.org/10.1007/s40596-019-01127-6

Fagan, J., Frye, V., Calixte, R., Jain, S., Molla, L., Lawal, A., Mosley, M. P., Greene, E., Mayer, K. H., & Zingman, B. S. (2020). "It's like plan B but for HIV!" design and evaluation of a media campaign to drive demand for PEP. *AIDS and Behavior, 24*(12), 3337–3345. https://doi.org/10.1007/s10461-020-02906-1

Fancher, R. T. (2017). *Health and suffering in America: The context and content of mental health care*. Routledge.

Farrington-Douglas, J. (2022, May 15). *Time to drop "lifestyle" out of health policy*. The Health Policy Partnership. https://www.healthpolicypartnership.com/time-to-drop-lifestyle-out-of-health-policy

Gara, M. A., Minsky, S., Silverstein, S. M., Miskimen, T., & Stakowski, S. M. (2019). A naturalistic study of racial disparities in diagnoses at an outpatient behavioral health clinic. *Psychiatric Services, 70*(2), 130–134. https://doi.org/10.1176/appi.ps.201800223

Gaston, G. B., Earl, T. R., Nisanci, A., & Glomb, B. (2016). Perception of mental health services among black Americans. *Social Work in Mental Health, 14*(6), 676–695. https://doi.org/10.1080/15332985.2015.1137257

Good, J. J., Woodzicka, J. A., & Wingfield, L. C. (2010). The effects of gender stereotypic and counter-stereotypic textbook images on science performance. *Journal of Social Psychology, 150*(2), 132–147. https://doi.org/10.1080/00224540903366552

Gotlieb, R., Praska, C., Hendrickson, M. A., Marmet, J., Charpentier, V., Hause, E., Allen, K. A., Lunos, S., & Pitt, M. B. (2022). Accuracy in patient understanding of common medical phrases. *JAMA Network Open, 5*(11), e2242972. https://doi.org/10.1001/jamanetworkopen.2022.42972

Harrington, N. G., Francis, D. B., & Occa, A. (2022). Theoretical and methodological matters in health communication: Navigating current and future directions. In T. L. Thomson & N. G. Harrington (Eds.), *The Routledge handbook of health communication* (3rd ed., pp. 17–32). Routledge. https://doi.org/10.4324/9781003043379

Harris, C. A., Blencowe, N., & Telem, D. A. (2017). What is in a pronoun? Why gender-fair language matters. *Annals of Surgery, 266*(6), 932–933. https://doi.org/10.1097/sla.0000000000002505

Haskard-Zolnierek, K., Snyder, M., Hernandez, R.-K., & Thompson, T. L. (2021). Patient-provider communication and health outcomes. In T. L. Thomson & N. G. Harrington (Eds.), *The Routledge handbook of health communication* (3rd ed., pp. 213–226). Routledge. https://doi.org/10.4324/9781003043379

Henderson, C., Evans-Lacko, S., & Thornicroft, G. (2013). Mental illness stigma, help seeking, and public health programs. *American Journal of Public Health, 103*(5), 777–780. https://doi.org/10.2105/AJPH.2012.301056

Henderson, E. R., Goldbach, J. T., & Blosnich, J. R. (2022). Social determinants of sexual and gender minority mental health. *Current Treatment Options in Psychiatry, 9*, 229–245. https://doi.org/10.1007/s40501-022-00269-z

Holder, H. D., & Treno, A. J. (1997). Media advocacy in community prevention: News as a means to advance policy change. *Addiction, 92*(S2), S189–S199. https://doi.org/10.1111/j.1360-0443.1997.tb02991.x

Hottes, T. S., Bogaert, L., Rhodes, A. E., Brennan, D. J., & Gesnik, D. (2016). Lifetime prevalence of suicide attempts among sexual minority adults by study sampling strategies: A systematic review and meta-analysis. *American Journal of Public Health, 106*, e1–e12. https://doi.org/10.2105/AJPH.2016.303088

Hsieh, E., & Kramer, E. M. (2021). *Rethinking culture in health communication: Social interactions as intercultural encounters*. Wiley-Blackwell.

Huang, K., Calzada, E., Cheng, S., & Brotman, L. M. (2012). Physical and mental health disparities among young children of Asian immigrants. *Journal of Pediatrics, 160*(2), 331–336. https://doi.org/10.1016/j.jpeds.2011.08.005

Ivey-Stephenson, A. Z., Crosby, A. E., Jack, S. P. D., Haileyesus, T., & Sedacca-Kresnow, M. (2017). Suicide trends among and within urbanization levels by sex, race/ethnicity, age group, and mechanism of death—United States, 2001–2015. *MMWR Surveillance Summaries, 66*(18), 1–16. http://dx.doi.org/10.15585/mmwr.ss6618a1

Jiang, S. (2017). Pathway linking patient-centered communication to emotional well-being: Taking into account patient satisfaction and emotion management. *Journal of Health Communication, 22*(3), 234–242. https://doi.org/10.1080/10810730.2016.1276986

Kagawa-Singer, M., & Kassim-Lakha, S. (2003). A strategy to reduce cross-cultural miscommunication and increase the likelihood of improving health outcomes. *Academic Medicine, 78*(6), 577–587. https://doi.org/10.1097/00001888-200306000-00006

Kessell, E. R., Alvidrez, J., McConnell, W. A., & Shumway, M. (2009). Effect of racial and ethnic composition of neighborhoods in San Francisco on rates of mental health-related 911 calls. *Psychiatric Services, 60*(10), 1376–1378. https://doi.org/10.1176/ps.2009.60.10.1376

Kiing, J. S. H., Rajgor, D., & Toh, T.-H. (2016). Topical review: Mind your language—Translation matters (a narrative review of translation challenges). *Journal of Pediatric Psychology*, *41*(10), 1110–1119. https://doi.org/10.1093/jpepsy/jsw036

Korr, M. (2020). Martha H. Mowry, MD: Pioneer in medicine, suffrage movement. *Rhode Island Medical Journal*, *103*(1), 74–75. http://www.rimed.org/rimedicaljournal/2020/02/2020-02-74-heritage.pdf

Kreps, G. L. (2019). The chilling influences of social stigma on mental health communication: Implications for promoting health equity. In L. R. Lippert, R. D. Hall, A. E. Miller-Ott, & D. C. Davis (Eds.), *Communicating mental health: History, contexts, and perspectives* (pp. 11–27). Lexington Books.

Krist, A. H., Tong, S. T., Aycock, R. A., & Longo, D. R. (2017). Engaging patients in decision-making and behavior change to promote prevention. *Studies in Health Technology and Informatics*, *37*(2), 105–122. https://doi.org/10.3233/978-1-61499-790-0-284

Lawhorn, C., Stirratt, M. J., & Rausch, D. M. (2022). Turning the tide in HIV through health communication research. *Journal of the International AIDS Society*, *25*(6), e25955. https://doi.org/10.1002/jia2.25955

Lawrence, R. E., Rasinski, K. A., Yoon, J. D., & Curlin, F. A. (2015). Physician race and treatment preferences for depression, anxiety, and medically unexplained symptoms. *Ethnicity & Health*, *20*(4), 354–364. https://doi.org/10.1080/13557858.2014.921893

Leavitt, R. A., Ertl, A., Sheats, K., Petrosky, E., Ivey-Stephenson, A., & Fowler, K. A. (2018). Suicides among American Indian/Alaska natives—National Violent Death Reporting System, 18 states, 2003–2014. *MMWR Morbidity and Mortality Weekly Report*, *67*, 237–242. http://dx.doi.org/10.15585/mmwr.mm6708a1

Lindsay, S. L., & Vuolo, M. (2021). Criminalized or medicalized? Examining the role of race in responses to drug use. *Social Problems*, *68*(4), 942–963. https://doi.org/10.1093/socpro/spab027

Lindsey, M. A., Sheftall, A. H., Xiao, Y., & Joe, S. (2019). Trends of suicidal behaviors among high school students in the United States: 1991–2017. *Pediatrics*, *144*(5), e20191187. https://doi.org/10.1542/peds.2019-1187

Lutanco-Chua, J. (2022, July 13). *5 celebrities who are taking mental health breaks*. MindNation. https://blog.mindnation.com/2022/07/13/mental-health-breaks

Magana, D. (2019). Cultural competence and metaphor in mental healthcare interactions: A linguistic perspective. *Patient Education and Counseling*, *102*(12), 2192–2198. https://doi.org/10.1016/j.pec.2019.06.010

Marshall, G. N., Schell, T. L., & Miles, J. N. V. (2009). Ethnic differences in posttraumatic distress: Hispanics' symptoms differ in kind and degree. *Journal of Consulting and Clinical Psychology*, *77*(6), 1169–1178. https://doi.org/10.1037/a0017721

McGinty, E., Pescosolido, B., Kennedy-Hendricks, A., & Barry, C. L. (2018). Communication strategies to counter stigma and improve mental illness and substance use disorder policy. *Psychiatric Services*, *69*(2), 136–146. https://doi.org/10.1176/appi.ps.201700076

Meffert, S. M., Lawhorn, C., Ongeri, L., Bukusi, E., Campbell, H. R., Goosby, E., Bertozzi, S. M., & Kahonge, S. N. (2021). Scaling up public mental health care in sub-Saharan Africa: Insights from infectious disease. *Global Mental Health*, *8*, e41. https://doi.org/10.1017/gmh.2021.41

Merikangas, K. R., He, J. P., Burstein, M., Swanson, S. A., Avenevoli, S., Cui, L., Benjet, C., Georgiades, K., & Swendsen, J. (2010). Lifetime prevalence of mental disorders in U.S. adolescents: Results from the National Comorbidity Survey Replication–Adolescent Supplement (NCS-A). *Journal of the American Academy of Child & Adolescent Psychiatry*, *49*(10), 980–989. https://doi.org/10.1016/j.jaac.2010.05.017

Muvuka, B., Combs, R. M., Ali, N. M., Scott, H., & Williams, M. T. (2020). Depression is real: Developing a health communication campaign in an urban African American community. *Progress in Community Health Partnerships: Research, Education, and Action*, *14*(2), 161–172. https://doi.org/10.1353/cpr.2020.0029

National Academies of Sciences, Engineering, and Medicine. (2019). *Fostering healthy mental, emotional, and behavioral development in children and youth: A national agenda*. The National Academies Press. https://doi.org/10.17226/25201

Neff, J., Knight, K. R., Satterwhite, S., Nelson, N., Matthews, J., & Holmes, S. M. (2017). Teaching structure: A qualitative evaluation of a structural competency training for resident physicians. *Journal of General Internal Medicine*, *32*(4), 430–433. https://doi.org/10.1007/s11606-016-3924-7

Park, M., Chesla, C. A., Rehm, R. S., & Chun, K. M. (2011). Working with culture: Culturally appropriate mental health care for Asian Americans. *Journal of Advanced Nursing*, *67*(11), 2373–2382. https://doi.org/10.1111/j.1365-2648.2011.05671.x

Peinado, S., Treiman, K., Uhrig, J. D., Taylor, J. C., & Stryker, J. E. (2020). Effectively communicating about HIV and other health disparities: Findings from a literature review and future directions. *Frontiers in Communication*, *5*, 539174. https://doi.org/10.3389/fcomm.2020.539174

Perez-Stable, E. J., Alvidrez, J., & Hill, C. V. (2021). Definitions, principles, and concepts for minority health and health disparities research. In I. Dankwa-Mullan, E. J. Perez-Stable, K. L. Gardner, X. Zhang, & A. M. Rosario (Eds.), *The science of health disparities research* (pp. 1–12). Wiley Blackwell. https://doi.org/10.1002/9781119374855.ch1

Petty, J., Metzl, J. M., & Keeys, M. R. (2017). Developing and evaluating an innovative structural competency curriculum for pre-health students. *Journal of Medical Humanities*, *38*(4), 459–471. https://doi.org/10.1007/s10912-017-9449-1

President's New Freedom Commission on Mental Health. (2003). *Achieving the promise: Transforming mental health care in America*. US Department of Health and Human Services. https://govinfo.library.unt.edu/mentalhealthcommission/reports/FinalReport/FullReport-1.htm

Raifman, J., Charlton, B. M., Arrington-Sanders, R., Chan, P. A., Rusley, J., Mayer, K. H., Stein, M. D., Austin, S. B., & McConnell, M. (2020). Sexual orientation and suicide attempt disparities among US adolescents: 2009–2017. *Pediatrics, 145*(3), e20191658. https://doi.org/10.1542/peds.2019-1658

Ruben, B. D. (2016). Communication theory and health communication practice: The more things change, the more they stay the same. *Health Communication, 31*(1), 1–11. https://doi.org/10.1080/10410236.2014.923086

Schiavo, R. (2014). *Health communication: From theory to practice* (2nd ed.). John Wiley & Sons.

Schmid, K. L., Rivers, S. E., Latimer, A. E., & Salovey, P. (2008). Targeting or tailoring? Maximizing resources to create effective health communications. *Marketing Health Services, 28*(1), 32–37. PMID: 18389854.

Schulz, P. J., & Jiang, S. (2021). Theoretical frameworks of provider-patient interaction. In T. L. Thompson & P. J. Schulz (Eds.), *Health communication theory* (pp. 108–130). Wiley/Blackwell.

Sedgwick, C., Belmonte, L., Margolis, A., Shafer, P. O., Pitterle, J., & Gidal, B. E. (2021). Extending the reach of science—talk in plain language. *Epilepsy & Behavior Reports, 16*, 100493. https://doi.org/10.1016/j.ebr.2021.100493

Selvarajah, S., Deivanayagam, T. A., Lasco, G., Scafe, S., White, A., Zembe-Mkabile, W., & Devakumar, D. (2020). Categorization and minoritisation. *BMJ Global Health, 5*(12), e004508. https://doi.org/10.1136/bmjgh-2020-004508

Shadravan, S. M., Edwards, M. L., & Vinson, S. Y. (2021). Dying at the intersections: Police-involved killings of Black people with mental illness. *Psychiatric Services, 72*(6), 623–625. https://doi.org/10.1176/appi.ps.202000942

Shim, R. S., Kho, C. E., & Murray-Garcia, J. (2018). Inequities in mental health and mental health care: A review and future directions. *Psychiatric Annals, 48*(3), 138–142. https://doi.org/10.3928/00485713-20180213-01

Skierkowski, D. D., Florin, P., Harlow, L. L., Machan, J., & Ye, Y. (2019). A readability analysis of online mental health resources. *American Psychologist, 74*(4), 474–483. https://doi.org/10.1037/amp0000324

Sloat, S. (2022, June 1). Mental health care should be available for all, not a luxury. *Scientific American, 326*, 6. https://www.scientificamerican.com/article/mental-health-care-should-be-available-for-all-not-a-luxury

Sotto-Santiago, S. (2019). Time to reconsider the word minority in academic medicine. *Journal of Best Practices in Health Professions Diversity, 12*(1), 72–83. https://www.jstor.org/stable/26894228

Street, R. L. (2019). Mapping diverse measures of patient-centered communication onto the conceptual domains of patient-centered care. *Patient Education and Counseling, 102*(7), 1225–1227. https://doi.org/10.1016/j.pec.2019.05.011

Stuart, H. (2016). Reducing the stigma of mental illness. *Global Mental Health, 3*, e17. https://doi.org/10.1017/gmh.2016.11

Sussman, S., Kattari, S. K., Baezconde-Garbanati, L., & Glackin, S. N. (2020). Commentary: The problems of grouping all adversity into a special populations label. *Evaluation & the Health Professions, 43*(1), 66–70. https://doi.org/10.1177/0163278719882738

Tambling, R. R., D'Aniello, C., & Russell, B. S. (2021). Mental health literacy: A critical target for narrowing racial disparities in behavioral health. *International Journal of Mental Health and Addiction, 21*(3), 1867–1881. https://doi.org/10.1007/s11469-021-00694-w

Taylor, R. E., & Kuo, B. C. H. (2019). Black American psychological help-seeking intention: An integrated literature review with recommendations for clinical practice. *Journal of Psychotherapy Integration, 29*(4), 325–357. https://doi.org/10.1037/int0000131

Treisman, R. (2023, March 17). *7 deputies and 3 others face murder charges in a Black man's death at mental hospital.* NPR. https://www.npr.org/2023/03/16/1163933779/irvo-otieno-police-killing-virginia-hospital

US Department of Health and Human Services. (2001). *Mental health: Culture, race, and ethnicity: A supplement to mental health: A report of the Surgeon General.* Substance Abuse and Mental Health Services Administration.

US Department of Health and Human Services. (2022). *Healthy people 2030: Health communication.* https://health.gov/healthypeople/objectives-and-data/browse-objectives/health-communication

Van Beveren, L., Rutten, K., Roets, G., & Buysse, A. (2023). Critical cultural disability studies and mental health: A rhetorical perspective. *Disability & Society, 38*(2), 342–361. https://doi.org/10.1080/09687599.2021.1918539

Viswanath, K. (2006). Public communications and its role in reducing and eliminating health disparities. In G. E. Thomson, F. Mitchell, & M. B. Williams (Eds.), *Examining the health disparities research plan of the National Institutes of Health: Unfinished business. Appendix G* (pp. 212–253). National Academies Press. https://www.ncbi.nlm.nih.gov/books/NBK57046

Viswanath, K., McCloud, R. F., & Bekalu, M. A. (2021). Communication, health, and equity: Structural influences. In T. L. Thomson & N. G. Harrington (Eds.), *The Routledge handbook of health communication* (3rd ed., pp. 426–440). Routledge. https://doi.org/10.4324/9781003043379

White, A., & Chanoff, D. (2011). *Seeing patients: Unconscious bias in health care.* Harvard University Press.

Williams, D. R., González, H. M., Neighbors, H., Nesse, R., Abelson, J. M., Sweetman, J., & Jackson, J. S. (2007). Prevalence and distribution of major depressive disorder in African Americans, Caribbean Blacks, and non-Hispanic Whites: Results from the National Survey of American Life. *Archives of General Psychiatry, 64*(3), 305–315. https://doi.org/10.1001/archpsyc.64.3.305

Woods-Giscombe, C., Robinson, M. N., Carthon, D., Devane-Johnson, S., & Corbie-Smith, G. (2016). Superwoman schema, stigma, spirituality, and culturally sensitive providers: Factors influencing African American women's use of mental health services. *Journal of Best Practices in Health Professions Diversity, 9*(1), 1124–1144. https://www.jstor.org/stable/26554242

Xiao, Y., & Lu, W. (2021). Temporal trends and disparities in suicidal behaviors by sex and sexual identity among Asian American adolescents. *JAMA Network Open, 4*(4), e214498–e214498. https://doi.org/10.1001/jamanetworkopen.2021.4498

Xie, H. (2013). Strengths-based approach for mental health recovery. *Iranian Journal of Psychiatry and Behavioral Sciences, 7*(2), 5–10. PMID: 24644504.

Yang, L., & Benson, J. M. (2016). The role of culture in population mental health: Prevalence of mental disorders among Asian and Asian American populations. In J. Y. Chiao, S. Li, R. Seligman, & R. Turner (Eds.), *The Oxford handbook of cultural neuroscience* (pp. 339–354). Oxford University Press.

Yohanna, D. (2013). Deinstitutionalization of people with mental illness: Causes and consequences. *AMA Journal of Ethics, 15*(10), 886–891. https://doi.org/10.1001/virtualmentor.2013.15.10.mhst1-1310

17

Affinity and Advocacy: Online Communities for People Experiencing Mental Health Conditions

Frances J. Griffith and Sydney C. Simmons
Yale School of Medicine

About 970 million people globally are experiencing mental health challenges, and access to care continues to be limited (World Health Organization [WHO], 2022). The discrepancy between demand and mental health care availability grew during the COVID-19 pandemic, which increased mental health concerns and further strained resources (Moreno et al., 2020). Factors contributing to insufficient mental health care for adults and adolescents include a lack of providers, especially in rural areas (Steiner et al., 2023); the cost of mental health care depending on insurance status and coverage (Rowan et al., 2013); long wait lists for treatment (American Psychological Association, 2022; Furukawa et al., 2014); and external and self-stigma that may prevent help-seeking (Corrigan et al., 2014). Although increased telehealth has made care more accessible, many still lack internet connectivity sufficient for synchronous video conferencing (Patel et al., 2023). Other barriers to care include limited availability of providers who speak an individual's preferred language or engage in culturally competent practices for those with minoritized identities (Naz et al., 2019).

Online peer communities may offer social support and other benefits for individuals facing barriers to care. There are a variety of online mental health resources (e.g. telehealth services, phone-based applications, closed online support groups), but public online forums uniquely offer users access to a broader base of peers who also self-identify with mental health conditions (MHCs). Through these online communities, individuals can seek emotional, informational, and instrumental support without cost, geographic restrictions, or hurdles to community entry (Steiner et al., 2023). Further, given the potential for full or partial anonymity, users can access support with a reduced likelihood of stigma from family, friends, or employers (Moore et al., 2016). Online communities may also enable users to engage in advocacy to increase mental health awareness and reduce mental health stigma and stigma toward other identities, such as minoritized race, ethnicity, gender, or sexual identity (Sangeorzan et al., 2019).

Current Review

Recent scholarship has seen a significant upsurge in publications about online mental health communities. Some articles have mapped peer networks within communities (e.g. Lu et al., 2021), whereas other research has analyzed the thematic content of online community discussions (e.g. Park et al., 2018). A small number of literature reviews have begun to summarize aspects of these findings,

The Handbook of Mental Health Communication, First Edition.
Edited by Marco C. Yzer and Jason T. Siegel.

such as peer interactions (Storman et al., 2022), classification of diagnoses via linguistic markers (Boettcher, 2021), and connections between symptoms and engagement in online communities (Bizzotto et al., 2023). However, a comprehensive review of research on naturalistic interactions in online mental health communities is needed to understand the potential benefits of these communities, including findings related to *thematic content* (what is being shared), *peer interaction* (how it is being shared), and *community affordances* (what users derive from sharing). The current chapter undertook a scoping literature review and a topic modeling analysis of recent literature to systematically characterize extant findings. These results can inform how online peer mental health communities are operating in the gap between mental health care resources and unmet needs.

Methods

Scoping Review

Eligibility Criteria

For the current scoping review, we considered peer-reviewed journal articles examining peer-to-peer interactions about self-identified MHCs. We defined MHCs as symptoms and experiences consistent with diagnoses in the *Diagnostic and Statistical Manual of Mental Disorders, Fifth Edition, Text Revision* (American Psychiatric Association, 2022). To be eligible, articles needed to be published in 2000 or later and written in English. Conference papers, preprints, dissertations/theses, and review articles were not considered. Most of the participant or user sample needed to self-identify with MHCs as opposed to self-reporting temporary stress, a physical health condition, trauma without posttraumatic stress, nonclinical substance use, or a loved one with an MHC. Further, most participants or users needed to post about their experiences with MHCs in an open online community composed of peers, such as a social media site or open forum. We excluded studies focused on closed online support groups or one-on-one interactions. Studies testing digital mental health interventions were not considered, and we also eliminated studies reporting peer interactions in the context of mental health provider websites, phone- or web-based applications, or forums moderated by mental health care providers. Eligible studies also needed to systematically examine peer-to-peer interactions as a primary research focus; therefore, we excluded studies chiefly seeking to detect diagnoses or risks through linguistic markers in posts.

Search Strategy

To develop a comprehensive search strategy, we used the *citationchaser* software (Haddaway et al., 2021) to extract the references and citing articles of three articles known to be relevant to the scoping review (i.e. Griffith & Stein, 2021; Moore et al., 2016; Pretorius et al., 2019). Both references and citing articles were screened using Covidence software (Veritas Health Innovation, 2023) by a single screener. After the citation analysis, we developed focused search strategies using keywords in the titles, abstracts, and Medical Subject Headings (MeSH) terms of the included studies. On August 1, 2023, a search of the following databases was completed: Ovid MEDLINE, Embase (Ovid), and American Psychological Association PsycInfo (Ovid). The searches were limited to English-language articles. No date limit was applied, but one was later implemented in the eligibility criteria (described previously). Search terms included those related to mental health (e.g. "mental illness," "mental health," "depression"), online communities (e.g. "internet," "online," "Reddit"), and peer interactions (e.g. "peer," "community," "social support").

Data Extraction

Two screeners independently screened 10% of the abstracts returned from the search to evaluate interrater agreement on relevance and reconcile conflicts. The remaining abstracts were each screened by a single screener. Of those articles moved to full-text review, 10% were again independently screened by the two screeners to evaluate interrater agreement on exclusion and reconcile conflicts. A single screener reviewed the remaining full texts. Data were extracted from the retained articles, including the title, author(s), year, country, online setting, study aims, study design, diagnostic focus, sample demographics, inclusion criteria, sample size of participants/users, and sample size of posts (if collected). Additionally, findings related to thematic content, peer interaction, and the affordances or drawbacks of online communities for users were collected.

Topic Modeling Analysis

To further characterize the scope of recent literature about online peer interactions, we conducted Latent Dirichlet Allocation (LDA) using the titles, abstracts, and keywords of included articles. LDA is a topic modeling approach that uses Bayesian probabilistic models to estimate the likelihood that given words are in a topic and that given topics are in a document (Blei et al., 2003). The order of words, however, is not considered (i.e., a "bag of words" approach), and the relatedness of words is based on their co-occurrence within documents. Topic modeling with LDA is a common approach to literature reviews across multiple disciplines (e.g. Madzík & Falát, 2022; Moro et al., 2015), and it enables primary topics in extant literature to be compared with other salient literature variables (e.g. publication years, journals; Ponweiser, 2012). The current LDA was conducted with the ***topicmodels*** package version 2-14 (Grün & Hornik, 2023) in the programming language R (R Core Team, 2023). Because LDA requires an a priori determination of the number of topics (*k*), we evaluated potential models (different *k*-values) using three model selection methods (Arun et al., 2010; Cao et al., 2009; Griffiths et al., 2004) with the *ldatuning* package (Nikita, 2020). We reviewed the most likely terms within each topic to label and characterize those topics. Further, the most likely topics in each document were considered to examine the distribution of topics across the included sources.

In addition to summarizing topics across included articles with LDA, we conducted a subsequent analysis to assess whether topics were associated with self-identified diagnostic communities in the articles. Diagnoses were selected as a salient factor for topical comparison because they are important identities and features of online mental health communities. Forums or threads are often labeled by diagnostic categories (Park et al., 2018), community members strive to maintain authenticity as having particular diagnoses (Wiggins et al., 2016), and self- and other-diagnosis support is a central feature of peer interaction (Giles & Newbold, 2011). We used a chi-square analysis to determine whether the most likely topic for each source was associated with that source's primary diagnostic focus (e.g. depression/suicidality, substance use disorders, eating disorders, or multiple diagnoses).

Results

Scoping Review

The literature search resulted in 58 included sources (see Figure 17.1). The initial search of references and citing articles of the three known articles yielded 674 sources. Relevant abstracts from this set were used to inform the database search, which resulted in 1,684 additional sources. Of the 2,358 total sources, 96 were eliminated as duplicates, and 2,160 were screened as irrelevant during the abstract review. Therefore, the full texts of 102 sources were reviewed. A total of 44 sources were excluded, and the most common reason for exclusion was a focus on the incorrect population (i.e., participants not identifying with MHCs or with primarily medical conditions; $n = 14$ sources). The full-text review resulted in 58 included, peer-reviewed articles focusing on peer interactions in online mental health communities.

The included articles were published from 2009 to 2023, and over 60% were published in 2020 or later (see Tables 17.1–17.4). Over three fourths of articles ($n = 46$, 79%) used only secondary analysis of data scraped from online mental health communities, including posts and comments. Ten articles (17%) used only primary data collection, including interviews and surveys with participants who use online mental health communities. A small proportion ($n = 2$, 3%) used a combination of primary and secondary data analysis. The majority of articles ($n = 30$, 52%) focused on online communities founded

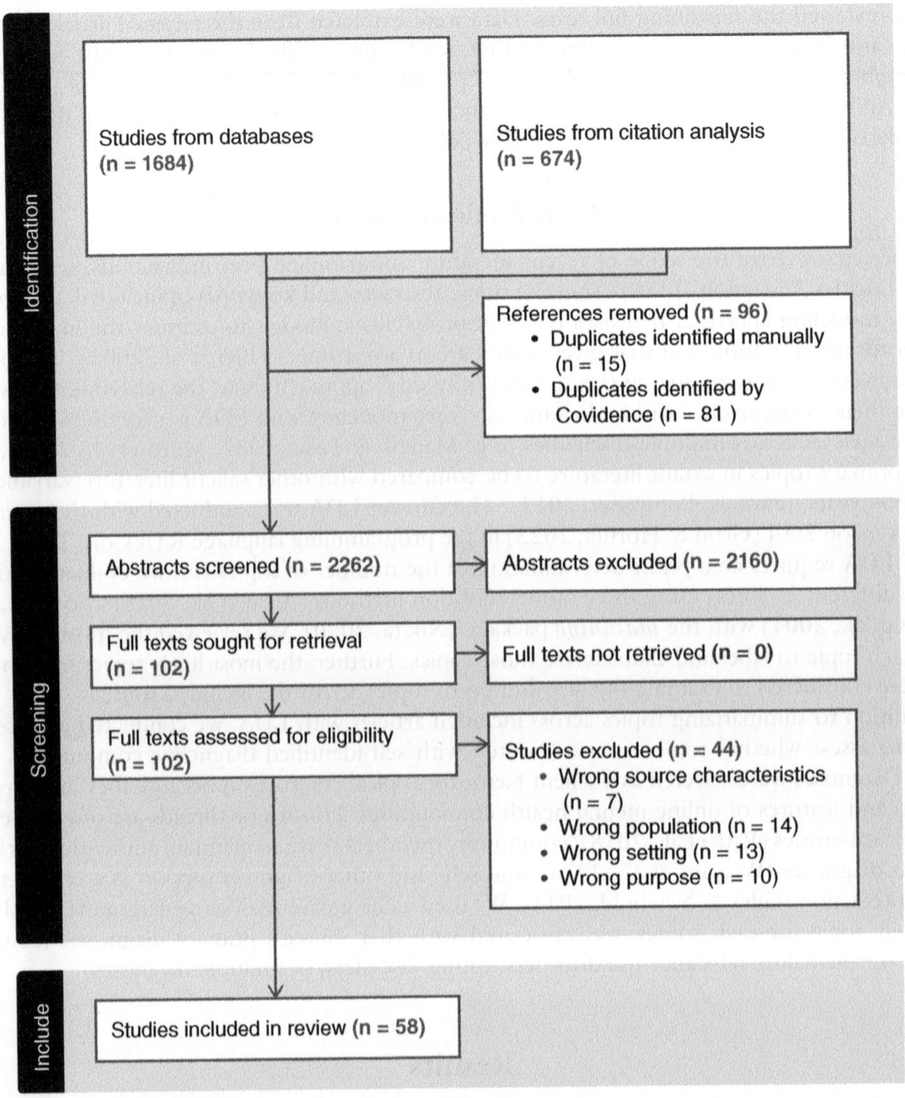

Figure 17.1 Literature search and data extraction for scoping review.
Note. This figure shows the literature search and data extraction process for the scoping review of sources about online mental health communities.

in the United States or with primarily US-based users. Following the United States, Chinese online communities were the most common focus of articles (n = 10, 17%), followed by the United Kingdom (n = 8, 14%), the Netherlands (n = 3, 5%), multiple countries (n = 3, 5%), Australia (n = 2, 3%), Korea (n = 1, 2%), and Hungary (n = 1, 2%).

The largest proportion of articles exclusively focused on mental health communities on the social media platform Reddit (n = 13, 22%). Almost as many sources (n = 12, 21%) did not identify the online setting of the online communities they studied. Eleven sources (19%) focused on online communities across multiple platforms or websites, and small groups of articles focused on online communities on other single platforms, such as Instagram, YouTube, and Sina Weibo. Less than half of the articles (n = 24, 41%) described the demographics of participants or users. All these articles noted the inclusion of adults, and a small proportion (n = 6, 10%) included adolescents. Seven articles (12%) included both men and women (or boys and girls), seven (12%) focused exclusively on women or girls, two (3%) included gender-diverse participants, and one (2%) focused on only men. The remaining seven

Table 17.1 Depression, Suicidality: Source Characteristics (n = 31)

Source	*Country*	*Online setting*	*Research design*	*Diagnoses, symptoms*	*Sample*	*Users n*	*Posts n*	*Primary post theme findings*	*Primary peer interaction findings*
Alang & Fomotar (2015)	US	U/I forum	Secondary	Depression	Peri/postnatal women; lesbians	NS	236 P, 1,185 C	Medications, comorbid conditions, perseverance, treatment reluctance	Peers enable disclosure and companionship
Biester et al. (2022)	US	Reddit	Secondary	Depression	NS	5,854 forum, 5,854 control	NS	Increased language markers prior to depression claim (e.g. anxiety) decrease after to match control users.	Posting depression claims while seeking help from peers is associated with greater change in language.
Feldhege et al. (2020)	US	Reddit	Secondary	Depression	NS	20,037	16,291 P, 71,543 C	Feelings, Reddit community, motivation, time	Topics of feelings, support, small talk received more upvotes, comments from peers.
Gough (2016)	UK	U/I forums	Secondary	Depression	Men	NS	676 P	Authenticity through official diagnosis, symptoms, or assessments	Peers offer social support for official diagnoses, detailed accounts.
Hale (2019)	US	Imgur	Secondary	Depression	NS	NS	20 P, 1,530 C	Peer support	Peer comments were supportive, including reassurance, information.
Horne & Wiggins (2009)	UK	U/I forums	Secondary	Suicidality	NS	NS	42 P, 287 C	Authenticity of suicidality through narrative, content outside of depression, rationality	Users may not ask for help directly but receive supportive replies at suicide crisis points.
Jiang et al. (2020)	US	Reddit	Secondary; Survey	Suicidality	NS	491	21,430 P, 129,008 C	Psychological pain; relationship, academic, financial stress; diagnoses	Peers asked questions, gave support, academic encouragement.
Johnson et al. (2021)	US	YouTube	Secondary	Depression	US adults; Black	50	50 P (videos)	Discrimination as barrier, factor; depression management, advocacy, positive treatment experiences	Users found informal support, pathways to mental health care online.
Kim et al. (2022)	KR	Momsholic	Secondary	Depression	Peri/postnatal women	NS	1,676 P	Emotion-, problem-focused coping strategies	Users provided support more often than seeking.

(*Continued*)

Table 17.1 (Continued)

Source	*Country*	*Online setting*	*Research design*	*Diagnoses, symptoms*	*Sample*	*Users n*	*Posts n*	*Primary post theme findings*	*Primary peer interaction findings*
Liu & Wang (2021)	CN	U/I forum	Interviews; survey	Depression	Adults, youth; men, women	272	NA	NA	Effects of users' social empowerment on forum use is mediated by self-efficacy and expectation confirmation.
Liu & Kong (2021)	CN	U/I forum	Secondary	Depression	NS	NS	47,307 P	Social experiences, emotional expression	Users' social, emotional content was reinforced.
Lu et al. (2019)	CN	SunForum	Secondary	Depression	NS	197	31,440 P	Ties, trust, shared identity, expertise, shared values	Social capital predicted users' disclosure.
Lu et al. (2020)	CN	Sunshine Project	Secondary	Depression	Men, women; age NS	244	465,337 P	Information, emotional and socializing support, shared identity, trust	Information, support, trust, shared identity reduced depression, but not socializing.
Lu et al. (2021)	CN	U/I forum	Secondary	Depression	Men, women, age NS	1,077	74,986 P	NS	Users' reciprocity, transitivity effected informational, emotional support networks.
Moore et al. (2016)	UK	Mumsnet	Secondary	Depression	Peri/postnatal women	NS	102 P, 1,444 C	Stigma, negative experiences of offline disclosure	Peers provided healthcare suggestions, reassurance, advocacy.
Nemeth et al. (2021)	Various	Various	Secondary	Depression	NS	20,000	67,857 P	Attributions, self-disclosure related to personal struggles	Users consulted peers for information and received therapeutic interactions.
Nimrod (2012)	Various	Various	Secondary	Depression	NS	73,046	15,770 P, 133,446 C	Coping, causes, life, symptoms, mental health care, medication, work, relationships, suicide.	Peers offered knowledge, experience, suggestions, and helped empower users.
Nimrod (2013)	Various	U/I forums	Survey	Depression	Adults, youth	793	NA	NA	Users interested in many online topics reported increased online support, offline improvement.
Pan et al. (2020)	US	Depression Forums	Secondary	Depression	NS	2,061	62,274 C	Self-referent words, negative emotions representing health condition, states	Users' network position is associated with peers' communication accommodation.

Shi & Khoo (2023)	CN	Sina Weibo	Secondary	Depression	NS	221 forum, 1,683 friends	NS	Self-disclosure attributes, e.g. negative emotions, biological processes	Users' network position and disclosure attributes impact social support.
Sik (2021)	HU	U/I forums	Secondary	Depression	NS	NS	NS	Self-narratives, narrative interpretation, mental health care suggestions	Users' experience level affects roles (e.g. asking, suggesting)
Smit et al. (2021)	NL	Depression Connect	Interviews	Depression	Adults	15	NA	NA	Supporting peers enhanced user self-efficacy, empowerment.
Smit et al. (2022)	NL	Depression Connect	Survey	Depression	Adults; women, men	301	NA	NA	Type, intensity of engagement did not affect positive outcomes.
Tang et al. (2020)	CN	Sina Weibo, Baidu Tieba	Secondary	Depression	NS	92,338 SW, 34,490 BT	587,730 SW C, 249,086 BT P	Negative emotions (esp. on SW)	Less social support, information for users on SW
Tang, Yu, & Yao (2021)	CN	Sina Weibo	Secondary	Depression	NS	1,548	242,788 P, 67,987 C	Positive, negative emotions	Emotional contagion, esp. positive, occurs.
Tang, Yao, & Yu (2021)	CN	Sina Weibo, Baidu Tieba	Secondary	Depression	NS	NS	10,000 SW C, 10,000 BT P	Positive (esp. BT), negative (esp. SW) emotions	Users with positive emotions give more support, responses increase engagement.
Tao & Jacobs (2019)	US	Facebook	Secondary	Depression, suicidality	Young adults	NS	156 P, 445 C	Symptom disclosure	Peers offered support with very few negative reactions.
Wang et al. (2021)	CN	Sina Weibo	Secondary	Depression	NS	39,071	203,659 P, 1,712,840 control P	More emotionality (compared to control)	Forum posts get more peer comments than control posts.
Wiggins et al. (2016)	UK	U/I forum	Secondary	Suicidality	NS	NS	80 P, 527 C	Suicidality (changes over time)	Users seek support for crises while maintaining authenticity.
Zingg et al. (2021)	US	What to Expect, BabyCenter	Secondary	Depression	Peri/postnatal women	NS	62,015 P	Medication, support, disclosure, family/friends, breastfeeding. Positive, negative emotions.	Peers provide emotional, appraisal-based, instrumental, and informational support.
Zingg et al. (2023)	US	What to Expect, BabyCenter	Secondary, Interviews, Focus groups	Depression	Peri/postnatal women	28	1,424 P	Physical, mental health; support; medication; mother/infant; family and friends; doctor/patient	Peers provide emotional, appraisal, instrumental, informational support.

Note. Some sources included the comments without specifying the number. BT, Baidu Tieba; C, comments; CN, China; HU, Hungary; KR, South Korea; NA, not applicable; NS, not specified; P, posts; SW, Sina Weibo; U/I, unidentified; UK, United Kingdom; US, United States.

Table 17.2 Multiple Mental Health Communities: Source Characteristics (n = 18)

Source	*Country*	*Online setting*	*Research design*	*Diagnoses, symptoms*	*Sample*	*Users n*	*Posts n*	*Primary post theme findings*	*Primary peer interaction findings*
Chen & Yu (2021)	US	Reddit	Secondary	Various	NS	46,256 with comments, 14,238 without	106,155 P, 396,352 C	Social support, empathy	Users with support were more likely to post, give support; those getting empathy gave empathy.
Giles & Newbold (2011)	UK	Face the Issue, Addicted	Secondary	Various	NS	10	21 P	Ambivalence toward health professionals, self-diagnosis	Peers may offer diagnostic information, support.
Giles & Newbold (2013)	UK	Depression Tribe, No More Panic	Secondary	Depression, Panic Disorder	NS	6	10 P	Diagnostic criteria, personal disclosure	Users strengthen membership by help-seeking, and disclosure is used to help others.
Griffith et al. (2021)	US	Instagram	Secondary	Various	NS	461	1,000 P (100 per hashtag)	Emotional content in art; diagnostic symptoms, art techniques; art sales, art techniques	Peers highly reinforced posts showing functional art from artists describing their sobriety.
Griffith & Stein (2021)	US	Tumblr	Secondary	Various	NS	14,626	1–554 P per user	Emotions and cognitions about mental health; interpersonal loss, change; different themes by diagnosis	Users posted more with more reinforcement, those using #autistic and #anorexia received the most reinforcement.
Kang et al. (2022)	AU	SANE	Secondary	Various	NS	2,357	70,179 P	Resilience, including self-efficacy, adaptive capacity	Users achieved learning, belonging, social capital.
Lee et al. (2020)	US	Instagram	Secondary	Various	Men, women; age NS	NS	758 P	Wellness practices, anxiety, depression	Users seek support more often when they describe diagnoses.
Merchant et al. (2022)	US	U/I forums	Survey	Various	Adults; men, women; mostly White	369	NA	NA	Users reported more benefits the more they used peer forums.
Mickles & Weare (2020)	US	YouTube	Interviews	Various	Adults; men, women	10	NA	NA	Users disclosed experiences to encourage others, build community.

Moore & Ayers (2016)	UK	U/I forums	Interviews	Various	Peri/postnatal women; mostly White	15	NA	NA	Peers provided social support, shared understanding.
Naslund et al. (2014)	US	YouTube	Secondary	Schizophrenia, schizoaffective, and bipolar disorders	NS	NS	19 P (videos), 3,044 C	Minimized isolation, hope; reciprocity; coping strategies; medication; mental health care	Peers provided hope, support, shared strategies and experiences with medication and care.
Park et al. (2018)	US	Reddit	Secondary	Anxiety, depression, PTSD	NS	41,967	7,410 P, 132,599 C	Sleep, work, medication, treatment issues; depression contexts. Varied by diagnosis.	Users expressed positive emotion and gratitude to peers across diagnostic groups.
Prescott et al. (2020)	UK	18%	Survey	Various	Adults, youth; men, women, NB	128	NA	NA	Peers help users increase self-efficacy and seek mental health care.
Sangeorzan et al. (2019)	US	YouTube	Secondary	Severe, persistent conditions	NS	28	30 P (videos)	Reduced isolation, fighting stigma, therapeutic effects	Peers give support, and vlogging increases self-efficacy, reduces stigma.
Sit et al. (2022)	US	Reddit	Secondary	Various	Young adults, youth	NS	98 P	Navigating psychiatric issues, offline disclosure, treatment barriers, treatment experiences	Users sought advice on peer support, diagnosis definitions, and gave treatment suggestions.
Steiner et al. (2023)	AU	SANE, Beyond Blue, ReachOut	Secondary	Various	Rural residents	30	3,000 P	Challenges, including relationships, lack of hope and agency, service inaccessibility.	Users gain social capital, belonging, knowledge through questions and advice-seeking.
van de Beek et al. (2023)	NL	marokko.nl	Secondary	Various	Moroccan-Dutch young adults, youth	NS	22 P, 2,162 C	Isolation, discrimination, cultural challenges, mental health explanations.	Peers gave support, remedy suggestions, mental health explanations.
Yoo et al. (2019)	US	Reddit	Secondary	Bipolar disorder, depression	NS	NS	5,409 P	Sleep, financial issues; negative emotion; medication; suicidality	Peers gave advice, sympathetic responses to suicidality.

Note. Some sources included the comments without specifying the number. AU, Australia; C, comments; NA, not applicable; NB, nonbinary; NL, Netherlands; NS, not specified; P, posts; U/I, unidentified; UK, United Kingdom; US, United States.

Table 17.3 Substance Use Disorders: Source Characteristics (n = 5)

Source	*Country*	*Online setting*	*Research design*	*Diagnoses, symptoms*	*Sample*	*Users n*	*Posts n*	*Primary post theme findings*	*Primary peer interaction findings*
Arshonsky et al. (2022)	US	Reddit	Secondary	Opioid use disorder	NS	NS	1,000 P, 1000 C	Coping skills (e.g. mindfulness) and health habits (e.g. exercise)	Posting to peers enables coping.
Bailey et al. (2020)	US	Twitter, Reddit	Secondary	Alcohol use disorder	NS	302 Twitter, 76,183 friends, 1,074 Reddit	274,595 P, 14,921,997 friends' P	Recovery topics (e.g. AA programs, sobriety) and relapse topics (e.g. alcohol, struggles)	Peers served as advice givers and encouragers. Online socialization was a recovery predictor.
D'Agostino et al. (2017)	US	Reddit	Secondary	Opioid use disorder	NS	73	100 P, 511 C	Opioid use disorder symptoms (e.g. social problems), sobriety status, other substances, medical help	Posts sought advice and support, and comments provided at least one therapeutic factor and information.
El-Bassel et al. (2022)	US	Reddit	Secondary	Opioid use disorder	NS	2,342	525 P, 9,284 C	Recovery, medication and access barriers, withdrawal	Users wrote social words and asked for information or help.
Sowles e al. (2017)	US	Reddit	Secondary	Cannabis use disorder	NS	91	100 P	Seeking advice, support	Most posts seeking support received it.

Note. Some sources included the comments without specifying the number. C, comments; NS, not specified; P, posts; US, United States.

Table 17.4 Eating Disorders: Source Characteristics (n = 4)

Source	*Country*	*Online setting*	*Research design*	*Diagnoses, symptoms*	*Sample*	*Users n*	*Posts n*	*Primary post theme findings*	*Primary peer interaction findings*
Feuston et al. (2022)	US	Various	Interviews	Eating disorders	Adults; transgender; mostly White	14	NA	NA	Trans people are marginalized in eating disorder spaces, must parse identities.
Park et al. (2022)	US	Reddit	Secondary	Eating disorders	NS	NS	167 P, 9,883 C	Emotional and informational support, eating disorder questions	Peers gave more empathy to posts seeking emotional support.
Sowles et al. (2018)	US	Reddit	Secondary	Eating disorders	NS	NS	125 P, 115 C	Eating and shape concerns	Peers often offered esteem and support.
Yeshua-Katz & Martins (2012)	US	U/I blogs	Interviews	Anorexia	Adults, youth; women, girls; mostly White	33	NA	NA	Peers gave support with coping but may encourage disordered eating.

Note. Some sources included the comments without specifying the number. C, comments; NA, not applicable; NS, not specified; P, posts; U/I, unidentified; US, United States.

articles (12%) that reported demographics did not describe participants' gender. Only five articles (9%) noted the primary racial identity of participants, including four (7%) with primarily White participants and one (2%) with primarily Black participants.

Online Depression Communities

Among reviewed articles, the majority (n = 31, 53%) described online mental health communities focusing on depression and suicidality (see Table 17.1). Twenty-six of these articles (84% of depression-focused sources)[1] reported findings related to the *thematic content* of scraped posts and comments. Within depression-focused sources, 13 articles (42%) discussed the symptoms that users posted, including their narrative attempts to establish the authenticity of their diagnoses within the communities. Among other themes found were positive and negative emotional content (n = 9, 29% of depression-focused articles); mental health care and medication experiences, questions, and suggestions (n = 6, 19%); online relationships (n = 6, 19%); offline relationships (n = 5, 16%); coping, motivation, and perseverance (n = 4, 13%); life and work stressors (n = 3, 10%); and stigma and advocacy (n = 2, 6%).

Sources related to depression also reported their systematic evaluation of online *peer interactions* and *community affordances*. As shown in Table 17.1, most depression-focused articles (n = 21, 68%) discussed the provision of social support among peers, including emotional, instrumental, and informational support, but one article (3%) found that insufficient forum moderation resulted in less social support. Eight articles reported findings on the association between user characteristics (e.g. self-efficacy, online network position, interest in topics) and these users' peer interactions and affordances (e.g. social capital, empowerment, support, networks, and communication accommodation). Three articles (10%) reported which topics received more reinforcement from other users (e.g. comments, likes), including emotional content.

Multiple Online Mental Health Communities

After articles focused on depression communities, articles examining multiple mental health communities were the second-largest group (n = 18, 31% of 58 included articles; see Table 17.2). These studies each examined two or more online communities with different diagnostic foci, including mood, anxiety, schizophrenia spectrum, and posttraumatic stress disorders. Over three fourths of these articles (n = 14, 78%) discussed the *thematic content* of scraped posts and comments. Themes included users' disclosure of symptoms (n = 7, 39% of multiple community sources); experiences with mental health care, including lack of access (n = 6, 33%); coping and resilience (n = 4, 22%); offline relationships with a focus on interpersonal challenges (n = 4, 22%); online relationships (n = 3, 17%); emotions (n = 3, 17%); stigma (n = 3, 17%); and life stressors (n = 2, 11%).

All sources that discussed multiple mental health communities described their findings related to *peer interactions* and *community affordances*. Most of these articles (n = 14, 78%) described social support given to users by peers, including emotional, informational, and instrumental support. This social support afforded users with social capital, belonging, and empowerment. Seven articles (39%) discussed strategies used by community members to obtain social support, including seeking advice, being more active in the community, and expressing gratitude to peers. Two articles (11%) described what peers reinforced (i.e., through likes, comments, and reposts), including descriptions of particular user traits, such as sobriety and diagnoses of anorexia and autism.

Online Substance Use Disorder Communities

A smaller group of sources (n = 5, 9%) studied online communities formed around recovery from substance use disorders, including alcohol, opioid, and cannabis use disorders (see Table 17.3). All substance use-focused sources reported *thematic content* of scraped posts and comments. Four articles (80% of substance use-focused sources) discussed users' coping strategies that supported their recovery and sobriety. Other themes included symptoms, such as withdrawal and psychological effects associated with relapse (n = 3, 60% of substance use-focused articles), and experiences with mental health care (n = 3, 60%). All five articles reported findings about *peer interaction* and *community affordances* from substance use disorder communities. For example, all articles noted strategies participants or users employed in online communities to gain social support and enhance recovery, such as seeking advice and socialization. Three articles (60%) discussed the social support provided in these communities, including informational and emotional support.

Online Eating Disorder Communities

The smallest group of sources (n = 4, 7%) studied online eating disorder communities (see Table 17.4). Only two of these sources (50% of eating disorder-focused sources) reported ***thematic contact*** of scraped posts and comments, which included symptoms, such as eating patterns and shape concerns, and themes related to online community relationships. All four sources reported findings related to ***peer interactions*** and ***community affordances***. Three of the four sources (75%) described social support offered by peers with an emphasis on emotional support. However, two of the four sources (50%) highlighted potentially harmful interactions in online eating disorder communities, including the marginalization of transgender users in primarily cisgender groups and the encouragement of disordered eating in proanorexia spaces.

Topic Modeling Analysis

Our LDA of 58 article abstracts focusing on peer interactions in online mental health communities included nine topics: ***Stigma and treatment content***; ***Emotional content***; ***Support seeking about symptoms***; ***Depression discussions***; ***Resilience from communities***; ***Support, empowerment from communities***; ***Network communication analysis***; ***Topic modeling approaches***; ***Recovery prediction*** (see Figure 17.2, Table 17.5). We determined that nine was the best number of topics during the model selection process using three methods (Arun et al., 2010; Cao et al., 2009; Griffiths et al., 2004; Nikita, 2020). Topics were named based on the 10 terms most likely to be included in each of these topics. These topics were significantly associated with the type of online mental health community—depression, substance use, eating disorder, or multiple communities—described in the article ($X^2 = 57.17$, $p < 0.001$).

The most common topics across article abstracts related to thematic content in posts and comments. Eleven of the 58 articles (19%) were most likely to contain the topic ***stigma and treatment content***. Abstracts characterized by this topic described thematic results that focused on users' experiences of mental health care and stigmatization. This topic was most common among articles about online depression communities (n = 5, 16% of these 31 articles) and about multiple online mental health communities (n = 5, 28% of these 18 articles). The topic ***emotional content*** occurred in 10 of the 58 articles (17%). This topic was found most often in depression-focused articles (n = 9, 29% of these 31 articles) and was also the most frequent topic among depression-focused articles as a group. Abstracts containing ***emotional content*** described thematic findings related to feelings and sentiment (i.e. positive and negative emotions) within scraped posts and comments.

The next most common topics across article abstracts were those related to seeking and obtaining community affordances through peer interaction. The topic ***support seeking about symptoms*** occurred across articles focusing on each type of community, but it was most often found in articles about substance use disorder communities. This topic described articles' results related to online disclosure and support seeking about a variety of mental health symptoms. This was the most frequent topic among substance use-focused articles as a group (n = 4, 80% of these five articles) and eating disorder-focused articles as a group (n = 2, 50% of these four articles). The topic ***depression discussions*** was most likely in 7 of the 58 articles (12%) and was most often found in depression-focused articles (n = 6, 19% of these 31 articles). This topic focused on articles' results related to online disclosure, questions, and replies about depression and suicide. Seven articles (12% of 58 articles) were most likely to contain the topic ***resilience from communities***, and this topic was most frequent among articles about multiple mental health communities as a group (n = 6, 33% of these 18 articles). Abstracts characterized by this topic shared how online communities enhance wellness and coping. The topic ***support, empowerment from communities*** was found among 6 articles (10% of all 58) and was most often found among depression-focused articles (n = 4, 13% of these 31 articles). This topic contained articles' results related to building social capital through online communities.

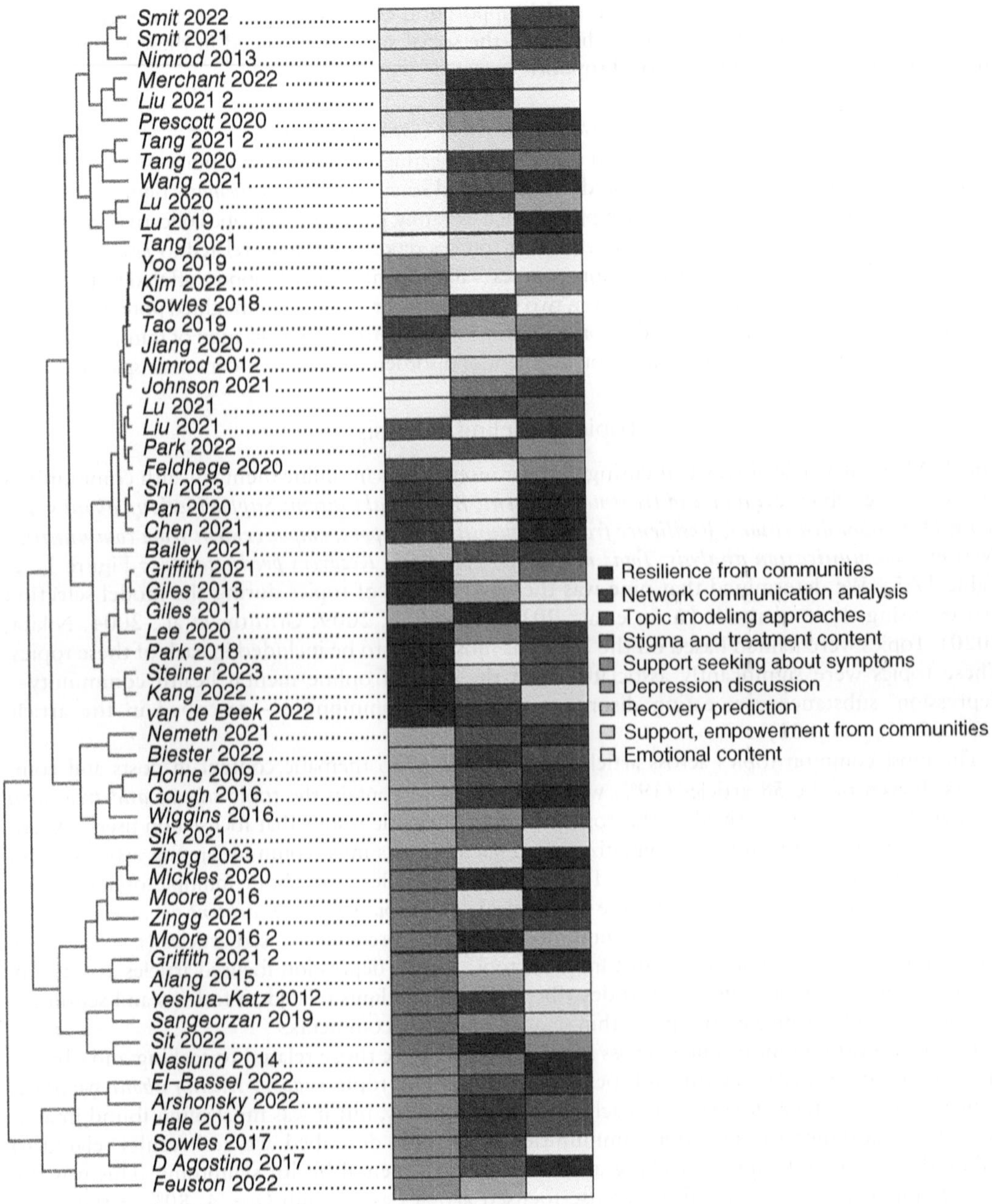

Figure 17.2 Latent Dirichlet Allocation topics and terms.
Note. This figure shows the three most likely topics for each peer-reviewed source (from left to right) across nine topics from the topic modeling analysis.

The least common of the nine topics in abstracts were those related to methodology and analysis in articles. The topic ***network communication analysis*** was most likely in 4 of the 58 articles (7%) and was most often found in depression-focused articles (n = 3, 10% of these 31 articles). Abstracts containing this topic detailed their analysis of online social networks within mental health communities, including users' structural network position and network communication. Three articles (5% of 58) contained the topic of ***topic modeling approaches***, and these were all

Table 17.5 Topics from Latent Dirichlet Allocation

Topic	*Topic type*	*Frequent terms (stemmed)*	*Articles n (%)*
Stigma and treatment content	Thematic content	ill, provid, experi, disclosur, stigma, forum, need, care, respons, treatment, women, media, ppd, youtub, disclos	11 (19%)
Emotional content	Thematic content	communiti, depress, onlin, support, emot, member, inform, effect, posit, result, differ, particip, help, negat, peopl	10 (17%)
Support seeking about symptoms	Thematic content	disord, use, support, post, comment, content, eat, people, reddit, media, individu, provid, sever, opioid, seek	9 (16%)
Depression discussions	Peer interaction	onlin, forum, depress, suicide, discuss, discours, analysi, ident, share, work, function, men, quality, issu, suggest	7 (12%)
Resilience from communities	Peer interaction	health, mental, forum, resili, share, analysi, studi, condit, discuss, text, common, service, theme, method, challeng	7 (12%)
Support, empowerment from communities	Peer interaction	onlin, studi, support, peer, engag, use, user, community, group, explor, aim, empower, particip, benefit, connect	6 (10%)
Network communication analysis	Methodology	social, user, support, network, analysi, receiv, onlin, examin, associ, use, repli, form, self-disclosur, chang, communic	4 (7%)
Topic modeling approaches	Methodology	topic, post, model, data, understand, relat, help, approach, indic, import, learn, develop, inform, analyz, experi	3 (5%)
Recovery prediction	Methodology	user, recoveri, rule, feature, model, word, predict, relaps, use, tweet, dataset, differ, linguist, captur, sober	1 (2%)

depression-focused articles (n = 3, 10% of these 31 articles). Abstracts containing this theme described their methods, including LDA, to model commonly occurring thematic topics among online posts and comments. The topic *recovery prediction* was most likely in only 1 of the 58 articles (2%), which was an article focused on substance use disorder communities (20% of these articles). This topic focused on a methodological approach whereby aspects of users' posts and online social networks are used to predict recovery from alcohol use disorder.

Discussion

The current review used a scoping literature review and topic modeling analysis to summarize multiple aspects of the extant literature on online peer mental health communities. Among 58 articles included after the scoping review, the largest group reported findings about online depression communities, followed by multiple mental health communities, substance use disorder communities, and eating disorder communities. Common thematic findings from the scoping review included mental health symptoms, mental health care and medications, coping strategies, and emotional content. Further, most articles described how online peers provided support to each other, including emotional, instrumental, and informational support. Findings also revealed characteristics or strategies of users that helped them obtain this support, such as seeking advice, being active and socializing, and showing interest in multiple topics. The topic modeling analysis identified nine topics across the 58 article abstracts: *Stigma and treatment content*; *Emotional content*; *Support seeking about symptoms*; *Depression discussions*; *Resilience from communities*; *Support, empowerment from communities*; *Network communication analysis*; *Topic modeling approaches*; and *Recovery prediction*.

Online Community Themes

Similar themes in posts—emerging in the scoping review and the topic modeling analysis—speak to users' ongoing unmet mental health needs. These needs reflect the general lack of access to and availability of mental health care (American Psychological Association, 2022). The most common topics from the LDA represent thematic findings from articles: ***stigma and treatment content*** and ***emotional content***. These are paralleled by the most common thematic findings from the scoping review: mental health symptoms, mental health care and medications, coping strategies, and emotional content. Themes related to symptoms and emotions show users' propensity to disclose their mental health experiences in online communities. Not only is written disclosure itself often therapeutic (Frattaroli, 2006), but it may be more beneficial when disclosed to an audience (Boniel-Nissim & Barak, 2013). Further, some users may feel safer disclosing to peers through anonymous or semianonymous accounts as an alternative to disclosing a stigmatized identity offline (van de Beek et al., 2023).

Frequent themes concerning mental health care, medication, and coping strategies imply that users need support finding and evaluating treatment options. In the context of the post-pandemic era, many users may lack access to providers (Moreno et al., 2020), especially if living in rural areas (Steiner et al., 2023). Such users may turn to peers to ask whether they should seek professional help and, if so, how to proceed. ***Stigma and treatment content*** was the most frequent LDA topic in articles about depression-focused communities. Some of the articles characterized by this topic described users who were reticent to seek help from providers due to previous or expected stigma (e.g., Alang & Fomotar, 2015; Moore et al., 2016). Similarly, users frequently shared coping strategies, which suggests that many are seeking psychoeducation and resources to navigate mental health challenges. Online communities may serve as a stopgap for those unable to get this information from mental health care providers. These recurrent themes across the literature speak to a global issue of users unable to access or hesitant to access mental health care from professionals.

These thematic findings have been replicated across multiple types of online communities and a large proportion of the extant literature. Similar results related to recent themes in both the scoping review and topic modeling analysis establish consistent content in what users share in online mental health communities (e.g. symptoms, emotions, treatment, and coping strategies). ***Topic modeling approaches*** as a methodology even emerged in the LDA as a recurrent topic across the 58 abstracts. Our review shows a level of saturation in thematic findings, which suggests that future research could seek to explore other aspects of online mental health communities that are less examined.

Online Community Interactions and Affordances

Findings related to social support also underscore potential benefits to users of online communities who may lack offline mental health care. Our scoping review revealed that most articles found evidence of online social support among peers. Further, ***support seeking about symptoms***, ***depression discussions***, ***resilience from communities***, and ***support, empowerment from communities*** were found as recurrent article topics using LDA. ***Support seeking about symptoms*** was the most common LDA topic in articles about both substance use- and eating disorder-focused communities, suggesting that users self-identifying with these stigmatized conditions may lack outlets to disclose their experiences offline. Users formed affinity communities based on identifying with the same stigmatized identity of having an MHC, which could afford emotional support, social capital, and feelings of belongingness to these users (e.g. Lu et al., 2019). In addition, communities offered instrumental and informational support, whereby users could obtain advice, suggestions, and direct help from other users (e.g. Kim et al., 2022). ***Resilience from communities*** was the most frequent topic in articles focused on multiple mental health communities, and, therefore, this phenomenon is relevant across communities regardless of diagnostic focus. Therefore, online communities may serve a variety of supportive needs for some users that may otherwise have been filled in offline relationships with family, friends, and mental health providers.

The fact that online communities can provide social support was well established across our scoping review and topic modeling, but the circumstances that promote social support are more emergent in the literature. A subset of articles examined what makes it more likely that users will receive social support online. Findings included personal characteristics of users like self-efficacy (e.g. Liu & Wang, 2021), aspects of users' social network(s) and their network position (e.g. Pan et al. 2020), and features of the online community's infrastructure like moderation level (e.g. Tang et al., 2020). The ***network communication analysis*** theme in the LDA epitomizes this new area of inquiry related to online communities. The varied nature of research questions and findings in this area highlights the need for more research to establish the most salient individual and structural factors that promote the successful acquisition of social support. Further research would help inform individual users seeking support in online communities about the best strategies to build and maintain online social capital.

Even more emergent in the literature is the study of online advocacy among peers with multiple marginalized identities. A limited number of articles pointed to the added usefulness of peer support to users experiencing MHCs as well as another marginalized identity, such as being LGBTQ+ (Alang & Fomotar, 2015) or a person of color (Johnson et al., 2021). Online communities may offer venues for advocacy and antiprejudice efforts for some of these users experiencing discrimination toward one or more of their identities in various offline contexts. Finding community members who share similar experiences of multiple marginalization may be especially challenging offline. Online communities may enable users to engage in discussions and advocacy unique to their shared, lived, and historical experiences (Johnson et al., 2021). Conversely, one article in our review found that transgender users with self-reported eating disorders faced online marginalization in eating disorder communities and had to strategize to obtain support for different facets of their identities (Feuston et al., 2022). Given these limited and conflicting findings, more research is needed to understand the experiences of online community members with multiple marginalized identities.

Future Directions and Limitations

Despite the informative findings of the current review, it had some limitations. The large proportion of articles focused on online depression communities may approximate the actual proportion of research about depression within this area. However, it may also reflect a bias in the search terms, and it is possible that more articles fitting review criteria with a focus on other mental health conditions may have been found with different terms. Further, in the LDA, the model selection process used established methods, but this is only an estimate of the best way to summarize documents. If a different number of topics were selected a priori, the foci of these topics may have differed.

Our review also revealed a variety of emergent areas where more research is needed about online mental health communities and how they serve unmet needs. As described previously, future research could further investigate understudied aspects of peer interactions in online mental health communities, including individual and structural factors that promote obtaining social support. Such research could systematically examine the relative effects of different features of online communities (e.g. anonymity, moderation, country of origin, or links to self-guided interventions). Also, more research should focus on the unique experience of users who face intersecting inequality via multiple stigmatized identities. In particular, interviews or focus groups with users who encounter multiple marginalization could reveal their motivations, needs, and challenges in online mental health spaces. Except for research studies about Chinese online depression communities, most of the extant research has focused on online communities founded in the West and the Global North. More research is needed that focuses on users from countries in the Global South, and participant samples should be more diverse in terms of gender, race, ethnicity, age, and socioeconomic status. Research with community samples experiencing MHCs could also investigate technology readiness, internet connectivity, and any barriers to accessing social support via online communities.

Further, our findings can inform online health promotion campaigns that seek to promote mental health awareness, mental health literacy, and prevention of mental health challenges. Common thematic content across studies of online peer mental health communities reveals topics consistently of interest to users, including mental health care, treatment, symptoms, emotion regulation, and mental health stigma. These topics could form engaging content in health promotion campaigns and provide knowledge of interest to users asking for informational support in these areas. If campaigns are native to particular websites or social media platforms that house active and stable online communities, these campaigns could also encourage users to join these forum discussions and offer strategies to seek support from peers online. Given the emergent research area of intersecting marginalized identities in online mental health communities, campaigns could also focus on representing people experiencing intersecting inequity, such as people of color experiencing depression or gender diverse people with disordered eating. Not only could this promote diverse and relatable representation in media, but it could also emphasize the nuance of mental health challenges to the public.

Conclusion

Using a scoping literature review and topic modeling analysis, the current review examined extant literature about online communities from multiple angles. Similar thematic findings repeatedly found within this research suggest that users lack sufficient access to mental health support or psychoeducational resources. Recent articles also show that online peer communities consistently support users in multiple ways, including providing emotional support, information, and direct help. This results in increased social capital, feelings of belongingness, and empowerment for many users. Given the gap between available mental health care and consumer needs in the postpandemic era, as well as the prevalence of stigma, many users may be looking to these communities for help unavailable elsewhere. Future research could inform individual strategies and platform structures that would best support a variety of users to maximize benefits from online communities.

Acknowledgments

The authors would like to thank Melissa C. Funaro, Clinical Research & Education Librarian of the Cushing/Whitney Medical Library, for help with the literature searches and technical support and Daniel Griffith for his consultation on analyses conducted in R.

Note

1 Percentages reported in sections about specific diagnosis-focused online communities refer to the percentage of the subset of articles about those communities.

References

Alang, S. M., & Fomotar, M. (2015). Postpartum depression in an online community of lesbian mothers: Implications for clinical practice. *Journal of Gay & Lesbian Mental Health*, *19*(1), 21–39. https://doi.org/10.1080/19359705.2014.910853

American Psychiatric Association. (2022). *Diagnostic and statistical manual of mental disorders: DSM-5-TR* (5th ed., text rev.). American Psychiatric Association Publishing.

American Psychological Association. (2022). *Psychologists struggle to meet demand amid mental health crisis: 2022 COVID-19 practitioner impact survey*. https://www.apa.org/pubs/reports/practitioner/2022-covid-psychologist-workload

Arshonsky, J., Krawczyk, N., Bunting, A. M., Frank, D., Friedman, S. R., & Bragg, M. A. (2022). Informal coping strategies among people who use opioids during COVID-19: Thematic analysis of reddit forums. *JMIR Formative Research*, *6*(3), e32871. https://doi.org/10.2196/32871

Arun, R., Suresh, V., Veni Madhavan, C. E., & Narasimha Murthy, M. N. (2010). On finding the natural number of topics with latent Dirichlet allocation: Some observations. In M. J. Zaki, J. X. Yu, B. Ravindran, & V. Pudi (Eds.), *Lecture notes in computer science: Vol. 6118. Advances in knowledge discovery and data mining* (pp. 391–402). Springer. https://doi.org/10.1007/978-3-642-13657-3_43

Bailey, S., Zhang, Y., Ramesh, A., Golbeck, J., & Getoor, L. (2020). A structured and linguistic approach to understanding recovery and relapse in AA. *ACM Transactions on the Web (TWEB)*, *15*(1), 1–35. https://doi.org/10.1145/3423208

Biester, L., Pennebaker, J., & Mihalcea, R. (2022). Emotional and cognitive changes surrounding online depression identity claims. *PLoS One*, *17*(12), e0278179. https://doi.org/10.1371/journal.pone.0278179

Bizzotto, N., Marciano, L., de Bruijn, G. J., & Schulz, P. J. (2023). The empowering role of web-based help seeking on depressive symptoms: Systematic review and meta-analysis. *Journal of Medical Internet Research*, *25*, e36964. https://doi.org/10.2196/36964

Blei, D. M., Ng, A. Y., & Jordan, M. I. (2003). Latent Dirichlet allocation. *Journal of Machine Learning Research*, *3*, 993–1022.

Boettcher, N. (2021). Studies of depression and anxiety using reddit as a data source: Scoping review. *JMIR Mental Health*, *8*(11), e29487. https://doi.org/10.2196/29487

Boniel-Nissim, M., & Barak, A. (2013). The therapeutic value of adolescents' blogging about social-emotional difficulties. *Psychological Services*, *10*(3), 333–341. https://doi.org/10.1037/a0026664

Cao, J., Xia, T., Li, J., Zhang, Y., & Tang, S. (2009). A density-based method for adaptive LDA model selection. *Neurocomputing*, *72*(7–9), 1775–1781. https://doi.org/10.1016/j.neucom.2008.06.011

Chen, Y., & Xu, Y. (2021). Exploring the effect of social support and empathy on user engagement in online mental health communities. *International Journal of Environmental Research and Public Health*, *18*(13), 6855. https://doi.org/10.3390/ijerph18136855

Corrigan, P. W., Druss, B. G., & Perlick, D. A. (2014). The impact of mental illness stigma on seeking and participating in mental health care. *Psychological Science in the Public Interest*, *15*(2), 37–70. https://doi.org/10.1177/1529100614531398

D'Agostino, A. R., Optican, A. R., Sowles, S. J., Krauss, M. J., Escobar Lee, K., & Cavazos-Rehg, P. A. (2017). Social networking online to recover from opioid use disorder: A study of community interactions. *Drug and Alcohol Dependence*, *181*, 5–10. https://doi.org/10.1016/j.drugalcdep.2017.09.010

El-Bassel, N., Hochstatter, K. R., Slavin, M. N., Yang, C., Zhang, Y., & Muresan, S. (2022). Harnessing the power of social media to understand the impact of COVID-19 on people who use drugs during lockdown and social distancing. *Journal of Addiction Medicine*, *16*(2), e123–e132. https://doi.org/10.1097/ADM.0000000000000883

Feldhege, J., Moessner, M., & Bauer, S. (2020). Who says what? Content and participation characteristics in an online depression community. *Journal of Affective Disorders*, *263*, 521–527. https://doi.org/10.1016/j.jad.2019.11.007

Feuston, J. L., Devito, M. A., Scheuerman, M. K., Weathington, K., Benitez, M., Perez, B. Z., Sondheim, L., & Brubaker, J. R. (2022). "Do you ladies relate?": Experiences of gender diverse people in online eating disorder communities. *Proceedings of the ACM on Human-Computer Interaction*, *6*(CSCW2), 1–32. https://doi.org/10.1145/3555145

Frattaroli, J. (2006). Experimental disclosure and its moderators: A meta-analysis. *Psychological Bulletin*, *132*(6), 823. https://doi.org/10.1037/0033-2909.132.6.823

Furukawa, T. A., Noma, H., Caldwell, D. M., Honyashiki, M., Shinohara, K., Imai, H., Hunot, V., & Churchill, R. (2014). Waiting list may be a nocebo condition in psychotherapy trials: A contribution from network meta-analysis. *Acta Psychiatrica Scandinavica*, *130*(3), 181–192. https://doi.org/10.1111/acps.12275

Giles, D. C., & Newbold, J. (2011). Self- and other-diagnosis in user-led mental health online communities. *Qualitative Health Research*, *21*(3), 419–428. https://doi.org/10.1177/1049732310381388

Giles, D. C., & Newbold, J. (2013). "Is this normal?" The role of category predicates in constructing mental illness online. *Journal of Computer-Mediated Communication*, *18*(4), 476–490. https://doi.org/10.1111/jcc4.12022

Gough, B. (2016). Men's depression talk online: A qualitative analysis of accountability and authenticity in help-seeking and support formulations. *Psychology of Men & Masculinity*, *17*(2), 156–164. https://doi.org/10.1037/a0039456

Griffith, F. J., & Stein, C. H. (2021). Behind the hashtag: Online disclosure of mental illness and community response on Tumblr. *American Journal of Community Psychology*, *67*(3–4), 419–432. https://doi.org/10.1002/ajcp.12483

Griffith, F. J., Stein, C. H., Hoag, J. E., & Gay, K. N. (2021). #MentalHealthArt: How Instagram artists promote mental health awareness online. *Public Health*, *194*, 67–74. https://doi.org/10.1016/j.puhe.2021.02.006

Griffiths, T. L., Steyvers, M., Blei, D. M., & Tenenbaum, J. B. (2004). Integrating topics and syntax. *Advances in Neural Information Processing Systems*, *17*, 537–544.

Grün, B., & Hornik, K. (2023). *Topicmodels: Topic Models*. R package version 0.2-14. https://CRAN.R-project.org/package=topicmodels

Haddaway, N. R., Grainger, M. J., & Gray, C. T. (2021). *citationchaser: An R package and shiny app for forward and backward citations chasing in academic searching*. https://doi.org/10.5281/zenodo.4543513

Hale, B. J. (2019). Responding to depression-related Imgur posts: A content analysis of social support and non-bona fide features in user-generated comments. *Digital Health*, *5*, 2055207619890476. https://doi.org/10.1177/2055207619890476

Horne, J., & Wiggins, S. (2009). Doing being "on the edge": Managing the dilemma of being authentically suicidal in an online forum. *Sociology of Health and Illness*, *31*(2), 170–184. https://doi.org/10.1111/j.1467-9566.2008.01130.x

Jiang, M., Ammerman, B. A., Zeng, Q., Jacobucci, R., & Brodersen, A. (2020). Phrase-level pairwise topic modeling to uncover helpful peer responses to online suicidal crises. *Humanities and Social Sciences Communications*, *7*(1), 1–13. https://doi.org/10.1057/s41599-020-0513-5

Johnson, K. F., Brookover, D. L., Borden, N. J., Worth, A., Temple, P., & Mahan, L. B. (2021). What YouTube narratives reveal about online support, counseling entrance, and how black Americans manage depression symptomatology. *Informatics for Health & Social Care*, *46*(1), 84–99. https://doi.org/10.1080/17538157.2020.1865967

Kang, Y.-B., McCosker, A., Kamstra, P., & Farmer, J. (2022). Resilience in web-based mental health communities: Building a resilience dictionary with semiautomatic text analysis. *JMIR Formative Research*, *6*(9), e39013. https://doi.org/10.2196/39013

Kim, H. S., Chung, M. Y., Rhee, E. S., & Kim, Y. (2022). Is it reciprocating or self-serving? Understanding coping strategies for postpartum depression in an online community for Korean mothers. *Health Care for Women International*, *43*(12), 1464–1481. https://doi.org/10.1080/07399332.2022.2037604

Lee, N., Buchanan, K., & Yu, M. (2020). Each post matters: A content analysis of #mentalhealth images on Instagram. *Journal of Visual Communication in Medicine*, *43*(3), 128–138. https://doi.org/10.1080/17453054.2020.1781535

Liu, J., & Kong, J. (2021). Why do users of online mental health communities get likes and reposts: A combination of text mining and empirical analysis. *Healthcare*, *9*(9), 1133. https://doi.org/10.3390/healthcare9091133

Liu, J., & Wang, J. (2021). Users' intention to continue using online mental health communities: Empowerment theory perspective. *International Journal of Environmental Research and Public Health*, *18*(18), 9427. https://doi.org/10.3390/ijerph18189427

Lu, Y., Luo, S., & Liu, X. (2021). Development of social support networks by patients with depression through online health communities: Social network analysis. *JMIR Medical Informatics*, *9*(1), e24618. https://doi.org/10.2196/24618

Lu, Y., Pan, T., & Deng, S. (2019). What drives patients affected by depression to share in online depression communities? A social capital perspective. *Healthcare*, *7*(4), 133. https://doi.org/10.3390/healthcare7040133

Lu, Y., Pan, T., Liu, J., & Wu, J. (2020). Does usage of online social media help users with depressed symptoms improve their mental health? Empirical evidence from an online depression community. *Frontiers in Public Health*, *8*, 581088. https://doi.org/10.3389/fpubh.2020.581088

Madzík, P., & Falát, L. (2022). State-of-the-art on analytic hierarchy process in the last 40 years: Literature review based on latent Dirichlet allocation topic modelling. *PLoS One*, *17*(5), e0268777. https://doi.org/10.1371/journal.pone.0268777

Merchant, R., Goldin, A., Manjanatha, D., Harter, C., Chandler, J., Lipp, A., Nguyen, T., & Naslund, J. A. (2022). Opportunities to expand access to mental health services: A case for the role of online peer support communities. *Psychiatric Quarterly*, *93*(2), 613–625. https://doi.org/10.1007/s11126-022-09974-7

Mickles, M. S., & Weare, A. M. (2020). Trying to save the game(r): Understanding the self-disclosure of YouTube subscribers surrounding mental health in video-game vlog comments. *Southern Communication Journal*, *85*(4), 231–243. http://dx.doi.org/10.1080/1041794X.2020.1798494

Moore, D., & Ayers, S. (2016). Virtual voices: Social support and stigma in postnatal mental illness internet forums. *Psychology, Health & Medicine*, *22*(5), 546–551. https://doi.org/10.1080/13548506.2016.1189580

Moore, D., Ayers, S., & Drey, N. (2016). A thematic analysis of stigma and disclosure for perinatal depression on an online forum. *JMIR Mental Health*, *3*(2), e18. https://doi.org/10.2196/mental.5611

Moreno, C., Wykes, T., Galderisi, S., Nordentoft, M., Crossley, N., Jones, N., & Arango, C. (2020). How mental health care should change as a consequence of the COVID-19 pandemic. *Lancet Psychiatry*, *7*(9), 813–824. https://doi.org/10.1016/S2215-0366(20)30307-2

Moro, S., Cortez, P., & Rita, P. (2015). Business intelligence in banking: A literature analysis from 2002 to 2013 using text mining and latent Dirichlet allocation. *Expert Systems with Applications*, *42*(3), 1314–1324. https://doi.org/10.1016/j.eswa.2014.09.024

Naslund, J. A., Grande, S. W., Aschbrenner, K. A., & Elwyn, G. (2014). Naturally occurring peer support through social media: The experiences of individuals with severe mental illness using YouTube. *PLoS One*, *9*(10), e110171. https://doi.org/10.1371/journal.pone.0110171

Naz, S., Gregory, R., & Bahu, M. (2019). Addressing issues of race, ethnicity and culture in CBT to support therapists and service managers to deliver culturally competent therapy and reduce inequalities in mental health provision for BAME service users. *Cognitive Behaviour Therapist*, *12*, e22. https://doi.org/10.1017/S1754470X19000060

Nemeth, R., Sik, D., & Katona, E. (2021). The asymmetries of the biopsychosocial model of depression in lay discourses—Topic modelling online depression forums. *SSM–Population Health*, *14*, 100785. https://doi.org/10.1016/j.ssmph.2021.100785

Nikita, M. (2020). *ldatuning: Tuning of the Latent Dirichlet Allocation models parameters R package version 1.0.2.* https://CRAN.R-project.org/package=ldatuning

Nimrod, G. (2012). From knowledge to hope: Online depression communities. *International Journal on Disability and Human Development*, *11*(1), 23–30. https://doi.org/10.1515/IJDHD.2012.009

Nimrod, G. (2013). Online depression communities: Members' interests and perceived benefits. *Health Communication*, *28*(5), 425–434. https://doi.org/10.1080/10410236.2012.691068

Pan, W., Feng, B., & Shen, C. (2020). Examining social capital, social support, and language use in an online depression forum: Social network and content analysis. *Journal of Medical Internet Research*, *22*(6), e17365. https://doi.org/10.2196/17365

Park, A., Conway, M., & Chen, A. T. (2018). Examining thematic similarity, difference, and membership in three online mental health communities from reddit: A text mining and visualization approach. *Computers in Human Behavior*, *78*, 98–112. https://doi.org/10.1016/j.chb.2017.09.001

Park, E., Kim, W. H., & Kim, S. B. (2022). What topics do members of the eating disorder online community discuss and empathize with? An application of big data analytics. *Healthcare*, *10*(5), 928. https://doi.org/10.3390/healthcare10050928

Patel, M., Berlin, H., Rajkumar, A., Krein, S. L., Miller, R., DeVito, J., & Peahl, A. F. (2023). Barriers to telemedicine use: Qualitative analysis of provider perspectives during the COVID-19 pandemic. *JMIR Human Factors*, *10*(1), e39249. https://doi.org/10.2196/39249

Ponweiser, M. (2012, May). *Latent Dirichlet allocation in R*. WU Working Papers No. 2. WU Vienna University of Economics and Business. https://doi.org/10.57938/533618e5-dcd9-4c8f-913a-2339fa145c71

Prescott, J., Rathbone, A. L., & Hanley, T. (2020). Online mental health communities, self-efficacy and transition to further support. *Mental Health Review Journal*, *25*(4), 329–344. https://doi.org/10.1108/MHRJ-12-2019-0048

Pretorius, C., Chambers, D., & Coyle, D. (2019). Young people's online help-seeking and mental health difficulties: Systematic narrative review. *Journal of Medical Internet Research*, *21*(11), e13873. https://doi.org/10.2196/13873

R Core Team. (2023). *R: A language and environment for statistical computing*. R Foundation for Statistical Computing. https://www.R-project.org

Rowan, K., McAlpine, D. D., & Blewett, L. A. (2013). Access and cost barriers to mental health care, by insurance status, 1999–2010. *Health Affairs*, *32*(10), 1723–1730. https://doi.org/10.1377/hlthaff.2013.0133

Sangeorzan, I., Andriopoulou, P., & Livanou, M. (2019). Exploring the experiences of people vlogging about severe mental illness on YouTube: An interpretative phenomenological analysis. *Journal of Affective Disorders*, *246*, 422–428. https://doi.org/10.1016/j.jad.2018.12.119

Shi, J., & Khoo, Z. (2023). Online health community for change: Analysis of self-disclosure and social networks of users with depression. *Frontiers in Psychology*, *14*, 1092884. https://doi.org/10.3389/fpsyg.2023.1092884

Sik, D. (2021). From lay depression narratives to secular ritual healing: An online ethnography of mental health forums. *Culture, Medicine and Psychiatry*, *45*(4), 751–774. https://doi.org/10.1007/s11013-020-09702-5

Sit, M., Elliott, S. A., Wright, K. S., Scott, S. D., & Hartling, L. (2022). Youth mental health help-seeking information needs and experiences: A thematic analysis of reddit posts. *Youth and Society*, *56*(1), 24–41. https://doi.org/10.1177/0044118X221129642

Smit, D., Vrijsen, J. N., Broekman, T., Groeneweg, B., & Spijker, J. (2022). User engagement within an online peer support community (Depression Connect) and recovery-related changes in empowerment: Longitudinal user survey. *JMIR Formative Research*, *6*(11), e39912. https://doi.org/10.2196/39912

Smit, D., Vrijsen, J. N., Groeneweg, B., Vellinga-Dings, A., Peelen, J., & Spijker, J. (2021). A newly developed online peer support community for depression (Depression Connect): Qualitative study. *Journal of Medical Internet Research*, *23*(7), e25917. https://doi.org/10.2196/25917

Sowles, S. J., Krauss, M. J., Gebremedhn, L., & Cavazos-Rehg, P. A. (2017). "I feel like I've hit the bottom and have no idea what to do": Supportive social networking on reddit for individuals with a desire to quit cannabis use. *Substance Abuse*, *38*(4), 477–482. https://doi.org/10.1080/08897077.2017.1354956

Sowles, S. J., McLeary, M., Optican, A., Cahn, E., Krauss, M. J., Fitzsimmons-Craft, E. E., Wilfley, D. E., & Cavazos-Rehg, P. A. (2018). A content analysis of an online pro-eating disorder community on reddit. *Body Image*, *24*, 137–144. https://doi.org/10.1016/j.bodyim.2018.01.001

Steiner, A., Farmer, J., Kamstra, P., Carlisle, K., McCosker, A., & Kilpatrick, S. (2023). Online mental health forums and rural resilience: Mixed methods study and logic model. *JMIR Mental Health*, *10*, e47459. https://doi.org/10.2196/47459

Storman, D., Jemioło, P., Swierz, M. J., Sawiec, Z., Antonowicz, E., Prokop-Dorner, A., Gotfryd-Burzyńska, M., & Bala, M. M. (2022). Meeting the unmet needs of individuals with mental disorders: Scoping review on peer-to-peer web-based interactions. *JMIR Mental Health*, *9*(12), e36056. https://doi.org/10.2196/36056

Tang, J., Yao, X., & Yu, G. (2021). Exploring the online behavior of users of online depression-focused communities: Comparing communities with different management types. *Psychology Research and Behavior Management*, *14*, 1707–1724. https://doi.org/10.2147/PRBM.S323027

Tang, J., Yu, G., & Yao, X. (2020). A comparative study of online depression communities in China. *International Journal of Environmental Research and Public Health*, *17*(14), 1–13. https://doi.org/10.3390/ijerph17145023

Tang, J., Yu, G., & Yao, X. (2021). Emotional contagion in the online depression community. *Healthcare*, *9*(12), 1609. https://doi.org/10.3390/healthcare9121609

Tao, L., & Jacobs, L. (2019). "Inbox me, please": Analysing comments on anonymous Facebook posts about depression and suicide. *Journal of Psychology in Africa*, *29*(5), 491–498. https://doi.org/10.1080/14330237.2019.1665903

van de Beek, M. H., Landman, E., Veling, W., Schoevers, R. A., & van der Krieke, L. (2023). Discussing the unspoken: A qualitative analysis of online forum discussions on mental health problems in young Moroccan-Dutch migrants. *Transcultural Psychiatry*, *60*(1), 86–98. https://doi.org/10.1177/13634615221105118

Veritas Health Innovation. (2023). *Covidence systematic review software* [Computer software]. www.covidence.org.
Wang, X., Tian, X., Pan, X., Wei, D., & Qi, Q. (2021). What happens when people with depression gather online? *International Journal of Environmental Research and Public Health*, *18*(16), 8762. https://doi.org/10.3390/ijerph18168762
Wiggins, S., McQuade, R., & Rasmussen, S. (2016). Stepping back from crisis points: The provision and acknowledgment of support in an online suicide discussion forum. *Qualitative Health Research*, *26*(9), 1240–1251. https://doi.org/10.1177/1049732316633130
World Health Organization. (2022). *Mental disorders*. https://www.who.int/news-room/fact-sheets/detail/mental-disorders
Yeshua-Katz, D., & Martins, N. (2012). Communicating stigma: The pro-ana paradox. *Health Communication*, *28*(5), 499–508. https://doi.org/10.1080/10410236.2012.699889
Yoo, M., Lee, S., & Ha, T. (2019). Semantic network analysis for understanding user experiences of bipolar and depressive disorders on reddit. *Information Processing and Management*, *56*(4), 1565–1575. https://doi.org/10.1016/j.ipm.2018.10.001
Zingg, A., Singh, T., Franklin, A., Ross, A., Selvaraj, S., Refuerzo, J., & Myneni, S. (2023). Digital health technologies for peripartum depression management among low-socioeconomic populations: Perspectives from patients, providers, and social media channels. *BMC Pregnancy and Childbirth*, *23*(1), 411. https://doi.org/10.1186/s12884-023-05729-9
Zingg, A., Singh, T., & Myneni, S. (2021). Analysis of online peripartum depression communities: Application of multilabel text classification techniques to inform digitally-mediated prevention and management. *Frontiers in Digital Health*, *3*, 653769. https://doi.org/10.3389/fdgth.2021.653769

18

Well-Being Among Physicians in Training: Barriers to Treatment and Efforts to Increase Help Seeking for Depression

Sabrina Menezes[1] and Gregory Guldner[2]
[1] Claremont Graduate University
[2] HCA Healthcare

This chapter will provide a broad overview of help seeking for depression among resident physicians by describing what medical residency is, discussing depression as it relates to residents, and describing barriers that impede residents from seeking help. We will also cover attempts to increase help seeking in this population and suggestions for future research. When describing efforts to influence help seeking, this chapter will focus mainly on programs that target the utilization of mental health services (and measure this outcome). This chapter will conclude with some thoughts on how mental health communication research could be used for this purpose.

Life as a Resident Physician

Residency is the interim period (typically three to seven years) when physicians must balance roles as learners and professionals. Residents have graduated from medical school and hold a medical degree but are still training to become independent doctors in their chosen specialty. During this period, these physicians practice medicine under the supervision of more experienced physicians, including more senior residents, working in hospitals and other medical arenas. Depending on the specialty, duties may include interviewing and examining patients, developing treatment plans, ordering medications and diagnostic tests, interpreting data from images and labs, documenting care in the medical record, and, for some specialties, performing surgeries or procedures. As such, residency is known as a time when residents must work difficult and long hours (Dyrbye et al., 2014; Prins et al., 2007; Temple, 2014). Residents can work up to 80 hours a week, according to the Accreditation Council for Graduate Medical Education (ACGME, 2022), and in the Medscape Residents Salary and Debt Report (Robbins, 2023), most residents report working at least one to five night shifts a month. Despite this, residents report making $67,400 a year on average, and only 24% say they feel their pay is fair. Here, it is also essential to keep in mind that the average resident is heavily in debt from medical school. In the Medscape survey (Robbins, 2023), and a similar survey from the Association of American Medical Colleges (AAMC, 2022), more than 49% of those who graduated medical school had over $200,000 in debt related to their schooling.

The Handbook of Mental Health Communication, First Edition.
Edited by Marco C. Yzer and Jason T. Siegel.

Depression in Resident Physicians

Millions of adults around the world suffer from depression each year (National Institute to Mental Health [NIMH], 2017; World Health Organization [WHO], 2020). Unfortunately, depression rates are even higher for those in the medical field, including physicians in training (Joules et al., 2014). A review of several studies (Mata et al., 2015) suggests that the percentage of residents with depression ranges from 20.9% to 43.2% depending on how depression is measured. Mata et al. (2015) also found that the rate of depression among residents increases yearly, and the start of residency marks a significant emergence of symptoms. Furthermore, the more hours residents put in, the greater their chance of developing moderate to severe symptoms of depression (Fang et al., 2022).

Research shows that depression is associated with myriad adverse outcomes, such as poor work performance (Harvey et al., 2011), cardiovascular disease (Van der Kooy et al., 2007), neurocognitive deficits (Jaeger et al., 2006), and suicide (Brown et al., 2000). Similarly, just as residents are at potentially greater risk of developing depression due to their profession, they also experience several unique impacts on their personal and work lives if they experience depression. Depression in residents has been linked to problems such as medical errors, trouble coping with work stress, more days off, and even leaving medical training altogether (Joules et al., 2014). Similarly, Fahrenkopf et al. (2008) found that residents with depression make significantly more medication mistakes (i.e., "any error in the ordering, transcription, or administration of a medication," p. 2). Unfortunately, depression also can lead to tragedies such as suicide (Shanafelt et al., 2021), the second leading cause of death for resident physicians and the first cause of death for male residents (Yaghmour et al., 2017).

Barriers to Help Seeking

Depression is treatable (NIMH, 2017), but many people do not seek help (Pratt & Brody, 2014). Research shows that those with more severe depressive symptoms experience worse help-seeking attitudes, expectations, and intentions (Hollar & Siegel, 2023; Siegel et al., 2015; Siegel et al., 2017). In the general population, barriers to mental health treatment include the desire to deal with problems on one's own, not thinking one needs help, and stigma (Mojtabai et al., 2011). In resident physicians, additional barriers unique to their profession may exacerbate the problem. Below is a discussion of some of these barriers to help better understand why residents are hesitant to seek care for depression.

Knowledge

Ey et al. (2013) found that resident physicians are reluctant to seek help based on perceptions that help seeking is ineffective. Moreover, higher levels of depressive symptomatology are associated with less favorable help-seeking outcome expectations (Siegel et al., 2024). Along with this, knowing where to seek help could also be a roadblock on the path to help seeking. Levy et al. (2019a; 2019b) found that about 30% of residents in their study did not know where to seek help, even though over 92% of their program directors knew where to refer residents, and those with moderate or higher depressive symptoms were more likely not to know where to seek help. Residents also can have trouble recognizing symptoms of depression in themselves, therefore preventing them from realizing that they need assistance in the first place (Hochberg et al., 2013). Altogether, resident physicians are less likely to seek help for depression if they do not know they have depression, are not knowledgeable on how help seeking can improve their lives, and do not understand how to seek help.

Stigma

Stigma is often recognized as a barrier to anyone seeking help for depression (Mojtabai et al., 2011). Resident physicians have similar perceptions to the general population, but these thoughts and fears could be amplified based on their role as doctors. Studies have long reported stigmatization as a barrier to help seeking among residents (Clement et al., 2015; Ey et al., 2013; George et al., 2014; Rubanovich et al., 2022). More specifically, some doctors have expressed views that depression is embarrassing and a sign of weakness (Wijeratne et al., 2021) and believed they should handle problems independently (Clough et al., 2019; Guille et al., 2010). They also were concerned that if they did seek help, others would judge them for it (Clough et al., 2019).

One reason doctors, including residents, have negative beliefs about depression and help seeking stems from doctors viewing their role in society as caretakers. Thompson et al. (2001) found that physicians expressed discomfort with taking on the patient role and felt they needed to advance an image of perfect health to their colleagues and patients. Along with this, it has been suggested that physicians have an enhanced sense of responsibility (see Gabbard, 1985 for more on this), which could be beneficial for professional purposes, but ultimately makes them less likely to seek outside help. Thus, along with general preconceived notions about depression and help seeking, a barrier specific to this population is stigmatization regarding what it means to be a doctor.

Confidentiality

Another barrier to help seeking for resident physicians is confidentiality concerns (Clement et al., 2015; Ey et al., 2013; George et al., 2014; Guille et al., 2010; Rubanovich et al., 2022). In a systematic review of the literature on stigma and help seeking, Clement et al. (2015) found that health professionals were more likely to report concerns for privacy than other groups. In residents specifically, Guille et al.s' (2010) multi-site study showed that over 50% of residents were concerned about confidentiality. A qualitative study reported that participants were concerned colleagues would review their medical records and see that they have sought care, given physicians have access to medical health records (George et al., 2014). It was also mentioned here that there is difficulty finding someone to help who is not someone they know (e.g., a mentor or physician). This may be of particular concern to resident physicians who worry that they will interact in a teaching or professional role with the very mental health providers that would be treating them outside of work. The following two barriers further expand upon why confidentiality is such an essential barrier to address in this population.

Career Implications

As mentioned, a hurdle to help seeking in this population is disquietude around their help seeking and mental health status documented for fear that it will be revealed. Resident physicians are particularly concerned that it could negatively impact their career trajectory. Dyrbye et al. (2021) suggested that residents are reluctant to take any medical leave whatsoever due to career concerns and believe it would be challenging to request time off from a supervisor for a medical appointment, let alone a mental health appointment, which people are more hesitant to disclose (Kowalski & Peipert, 2019). Similarly, Dunn et al. (2009) found that residents expressed trepidation that their position in their training program would be jeopardized if their supervisor or director were to learn they sought help for a mental health problem.

Licensing

A physician study showed that about 40% of doctors would be concerned about their medical license if they were to seek help for mental health problems (Dyrbye et al., 2017). This is because some states ask questions about mental health (and treatments for such) on licensing applications, along with many other questions determining their eligibility to practice (Dyrbye et al., 2017; Welcher et al., 2019). In turn, there have been efforts to remedy this, such as those by the Dr. Lorna Breen Heroes Foundation (Feist et al., 2020) and updated recommendations by the Federation of State Medical Boards (2018), resulting in changes to some states licensing questions. However, applications in other states remain problematic (Welcher et al., 2019). Saddawi-Konefka et al. (2021) found that 69% of states examined still ask questions that could require disclosure of mental health disorders, and only one of the 54 states (including four US territories) were in line with all four of the recommendations from the Federation of State Medical Boards (2018) regarding mental health questions in licensing applications.

Available Resources

Even if physicians have adequate knowledge to seek care for depression and desire to, regardless of the barriers mentioned above, they can still lack the resources to do so. To illustrate, Wu et al. (2021) found that the two most significant barriers to seeking counseling for internal medicine residents they surveyed were time and money.

Time

Time was found to be one of the biggest barriers to help seeking across several studies (Cedfeldt et al., 2015; Ey et al., 2013; George et al., 2014; Guille et al., 2010; Rosen et al., 2000). This is unsurprising given that US resident physicians can work up to 80 hours a week (ACGME, 2022), and residency is well known as a time when physicians must balance patient care, administrative work, and education. Along these same lines, given the limited flexibility in the schedule of resident physicians, if they do not have access to convenient services when they need them, they will be less likely to seek help. Guille et al. (2010) found that over 60% of residents said not having convenient access to care was a barrier to seeking help.

Money

Wu et al. (2021) found that money is one of the highest-ranking barriers to professional help seeking. Similarly, Guille et al. (2010) showed that over 50% of residents with depression surveyed agreed or strongly agreed that cost was a barrier to treatment. Cost is likely an extensive consideration for residents considering that residents have already paid high costs to get where they are in their careers. As a reminder, over 49% of medical school graduates have more than $200,000 in debt (AAMC, 2022; Robbins, 2023), and the average salary for residents is $67,400 (Robbins, 2023).

Impact on Coworkers and Patients

Residents are likely also concerned about finding adequate coverage for their responsibilities when attending mental health appointments without negatively impacting others. Typically, when resident physicians take time off during a work day, patient care needs remain unchanged, requiring the rest of the resident team to manage an even greater workload. A study by Cedfeldt et al. (2015) found that a barrier to using a time off policy for health appointments was concern about the impact their time off would have on their colleagues' workload. They also saw that they were somewhat worried about the repercussions for patients as well. Though few studies assess this impact as a barrier to help seeking, it has been discussed in multiple publications (Meeks et al., 2019; Stergiopoulos et al., 2021).

Attempts to Influence Help seeking for Depression in Resident Physicians

Given the high rates of depression in residents and the barriers that impede them from seeking help, there have been efforts to address this in residency programs. This next section (also, see Appendix Table 18.A.1) will dive into programs that showed influence on utilization of mental health services given its relevance and importance to this topic. As will be seen in this next section, resident data is often provided in conjunction with fellows (those completing sub-specialty training after residency; Miloslavsky & Dua, 2022), and thus will sometimes be reported as such.

Programs Measuring Utilization of Services

Approaches to increase help seeking among residents with depression are still relatively scarce. However, there are some initiatives enacted in residency programs to influence their use of mental health services overall. One program that saw modest success in influencing this was the UCLA Mental Health Program for Physicians in Training (Borenstein, 1985; Borenstein & Cook, 1982). They attempted to improve their program members' mental health and encourage help seeking by increasing the availability of services to interns, residents, and faculty. In doing so, they created an off-site clinic of volunteer UCLA providers with broad mental health specialties. These services were of no cost to residents in the short term and often were discounted for those who needed long-term care. Additionally, records for these services were kept separate from the hospital to avoid concerns that counseling would impact their training status or broader career. When looking at initial data for use of their program, they saw a rate of 7.9% utilization for residents, indicating a relatively small uptake of services (Borenstein, 1985) but as will be discussed later, they did not have a comparison group to rule out possible trend effects.

The House Officer Mental Health Program (Pitt et al., 2004), was modeled after the UCLA effort (Borenstein, 1985; Borenstein & Cook, 1982) by building counseling services separate from the training program. In doing so, they provided five free visits, then continued treatment through insurance. To promote the program, they advertised via email, presentations, posters, and flyers, and had psychiatrists meet with residency directors to provide guidance on identifying and referring struggling residents. The results of this program indicated that it was able to successfully build upon its predecessor, reporting that twice as many residents used services in the first year than the employee assistance program in previous years (based on a 10-year average), and utilization increased with every passing year. Both this and the previous UCLA program found that many of those who sought help continued to follow-up appointments (Borenstein, 1985; Pitt et al., 2004), indicating that once residents initially saw someone for their mental health issues, it led to greater help seeking thereafter. However, again no true comparison group was used.

Another tool that has been used to increase the number of residents that seek help is an interactive screener. This screener was created by the American Foundation for Suicide Prevention (AFSP) and implemented in undergraduates (Garlow et al., 2008; Haas et al., 2008), but has since been used in physician populations (Mortali & Moutier, 2018). The interactive screener is a confidential online survey with mental health measures (such as those for depression). After physicians complete the survey, their responses are sent to a counselor, who then provides an assessment based on their answers. Counselors can also answer respondents' questions in their assessment and invite physicians to chat anonymously with a counselor online. They can also make in-person appointments if they choose to (those classified as most distressed are encouraged to).

The Suicide Prevention and Depression Awareness Program (later described as the Healer Education, Assessment and Referral [HEAR] Program; Zisook et al., 2016) at the University of California, San Diego School of Medicine (UCSD) is one of the programs that used this screener for residents (in addition to medical students and fellows). They distributed the AFSP screener along with educational modules on physician mental health and help seeking, including a PowerPoint presentation, an AFSP video, information on the interactive screening, and discussion time. In the first year of this program, only 8% of residents and fellows completed the screener (a later estimate showed 17% total completion for residents and fellows from 2009 to 2014; Zisook et al., 2016), and of the 8%, a notable portion talked to the counselor online (33%). They also reported that 14% met with a professional in-person (Moutier et al., 2012).

Similar results were also obtained by Mortali and Moutier (2018) using secondary data obtained from medical schools. Based on the resident/fellow samples they collected who completed the screener, 82.4% looked at the assessment by the counselor, a little over 37% of this group talked with the counselor online, and 48.3% asked for a face-to-face appointment or referral. Those most distressed also had higher rates of engagement with the program than those in lower distress categories. Altogether, these results indicate a concentrated effort should be advanced to encourage residents to fill out the screener, and once residents engage with this format it can lead those most distressed to engage with professional help to greater degrees.

Also notable when discussing help-seeking approaches is a resident wellness program (Ey et al., 2013, 2016) that included elements of the previous programs noted earlier (Borenstein, 1985; Borenstein & Cook, 1982; Moutier et al., 2012; Pitt et al., 2004). It made professional psychologists and psychiatrists free and available to residents and fellows while keeping counseling records separate from the training hospital's records. They also told the residents they did not have to report their use of counseling to the state medical board and could use these services as much as they desired. On top of that, this program grew to include many elements, such as get-togethers, support groups in specific residency programs, coaching, workshops about help-seeking benefits and suicide, and interactive screening (as used in Moutier et al., 2012). The combination of all these efforts appeared to result in the utilization of mental health services increasing from 5.2% to 12% between 2004–2005 and 2009–2010 (Ey et al., 2013), and even more so, to a high of 24.7% in 2013–2014 (Ey et al., 2016), indicating greater help seeking over time. Ey et al. (2013) were also among the few studies to measure both barriers to seeking care through the program and utilization. They found that while 88% of those surveyed knew of the resident wellness program, over 65% of residents and fellows divulged time as a remaining barrier to using services. Additionally, time, confidentiality, stigma, and concerns about helpfulness were related to being less likely to use the resident wellness program (Ey et al., 2013), indicating that there are still gaps between the program's intentions and its actual impact on barriers. However, more follow-up is needed, as Ey et al. (2016) did not report barriers to use, and there were no comparison groups across both studies (i.e., Ey et al., 2013, 2016).

The opt-out method is another intervention for increasing the utilization of mental health services that diverges from past efforts. Typically, residents choose to schedule a mental health appointment unless they are mandated to do so due to extreme circumstances or remediation plans (Sofka et al., 2018). In contrast, opt-out programs automatically schedule residents for an appointment with a mental health professional. Then residents can opt-out if they do not want to attend (Guldner et al., 2024; Sofka et al., 2018, 2021). When this novel program was first put into practice at West Virginia University with internal medicine residents, they scheduled opt-out appointments for residents with counselors at the Faculty and Staff Assistance Program (FSAP) when they were already working outpatient shifts or electives, so they did not have to use any paid time off or sick days. They also had separate records from the hospital where they worked, and all appointments were completely free. Notably, 93% attended the scheduled appointments, and only 7% chose to opt-out. Furthermore, after four-years of the program, the number of opt-outs was even lower (3.3%), and there was a significant increase in self-scheduled visits from 2014–2015 to 2018–2019 (Sofka et al., 2021). Similar to Ey et al. (2013), Sofka et al. (2018) were one of the rare few to measure barriers along with utilization, finding that residents viewed the opt-out services as vastly convenient, with a mean of 7.8 on a scale of 1 (*not convenient*) to 9 (*very convenient*). Residents also appeared unbothered if colleagues found out they attended an appointment, with a mean of 7.9 on a scale of 1 (*very embarrassed*) to 9 (*not at all embarrassed*).

Likewise, an opt-out approach was employed to encourage residents to seek help at a large training hospital (Kevern et al., 2023). Similar to Sofka et al. (2018, 2021), this program scheduled residents for free appointments during protected time when they were relieved from clinical duties, without having to use personal time off. Appointments in this intervention were also telehealth for added convenience. As a result of these efforts, 59% of residents attended their scheduled appointments, and 34% of residents who kept their scheduled therapy sessions attended further appointments. Moreover, residents who completed a meeting with a mental health professional were surveyed on their experience. Of those who responded to the survey, 80% reported the appointments increased their willingness to use services for their mental health, and 98% said these opt-out appointments should be extended to future residents. Furthermore, 94% said this initiative signified their program cared for them, and 96% were highly satisfied and thought the appointment was worthwhile. No comparison group was implemented in this study, though the authors suggested there was an increase in mental health appointments at their wellness office, with 10% of all mental health sessions during the 2020-2021 academic year attributed to the opt-out program.

An opt-out intervention also was used with emergency medicine, family medicine, and internal medicine residents at Riverside Community Hospital in Riverside, California, which was compared to a traditional opt-in approach. Like the previous two opt-out approaches, these appointments were during protected time. These appointments were also telehealth for convenience and utilized third-party therapists to make residents feel more comfortable speaking with them. Similarly, therapists introduced themselves virtually to residents at the beginning of the program to reduce stigma. This initiative showed that 55% of residents retained their pre-scheduled appointment, and 39% initiated at least one more appointment (Guldner et al., 2024), whereas in the traditional opt-in condition, only 6% of residents scheduled an appointment. Altogether, these results, along with those of Sofka et al. (2018, 2021) and Kevern et al. (2023), suggest that not only did this approach successfully influence residents' use of pre-scheduled appointments at high rates, but it also influenced their likelihood to schedule appointments independently.

Discussion

As seen in the previous section, programs to increase help seeking in residents have used various methods, such as mental health clinics, interactive screening, education, and automatically scheduled appointments. There were also those that encompassed multiple of these methods (i.e., screening, mental health clinics, etc.). Each of these programs also intentionally reduced barriers to help seeking through their program. For instance, several of these programs placed counseling services off-site and off the training hospital's records to protect confidentiality (Borenstein, 1985; Borenstein & Cook, 1982; Ey et al., 2013; Guldner et al., 2024; Pitt et al., 2004; Sofka et al., 2018). Also, time was primarily addressed by carving out hours during the workday to seek care or creating around-the-clock services and cost was zeroed in on by making services low-cost to free (Borenstein, 1985; Borenstein & Cook, 1982; Ey et al., 2013; Guldner et al., 2024; Kevern et al., 2023; Pitt et al., 2004; Sofka et al., 2018, 2021).

In evaluating the success of these approaches, multiple programs showed that utilization increased after their program was enacted compared to records from previous time points (Ey et al., 2013; Pitt et al., 2004). Several also showed increases over time (Ey et al., 2013, 2016; Pitt et al., 2004; Sofka et al., 2021) or that many who sought help through their program continued to seek care (Borenstein, 1985; Guldner et al., 2024; Kevern et al., 2023; Pitt et al., 2004). These results indicate that these programs did indeed have some influence for the better on resident help seeking. However, not all these programs reported utilization in reference to previous time points (Borenstein, 1985; Mortali & Moutier, 2018; Moutier et al., 2012), and only one covered had a comparison group (Guldner et al., 2024).

Methodological Limitations of Past Approaches

Many programs for resident help seeking targeted barriers to help seeking, yet very few approaches explicitly measured their program's impact on barriers. On the contrary, studies that measured utilization rarely assessed the barriers to seeking help through their program. In the same way, studies that assessed barriers often did not measure utilization directly. For instance, Cedfeldt et al. (2015)

reported on a wellness time off policy and surveyed residents about barriers and their use of the policy but had no direct measures of actual mental health service utilization. Similarly, Vaa Stelling and West (2021) showed promising survey results in response to faculty discussing their mental health struggles but again did not measure actual help seeking (see Appendix Table 18.A.1 for more information on these studies).

Studies that measure both barriers and utilization should be conducted, and mediation analyses should be used to understand how impacting these barriers is associated with later influence on residents' use of services. Doing so can provide more explicit guidance regarding where residency programs should place their resources to increase help seeking and where their efforts are in vain. With this, it is also vital that more approaches employ control and comparison groups to ensure their efforts genuinely impact utilization outcomes and result in more significant effects than standard care practices alone. This aligns with past calls by scholars for a more theoretically driven, well-constructed methodology in interventions for healthcare workers' well-being (Cairns et al., 2021; Eskander et al., 2021).

Finally, it is essential to consider the variation in influence programs may have depending on the characteristics of residents. Several efforts discussed found their results differed based on demographics (Cedfeldt et al., 2015; Ey et al., 2013; Pitt et al., 2004). For example, Ey et al. (2013) found that women and primary care residents were most concerned about taking a break to use services; men were worried about whether help seeking would be effective, and racial/ethnic minorities were more uneasy about confidentiality. This suggests that addressing the unique barriers influencing specific groups rather than generalizing interventions across many residents could improve help-seeking approaches. Likewise, it would be remiss not to mention that several of these programs were conducted to increase a specific group of residents' mental health and thus focused on resident populations at singular institutions. Given that there were differences found between subgroups within these singular groups, more data are needed across multiple different residents before conclusions are drawn.

Similarly, few programs in this chapter considered depressive symptomatology when designing their approach. Yet, previous theories imply that those with depression process information about themselves, the future, and their surroundings in a negative light (Beck et al., 1987), which can make it harder for them to pursue care, given that they are more likely to view help seeking in this same fashion (Keeler & Siegel, 2016). Also, Lienemann et al. (2013) found that public service announcements designed to help those with depression backfired, resulting in greater self-stigma after viewing (which was associated with a reduced likelihood to seek help), showing how vital it is to take depressive symptomatology into account.

Suggestions from Mental Health Communication Research

As mentioned, those with depressive symptoms typically process information differently from those without (Beck et al., 1987; Keeler & Siegel, 2016; Lienemann et al., 2013), yet very few programs to influence help seeking in residents mentioned how their approach circumvented the negative schema that dissuades people with depression from seeking care. This lack of acknowledgment may be in part due to the minimal research on which communication methods work best for resident populations. As such, future efforts must look to previously developed methods in other fields, namely mental health communication (Siegel et al., 2017). Research here shows that certain messaging works better for those with depression, like other-directed messages (e.g., "Do you know someone who is feeling distressed? Feeling hopeless? They might be depressed.") as opposed to self-directed messages (e.g., "Are you feeling distressed? Feeling hopeless? You might be depressed."; Siegel et al., 2015, p. 253). Moreover, Lienemann and Siegel (2018) saw that using the same motivation (object-appraisal versus social-adjustive) in messaging as the one behind someone's attitude toward help seeking can increase outcome expectations, attitudes, and intentions toward seeking help for depression.

These concepts could be applied when distributing information or advertising about services provided as part of these help-seeking programs. For instance, in Moutier and colleagues (2012), the initial number of residents who participated in the interactive screening was minimal. However, once residents completed the screener, a notable portion engaged with the counselor. Using mental health communication strategies (e.g., overheard techniques, self-distancing, attitude function matching, etc.) when discussing the screener during educational modules or in other advertising efforts could increase the number of struggling residents who complete the screener from the start, thus putting more residents in contact with the counselor. More research using these communication concepts on residents is needed.

Conclusion

Resident physicians are more vulnerable to depression than the general population due to specific job strains (Joules et al., 2014) and face consequences to their personal and professional lives (Fahrenkopf et al., 2008; Joules et al., 2014; Shanafelt et al., 2021; Yaghmour et al., 2017). Despite this, many residents do not seek help for their depression. As such, there have been efforts to reduce barriers to help seeking and increase the number of residents who receive mental health care for depression. These programs have seen varying degrees of success; notably, the opt-out approach was helpful for substantial increases in help seeking (Guldner et al., 2024; Kevern et al., 2023; Sofka et al., 2018, 2021).

Nevertheless, it is essential to remember that only a few of the papers covered in this chapter measured barrier-related outcomes and did not assess whether reducing specific barriers led to increased utilization rates. Thus, more work is needed to examine the specific mechanisms of these programs' effects on help seeking for resident physicians. Similarly, there should be more careful methodology employed to examine the true effectiveness of these programs, such as employing comparison groups. More approaches should also take heed of previously developed communication methods for those experiencing depression to have a greater influence on struggling residents.

Disclaimer

This research was supported (in whole or in part) by HCA Healthcare and/or an HCA Healthcare affiliated entity. The views expressed in this publication represent those of the author(s) and do not necessarily represent the official views of HCA Healthcare or any of its affiliated entities.

References

Accreditation Council for Graduate Medical Education. (2022). *ACGME Common Program Requirements; Residency.* https://www.acgme.org/globalassets/PFAssets/ProgramRequirements/CPRResidency_20 22v2.pdf

Association of American Medical Colleges. (2022). *Medical student education: Debt, costs, and loan repayment fact card for the class of 2022.* https://store.aamc.org/downloadable/download/sample/sample_id/575

Beck, A. T., Rush, A., John, S., Brian, F., & Emery, G. (1987). *Cognitive therapy of depression.* Guilford Press.

Borenstein, D. B. (1985). Should physician training centers offer formal psychiatric assistance to house officers? A report on the major findings of a prototype program. *The American Journal of Psychiatry, 142*(9), 1053–1057. https://doi.org/10.1176/ajp.142.9.1053

Borenstein, D. B., & Cook, K. (1982). Impairment prevention in the training years: A new mental health program at UCLA. *JAMA, 247*(19), 2700–2703. https://doi.org/10.1001/jama.1982.03320440048034

Brown, G. K., Beck, A. T., Steer, R. A., & Grisham, J. R. (2000). Risk factors for suicide in psychiatric outpatients: A 20-year prospective study. *Journal of Consulting and Clinical Psychology, 68*(3), 371–377. https://doi.org/10.1037/0022-006X.68.3.371

Cairns, P., Aitken, G., Pope, L., Cecil, J. E., Cunningham, K., Ferguson, J., Gibson-Smith, K., Gordon, L., Peter, J., Laidlaw, A. H., Scanlan, G., Tooman, T., Wakeling, J., & Walker, K. A. (2021). Interventions for the well-being of healthcare workers during a pandemic or other crisis: Scoping review. *BMJ Open*, *11*(8), e047498. http://dx.doi.org/10.1136/bmjopen-2020-047498

Cedfeldt, A. S., Bower, E., Flores, C., Brunett, P., Choi, D., & Girard, D. E. (2015). Promoting resident wellness: Evaluation of a time-off policy to increase residents' utilization of health care services. *Academic Medicine*, *90*(5), 678–683. https://doi.org10.1097/ACM.0000000000000541

Clement, S., Schauman, O., Graham, T., Maggioni, F., Evans-Lacko, S., Bezborodovs, N., Morgan, C., Rüsch, N., Brown, J. S., & Thornicroft, G. (2015). What is the impact of mental health-related stigma on help-seeking? A systematic review of quantitative and qualitative studies. *Psychological Medicine*, *45*(1), 11–27. https://doi.org/10.1017/S0033291714000129

Clough, B. A., March, S., Leane, S., & Ireland, M. J. (2019). What prevents doctors from seeking help for stress and burnout? A mixed-methods investigation among metropolitan and regional-based Australian doctors. *Journal of Clinical Psychology*, *75*(3), 418–432. https://doi.org/10.1002/jclp.22707

Dunn, L. B., Hammond, K. A. G., & Roberts, L. W. (2009). Delaying care, avoiding stigma: Residents' attitudes toward obtaining personal health care. *Academic Medicine*, *84*(2), 242–250. https://doi.org/10.1097/ACM.0b013e31819397e2

Dyrbye, L. N., Leep Hunderfund, A. N., Winters, R. C., Moeschler, S. M., Vaa Stelling, B. E., Dozois, E. J., Satele, D. V., & West, C. P. (2021). The relationship between burnout and help-seeking behaviors, concerns, and attitudes of residents. *Academic Medicine*, *96*(5), 701–708. https://doi.org/10.1097/ACM.0000000000003790

Dyrbye, L. N., West, C. P., Satele, D., Boone, S., Tan, L., Sloan, J., & Shanafelt, T. D. (2014). Burnout among US medical students, residents, and early career physicians relative to the general US population. *Academic Medicine*, *89*(3), 443–451. https://doi.org/10.1097/ACM.0000000000000134

Dyrbye, L. N., West, C. P., Sinsky, C. A., Goeders, L. E., Satele, D. V., & Shanafelt, T. D. (2017). Medical licensure questions and physician reluctance to seek care for mental health conditions. *Mayo Clinic Proceedings*, *92*(10), 1486–1493. https://doi.org/10.1016/j.mayocp.2017.06.020

Eskander, J., Rajaguru, P. P., & Greenberg, P. B. (2021). Evaluating wellness interventions for resident physicians: A systematic review. *Journal of Graduate Medical Education*, *13*(1), 58–69. https://doi.org/10.4300/JGME-D-20-00359.1

Ey, S., Moffit, M., Kinzie, J. M., & Brunett, P. H. (2016). Feasibility of a comprehensive wellness and suicide prevention program: A decade of caring for physicians in training and practice. *Journal of Graduate Medical Education*, *8*(5), 747–753. https://doi.org/10.4300/JGME-D-16-00034.1

Ey, S., Moffit, M., Kinzie, J. M., Choi, D., & Girard, D. E. (2013). "If you build it, they will come": Attitudes of medical residents and fellows about seeking services in a resident wellness program. *Journal of Graduate Medical Education*, *5*(3), 486–492. https://doi.org/10.4300/JGME-D-12-00048.1

Fahrenkopf, A. M., Sectish, T. C., Barger, L. K., Sharek, P. J., Lewin, D., Edwards, S., Wiedermann, B. L., & Landrigan, C. P. (2008). Rates of medication errors among depressed and burnt out residents: Prospective cohort study. *BMJ: British Medical Journal*, *336*(7642), 488. https://doi.org/10.1136/bmj.39469.763218.BE

Fang, Y., Lodi, S., Hughes, T. M., Frank, E., Sen, S., & Bohnert, A. S. (2022). Work hours and depression in US first-year physicians. *New England Journal of Medicine*, *387*(16), 1522–1524. https://doi.org/10.1056/NEJMc2210365

Federation of State Medical Boards. (2018). *Physician wellness and burnout*. https://www.fsmb.org/siteassets/advocacy/policies/policy-on-wellness-and-burnout.pdf

Feist, J. B., Feist, J. C., & Cipriano, P. (2020). Stigma compounds the consequences of clinician burnout during COVID-19: A call to action to break the culture of silence. *NAM Perspectives*. https://doi.org/10.31478/202008b

Gabbard, G. O. (1985). The role of compulsiveness in the normal physician. *JAMA*, *254*(20), 2926–2929. https://doi.org/10.1001/jama.1985.03360200078031

Garlow, S. J., Rosenberg, J., Moore, J. D., Haas, A. P., Koestner, B., Hendin, H., & Nemeroff, C. B. (2008). Depression, desperation, and suicidal ideation in college students: Results from the American Foundation for Suicide Prevention College Screening Project at Emory University. *Depression and Anxiety*, *25*(6), 482–488. https://doi.org/10.1002/da.20321

George, S., Hanson, J., & Jackson, J. L. (2014). Physician, heal thyself: A qualitative study of physician health behaviors. *Academic Psychiatry*, *38*, 19–25. https://doi.org/10.1007/s40596-013-0014-6

Guille, C., Speller, H., Laff, R., Epperson, C. N., & Sen, S. (2010). Utilization and barriers to mental health services among depressed medical interns: A prospective multisite study. *Journal of Graduate Medical Education*, *2*(2), 210–214. https://doi.org/10.4300/JGME-D-09-00086.1

Guldner, G., Siegel, J. T., Broadbent, C., Ayutyanont, N., Streletz, D., Popa, A., Fuller, J., & Sisemor, T. (2024). Use of an opt-out versus opt-in strategy for resident therapy substantially increases resident use of mental health services. *Journal of Graduate Medical Education*, *16*(2), 195–201. https://doi.org/10.4300/JGME-D-23-00460.1

Haas, A., Koestner, B., Rosenberg, J., Moore, D., Garlow, S. J., Sedway, J., Nicholas, L., Hendin, H., Mann, J. J., & Nemeroff, C. B. (2008). An interactive web-based method of outreach to college students at risk for suicide. *Journal of American College Health*, *57*(1), 15–22. https://doi.org/10.3200/JACH.57.1.15-22

Harvey, S. B., Glozier, N., Henderson, M., Allaway, S., Litchfield, P., Holland-Elliott, K., & Hotopf, M. (2011). Depression and work performance: An ecological study using web-based screening. *Occupational Medicine, 61*(3), 209–211. https://doi.org/10.1093/occmed/kqr020

Hochberg, M. S., Berman, R. S., Kalet, A. L., Zabar, S. R., Gillespie, C., & Pachter, H. L. (2013). The stress of residency: Recognizing the signs of depression and suicide in you and your fellow residents. *The American Journal of Surgery, 205*(2), 141–146.

Hollar, S. M., & Siegel, J. T. (2023). Increasing help-seeking among people with depression by self-distancing using mental time-travel. *Journal of Mental Health, 32*(3), 575–581. https://doi.org/10.1080/09638237.2022.2118684

Jaeger, J., Berns, S., Uzelac, S., & Davis-Conway, S. (2006). Neurocognitive deficits and disability in major depressive disorder. *Psychiatry Research, 145*(1), 39–48. https://doi.org/10.1016/j.psychres.2005.11.011

Joules, N., Williams, D. M., & Thompson, A. W. (2014). Depression in resident physicians: A systematic review. *Open Journal of Depression, 3*(3), 89–100. https://doi.org/10.4236/ojd.2014.33013

Keeler, A. R., & Siegel, J. T. (2016). Depression, help-seeking perceptions, and perceived family functioning among Spanish-dominant Hispanics and non-Hispanic whites. *Journal of Affective Disorders, 202*, 236–246. https://doi.org/10.1016/j.jad.2016.05.017

Kevern, T., Davies, D. R., Stiel, K., & Raaum, S. (2023). Impact of opt-out therapy appointments on resident physicians' mental health, well-being, stigma, and willingness to engage. *Journal of Graduate Medical Education, 15*(6), 734–737. https://doi.org/10.4300/JGME-D-22-00898.1

Kowalski, R. M., & Peipert, A. (2019). Public- and self-stigma attached to physical versus psychological disabilities. *Stigma and Health, 4*(2), 136–142. https://doi.org/10.1037/sah0000123

Levy, A. B., Nahhas, R. W., Sampang, S., Jacobs, K., Weston, C., Cerny-Suelzer, C., Riese, A., Munetz, M. R., & Shaw, J. (2019a). Characteristics associated with depression and suicidal thoughts among medical residents: Results from the DEPRESS-Ohio study. *Academic Psychiatry, 43*, 480–487. https://doi.org/10.1007/s40596-019-01089-9

Levy, A. B., Nahhas, R. W., Sampang, S., Jacobs, K., Weston, C., Cerny-Suelzer, C., Riese, A., Niedermier, J., Munetz, M. R., Shaw, J., & Mast, R. (2019b). Perceptions of residents and their training directors regarding wellness education, program support, and access to depression treatment: The DEPRESS-Ohio study. *Academic Psychiatry, 43*, 488–493. https://doi.org/10.1007/s40596-019-01067-1

Lienemann, B. A., & Siegel, J. T. (2018). Increasing help-seeking outcomes among people with elevated depressive symptomatology with public service announcements: An examination of functional matching and message sidedness. *Journal of Health Communication, 23*(1), 28–39. https://doi.org/10.1080/10810730.2017.1396630

Lienemann, B. A., Siegel, J. T., & Crano, W. D. (2013). Persuading people with depression to seek help: Respect the boomerang. *Health Communication, 28*(7), 718–728. https://doi.org/10.1080/10410236.2012.712091

Mata, D. A., Ramos, M. A., Bansal, N., Khan, R., Guille, C., Di Angelantonio, E., & Sen, S. (2015). Prevalence of depression and depressive symptoms among resident physicians: A systematic review and meta-analysis. *JAMA, 314*(22), 2373–2383. https://doi.org/10.1001/jama.2015.15845

Meeks, L. M., Ramsey, J., Lyons, M., Spencer, A. L., & Lee, W. W. (2019). Wellness and work: Mixed messages in residency training. *Journal of General Internal Medicine, 34*, 1352–1355. https://doi.org/10.1007/s11606-019-04952-5

Miloslavsky, E. M., & Dua, A. B. (2022). The transition from residency to fellowship: Enhancing training by increasing transparency. *Arthritis and Rheumatology, 74*(10), 1625. https://doi.org/10.1002/art.42158

Mojtabai, R., Olfson, M., Sampson, N. A., Jin, R., Druss, B., Wang, P. S., Wells, K. B., Pincus, H. A., & Kessler, R. C. (2011). Barriers to mental health treatment: Results from the national comorbidity survey replication. *Psychological Medicine, 41*(8), 1751–1761. https://doi.org/10.1017/S0033291710002291

Mortali, M., & Moutier, C. (2018). Facilitating help-seeking behavior among medical trainees and physicians using the interactive screening program. *Journal of Medical Regulation, 104*(2), 27–36. https://doi.org/10.30770/2572-1852-104.2.27

Moutier, C., Norcross, W., Jong, P., Norman, M., Kirby, B., McGuire, T., & Zisook, S. (2012). The suicide prevention and depression awareness program at the University of California, San Diego School of Medicine. *Academic Medicine, 87*(3), 320–326. https://doi.org/10.1097/ACM.0b013e31824451ad

National Institute of Mental Health. (2017). *Depression: Symptoms*. https://www.nami.org/About-Mental-Illness/Mental-Health-Conditions/Depression

Pitt, E., Rosenthal, M. M., Gay, T. L., & Lewton, E. (2004). Mental health services for residents: More important than ever. *Academic Medicine, 79*(9), 840–844. https://doi.org/10.1097/00001888-200409000-00005

Pratt, L. A., & Brody, D. J. (2014). Implications of two-stage depression screening for identifying persons with thoughts of self-harm. *General Hospital Psychiatry, 36*(1), 119–123. https://doi.org/10.1016/j.genhosppsych.2013.09.007

Prins, J. T., Gazendam-Donofrio, S. M., Tubben, B. J., Van der Heijden, F. M., Van de Wiel, H. B., & Hoekstra-Weebers, J. E. (2007). Burnout in medical residents: A review. *Medical Education, 41*(8), 788–800. https://doi.org/10.1111/j.1365-2923.2007.02797.x

Robbins. (2023). *Annual Income Rises, Pay Satisfaction High: Medscape Resident Salary & Debt Report 2023*. https://www.medscape.com/slideshow/2023-residents-salary-debt-report-6016676#1

Rosen, I. M., Christie, J. D., Bellini, L. M., & Asch, D. A. (2000). Health and health care among housestaff in four US internal medicine residency programs. *Journal of General Internal Medicine*, *15*(2), 116–121. https://doi.org/10.1046/j.1525-1497.2000.11218.x

Rubanovich, C. K., Zisook, S., & Bloss, C. S. (2022). Associations between privacy-related constructs and depression and suicide risk in health care professionals, trainees, and students. *Academic Medicine*, *97*(2), 239–246. https://doi.org/10.1097/ACM.0000000000004513

Saddawi-Konefka, D., Brown, A., Eisenhart, I., Hicks, K., Barrett, E., & Gold, J. A. (2021). Consistency between state medical license applications and recommendations regarding physician mental health. *JAMA*, *325*(19), 2017–2018. https://doi.org/10.1001/jama.2021.2275

Shanafelt, T. D., Dyrbye, L. N., West, C. P., Sinsky, C., Tutty, M., Carlasare, L. E., Wang, H., & Trockel, M. (2021). Suicidal ideation and attitudes regarding help seeking in US physicians relative to the US working population. *Mayo Clinic Proceedings*, *96*(8), 2067–2080. https://doi.org/10.1016/j.mayocp.2021.01.033

Siegel, J. T., Ellis, B., Riazi, G., Brafford, A., Guldner, G., & Wells, J. C. (2024). The paradox of the resident experiencing depression: Higher depression, less favorable help-seeking outcome expectations, and lower help-seeking intentions. *Social Science and Medicine*, *344*(6), 116593. https://doi.org/10.1016/j.socscimed.2024.116593

Siegel, J. T., Lienemann, B. A., & Rosenberg, B. D. (2017). Resistance, reactance, and misinterpretation: Highlighting the challenge of persuading people with depression to seek help. *Social and Personality Psychology Compass*, *11*, e12322. https://doi.org/10.1111/spc3.12322

Siegel, J. T., Lienemann, B. A., & Tan, C. N. (2015). Influencing help-seeking among people with elevated depressive symptomatology: Mistargeting as a persuasive technique. *Clinical Psychological Science*, *3*(2), 242–255. https://doi.org/10.1177/2167702614542846 cpx.sagepub.com

Sofka, S., Grey, C., Lerfald, N., Davisson, L., & Howsare, J. (2018). Implementing a universal well-being assessment to mitigate barriers to resident utilization of mental health resources. *Journal of Graduate Medical Education*, *10*(1), 63–66. https://doi.org/10.4300/JGMED-17-00405.1

Sofka, S., Lerfald, N., Reece, J., Davisson, L., Howsare, J., & Thompson, J. (2021). Universal well-being assessment associated with increased resident utilization of mental health resources and decrease in professionalism breaches. *Journal of Graduate Medical Education*, *13*(1), 83–88. https://doi.org/10.4300/JGME-D-20-00352.1

Stergiopoulos, E., Fragoso, L., & Meeks, L. M. (2021). Cultural barriers to help-seeking in medical education. *JAMA Internal Medicine*, *181*(2), 155–156. https://doi.org/10.1001/jamainternmed.2020.7567

Temple, J. (2014). Resident duty hours around the globe: Where are we now? *BMC Medical Education*, *14*(1), 1–5. https://doi.org/10.1186/1472-6920-14-S1-S8

Thompson, W. T., Cupples, M. E., Sibbett, C. H., Skan, D. I., & Bradley, T. (2001). Challenge of culture, conscience, and contract to general practitioners' care of their own health: Qualitative study. *BMJ: British Medical Journal*, *323*(7315), 728–731. http://www.jstor.org/stable/25467991

Vaa Stelling, B. E., & West, C. P. (2021). Faculty disclosure of personal mental health history and resident physician perceptions of stigma surrounding mental illness. *Academic Medicine*, *96*(5), 682–685. https://doi.org/10.1097/ACM.0000000000003941

Van der Kooy, K., Van Hout, H., Marwijk, H., Marten, H., Stehouwer, C., & Beekman, A. (2007). Depression and the risk for cardiovascular diseases: Systematic review and meta-analysis. *International Journal of Geriatric Psychiatry: A Journal of the Psychiatry of Late Life and Allied Sciences*, *22*(7), 613–626. https://doi.org/10.1002/gps.1723

Welcher, C. M., Radabaugh, C. L., Aparicio, A., Chaudhry, H. J., Staz, M. L., Kirk, L. M., & Bresnahan, L. (2019). Programs and resources to alleviate concerns with mental health disclosures on physician licensing applications. *Journal of Medical Regulation*, *105*(2), 24–32. https://doi.org/10.30770/2572-1852-105.2.24

Wijeratne, C., Johnco, C., Draper, B., & Earl, J. (2021). Doctors' reporting of mental health stigma and barriers to help-seeking. *Occupational Medicine*, *71*(8), 366–374. https://doi.org/10.1093/occmed/kqab119

World Health Organization. (2020). *Depression: Key Facts*. https://www.who.int/news-room/fact-sheets/detail/depression

Wu, A., Radhakrishnan, V., Targan, E., Scarella, T. M., Torous, J., & Hill, K. P. (2021). Self reported preferences for help-seeking and barriers to using mental health supports among internal medicine residents: Exploratory use of an econometric best-worst scaling framework for gathering physician wellness preferences. *JMIR Medical Education*, *7*(4), e28623. https://doi.org/10.2196/28623

Yaghmour, N. A., Brigham, T. P., Richter, T., Miller, R. S., Philibert, I., Baldwin, D. C., Jr., & Nasca, T. J. (2017). Causes of death of residents in ACGME-accredited programs 2000 through 2014: Implications for the learning environment. *Academic Medicine*, *92*(7), 976. https://doi.org/10.1097/ACM.0000000000001736

Zisook, S., Young, I., Doran, N., Downs, N., Hadley, A., Kirby, B., McGuire, T., Moutier, C., Norcross, W., & Tiamson-Kassab, M. (2016). Suicidal ideation among students and physicians at a U.S. medical school: A healer education, assessment and referral (HEAR) program report. *OMEGA - Journal of Death and Dying*, *74*(1), 35–61. https://doi.org/10.1177/0030222815598045

Appendix

Table 18.A.1 Description of Program Elements and Outcomes

Program	*Approach*	*Barriers targeted*	*Outcomes on barriers*	*Utilization outcomes*
The UCLA mental health program for physicians in training Borenstein and Cook (1982), Borenstein (1985)	Created a mental health clinic to increase availability of services	*Confidentiality and Career Implications:* • Clinic placed off-campus. • Visits off official records. *Cost:* • Short-term treatment was of no charge. • Long-term care, offered either free or discounted. *Time:* • Drew upon many volunteer physicians from UCLA with a breadth of specialties to help maximize the likelihood that appointments would be prompt.	None	• Average yearly utilization over a two-year period = 7.9% for residents • 81.1% of residents suggested for continued care after the initial appointments, went on to receive further treatment.
The house officer mental health program Pitt et al. (2004)	Created a mental health clinic to increase availability of services	*Knowledge*: • Advertised the program via email, presentations, posters and flyers. • Psychiatrists met with residency directors to provide information on identifying residents who are struggling and how to refer them to treatment. *Confidentiality:* • Services separate from training programs. *Cost:* • First five visits free. Residents could continue treatment through their insurance after first five. *Time*: • Services available around the clock.	None	• Twice as many residents used services in the first year compared to the 10-year past average utilization rate of the employee assistance program. • Utilization increased with every passing year. • 1/3rd of residents chose to keep receiving treatment after the initial sessions. • No overall utilization rates reported

(*Continued*)

Table 18.A.1 (Continued)

Program	*Approach*	*Barriers targeted*	*Outcomes on barriers*	*Utilization outcomes*
The suicide prevention and depression awareness program Moutier et al. (2012), Zisook et al. (2016)	Interactive Screening Education modules on physician depression and help seeking (i.e., presentation, AFSP video, and discussion time)	*Knowledge:* • Screening to help-residents understand their mental health status. • Counselors could refer residents to other professionals and resources. • Educational elements to inform residents about depression, and help seeking. *Stigma:* • Said they hoped stigma would be reduced through exposure to program *Confidentiality:* • Anonymous screener survey. • Could talk anonymously with the counselor online. Licensing: • Discussed barriers to help seeking such as licensing in educational module.	None	• 8% of residents and fellows completed the screener in the first year. • 33% of residents and fellows who did the screener talked online with the counselor. • 14% of residents and fellows who completed the screener met in-person with the counselor. • Later it as found that 17% of residents and fellows completed the screener over a five-year period
Secondary data analysis of interactive screening data Mortali and Moutier (2018)	Analyzed Interactive Screening data from medical schools during the 2007–2013 period	*Confidentiality:* • Anonymous screener survey. • Could talk anonymously with the counselor online. • Counselors could refer residents to other professionals and resources. *Knowledge:* • Screening to help-residents understand their mental health status. • Could talk anonymously with the counselor online.	None	• 82.4% of residents/fellows looked at the assessment from the counselor. • 37.7% of residents/fellows who looked at the assessment, talked with the counselor online. • 48.3% of residents/fellows who conversed with the counselor online, asked for a face-face appointment or referral for another mental health professional.
Resident wellness program Ey et al. (2013, 2016)	Professional psychologists and psychiatrists were made available to residents. Workshops to teach residents about help seeking.	*Knowledge:* • Counselors could refer residents to other professionals and resources. • Provided screening services. *Cost:* • Services were of no charge to residents. • Did not need to go through their health insurance.	• 88% knew about the Resident Wellness Program • 67% said time was a barrier to the resident wellness program. • 27% said helpfulness was a barrier. • 27% said stigma was a barrier.	• Utilization of mental health services was about 5% in 2004–2005. • Utilization increased to a high of 24.7% in 2013–2014.

	Workshops to teach physicians about suicide. Resident get-togethers Support groups in specific residency programs (i.e., pediatric, neonatal, medical intensive care units, and psychiatry). Interactive screening.	*Confidentiality, Career Implications:* • Kept resident records of counseling services separate from the hospital's health record system. *Licensing:* • Told residents they did not have to report their use of services to the state medical board. *Time:* • Serviced available to residents all week. • Phone line for those who needed help after work hours. • Asked chief residents and program directors to be flexible during work hours.	• 24% said reportability was a barrier. • 21% said confidentiality was a barrier.	
Opt-out Sofka et al. (2018, 2021)	Scheduled residents for appointments with a counselor at FSAP	*Knowledge:* • Increased residents' familiarity with FSAP services. • Counselors could refer residents to other professionals and resources. *Stigma:* • Scheduled all residents for an appointment to normalize it. *Confidentiality:* • FSAP services were off-site. • Counseling used separate records from training hospital. *Cost:* • Free services. • Did not have to use their paid time-off. *Time:* • Scheduled a wellness day for residents on the day of their counseling appointment when they normally would be doing out-patients or electives. • Did not have to request time-off themselves.	• The mean score for convenience of the FSAP services was 7.8, where 1 was labeled "not convenient" and 9 was labeled "very convenient." • The mean score for feeling embarrassed if colleagues found out they attended FSAP was 7.9, where 1 was labeled "very embarrassed" and 9 was labeled "not embarrassed at all."	• Over two years 93% of the residents attended the appointments. • Over four years 3.3% of residents opted out of appointments. • There was a significant increase in self-scheduled visits from the 2014–2015 year to the 2018–2019 year.

(*Continued*)

Table 18.A.1 (Continued)

Program	*Approach*	*Barriers targeted*	*Outcomes on barriers*	*Utilization outcomes*
Opt-out Kevern et al. (2023)	Scheduled residents for appointments with a mental health professional	*Stigma:* • Scheduled all residents for an appointment to normalize it. *Confidentiality:* • Programs were not told which residents chose to attend the appointments. *Cost:* • Free opt-out appointment. *Time:* • Provided protected work hours for appointment. • Telehealth appointments for convenience.	• 94% of residents surveyed who attended a scheduled appointment thought the appointment showed the training program cared about their wellness.	• 59% of residents attended the scheduled appointments. • 34% of residents who attended an initial scheduled appointment went to further appointments. • 80% of residents surveyed who attended a scheduled appointment said it increased their willingness to use services for mental health. • 98% of residents surveyed who attended a scheduled appointment said that opt-out appointments should be offered to future residents. • 96% of residents surveyed who attended a scheduled appointment were highly satisfied and said it was worthwhile. • 10% of all mental health sessions at their wellness office during the 2020-2021 academic year were opt-out appointments.
Opt-out Guldner et al. (2024)	Scheduled residents for appointments with outside counselors	*Knowledge:* • Advertised the program through announcements, screensavers and flyers. • Described some of the help-seeking benefits through their program. *Stigma:* • Scheduled all residents for an appointment to normalize it. • Had therapists virtually give an introduction to residents. *Confidentiality:* • Used third-party therapists. *Licensing:* • Counseling did not have to be reported to licensing boards, as it was part of an educational curriculum. *Cost:* • Free services. • Did not have to use their paid time-off. *Time:* • Appointments made during protected educational time. • Telehealth appointments for convenience.	None	• 55% of residents attended their pre-scheduled appointment. • 39% of residents who attended their pre-scheduled appointment initiated at least one more appointment. • Compared to a traditional opt-out condition, where only 6% of residents scheduled an appointment.

Wellness time-off policy Cedfeldt et al. (2015)	Implemented a policy that gives residents four half-days off to take care of themselves and attend appointments for their health	*Knowledge:* • Communicated the policy. • Provided lists of clinics residents and fellows could visit. *Time:* • Gave them four half-days off for appointments.	• 89% of those that were surveyed said they know about the policy. • 64% of those surveyed who used the policy said it was very easy or easy to use. • 50.9% of those who used the policy said there were no barriers to using the time-off policy. • 31.5% of those who used the policy reported concerns about how their time off would impact their co-workers. • Of those who did not use the policy, 42.5% were concerned how their time off work impact their co-workers, and 43.4% said they did not need to use the policy.	• No direct measures. • Self-reports show about 50% said they utilized the policy, and 9.7% of residents self-reported that they used it for counseling.
Faculty discourse Vaa Stelling and West (2021)	Faculty members gave talks about their mental health experiences and help seeking during a conference and had discussion time	*Knowledge:* • Gave information to residents on local mental health resources. • Faculty members discussed how they sought help and what worked for them. *Stigma:* • Important figures in the program discussing their own struggles with mental health.	• 89.7% surveyed agreed their knowledge of resources at their hospital organization increased. • 97.4% agreed that this approach helps reduce stigma.	• No direct measures. • Self-reports show 84.6% agreed they would be more likely to access mental health resources and 97.4% of residents said they contemplated their mental health afterward.

19

Communication, Equity, and Mental Well-Being: The Road Ahead

Laura Marciano, Ava Kikut-Stein, and K. Viswanath
Harvard University, Dana-Farber Cancer Institute

Three Streams of Thought

Concerns with mental health emerged on the global agenda recently, even to the extent of being dubbed an "epidemic," as highlighted in the World Health Organization's (WHO's) Comprehensive Mental Health Action Plan, 2013–2030 (WHO, 2021a). Although there are many reasons for this, one might speculate that the COVID-19 pandemic and centrality of digital media in the information ecosystem have plausibly contributed to the topic's current visibility and public concern. Yet, stressors such as poverty, discrimination, and constrained life chances have always been part of the lived experiences of many individuals in underserved and underresourced communities. As the field of mental health communication advances and evolves, it is critical that three parallel streams of thought are integrated in this area: a focus on well-being in addition to illness, consideration for social determinants of health, and the role of communication inequalities.

Beyond Mental Illness

The first stream of thought dates to the constitution of the WHO, which asserts that health is not "merely an absence of disease" but a "complete state of well-being—physical, mental and social" (WHO, 1946). The WHO accomplished three things by including this in its constitution more than seven decades ago. One, it argued for a more integrated conception of health that brings together the siloed dimensions ensuing from the specialization of medicine. Two, it averred that health should be conceived in more positive terms than focusing on deficits alone. Three, it explicitly included social health or well-being, an idea that is only now being recognized as an urgent public health concern.

Social Determinants

A second, relatively more recent, stream of thought centers on equity and shifts from putting the onus on the individual for their well-being to a focus on structural factors (Berkman & Kawachi, 2014). This model recognizes conditions that drive health fall under the umbrella term, "social determinants of health." More specifically, "social drivers of inequalities" (Viswanath, McCloud, & Bekalu, 2022) include "upstream factors," which are aspects of one's environment and life experiences, such as policies, culture, neighborhoods, segregation, and structural racism, and "downstream factors," that are

The Handbook of Mental Health Communication, First Edition.
Edited by Marco C. Yzer and Jason T. Siegel.

nonmedical individual-level characteristics, such as socioeconomic status, race, ethnicity, and gender (Braveman et al., 2011). At the heart of this framework is the idea that social conditions (upstream) can drive experiences of discrimination due to class, race, or gender and other factors (downstream) and have direct implications for mental health.

Communication Inequalities

A third, related area of work that is directly germane here is research that draws attention to communication inequalities. This body of work draws from research on social determinants of health but explicitly raises the issues of unequal access to, engagement with, processing of, and capacity to act on information, contributing to inequalities in health outcomes across different social groups (Viswanath, McCloud, & Bekalu, 2022). These latter arguments are elucidated in the Structural Influence Model (SIM; Viswanath et al., 2007), which focuses on multiple levels of social drivers that can influence individual communication factors, which in turn influence health (Viswanath, McCloud, & Bekalu, 2022) (see Figure 19.1). Exemplar social drivers include communication policies; communication institutions, including media companies and other types of organizations; community characteristics, such as distribution of resources and social power; and interpersonal factors such as social networks. All these drivers may contribute to communication inequalities (Viswanath, McCloud, & Bekalu, 2022).

Integrating Perspectives

This chapter considers mental health communication through the lens of these three interconnected areas of thought. First, we describe the potential contexts and mechanisms through which communication may influence both negative and positive mental health outcomes. Next, we consider key areas of mental health communication inequalities related to structural determinants. Finally, we draw on lessons learned in other areas of communication research to offer recommendations for mitigating inequalities in mental health communication research moving forward.

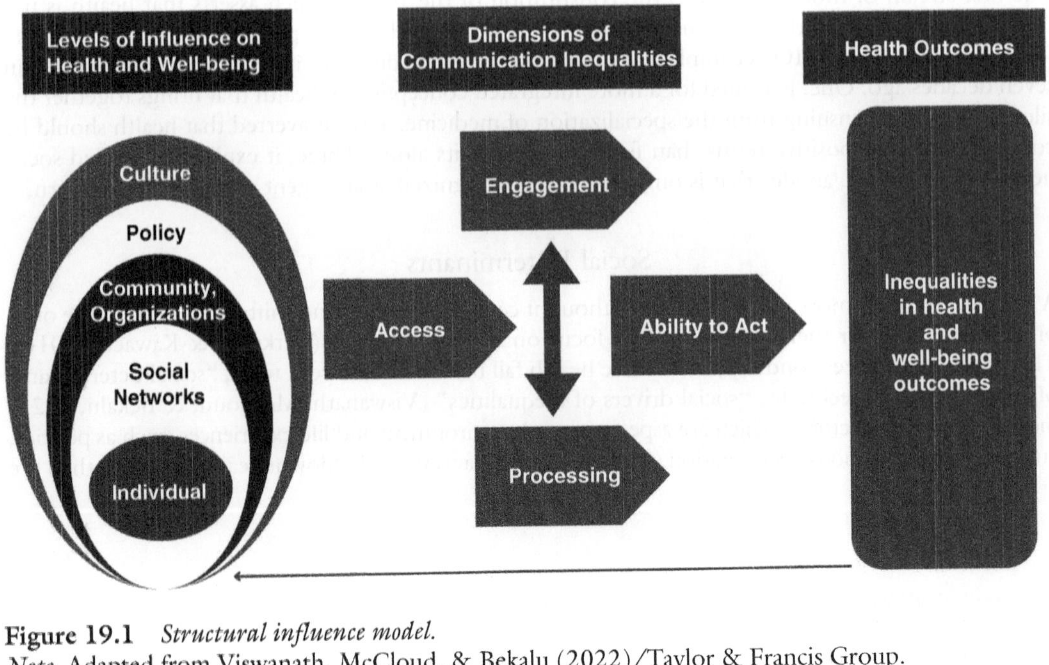

Figure 19.1 *Structural influence model.*
Note. Adapted from Viswanath, McCloud, & Bekalu (2022)/Taylor & Francis Group.

When Does Communication Influence Well-Being?

Supportive health communication is crucial in reducing stigma, promoting help-seeking behaviors, and fostering relationships that contribute to positive functioning. The latest figures from WHO show 6.9 million deaths since December 2019 (WHO, 2024). Public health communication guidelines during the pandemic encouraged creating a healthcare climate that supports people's intrinsic motivations and needs by, for example, identifying underlying rationale motivations and values, co-constructing communication material to understand needs, facilitators, and barriers, and building solidarity (Porat et al., 2020). Yet, little attention has been paid to communication inequalities during COVID-19 (Viswanath et al., 2020), and even less effort has been dedicated to mental health communication and how it was aggravated by structural inequities after the pandemic. For example, the evolving nature of science leading to changes in guidelines, competing priorities faced by those from lower socioeconomic positions, and racism (e.g. attacks on Asian Americans) could have contributed to stress and poor psychological health as well as physical health. Physical distancing guidelines might have contributed to social isolation and social ill-being for those whose work or school moved online. Meanwhile, many individuals in blue-collar occupations faced added pressure to work in conditions that heightened their risk of exposure to the virus. Both physical isolation and in-person work demands may affect information exposure and the ways in which individuals respond to public health messaging. Thus, COVID-19 is an excellent illustration of how communication inequalities can stem from structural forces and affect cross-group differences in physical, social, and psychological well-being (McCloud et al., 2024).

The COVID-19 pandemic shed light on another way communication can negatively affect well-being: through the spread of health misinformation. An umbrella review of 31 reviews (Wang et al., 2022) showed that social media platforms (including Twitter, Facebook, YouTube, and Instagram) spread between 0.2% and 28.8% of health-related misinformation, with adverse consequences, such as fostering fear and panic (Borges do Nascimento et al., 2022), negatively influencing attitudes toward healthy behaviors (Wang et al., 2022), and potentially reducing the likelihood of engaging in recommended public health behaviors, such as vaccination (Bekalu & Viswanath, 2024; Primack et al., 2021; Viswanath et al., 2021).

The role of misinformation becomes more relevant when it concerns mental health challenges, as it can increase physiological activations, protract negative mood (Feuerriegel et al., 2022), and even increase users' anxiety (Verma et al., 2022). Misinformation on social media has the potential to be harmful (Frenkel & Alba, 2021; Goel & Frenkel, 2019) especially if spread through communication with friends and family (Frenkel & Alba, 2021), and if it leads to misconceptions about mental health. Indeed, exposure to mental health misinformation has been associated with agreement with misinformation among members of online mental health communities (Bizzotto, de Bruijn et al., 2023a). These effects were heightened among those within communities that were led by peers rather than by experts and among those with low mental health literacy (Bizzotto, de Bruijn et al., 2023a). As illustrated in this example, information and misinformation exposure has the potential to influence how we think about mental health and well-being. Yet, effects may be moderated by socially driven environmental factors, like contact with experts, and individual-level factors, such as literacy and skills, which differ across groups.

How Does Communication Influence Well-Being?

Although social and individual-level variables may moderate communication effects, they may also mediate the relationship between communication and mental health. In particular, engagement with media may influence social connectedness, resilience, and coping skills, which are all predictors of well-being.

The need for social connection is rooted in human biology and lasts throughout our entire life. Well-being states are reached when social integration (i.e. a sense of belonging, ties or connections to society) is present. We know, for example, that good-quality social connections foster happiness while diminishing loneliness (Waldinger & Schulz, 2023) and act as a "social buffer" in stressful situations (Holt-Lunstad, 2022). Social support is an important protective factor against depression, especially in young adults (Rueger et al., 2016), although sources of effective social support vary from family to friends and peers (Holt-Lunstad & Proctor, 2024).

On the other hand, the lack of social support and peer rejection predicts the onset of depressive symptomatology (Nolan et al., 2003; Prinstein & Aikins, 2004; Sentse et al., 2010; Shochet et al., 2011; Witvliet et al., 2010; Young et al., 2005). Human beings experience distress when social connections are lacking or damaged and social pain shares the same neural emotional response as physical pain (Cacioppo & Patrick, 2008). The effects of poor social connection on adverse mental and physical health have been shown in prospective studies and summarized in several meta-analyses (e.g. Boehm & Kubzansky, 2012; Cohen, 2004; Holt-Lunstad et al., 2010; Roelfs et al., 2011; Shor & Roelfs, 2015). In fact, one meta-analysis showed that social isolation and loneliness were significantly associated with both morbidity and mortality (Holt-Lunstad et al., 2015).

Hence, the effects of communication on illness and well-being might pass through social experiences, for example, by shaping social support and resilience. A review of 48 studies (Bizzotto, Marciano et al., 2023b) indicated that younger generations (e.g. Gen Z) participate in online mental health support groups more than older generations, and web-based help-seeking behaviors augment feelings of empowerment. Having a wide network of peer relationships perceived as supportive makes the environment more conducive to positive, socially rewarding experiences (Durlak et al., 2011). Stewart et al. (2013) showed that friendship communication is supportive and receptive when one encourages a positive reappraisal of a stressful event and promotes positive affect, whereas media communication encourages ruminating on negative outcomes that protracted the stress response and negative feelings.

Relatedly, the extent to which digital media serves as an effective coping mechanism or tool for building coping mechanisms is still an open question. Wolfers and Schneider (2020) report that, although engagement with digital media content can encourage external coping strategies (like seeking support, exercise, or meditation), it may also be used as a coping mechanism in itself. That is, relief may be obtained from avoiding personal problems through the compulsive consumption of media. The repetitive use of media to escape becomes particularly problematic when this coping strategy is regarded as the only option ("coping inflexibility"). This is specifically important to consider during the developmental years, like the adolescent period, during which young people report high levels of screen and social media time, but their coping styles are still underdeveloped (Holt et al., 2005). In short, although there is more work to be done in this area, communication is likely to have a profound impact on mental illness and well-being by shaping how social integration is fulfilled and maintained and how we make sense of and respond to life challenges. Yet, information exposure and effects cannot be isolated from other factors and social determinants in one's environment.

Mental Health Communication Inequalities

Equity and Well-Being: Where Does Communication Fit in?

Researching mental health communication calls us to reflect on how offline determinants of positive functioning can be translated into the communication world. Health inequalities are rooted in many social factors, including housing, education, jobs, and means of communication, which can largely influence the mental health of minorities and populations living in poverty (Koh et al., 2010). For example, a report from 113 countries showed that socioeconomic inequalities not only influence the prevalence of common mental health disorders (with lower rates for higher household income) but, together with experiencing stigma and lower trust, may also affect willingness to talk to a mental health professional and the likelihood of finding a treatment helpful (Henking, 2022). However, poverty is more than low income; it encompasses nonmonetary facets such as social exclusion and vulnerability, as well as denial of opportunities and absence of choice (Saxena et al., 2007). People with mental health illnesses still largely struggle from experiencing stigma and marginalization for their diagnosis, to the point that mental health consequences of experiencing stigma could be perceived as worse than the condition itself (Lancet, 2016).

In this dynamic, communication inequalities (Spanakis et al., 2024), may influence mental ill-being and well-being status. Access alone is not sufficient. The quality of access matters too. For example, people experiencing similar communication access, skills, and activities may still report diverse well-being outcomes. Many groups experiencing digital inequalities also lack proper mental health support and access to other health resources (Viswanath & Kreuter, 2007). Mental health communication pathways should be designed to overcome inequities and foster people's well-being and their striving for virtue by fulfilling the human needs of autonomy, competence, and relatedness (Ryan & Deci, 2000) rather than exacerbating disparities. Yet, there has been limited attention to inequalities in communication (social and mass media) that can exacerbate stigma and inequalities in health outcomes (Viswanath et al., 2020).

Four Key Areas of Communication Inequalities

As explained earlier, the SIM in communication draws attention to the relationship between multilevel factors that influence health and dimensions of communication: access/exposure, engagement, processing and acting on information (Viswanath, McCloud, & Bekalu, 2022). For example, structural factors such as physical environments, structural racism (Bailey, 2024), and socioeconomic factors influence the relationships between media and mental health. Drawing from the SIM, four areas of potential inequalities include (a) exposure to media content that can harm mental health, (b) adverse mental health effects because of media exposure, (c) lower exposure to beneficial mental health promotion and resource information, and (d) higher risk of unintended adverse mental health effects because of mental health promotion messaging.

Exposure to Harmful Content

In general, cross-group differences in media exposure parallel broader structural inequalities and unmet mental health needs. For example, in the United States, more than half of Black and Hispanic/Latino teens report spending time online "almost constantly" (respectively, 56% and 55% compared to 37% of non-Hispanic White teens; Vogels et al., 2022). Environmental factors, including limited safe spaces for social gathering and entertainment, may contribute to a higher need for virtual gathering spaces and messaging platforms among racial and ethnic minority youth in urban and lower-resourced settings. Due to structural racism, poverty and gun violence disproportionately affects neighborhoods that are poorer and racially segregated (Creamer, 2020; Johnson et al., 2021). In 2021, Black and Hispanic/Latino high school students were twice as likely as non-Hispanic White high school students to have witnessed a violent crime in their neighborhoods (respectively, 29.3% and 26.2% compared to 14.8%) and to report missing school due to feeling unsafe getting to school (12.1% and 11.3% compared to 6.6%; Centers for Disease Control and Prevention [CDC], 2021). Compounding the presence of violence, access to urban vegetation and green spaces, such as city parks, greenways, and gardens, which is associated with positive mental health outcomes (Beyer et al., 2014), is unevenly distributed by race and socioeconomic status. Overall, urban vegetation and green space are scarce in urban neighborhoods that are majority racial/ethnic minority and lower income compared to those that are majority White and higher income (Dai, 2011; Nesbitt et al., 2019). In communities with unsafe physical environments, in-person social gathering, and mental health, social media offers virtual opportunities for entertainment, connection, and coping.

Although media exposure per se is not a risk factor for adverse mental health outcomes, higher ***total*** exposure may be connected to a higher probability of ***harmful*** content exposure. Stressors in one's physical environment may contribute to exposure to media content that threatens mental health. For example, individuals living in neighborhoods with high rates of gun violence and police brutality may witness videos or images of these incidents on the news and on social media (Motley et al., 2020). One study of Black teens living in neighborhoods disproportionately affected by violent crime described how participants' online environments "mirrored the harsh social realities of their communities," thus exacerbating feelings of unsafety and threats to well-being (Stevens et al., 2017). In addition to first-hand experiences with violence, second-hand exposure to traumatic events online has been associated with symptoms of depression and posttraumatic stress disorder (PTSD; Tynes et al., 2019).

This brief review suggests that all the attention to exposure to "harmful content" and time spent online or with media paints an incomplete picture of media exposure and mental health when it is divorced from the structural conditions in which people live their lives. Neighborhood conditions may impel people to spend time on media, increasing the potential for exposure to all kinds of content including harmful content. The reciprocal relationship between social conditions, such as structural racism and neighborhood violence, media use and exposure, and psychological and social well-being remain unexplored. Any efforts to regulate media content without addressing the larger social conditions may seem feasible but will fail to truly mitigate inequalities.

Effects of Exposure to Harmful Content

In addition to inequalities in the volume and types of media exposure, structural inequalities may affect cross-group differences in the *effects* of media exposure. One of the earliest examples of exposure to harmful content and its impact on cognitive and affective outcomes was explicated through the *Cultivation Hypothesis* that proposed how exposure to televised violence is likely to increase fear of victimization (Gerbner et al., 1994). Although the authors did not explicitly frame *Cultivation* in terms of communication inequalities, and in fact argued that effects are uniform if one is a heavy user, a meta question is the extent to which heavy exposure to harmful content whether on television, video games and social media (a) is more likely among certain groups and (b) affects different groups differently. Given the variation in the use of and exposure to mass and digital media among different socioeconomic, racial, and ethnic groups, it is imperative to do more work in this area.

The ways in which media institutions portray race and racial stereotypes, an example of structural racism, is relevant to explaining media content and media effects (Bailey, 2024; Bailey et al., 2017). For example, systemic racism and trauma may contribute to internalization of related media content. Prior work has shown that identification with the victim of a witnessed violent crime is associated with personalization and negative emotional reactions (Becker-Blease et al., 2008). Witnessing police violence on social media was associated with increased feelings of sadness, anger, and fear among Black men (Motley et al., 2020). Similarly, exposure to traumatic events online has been associated with PTSD and depressive symptoms among Black and Hispanic/Latino youth (Tynes et al., 2019). The risks of these adverse mental health outcomes are higher among those who live close to the area of the crime (Pine et al., 2005) or have experienced similar violence (Moore et al., 2016). In addition, groups who are at higher risk of social isolation, like those living in rural communities or isolated urban settings, recent immigrants, and older people, may have limited opportunities to socially process the media they consume (Umberson & Donnelly, 2023) and may experience more emotional distress as a result of harmful media, such as online fraud (Kemp & Erodes Pérez, 2023). In general, similar factors that contribute to adverse mental health outcomes in the offline world, including structural racism, social isolation, and lack of social support, may exacerbate the risks of harmful media content for mental health.

Exposure to Beneficial Content

Just as harmful media effects can mirror general mental health risks in one's physical environment, access to beneficial media content mirrors access to health resources more generally. As with other health resources, access to mental health counseling and support is limited in lower socioeconomic status, racial, and ethnic minority communities compared to higher socioeconomic status and majority-White communities (Cook et al., 2017; Rodgers et al., 2022). Yet, even when mental health resources are available, there are inequalities in resource use (Dobalian & Rivers, 2008). For example, although conversations with physicians offer opportunities for information sharing about mental health resources, treatments, and coping strategies, Black and Hispanic/Latino patients are 40% less likely than White and non-Hispanic patients to have a mental health concern addressed during a primary care visit (Rotenstein et al., 2023). Further, low-income households are less likely to have internet at home, due to both costs and lack of broadband infrastructure, and are more likely to rely on cellphones for internet use (Anderson, 2019; Dolcini et al., 2021), a phenomenon characterized as "smartphone dependency" (Gelles-Watnick, 2024). Smartphone-only internet access limits health information access; it raises challenges for connectivity, speed, and compatibility between devices and health delivery platforms (Dolcini et al., 2021). These inequalities may contribute to disparities in support resource use (Matthews et al., 2023). Although current policy initiatives are focused on addressing the need for broadband access in rural areas, there remains an unmet need to expand broadband access in poorer urban neighborhoods (Porter, 2021, Viswanath, McCloud and Bekalu, 2022).

Effects of Exposure to Beneficial Content

A fourth, and final, area of mental health communication inequalities is the disproportionate adverse effects of well-intended mental health communication. Although increasing access to available resources, and information about these resources, is critical, attention should also be paid to the potential for systems of support to perpetuate inequalities. In particular, in Black communities, mental illness has been historically criminalized (Beckmann et al., 2019). Individuals may refrain from seeking mental health support due to past individual or community experiences with racial discrimination and criminalization. A similar challenge arises for youth mental health support, as mandated reporter policies have long had harsher consequences for Black families compared to White families (Inguanta & Sciolla, 2021; Roberts, 2022). For example, Black children are three times as likely as White children to have had contact with child protective services (Maloney et al., 2017) and face 44% higher odds of foster care placement (Knott & Donovan, 2010). Black youth may be uncomfortable using available support resources, and confiding in a school counselor, teacher, helpline operator, or other mandated reporter, for fear of separation from parents (Lindsey et al., 2013). Thus, communication interventions promoting available mental health support should consider the potential for the resources themselves to perpetuate harm. Transparency around the requirements of mandated reporting (i.e. what kind of information must be reported and what kind cannot be shared), for example, may help rebuild trust and self-efficacy around resource use.

Promoting Equity in Mental Health Communication: Some Desiderata

Public and policy discourses in communication on mental well-being have, one may argue, failed by focusing on "illness" and "deficits" instead of defining health in more positive terms and focusing on assets and resilience. Such failure has extracted a considerable price in the form of misplaced policy and research priorities that are misaligned with the real needs, perpetuating inequalities and developing and implementing interventions that increase stigma and labeling. Three streams of thought shape the argument of this essay: a focus on well-being, social determinants, and communication inequalities. Drawing from these areas of thought, we believe that it is time to reframe the conversation in three important ways.

First, we contend that scholarship and practice may focus not just on mental illness or absence and treatment of illness but take a more integrated approach to health and well-being by connecting it to other dimensions of health: Physical and social well-being in line with the WHO's definition of health. The recent attention by the US Surgeon General to the "loneliness crisis" provides a policy window on developing an aggressive and active agenda for research and practice around social well-being (Office of the Surgeon General, 2023). Attributing social problems to social media is insufficient and even misleading. Is it likely that social drivers of inequities, for example, residential segregation and lack of neighborhood safety, lead people to spend more time with media or online, and therefore harmful content, leading to mental health communication inequalities including psychological and social well-being? Empirical evidence is sorely needed to shed light on this issue. Otherwise, not only will social well-being remain underexplored but also any policies and practices designed to improve well-being, especially through social media, may prove more harmful than beneficial. At the end of the day, drawing on communication science to explain harmful or beneficial psychological and social well-being outcomes requires that attention is also paid to the lived reality of those who suffer disproportionately from disease burden to ensure equity in mental health.

A second imperative is to improve research examining and addressing social determinants of health. Key to this imperative is reducing ***data absenteeism***. In general, individuals in communities that are overaffected by health inequalities are underrepresented in health and science communication research, limiting knowledge on how to prevent, detect, and treat mental illness and mental health communication inequalities (Lee & Viswanath, 2020; Viswanath, McCloud, Lee, & Bekalu, 2022). Just as structural inequalities contribute to inequitable distribution of well-being, health resources, information, and impact, they also contribute to limitations in the data needed to understand and address these issues. There is now a need to further research vulnerability factors that moderate the emotional responses in specific groups of users, considering different ages and contexts, and more consideration should be given to social media markets in low-income countries (LICs; Bekalu et al., 2023) and specific users at risk of developing negative outcomes. In particular, a bibliometric and thematic analysis covering the last 60 years (Mheidly & Fares, 2020) showed that, in LICs, health communication is mainly focused on promoting HIV awareness and prevention, followed by communication on infectious diseases. However, mental health communication is still largely undeveloped. The poorest countries use the lowest percentages of health budgets for mental health, and available scarce resources are also inequitably distributed among LICs, regions, and communities. In economically deprived contexts, those who have the highest need for mental health care also have the lowest access to it (Saxena et al., 2007). Moving forward, inclusive and equity-focused data collection practices are critical for addressing mental health communication needs and inequalities (Branquinho et al., 2020; Jones et al., 2020; Wallerstein & Duran, 2010).

Finally, our years of work on social change shows that participatory and inclusive approaches go hand in hand with asset-oriented approaches, supporting inclusive data collection practices, understanding social determinants of health, and addressing communication inequalities. Through community-based participatory research (CBPR), communities co-define the challenges and the solutions to improving health and well-being, including mental health. The long-established program of research in community-based participatory approaches in public health and its application in health communication shows pathways by which partnership with and engagement of community-based organizations could help address inequalities by drawing on community assets and developing and implementing appropriate and localized solutions (Kaholokula et al., 2024). Although we know a lot about mental health, communication can be instrumental in the translation of knowledge to influence practice or policy (Ramanadhan & Viswanath, 2018). For example, in one CBPR program, Black teens in West Philadelphia identified mental health as a priority in their peer communities, researched available resources, and created campaign messages sharing resource information with peers (Kikut, 2023). Youth in this program reported stronger mental health coping skills, a sense of support, and media literacy skills due to participating in CBPR. Teens in the broader community reported higher self-efficacy and intention to use the recommended resource as a result of viewing messages created by their peers (Kikut-Stein et al., 2024). This example suggests participatory approaches offer promise for both informing mental health communication knowledge and applying what is known in the field to addressing community-identified challenges.

Concluding Thoughts

This chapter draws on an asset-oriented focus on well-being as well as illness, focus on social determinants, and recognition of communication inequalities. These three streams impel us to focus beyond “mental illness” and health to a broader conception of equity-centered well-being—psychological, physical, and social. Attention could expand beyond illness to more positive conceptions, including hedonic (e.g. life satisfaction and positive emotions, Ryan & Deci, 2001) and eudemonic well-being (e.g. autonomy, personal growth, self-acceptance, life purpose, mastery, and positive relatedness; Ryff, 1989). However, we argue that a focus on purely individual well-being, hedonic or eudemonic, is still an incomplete conception of well-being without paying attention to social factors that influence them. For example, although underexplored, social health—such as connections to the community, access to social capital, and social integration—buffer the impact of stressors on individual psychological states and overall health (Berkman et al., 2000; Kawachi & Berkman, 2014; Moore & Kawachi, 2017). These ideas become relevant as practitioners, policy makers, and scholars increasingly pay attention to the health consequences of social isolation, loneliness, and communication. Social factors are also relevant in the context of how social networks, social support, and media use can buffer such consequences (Holt-Lunstad et al., 2015; Marciano et al., 2024; Valente, 2024). In summary, there is a critical need for a focus beyond illness to well-being in *all* its dimensions, for centering equity to understand the roles of communication in psychological well-being, and for drawing on the expertise of diverse communities in addressing mental health communication needs and inequalities.

References

Anderson, M. (2019, June 13). *Mobile technology and home broadband 2019.* Pew Research Center: Internet, Science & Tech. https://www.pewresearch.org/internet/2019/06/13/mobile-technology-and-home-broadband-2019

Bailey, Z. (2024). Race, health and equity. In K. Glanz, B. K. Rimer, & K. Viswanath (Eds.), *Health behavior: Theory, research, and practice* (6th ed.). Wiley.

Bailey, Z. D., Krieger, N., Agénor, M., Graves, J., Linos, N., & Bassett, M. T. (2017). Structural racism and health inequities in the USA: Evidence and interventions. *Lancet, 389*(10077), 1453–1463. https://doi.org/10.1016/S0140-6736(17)30569-X

Becker-Blease, K. A., Finkelhor, D., & Turner, H. (2008). Media exposure predicts children's reactions to crime and terrorism. *Journal of Trauma & Dissociation, 9*(2), 225–248. https://doi.org/10.1080/15299730802048652

Beckmann, D., Shtasel, D., & Myrick, K. (2019). Mental illness, addiction, and incarceration: Breaking the cycle. In M. M. Medlock, D. Shtasel, N. H. T. Trinh, & D. R. Williams (Eds.), *Racism and psychiatry* (pp. 71–86). Springer International Publishing. https://doi.org/10.1007/978-3-319-90197-8_5

Bekalu, M., & Viswanath, K. (2024). Social media and health. In K. Glanz, B. K. Rimer, & K. Viswanath (Eds.), *Health behavior: Theory, research, and practice* (6th ed.). Wiley.

Bekalu, M. A., Sato, T., & Viswanath, K. (2023). Conceptualizing and measuring social media use in health and well-being studies: Systematic review. *Journal of Medical Internet Research, 25*, e43191.

Berkman, L., & Kawachi, I. (2014). A historical framework for social epidemiology. In L. Berkman, I. Kawachi, & M. M. Glymour (Eds.), *Social epidemiology* (pp. 1–16). Oxford University Press. https://doi.org/10.1093/med/9780195377903.003.0001

Berkman, L. F., Glass, T., Brissette, I., & Seeman, T. E. (2000). From social integration to health: Durkheim in the new millennium. *Social Science & Medicine, 51*(6), 843–857. https://doi.org/10.1016/S0277-9536(00)00065-4

Beyer, K., Kaltenbach, A., Szabo, A., Bogar, S., Nieto, F., & Malecki, K. (2014). Exposure to neighborhood green space and mental health: Evidence from the Survey of the Health of Wisconsin. *International Journal of Environmental Research and Public Health, 11*(3), 3453–3472. https://doi.org/10.3390/ijerph110303453

Bizzotto, N., de Bruijn, G.-J., & Schulz, P. J. (2023a). Buffering against exposure to mental health misinformation in online communities on Facebook: The interplay of depression literacy and expert moderation. *BMC Public Health, 23*(1), 1577. https://doi.org/10.1186/s12889-023-16404-1

Bizzotto, N., Marciano, L., de Bruijn, G.-J., & Schulz, P. J. (2023b). The empowering role of web-based help-seeking on depressive symptoms: Systematic review and meta-analysis. *Journal of Medical Internet Research, 25*, e36964. https://doi.org/10.2196/36964

Boehm, J. K., & Kubzansky, L. D. (2012). The heart's content: The association between positive psychological well-being and cardiovascular health. *Psychological Bulletin, 138*(4), 655–691. https://doi.org/10.1037/a0027448

Borges do Nascimento, I. J., Pizarro, A. B., Almeida, J. M., Azzopardi-Muscat, N., Gonçalves, M. A., Björklund, M., & Novillo-Ortiz, D. (2022). Infodemics and health misinformation: A systematic review of reviews. *Bulletin of the World Health Organization, 100*(9), 544–561. https://doi.org/10.2471/BLT.21.287654

Branquinho, C., Tomé, G., Grothausen, T., & Gaspar de Matos, M. (2020). Community-based youth participatory action research studies with a focus on youth health and well-being: A systematic review. *Journal of Community Psychology, 48*(5), 1301–1315. https://doi.org/10.1002/jcop.22320

Braveman, P., Egerter, S., & Williams, D. R. (2011). The social determinants of health: Coming of age. *Annual Review of Public Health, 32*, 381–398. https://doi.org/10.1146/annurev-publhealth-031210-101218

Cacioppo, J. T., & Patrick, W. (2008). *Loneliness: Human nature and the need for social connection.* W. W. Norton & Co.

Centers for Disease Control and Prevention. (2021). *1991–2021 high school youth risk behavior survey data.* Retrieved July 31, 2024, from https://nccd.cdc.gov/Youthonline/App/Default.aspx

Cohen, S. (2004). Social relationships and health. *American Psychologist, 59*(8), 676–684. https://doi.org/10.1037/0003-066X.59.8.676

Cook, B. L., Trinh, N.-H., Li, Z., Hou, S. S.-Y., & Progovac, A. M. (2017). Trends in racial-ethnic disparities in access to mental health care, 2004–2012. *Psychiatric Services, 68*(1), 9–16. https://doi.org/10.1176/appi.ps.201500453

Creamer, J. (2020). *Inequalities persist despite decline in poverty for all major race and Hispanic origin groups.* US Census Bureau.https://www.census.gov/library/stories/2020/09/poverty-rates-for-blacks-and-hispanics-reached-historic-lows-in-2019.html

Dai, D. (2011). Racial/ethnic and socioeconomic disparities in urban green space accessibility: Where to intervene? *Landscape and Urban Planning, 102*(4), 234–244. https://doi.org/10.1016/j.landurbplan.2011.05.002

Dobalian, A., & Rivers, P. A. (2008). Racial and ethnic disparities in the use of mental health services. *Journal of Behavioral Health Services & Research, 35*(2), 128–141. https://doi.org/10.1007/s11414-007-9097-8

Dolcini, M. M., Canchola, J. A., Catania, J. A., Song Mayeda, M. M., Dietz, E. L., Cotto-Negrón, C., & Narayanan, V. (2021). National-level disparities in internet access among low-income and Black and Hispanic youth: Current Population Survey. *Journal of Medical Internet Research, 23*(10), e27723. https://doi.org/10.2196/27723

Durlak, J. A., Weissberg, R. P., Dymnicki, A. B., Taylor, R. D., & Schellinger, K. B. (2011). The impact of enhancing students' social and emotional learning: A meta-analysis of school-based universal interventions. *Child Development, 82*(1), 405–432. https://doi.org/10.1111/j.1467-8624.2010.01564.x

Feuerriegel, S., Robertson, C., Pröllochs, N., Schwarzenegger, K., Pärnamets, P., & Van Bavel, J. J. (2022). *Negativity drives online news consumption [Registered Report Stage 1 Protocol].* https://doi.org/10.6084/m9.figshare.19657452.v1

Frenkel, S., & Alba, D. (2021, October 23). In India, Facebook grapples with an amplified version of its problems. *New York Times.* https://www.nytimes.com/2021/10/23/technology/facebook-india-misinformation.html

Gelles-Watnick, R. (2024, January 31). *Americans' use of mobile technology and home broadband.* Pew Research Center. https://www.pewresearch.org/internet/2024/01/31/americans-use-of-mobile-technology-and-home-broadband

Gerbner, G., Gross, L., Morgan, M., & Signorelli, N. (1994). Growing up with television: The cultivation perspective. In J. Bryant & D. Zillmann (Eds.), *Media effects: Advances in theory and research* (pp. 17–41). Lawrence Erlbaum Associates, Inc.

Goel, V., & Frenkel, S. (2019, April 1). In India election, false posts and hate speech flummox Facebook. *New York Times.* https://www.nytimes.com/2019/04/01/technology/india-elections-facebook.html

Henking, C. (2022). Inequalities in common mental health disorders: Understanding the predictors of lifetime prevalence, treatment utilisation, and helpfulness across 113 countries. *Lancet, 400*, S45. https://doi.org/10.1016/S0140-6736(22)02255-3

Holt, N. L., Hoar, S., & Fraser, S. N. (2005). How does coping change with development? A review of childhood and adolescence sport coping research. *European Journal of Sport Science, 5*(1), 25–39. https://doi.org/10.1080/17461390500076915

Holt-Lunstad, J. (2022). Social connection as a public health issue: The evidence and a systemic framework for prioritizing the "social" in social determinants of health. *Annual Review of Public Health, 43*(1), 193–213. https://doi.org/10.1146/annurev-publhealth-052020-110732

Holt-Lunstad, J., & Proctor, A. S. (2024). Social support and health. In K. Glanz, B. K. Rimer, & K. Viswanath (Eds.), *Health behavior: Theory, research, and practice* (6th ed.). Wiley.

Holt-Lunstad, J., Smith, T. B., Baker, M., Harris, T., & Stephenson, D. (2015). Loneliness and social isolation as risk factors for mortality: A meta-analytic review. *Perspectives on Psychological Science, 10*(2), 227–237. https://doi.org/10.1177/1745691614568352

Holt-Lunstad, J., Smith, T. B., & Layton, J. B. (2010). Social relationships and mortality risk: A meta-analytic review. *PLoS Medicine, 7*(7), e1000316. https://doi.org/10.1371/journal.pmed.1000316

Inguanta, G., & Sciolla, C. (2021). Time doesn't heal all wounds: A call to end mandated reporting laws. *Columbia Social Work Review, 19*(1), Article 1. https://doi.org/10.52214/cswr.v19i1.7403

Johnson, B. T., Sisti, A., Bernstein, M., Chen, K., Hennessy, E. A., Acabchuk, R. L., & Matos, M. (2021). Community-level factors and incidence of gun violence in the United States, 2014–2017. *Social Science & Medicine, 280*, 113969. https://doi.org/10.1016/j.socscimed.2021.113969

Jones, D. E., Lindquist-Grantz, R., & DeJonckheere, M. (2020). A review of mixed methods community-based participatory research applications in mental health. *Journal of Social, Behavioral, and Health Sciences, 14*(1), 254–288. https://doi.org/10.5590/JSBHS.2020.14.1.18

Kaholokula, J. K., Oetzel, J. G., Sinclair, K. A., & Tupai-Fiestone, R. (2024). Improving health through community engagement: Research & practice. In K. Glanz, B. K. Rimer, & K. Viswanath (Eds.), *Health behavior: Theory, research, and practice* (6th ed.). Wiley.

Kawachi, I., & Berkman, L. (2014). Social cohesion, social capital, and health. In L. Berkman, I. Kawachi, & M. M. Glymour (Eds.), *Social epidemiology* (pp. 290–319). Oxford University Press. https://doi.org/10.1093/med/9780195377903.003.0008

Kemp, S., & Erades Pérez, N. (2023). Consumer fraud against older adults in digital society: Examining victimization and its impact. *International Journal of Environmental Research and Public Health, 20*(7), 5404. https://doi.org/10.3390/ijerph20075404

Kikut, A. (2023). *What you know or who you trust? Examining the main and interactive effects of behavioral beliefs and source trust on prevention behaviors throughout the covid-19 pandemic with longitudinal survey, experimental, and youth participatory action research* [Doctoral dissertation]. University of Pennsylvania. https://repository.upenn.edu/handle/20.500.14332/59171

Kikut-Stein, A., Givan, K., Branson, P., Fishman, J., Baily, K., Paolicelli, M., Crockett, T., Morris, T., Adesipo, A., Allen, D., Blanco-Liz, A., Bonds, L., Brooks, N., Carriker, M., Francis, K., Jean Pierre, M., Konner, H., Morris, T., Myers, R., . . . Tan, A. (2024). Youth participatory action communication research: A model for developing youth-driven health campaigns. *Health Communication*, 1–16. https://doi.org/10.1080/10410236.2024.2386713

Knott, T., & Donovan, K. (2010). Disproportionate representation of African American children in foster care: Secondary analysis of the National Child Abuse and Neglect Data System, 2005. *Children and Youth Services Review*, *32*(5), 679–684. https://doi.org/10.1016/j.childyouth.2010.01.003

Koh, H. K., Oppenheimer, S. C., Massin-Short, S. B., Emmons, K. M., Geller, A. C., & Viswanath, K. (2010). Translating research evidence into practice to reduce health disparities: A social determinants approach. *American Journal of Public Health*, *100*(S1), S72–S80. https://doi.org/10.2105/AJPH.2009.167353

Lancet. (2016). The health crisis of mental health stigma. *Lancet*, *387*(10023), 1027. https://doi.org/10.1016/S0140-6736(16)00687-5

Lee, E. W. J., & Viswanath, K. (2020). Big data in context: Addressing the twin perils of data absenteeism and chauvinism in the context of health disparities research. *Journal of Medical Internet Research*, *22*(1), e16377. https://doi.org/10.2196/16377

Lindsey, M. A., Chambers, K., Pohle, C., Beall, P., & Lucksted, A. (2013). Understanding the behavioral determinants of mental health service use by urban, under-resourced Black youth: Adolescent and caregiver perspectives. *Journal of Child and Family Studies*, *22*(1), 107–121. https://doi.org/10.1007/s10826-012-9668-z

Maloney, T., Jiang, N., Putnam-Hornstein, E., Dalton, E., & Vaithianathan, R. (2017). Black–white differences in child maltreatment reports and foster care placements: A statistical decomposition using linked administrative data. *Maternal and Child Health Journal*, *21*(3), 414–420. https://doi.org/10.1007/s10995-016-2242-3

Marciano, L., Lin, J., Sato, T., Saboor, S., & Viswanath, K. (2024). Does social media use make us happy? A meta-analysis on social media and positive well-being outcomes. *SSM – Mental Health*, *6*, 100331. https://doi.org/10.1016/j.ssmmh.2024.100331

Matthews, S., Cantor, J. H., Brooks Holliday, S., Eberhart, N. K., Breslau, J., Bialas, A., & McBain, R. K. (2023). Mental health emergency hotlines in the United States: A scoping review (2012–2021). *Psychiatric Services*, *74*(5), 513–522. https://doi.org/10.1176/appi.ps.20220128

McCloud, R. F., Bekalu, M., & Viswanath, K. (2024). Public health communication and equity in the COVID-19 pandemic. In D. T. Duncan, I. Kawachi, & S. S. Morse (Eds.), *The social epidemiology of the COVID-19 pandemic*. Oxford University Press.

Mheidly, N., & Fares, J. (2020). Health communication in low-income countries: A 60-year bibliometric and thematic analysis. *Journal of Education and Health Promotion*, *9*, 163. https://doi.org/10.4103/jehp.jehp_384_20

Moore, S., & Kawachi, I. (2017). Twenty years of social capital and health research: A glossary. *Journal of Epidemiology & Community Health*, *71*(5), 513–517. https://doi.org/10.1136/jech-2016-208313

Moore, S. E., Robinson, M. A., Adedoyin, A. C., Brooks, M., Harmon, D. K., & Boamah, D. (2016). Hands up—Don't shoot: Police shooting of young black males: Implications for social work and human services. *Journal of Human Behavior in the Social Environment*, *26*(3–4), 254–266. https://doi.org/10.1080/10911359.2015.1125202

Motley, R. O., Chen, Y.-C., Johnson, C., & Joe, S. (2020). Exposure to community-based violence on social media among Black male emerging adults involved with the criminal justice system. *Social Work Research*, *44*(2), 87–97. https://doi.org/10.1093/swr/svaa002

Nesbitt, L., Meitner, M. J., Girling, C., Sheppard, S. R. J., & Lu, Y. (2019). Who has access to urban vegetation? A spatial analysis of distributional green equity in 10 US cities. *Landscape and Urban Planning*, *181*, 51–79. https://doi.org/10.1016/j.landurbplan.2018.08.007

Nolan, S., Flynn, C., & Garber, J. (2003). Prospective relations between rejection and depression in young adolescents. *Journal of Personality and Social Psychology*, *85*, 745–755. https://doi.org/10.1037/0022-3514.85.4.745

Pine, D. S., Costello, J., & Masten, A. (2005). Trauma, proximity, and developmental psychopathology: The effects of war and terrorism on children. *Neuropsychopharmacology*, *30*(10), 1781–1792. https://doi.org/10.1038/sj.npp.1300814

Porat, T., Nyrup, R., Calvo, R. A., Paudyal, P., & Ford, E. (2020). Public health and risk communication during COVID-19—Enhancing psychological needs to promote sustainable behavior change. *Frontiers in Public Health*, *8*, 573397. https://doi.org/10.3389/fpubh.2020.573397

Porter, E. (2021, June 1). A rural–urban broadband divide, but not the one you think of. *New York Times*. https://www.nytimes.com/2021/06/01/business/rural-urban-broadband-biden.html

Primack, B. A., Shensa, A., Sidani, J. E., Escobar-Viera, C. G., & Fine, M. J. (2021). Temporal associations between social media use and depression. *American Journal of Preventive Medicine*, *60*(2), 179–188. https://doi.org/10.1016/j.amepre.2020.09.014

Prinstein, M. J., & Aikins, J. W. (2004). Cognitive moderators of the longitudinal association between peer rejection and adolescent depressive symptoms. *Journal of Abnormal Child Psychology*, *32*(2), 147–158. https://doi.org/10.1023/B:JACP.0000019767.55592.63

Ramanadhan, S. R., & Viswanath, K. (2018). Engaging communities to improve health: Models, evidence, and the participatory knowledge translation (PaKT) framework. In E. B. Fisher, L. D. Cameron, A. J. Christensen, U. Ehlert, Y. Guo, B. Oldenburg, & F. J. Snoek (Eds.), *Principles and concepts of behavioral medicine: A global handbook* (pp. 679–711). Springer.

Roberts, D. E. (2022). *Torn apart: How the child welfare system destroys Black families—And how abolition can build a safer world*. Basic Books.

Rodgers, C. R. R., Flores, M. W., Bassey, O., Augenblick, J. M., & Cook, B. L. (2022). Racial/ethnic disparity trends in children's mental health care access and expenditures from 2010–2017: Disparities remain despite sweeping policy reform. *Journal of the American Academy of Child & Adolescent Psychiatry*, *61*(7), 915–925. https://doi.org/10.1016/j.jaac.2021.09.420

Roelfs, D. J., Shor, E., Kalish, R., & Yogev, T. (2011). The rising relative risk of mortality for singles: Meta-analysis and meta-regression. *American Journal of Epidemiology*, *174*(4), 379–389. https://doi.org/10.1093/aje/kwr111

Rotenstein, L. S., Edwards, S. T., & Landon, B. E. (2023). Adult primary care physician visits increasingly address mental health concerns: Study examines primary care physician visits for mental health concerns. *Health Affairs*, *42*(2), 163–171. https://doi.org/10.1377/hlthaff.2022.00705

Rueger, S. Y., Malecki, C. K., Pyun, Y., Aycock, C., & Coyle, S. (2016). A meta-analytic review of the association between perceived social support and depression in childhood and adolescence. *Psychological Bulletin*, *142*(10), 1017–1067. https://doi.org/10.1037/bul0000058

Ryan, R. M., & Deci, E. L. (2000). Self-determination theory and the facilitation of intrinsic motivation, social development, and well-being. *American Psychologist*, *55*(1), 68–78. https://doi.org/10.1037/0003-066X.55.1.68

Ryan, R. M., & Deci, E. L. (2001). On happiness and human potentials: A review of research on hedonic and eudaimonic well-being. *Annual Review of Psychology*, *52*(1), 141–166. https://doi.org/10.1146/annurev.psych.52.1.141

Ryff, C. D. (1989). Happiness is everything, or is it? Explorations on the meaning of psychological well-being. *Journal of Personality and Social Psychology*, *57*(6), 1069–1081. https://doi.org/10.1037/0022-3514.57.6.1069

Saxena, S., Thornicroft, G., Knapp, M., & Whiteford, H. (2007). Resources for mental health: Scarcity, inequity, and inefficiency. *Lancet*, *370*(9590), 878–889. https://doi.org/10.1016/S0140-6736(07)61239-2

Sentse, M., Lindenberg, S., Omvlee, A., Ormel, J., & Veenstra, R. (2010). Rejection and acceptance across contexts: Parents and peers as risks and buffers for early adolescent psychopathology. The TRAILS study. *Journal of Abnormal Child Psychology*, *38*(1), 119–130. https://doi.org/10.1007/s10802-009-9351-z

Shochet, I. M., Smith, C. L., Furlong, M. J., & Homel, R. (2011). A prospective study investigating the impact of school belonging factors on negative affect in adolescents. *Journal of Clinical Child and Adolescent Psychology*, *40*(4), 586–595. https://doi.org/10.1080/15374416.2011.581616

Shor, E., & Roelfs, D. J. (2015). Social contact frequency and all-cause mortality: A meta-analysis and meta-regression. *Social Science & Medicine*, *128*, 76–86. https://doi.org/10.1016/j.socscimed.2015.01.010

Spanakis, P., Wadman, R., Walker, L., Heron, P., Mathers, A., Baker, J., Johnston, G., Gilbody, S., & Peckham, E. (2024). Measuring the digital divide among people with severe mental ill health using the essential digital skills framework. *Perspectives in Public Health*, *144*(1), 21–30. https://doi.org/10.1177/17579139221106399

Stevens, R., Gilliard-Matthews, S., Dunaev, J., Woods, M. K., & Brawner, B. M. (2017). The digital hood: Social media use among youth in disadvantaged neighborhoods. *New Media & Society*, *19*(6), 950–967. https://doi.org/10.1177/1461444815625941

Stewart, J. G., Mazurka, R., Bond, L., Wynne-Edwards, K. E., & Harkness, K. L. (2013). Rumination and impaired cortisol recovery following a social stressor in adolescent depression. *Journal of Abnormal Child Psychology*, *41*(7), 1015–1026. https://doi.org/10.1007/s10802-013-9740-1

Tynes, B. M., Willis, H. A., Stewart, A. M., & Hamilton, M. W. (2019). Race-related traumatic events online and mental health among adolescents of color. *Journal of Adolescent Health*, *65*(3), 371–377. https://doi.org/10.1016/j.jadohealth.2019.03.006

Umberson, D., & Donnelly, R. (2023). Social isolation: An unequally distributed health hazard. *Annual Review of Sociology*, *49*(1), 379–399. https://doi.org/10.1146/annurev-soc-031021-012001

Valente, T. W. (2024). Social networks and health behavior. In K. Glanz, B. K. Rimer, & K. Viswanath (Eds.), *Health behavior: Theory, research, and practice* (pp. 205–222). Wiley.

Verma, G., Bhardwaj, A., Aledavood, T., De Choudhury, M., & Kumar, S. (2022). Examining the impact of sharing COVID-19 misinformation online on mental health. *Scientific Reports*, *12*(1), Article 1. https://doi.org/10.1038/s41598-022-11488-y

Viswanath, K., Bekalu, M., Dhawan, D., Pinnamaneni, R., Lang, J., & McLoud, R. (2021). Individual and social determinants of COVID-19 vaccine uptake. *BMC Public Health*, *21*(1), 818. https://doi.org/10.1186/s12889-021-10862-1

Viswanath, K., & Kreuter, M. W. (2007). Health disparities, communication inequalities, and eHealth. *American Journal of Preventive Medicine*, *32*(5 Suppl), S131–S133. https://doi.org/10.1016/j.amepre.2007.02.012

Viswanath, K., Lee, E. W. J., & Pinnamaneni, R. (2020). We need the lens of equity in COVID-19 communication. *Health Communication*, *35*(14), 1743–1746. https://doi.org/10.1080/10410236.2020.1837445

Viswanath, K., McCloud, R. F., & Bekalu, M. A. (2022). Communication, health and equity: Structural influences. In T. L. Thompson & N. G. Harrington (Eds.), *Routledge handbook of health communication* (3rd ed., pp. 426–440). Routledge.

Viswanath, K., McCloud, R. F., Lee, E. W., & Bekalu, M. A. (2022). Measuring what matters: Data absenteeism, science communication, and the perpetuation of inequities. *Annals of the American Academy of Political and Social Science, 700*(1), 208–219. https://doi.org/10.1177/00027162221093268

Viswanath, K., Ramanadhan, S., & Kontos, E. Z. (2007). Mass media. In S. Galea, et al. (Eds.), *Macrosocial determinants of population health* (pp. 275–294). Springer.

Vogels, E., Gelles-Watnick, R., & Massarat, N. (2022, August 10). *Teens, social media and technology*. Pew Research Center. https://www.pewresearch.org/internet/2022/08/10/teens-social-media-and-technology-2022

Waldinger, R., & Schulz, M. (2023). *The good life: Lessons from the world's longest scientific study of happiness*. Simon and Schuster.

Wallerstein, N., & Duran, B. (2010). Community-based participatory research contributions to intervention research: The intersection of science and practice to improve health equity. *American Journal of Public Health, 100*(S1), S40–S46. https://doi.org/10.2105/AJPH.2009.184036

Wang, Y., Thier, K., & Nan, X. (2022). *Is health misinformation harmful? A systematic review of the psychological and behavioral impact of beliefs in and exposure to health misinformation*. OSF Preprints. https://doi.org/10.31219/osf.io/7te56

Witvliet, M., Brendgen, M., van Lier, P. A. C., Koot, H. M., & Vitaro, F. (2010). Early adolescent depressive symptoms: Prediction from clique isolation, loneliness, and perceived social acceptance. *Journal of Abnormal Child Psychology, 38*(8), 1045–1056. https://doi.org/10.1007/s10802-010-9426-x

Wolfers, L. N., & Schneider, F. M. (2020). Using media for coping: A scoping review. *Communication Research, 48*(8), 1210–1234. https://doi.org/10.1177/0093650220939778

World Health Organization. (2021a). *Comprehensive mental health action plan, 2013–2030*. https://www.who.int/publications/i/item/9789240031029

World Health Organization. (1946). *Constitution*. https://www.who.int/about/governance/constitution

World Health Organization. (2024). *Coronavirus Disease (COVID-19)*. Acessed on November 29, 2024. Available at https://www.who.int/news-room/fact-sheets/detail/coronavirus-disease-(covid-19)

Young, J. F., Berenson, K., Cohen, P., & Garcia, J. (2005). The role of parent and peer support in predicting adolescent depression: A longitudinal community study. *Journal of Research on Adolescence, 15*(4), 407–423. https://doi.org/10.1111/j.1532-7795.2005.00105.x

Part V

Stigma Reduction

20

Stigmatizing Communication and Mental Health

Xun Zhu[1], Rachel A. Smith[2], and Ruth A. Osoro[2]

[1] University of Kentucky
[2] Pennsylvania State University

Stigma profoundly influences people living with mental illness. Mental illness stigma affects almost all aspects of life—from employment, health care, and housing to education and interpersonal relationships (Thornicroft et al., 2022), and influences experiences across the lifespan (Earnshaw et al., 2022). Some people living with mental illness are also members of other marginalized groups (Oexle & Corrigan, 2018) and experience compounded devaluation and discrimination associated with their intersecting, marginalized identities. For instance, members of racial or ethnic minority groups—who already bear the burden due to historical and contemporary injustice because of their group affiliation—are further marginalized when they endure prejudice and discrimination associated with mental illness (Gary, 2005).

Mental illness stigma also influences social systems: institutions, laws, and investments (Pescosolido & Martin, 2015). At the institutional level, stigma manifests as private and governmental policies that differentially target and adversely affect people living with mental illness (Corrigan et al., 2005). Additionally, stigma threatens basic human rights (World Health Organization [WHO], 2021). For example, over one-third of the countries in the United Nations deny people with mental illness the right to vote (Bhugra et al., 2016). Stigma also dampens investments. For decades, there has been a chronic underinvestment in mental health services by local, national, and international agencies, a problem that was exacerbated during the COVID-19 pandemic (Mahomed, 2020). Thus, mental illness stigma denies people opportunities for a life with quality and dignity, and compromises the institutions purported to serve, protect, and advocate for vulnerable groups.

Mental illness stigma is fundamentally connected with communication processes: message production, diffusion, and effects (e.g., Meisenbach & Hutchins, 2020; Smith, 2007; Thompson & Seibold, 1978; Zhu & Smith, 2021). Our goal for this chapter is to engage with research addressing the intersections of communication, stigma, and mental illness. This chapter prioritizes theories and research illuminating three points of intersection: (a) socializing stigmas within communities; (b) coping with stigmatizing experiences; and (c) expressing stigmas in social interaction, with an eye toward the implications of the multiple, intersecting identities for those communication processes. We conclude the chapter by considering the implications of these stigma processes for mental health communication. We start by defining mental illness stigma and related concepts.

Stigma of Mental Illness: A Moment on Definitions

Stigma is a robust topic of scholarship in mental health research. Indeed, over 400 measures of mental illness stigma have been developed since 2004 (Fox et al., 2018). Why so many measures? Part of the issue is the conceptual complexity of stigma (Link & Phelan, 2001), including its components

The Handbook of Mental Health Communication, First Edition.
Edited by Marco C. Yzer and Jason T. Siegel.

(e.g., attributes, stereotypes, antipathy, and discrimination; Rüsch et al., 2005) and levels of operation (e.g., personal, group, and institutional; Pescosolido & Martin, 2015). The conceptual complexity of stigma also reflects the multidisciplinary nature of stigma scholarship, with each discipline approaching the concept with distinct theoretical orientations (Link & Phelan, 2001).

For the sake of clarity, in this chapter, we use specific terms to refer to different aspects of the *stigma complex* (Pescosolido & Martin, 2015, p. 87). We use *public stigma* to refer to profoundly negative stereotypes about a group and its members that have diffused and normalized within a community (Rüsch et al., 2005; Smith, 2007). Stereotypes are simplified and fixed beliefs that act as default assumptions about a social group and its members (Ashmore & Del Boca, 1981). Not all stereotypes are stigmas; stereotypes constitutive of public stigma are profoundly derogatory (Corrigan, 2018). Public stigmas are socialized (created, spread, and eventually normalized) through communication (Smith, 2007). Scholars emphasize that public stigma is inherently built upon a power-laden process, where members of a dominant group create and normalize stigma while members of a stigmatized group struggle to manage social exclusion and resist it (Link & Phelan, 2001; Meisenbach & Hutchins, 2020). Public stigma is akin to a social fact (Durkheim, 1982)—a social construct that has its own regulatory force. If public stigma exists and people do not enforce it, they may experience social sanctioning; if people stigmatize others when a stigma is not in place, they may be punished for their dehumanizing behavior (Thompson & Seibold, 1978).

We use *associative stigma* to refer to moments in which communities extend a public stigma to those who interact with members of a stigmatized group (Mehta & Farina, 1988; also referred to as courtesy stigma; Goffman, 1963). For instance, a qualitative study of relatives of people in treatment for schizophrenia reported experiencing rejection, derogatory comments, ridicule, and discrimination from employers and landlords (Angermeyer & Matschinger, 2003). Similarly, service providers may experience backlash from their social networks and mockery of their jobs, which are associated with occupational burnout (Yanos et al., 2020).

Public and associative stigma may be *internalized*, becoming a defining part of a person's identity (Rüsch et al., 2005). Internalized stigma causes harm to people's identity and agency; it can exacerbate symptoms of mental illness and hamper adherence to treatment (Livingston & Boyd, 2010). Internalized stigma also negatively affects a range of factors critical for resilience, such as hope, empowerment, and self-worth (Livingston & Boyd, 2010).

Beyond personal and interpersonal levels, stigma can manifest at a broader, structural level. We use *structural stigma* to refer to "societal-level conditions, cultural norms, and institutional policies that constrain the opportunities, resources, and wellbeing of the stigmatized" (Hatzenbuehler & Link, 2014, p. 2). Structural stigma is rooted in related concepts such as institutional racism, which emphasizes the role of institutions, oppressive ideologies, and power in perpetuating injustice and marginalization (Hatzenbuehler, 2016).

Stigma is not the only complicated concept; we want to briefly consider definitions of mental illness and mental health. It is useful to separate mental illness and mental health into different dimensions of well-being. Mental illnesses are "health conditions involving changes in emotion, thinking or behavior" (American Psychiatric Association, n.d.). The term *mental illness* is not neutral: it denotes difference and dysfunction. Mental health refers to a "state of well-being in which the individual realizes his or her own abilities, can cope with the normal stresses of life, can work productively and fruitfully, and is able to make a contribution to his or her community" (WHO, 2021, p. 1). The dual-continua model (Keyes, 2002) conceptualizes mental health and mental illness on two separate dimensions, with each dimension ranging from little to abundant mental health or few to many mental issues. This dual-continua model invites us to consider a state of flourishing as high levels of mental health and few mental issues and languishing as low levels of both. Although this chapter focuses on the stigma of mental illness, efforts should also be made to promote robust mental health.

Socializing Public Stigma

Public stigmas are created, spread, and normalized through communication (e.g., Goffman, 1963; Pescosolido et al., 2008; Smith, 2007). Communication at all levels—face-to-face interactions, mediated encounters, and media programming—may include content that teaches people how to identify members of a stigmatized group and to mobilize the community to enact devaluation and discrimination (Pescosolido et al., 2008; Smith, 2007). Public stigma can result from intentional, blatant communication choices that dehumanize a social group and its members, such as those in Nazi propaganda leading up to the killing of hundreds of thousands of people living with mental illness (Fischer, 2012). However, problematic communication is not always intentional. People can unintentionally communicate about mental illness in a way that socializes others to devalue those living with it. Indeed, the very assignment of a diagnosis by psychiatrists can be inadvertently stigmatizing, indicating those who experience a set of symptoms are inherently different from and less than everyone else (Corrigan, 2007). Even communication efforts meant to decrease existing stigmas can exacerbate them. For example, campaigns seeking to debunk the myths of mental illness with factual information may inadvertently increase the perception of dangerousness (Dobson & Rose, 2022).

Media can play a key role in creating, spreading, and normalizing new stigmas. An extensive body of literature has examined the stigmatizing representation of people living with mental illness in various media sources, including traditional mass media and emerging social media (e.g., Corrigan et al., 2005; Klin & Lemish, 2008; Ross et al., 2019; Wahl, 2003). In media programming (e.g., television, film, podcasts), people living with mental illness are characterized as dangerous (Klin & Lemish, 2008), incompetent (Goulden et al., 2011), and "helpless, disempowered and child-like" (Olstead, 2002, p. 634). In addition, mental illness is treated as a source of ridicule (Klin & Lemish, 2008), often presented in connection with other stigmatizing attributes, such as risky health behaviors and maladaptive responses to adversity (Riles et al., 2021). Media programming rarely features the perspective of people with lived experiences, excluding their voices from public discourse and policy debates (Wahl, 2003).

In addition to the negative portrayals, media programming that depicts social acceptance and recovery is rare. A survey of over 3,000 articles from US newspapers with large circulations showed that only 4% addressed recovery (Corrigan et al., 2005). These problems are not limited to the United States (e.g., Hildersley et al., 2020; Ross et al., 2022). Further, media disproportionately connects mental illness with members of hegemonic majority groups. For example, popular films in the United States often portray mental illness as a challenge experienced by White, adult, and heterosexual males (Riles et al., 2021) and people from upper socioeconomic classes (Smith-Frigerio, 2018). The biased representation is problematic because it may lead audiences to believe that the typical picture of a person living with mental illness is characterized by the intersections of those identities (Smith-Frigerio, 2018, p. 392).

The critique that media plays a role in creating and diffusing stigmas is not new. Recent developments in communication scholarship have offered to understand how and why it happens. One such theory is the model of stigma communication (MSC; Smith, 2007; Smith et al., 2019). The MSC describes a *stigma frame* and the mechanisms that lead to the emergence of (new) public stigmas.

In the MSC, a stigma frame includes four types of content: marks, labels, etiology, and peril (Smith, 2007; Smith et al., 2019). *Marks* describe ways (often visual) to identify members of a stigmatized group (e.g., descriptions of symptoms, such as an uncontrollable twitch of facial muscles; Baldwin & Marcus, 2006); marks that are more visible and evoke disgust are easier to recognize and remember (Smith, 2007). *Labels* are linguistic terms used to reference a stigmatized group. Labels reify people into a homogenous and distinct entity characterized primarily, if not solely, by the group's stereotypes. *Etiology* describes how people become associated with a stigmatized group, centering on choice and control. People who are perceived to make choices that lead to a stigmatized condition are judged and punished more harshly (Jones et al., 1984). For example, despite myriad factors known to affect mental health (WHO, 2021), etiology content may imply that people are responsible for their mental illness. Etiology content may be conveyed through subtle word choices. For example, the Associated Press advises journalists to "avoid using *committed suicide* except in direct quotations from authorities" because the term *commit* implies an intentional, even criminal, act (Associated Press, 2016, p. xxvi). *Peril* presents the danger a stigmatized group poses to the rest of the community. For example, in children's television programming, characters with mental illness fail their tasks (Gerbner, 1995) and are referred to as twisted and deranged (Wilson et al., 2000). In a review of American cartoons from 1941 to 1990, Walter (2000) reported that every character with mental illness was depicted as cruel, amoral, and dangerous. Nonverbally, production decisions about music, sound effects, lighting, and camera shots can make a person or fictitious character appear dangerous, such as filming people living with mental illness in darker lighting and with awkward camera shots (Wilson et al., 2000). Peril content about people with mental illness is also prevalent in entertainment media, such as films and television shows (Smith et al., 2019) and video games (Ferrari et al., 2019).

According to the MSC, danger appraisal (a combination of perceived danger and felt threat) mediates the effects of exposure to a stigma frame on stigma-related outcomes (Smith et al., 2019). A stigma frame activates danger appraisal, which, in turn, facilitates stigma-related outcomes in those directly exposed to these messages. The outcomes of a stigma frame include stigma beliefs, behaviors to ostracize people labeled for a stigmatizing condition, and support for discriminatory policies (Ledford et al., 2022; Smith, 2012a, 2014; Smith et al., 2019).

Further distinguishing the MSC from other models of stigma is its unique focus on the social diffusion of stigma beliefs and the emergence of a public stigma (Smith, 2007). A stigma frame evokes reactions that promote the onward transmission of the message to others, leading to the diffusion of the stigma frame (Smith, 2007; Smith et al., 2019). Exposure and spread can include mediated and unmediated communication: for example, people can retransmit news stories they see online in person, broadcast the information through social media, or recount interpersonal conversations in online posts or in news stories.

According to the MSC, people share a stigma frame because the message is judged to have certain qualities that fulfill their psychological needs (Smith et al., 2019). Common ground, defined as the extent to which a message conveys common interest between senders and receivers, is an important judgment. Studies have found that stigma frames were judged as having common ground because they warned—albeit in a biased and inaccurate way—the larger community about the threat imposed by a stigmatized group (Ledford et al., 2022; Smith et al., 2019). Sharing messages built upon common ground facilitates social bonding with in-group members. Noticeably, studies have shown that although danger appraisal predicted stigma beliefs and stigmatizing acts, it was the message judgments, such as perceived common ground, that predicted how and with whom a stigma frame was shared (Smith et al., 2019). This suggests that while danger appraisal mounts a general reaction against a stigmatized group, message judgments pivot the responses to specific recipients in ways that facilitate social diffusion.

Communication scholars view the emergence of stigma as a fluid and dynamic process, but there is limited research on how stigma is (re)constructed in social interaction following initial media exposure. Theories of mass communication have long emphasized the indirect effects of mass media as people talk with other members of their community about the media messages (Katz & Lazarsfeld, 1955; Southwell & Yzer, 2007). Interpersonal conversations resulting from media exposure may amplify, alter, or even diminish the effects of media campaign messages (Jeong & Bae, 2018). In stigma scholarship, research is emerging to examine how the content of a stigmatizing frame changes through chains of interpersonal conversations. For example, Jacobs and Quinn (2022) presented participants with a news story about how a person living with mental illness stopped a theft in a shopping mall but was mistakenly identified as the shoplifter. Participants told the story to another participant who then retold it and so on, akin to the children's telephone game. The study found that participants not only focused more on aspects of the story consistent with negative stereotypes about people living with mental illness but also transformed the descriptions that challenged the stereotypes by making them more abstract and ambiguous. Scholars argue that the retransmission of a stigmatizing frame depends on the extent to which specific content helps interactants achieve psychological goals threatened by a stigmatized group (Zhu & Smith, 2016).

Coping with Stigma

For people living with mental illness, diagnosis is a critical moment that comes with benefits and risks. On one hand, a diagnosis is important for people to make sense of their symptoms, validate their experience, receive the appropriate treatment and interventions, and in some cases qualify for insurance and other social benefits (National Alliance on Mental Illness, 2023). On the other hand, a diagnosis is associated with labeling and its negative consequences on physical, psychological, and relational well-being (Link et al., 1989; O'Connor et al., 2022). Longitudinal evidence shows that the benefits of diagnosis and the damage of labeling appear to endure and are mutually unaffected. For example, Link et al. (2008) found that people who were diagnosed with severe mental illness experienced improvements in symptoms and social functioning one year after receiving the diagnosis. However, they also reported significantly higher public stigma and lower self-esteem. As Link and Phelan (2013) argued, labeling is part of a "package deal" (p. 575) that people living with mental illness have to confront while seeking help. The question is how people can effectively cope with stigma and its consequences associated with labeling.

Coping Strategies

A theory at the forefront of research examining how people cope with mental illness stigma is the modified labeling theory (MLT; Link et al., 1989). MLT posits that everyone is socialized to learn about stigmatized groups; as people are labeled, the public stigma becomes personally relevant, causing them to anticipate and worry about experiencing stigmatization. Out of the fear of being stigmatized, they engage in coping strategies aimed at preventing negative reactions. MLT identifies five coping strategies: secrecy (concealing labeling information), withdrawal (avoiding potential stigmatization), education (correcting stereotypes), challenge (confronting stigmatization), and distancing (disassociating with a stigmatized group). People may use a mixture of strategies to manage anticipated or enacted stigmatization (Link et al., 1989). These strategies are also used by confidants to whom people disclose their labeling conditions. For example, advice confidants of people living with mental illness were found to encourage their labeled loved ones not to tell other people, including health care providers, about their conditions (Smith & Hipper, 2010).

Communication scholarship further expands the strategies people use to manage stigmatization. The theory of stigma management communication (SMC) proposes a more nuanced catalog of coping strategies (Meisenbach, 2010). SMC predicts that people select coping strategies based on their beliefs in stigma's existence as well as their identification with a stigmatized group (Meisenbach, 2010). For example, people challenge stigmatization when they reject a public stigma and its relevance to the self. Challenging communication can take various forms, including questioning the credibility of those who enact stigma, highlighting logical fallacies in stigmatizing messages, denying the relevance of stigmatizing beliefs to themselves, or displaying the stigmata in interaction as a form of protest. SMC has been used to analyze communication responses to stigmatization due to mental health challenges (Jensen, 2018).

Media can provide an opportunity to vicariously learn about aspects of coping, such as disclosures, social support requests, and provision (Bandura, 2001). In addition, research has also begun to recognize the use of media as a strategy for coping with adverse situations, including discrimination and ostracism (Wolfers & Schneider, 2021). Using media, such as watching a movie or browsing social media posts, allows people to seek distraction from anxiety and stress (Nabi et al., 2017) and compensate for social support when other coping resources are limited or unavailable (Eden et al., 2020). For example, Black Americans experiencing higher levels of racial discrimination reported using social media more frequently to air their grievances, find community, and share coping resources (Miller et al., 2021). In the context of mental health, young adults who experience anxiety disorders turn to social media to seek information about anxiety and to cope with stigmatization when they do not have access to peer support or mental health services (Wolenski & Pettit, 2023).

Whereas the aforementioned strategies emphasize individual responses, emerging research has identified how people *collaboratively* cope with stigmatization. One line of work examines communal coping, which refers to communication processes involving multiple people jointly appraising a stressor and proactively acting upon it (Lyons et al., 1998). Communal coping occurs when people (a) share the ownership of a stressor, perceiving the problem as *ours* versus *mine* or *yours*, and (b) take actions aimed at reducing the negative impacts of the stressor based on shared resolve (Afifi et al., 2020). Although communal coping strategies may mirror those found in individual coping, the key distinction is that these strategies result from a joint effort: people involved in communal coping choose and enact the coping strategies through a cooperative decision-making and problem-solving process (Curtis et al., 2022).

A second line of work focuses on ally communication. In addition to stigmatizers and those who are stigmatized, Goffman (1963) described a third group consisting of people who do not fit the stigmatizing characterization but are sympathetic to and accepted by those who do (a.k.a. wise). Subsequent research shows that the wise group can be further divided into passive and active supporters (Smith, 2012b). Passive supporters tend to avoid direct confrontation with stigmatizers and instead to focus solely on support provision (e.g., expressing sympathy; Smith, 2012b). By contrast, active supporters use their social power to "challenge oppressive power structures—all at the risk of giving up the safety of their own privilege" (Jackson et al., 2020, p. 2); they engage in strategies directly targeting stigmatizers, such as confronting stigmatizers (Smith, 2012b) and social activism (Jackson et al., 2020).

Drawing from the scholarship addressing social justice activism, DeTurk (2011) identified a range of strategies for allyship communication, such as providing testimony from role models and developing rapport through humor. But not all action is affirming. Experiments show that messages containing identity-safety cues (i.e., one's identity is valued) result in stronger perceptions of allyship (Johnson et al., 2019), especially when those cues are from an ingroup member or when message recipients are aware of the public stigma (Pietri et al., 2018). Kam et al. (2022) examined supportive communication as a way to create allyship; the authors cautioned that the power differentials between support providers and receivers might reinforce the status of a stigmatized group as powerless and dependent on the dominant group.

Coping Effectiveness and Challenges

Although research has documented a rich repertoire of coping strategies, we know less about the effectiveness of these strategies in forestalling the negative consequences of mental illness stigma. The limited extant research suggests that individual-oriented coping strategies may be ineffective and in some cases can do more harm than good. Studies adopting the MLT showed that coping strategies—including secrecy, withdrawal, and education—had little effect on psychological distress and status loss (Link et al., 1991). Further, all three coping strategies were associated with smaller social networks, leaving labeled people with limited contacts to turn to for support (Link et al., 1991). Direct strategies, such as education and challenge, may antagonize others (Thoits, 2011), creating interpersonal tensions and inducing stress. Ranjit et al. (2022) found a similar negative effect when coping strategies are used by health care providers to manage associative stigma. Passive acceptance (e.g., ignoring when stigmatization occurs) was associated with more stress, while reducing offensiveness (e.g., shifting focus to a non-stigmatized identity) was linked to more severe depression (Ranjit et al., 2022).

Using media to cope with mental illness stigma may also come with risk. Given the prevalence of stigmatizing portrayals of mental illness on mass and social media (Klin & Lemish, 2008; Ross et al., 2019), people seeking relief may be incidentally exposed to more stigmatization and experience heightened stress. Further, some types of content in media may lead people to engage in behaviors that are stigmatized. For example, Myrick and Chen (2022) found that exposure to news about a member of a disliked outgroup becoming ill led to schadenfreude (i.e., pleasure at another's misery), which decreased willingness to perform recommended behaviors and thus might increase the risk of being stigmatized.

The available evidence suggests that communal coping may be effective in alleviating the negative effects of public and internalized stigma. Communal coping is thought to foster resilience by increasing self-efficacy in managing a stressor, facilitating reappraisal, and expanding shared resources with the community (Afifi et al., 2020). In married couples where one partner is labeled with a stigmatizing condition, research shows that communal coping reduces the discrepancy between desired and received support for the labeled person and their spouse, which, in turn, buffers stress experienced by both partners due to stigmatization (Smith et al., 2018). Research also shows that communal coping helps prevent labeled people and their partners from internalizing stigmatizing beliefs (Curtis et al., 2022).

But communal coping is not without challenges. For communal coping to occur, people need to disclose their labeled condition to potential allies. In the case of disclosing to conjointly cope with stigmatization, people do not just reveal personal information; they also need to mobilize other group members for collective appraisal and actions. Stigma scholarship has long focused on how people make disclosure decisions (Greene, 2009), but our understanding of the types of disclosures that not only reveal but also create a shared vision is only nascent. The disclosure quality model (DQM; Donovan et al., 2017) identifies three attributes that define a high-quality disclosure: *access to information* (i.e., willingly divulging personal information), *candor* (i.e., being honest and straightforward), and *relating to peers* (i.e., disclosing in a way that treats confidants as equal owners of the information). Applying the DQM to investigate the disclosure of mental illness in romantic relationships, Taniguchi-Dorios et al. (2023) found that access to information and candor consistently predicted disclosure quality. Higher disclosure quality was associated with stronger relational closeness and greater willingness to continue the conversation about mental illness (Taniguchi-Dorios et al., 2023)—the conditions theorized to facilitate communal coping (Afifi et al., 2020).

Involving allies to resist stigmatization raises another challenge. Research has identified a unique group called superficial allies (Davoudpour, 2023). Like allies, they are sympathetic to a stigmatized group and willing to challenge stigmatization when it occurs. However, they reject proximity to the stigmatized group, such as living in the same neighborhood or interacting interpersonally (Davoudpour, 2023). Although this paradoxical reaction may be a strategy by the allies to reduce the risk of being targeted by associative stigma, it may create uncertainty for people living with mental illness as to whom they can turn to for support without being stigmatized. It may also explain why people labeled with mental illness tend to avoid peripheral ties, such as coworkers, health care professionals, and neighbors, even though those weaker contacts can provide valuable information that may not be available through core networks (Perry & Pescosolido, 2015).

Expressing Stigma

Among the many actions people perform in relation to stigma, one action that receives arguably the least empirical attention is expressing stigma: verbal, nonverbal, and paraverbal behaviors that convey antipathy and enact devaluation or violence against a stigmatized group (Smith et al., 2016). To be clear, existing research has documented many forms of stigmatization experienced by people living with mental illness (e.g., Dickerson et al., 2002) and their allies (e.g., Yin et al., 2020). What is missing is, however, a theoretical understanding of the underlying dimensions that characterize the range of stigmatizing behaviors.

One way to consider stigmatization is as interpersonal influence (Smith & Bishop, 2019):

> an act of influence on the part of the stigmatizer to persuade a target to accept the stigmatizer's (a) belief about the existence of a social group, (b) belief that the target is a member of this social group, and (c) that the group has a marginalized status in the society at large. (p. 574).

Through this lens, we explore how the different communicative acts (e.g., name-calling, violence) may be understood as serving functions that facilitate the stigmatizer's persuasive goals. These acts of stigmatization can occur in face-to-face settings as well as in mass and emerging media.

Group Membership

If one function of stigmatizing communication is to persuade a target to accept the stigmatizer's belief about the existence of a social group and the target's membership within it, it may be useful to attend to messages that express those beliefs. For example, as noted earlier, labels are terms used to reference a group; the act of labeling locates someone as a group member. Name-calling, as a communicative act, involves the application of a label on the speech act's target (Samoilenko, 2016). Examples of name-calling identified in children's media programming on a popular streaming channel included crazy, nuts, insane, maniac, looney, lunatic, and psycho (Donohue & Swords, 2022). Out-group status may also be indicated more nuancedly through using selected pronouns (e.g., we vs. them) or manipulating the length and directness of eye contact during interaction (Kleck, 1968).

A third type of message appears in irrelevant (and often unsolicited) advice. People may ask for help with one topic but receive advice focused on a different social category. For example, in a qualitative study, adults seeking care in an emergency room reported being labeled, triaged, and treated as a psychiatric patient, regardless of their symptoms and needs. One patient shared, "I had a gallbladder attack and they took me off to psych" (Clarke et al., 2007, p. 128); another reported, "Once you are identified as a psych patient, even if you have a physical problem like a migraine, you are still treated as a psych patient" (p. 128). Unsolicited advice may also be given by ingroup members to reinforce a shared social identity (Vayreda & Antaki, 2009). In such instances, the stigmatizing communication expresses the provider's beliefs about which group membership is the most relevant for the target and frames the target's well-being through that social identity.

Marginalized Status

If a separate function of stigmatizing communication is to persuade a target to accept a marginalized status for a particular social group, two types of message content may appear: (a) devaluation (Smith et al., 2016) and (b) domination. A marginalized status is established when people are persuaded to believe that their group is low in value and power—that is, marginalized.

Devaluation refers to verbal and nonverbal acts that express a lack of worth as a human (Smith et al., 2016). Devaluation may dehumanize members of a group by denying a person's individuality or humanity (Haslam, 2006). Messages that deny a person's individuality may describe the members of a stigmatized group as lacking self-control, refinement, intelligence, and rationality, and in extreme cases, explicitly compare the group to animals (Boysen et al., 2020). This form of devaluation may also include weaponized uses of language that directly derogate, intimate, or insult people based on their group membership (Jones et al., 2016). Sometimes, these appeals happen in more subtle forms. For example, research shows that when disclosing a mental health challenge, veterans reported receiving unsolicited, intrusive advice about what it means to live with mental illness and how to fix the problem (Wilson et al., 2021). In contrast, messages that deny humanity may objectify a stigmatized group, portraying them as inert or instrumental (Haslam, 2006). For example, people living with mental illness experienced objectification when they were given orders with few explanations in a health care setting as if they were a machine (Birch et al., 2005).

Domineering communication conveys that the target of stigmatization is subordinate to the stigmatizer. Stigmatizers may use domineering language (e.g., extreme language) and nonverbal dominance (e.g., yelling) as they harass targets. Domineering communication (verbal and nonverbal) conveys the speaker's "intensity about the issue and they imply a relationship in which the hearer is subordinate" (Dillard, 2014, p. 183). A different manifestation appears through ostracism—being ignored, excluded, and/or rejected by others (Williams, 2001). Ostracism is a powerful, painful act that expels the target and strengthens the ostracizer's position and value. The silent treatment can be a powerful appeal that conveys a deeply marginalized status (Samoilenko, 2016). Power can also be communicated through what is or is not kept in public discourse and memory. Biased languages, such as derogatory labels and name-calling, may become routinized into "part of taken-for-granted, everyday discourse" (Ng, 2007, p. 106). Stigmatizing communication can also be used to erase targets from public memory, as seen in multiple examples of unmarked graves found next to long-stay institutions (Favert, 2006).

Directions for Future Research

Despite the advances in the scholarship on stigma communication, the extant work leaves many unanswered questions. We highlight four directions for future research. First, greater attention is needed to time and timing. Many stigma theories presume a longitudinal process. For example, the MSC conceptualizes stigma as an emergent social norm, where the stigmatizing characterization of a group spreads over time within a larger community through interactions (Smith, 2007). Coping is a dynamic process: People adapt their coping strategies in response to the distinct challenges and stressors imposed by stigmatization and their social networks. Strategies that are effective at one point may become maladaptive later. The ways people stigmatize others (e.g., specific insults and obscene gestures) may also evolve along with the changing norms, values, and laws. When we consider stigma as a longitudinal process, it is useful to distinguish two representations of time (Zhu, 2023). Stigma may be understood through a societal time metric where stigma waxes and wanes in response to historical, institutional, and cultural changes. In addition, stigma processes unfold through a personalized timeline, with the onset and trajectory of a stigmatizing experience varying across individuals. The two approaches can provide distinct yet complementary insights into the unfolding of stigma processes.

Second, research is also needed to understand how people use communication to confront stigmatization. For example, as people experience stigmatization, which forms of confrontation are most effective at stopping the encounter or allowing them to resist internalizing the stigmatizing attack? When and how do people (targets, bystanders, and allies) confront different forms of stigmatization? How does intersectionality affect the confrontation of and resistance to mental illness stigma?

Third, research on coping with stigma has shown that different coping strategies involve trade-offs, but evidence from allied fields suggests that the relationships among stigma, coping, and health may be more complex than previously understood. For example, research consistently demonstrates a pattern of "skin-deep resilience," where members of a marginalized group achieve upward mobility and good mental health at the expense of physical health (Chen et al., 2022). In one study, Brody et al. (2013) found that Black adolescents who were most resilient to mental health risks also experienced the highest level of allostatic load—a physiological sign of wear and tear on the body. Future research is needed to understand the potentially divergent effects of communication strategies for coping with mental illness stigma on health, relational, and social outcomes.

Fourth, and last, this chapter describes socializing, coping with, and expressing mental illness stigma as distinct communication processes, but, of course, these processes interact. Media coverage that depicts people living with mental illness in a stigma frame may drive the unmarked group to express stigma, blatantly or subtly, in interpersonal and mediated interactions. Exposure to stigmatization is inherently stressful, especially for groups who already endure adversity due to multiple marginalized identities. In the face of stigmatization, people undertake coping strategies to mitigate its negative effects. But, as described earlier, coping may be ineffective or even harmful, such as increasing stress (e.g., when challenging stigmatization creates intergroup intentions) or limiting the availability of resources for treatment and recovery (e.g., when secrecy reduces the size and diversity of support network). The heightened stress and resource reduction, in turn, can compromise mental and physical health, resulting in more stigmatization (Link et al., 2018). Consequently, the socialization and expression of stigma, coupled with coping efforts that inadvertently worsen the problem, may engender a vicious cycle of bidirectional effects that constrain people's ability to engage in behaviors for good mental health and put them at higher risk for stigmatization. Future research needs to examine the role of communication in these bidirectional effects of stigma and mental health.

Implications for Mental Health Communication

Disrupting the vicious cycle of mental illness stigma is challenging because it is distressingly easy to become entangled in the feedback loops that perpetuate stigmatization yet is extraordinarily difficult to extricate oneself from it. In theory, anyone may fall into the cycle of stigma, even if they do not directly experience stigmatization in social interactions (Link et al., 2018; Tomiyama, 2014). For example, people may experience the cascading outcomes of stigma when they anticipate social stereotypes and rejection. Due to associative stigma, people who provide services or support to those living with mental illnesses may become ensnared in the cycle (Yanos et al., 2020). Further, as media coverage frequently links mental illnesses with other stigmatized identities (Riles et al., 2021), people who are perceived to be characterized by those identities may experience stigmatization and inadvertently enter the cycle, even if they do not personally live with mental illnesses.

Different disciplines tend to emphasize different types of interventions to disrupt the stigma cycle. From a communication perspective, people designing informational materials or campaign interventions about mental illness should avoid content that cues stigma. One option is to use a checklist for stigmatizing language. This option has gained traction in academic journals and health agencies. Examples include *Inclusive Language Guide from American Psychological Association* (APA, 2023), *Writing Respectfully: Person-First and Destigmatizing Language from the National Institutes of Health* (NIH, 2023), and *Health Equity Guiding Principles for Inclusive Communication* from the Centers for

Disease Control and Prevention (CDC, 2023). Checklists for communicating with specific audiences are also available, such as guidance for clinicians on how to talk with patients about substance use disorder (CDC, 2022) and Addictionary—a glossary to educate the public and health professionals about addiction-related terms, with an emphasis on words that can induce stigma (Recovery Research Institute, 2023).

Importantly, the checklists for stigmatizing language should not be viewed as exhaustive or definitive. It is important to be mindful of the underlying assumptions that inform specific language choices. Consider, for instance, the language about disability (Dunn & Andrews, 2015). The social model of disability conceptualizes disability as a reflection of external barriers that inhibit people from full participation in social interaction. Guidance based on the social model recommends using person-first language (e.g., people living with disabilities) to underscore that a person's identity is not determined by their condition. By contrast, the diversity model places disability as an integral and celebrated aspect of identity, similar to gender and race. Guidance based on the diversity model recommends using identity-first language (e.g., disabled people) to emphasize that disability is a difference, not deviance (Dunn & Andrews, 2015). Given the diverse perspectives, communicators should consult established best practices while remaining flexible to adjust their language as needed.

In addition to changes in language, eliminating stigma requires interventions to dismantle the deeply ingrained beliefs that some groups are inherently inferior to others and to challenge the behaviors and social structures that express, normalize, and perpetuate such beliefs. Stigma reduction has been the subject of considerable research, yielding a rich repertoire of strategies for different components of mental illness stigma, segments of populations, and modes of interaction (e.g., Corrigan et al., 2012, 2015; Griffiths et al., 2014). Leveraging the multidimensional capabilities of media such as videos, music, and interactivity, communicators may design interventions that elicit stronger psychological responses that reduce stigma. For example, Hecht et al. (2022) found that videos featuring background music characterized by minor keys, slower tempos, and greater pitch variations evoked stronger empathetic feelings, which increased reflective thinking and reduced stigma toward people living with mental illness. Media may induce more complex responses for stigma reduction that may be otherwise difficult to achieve in brief, interpersonal encounters. For example, entertainment media may reduce stigma by creating eudaimonic appreciation—an experiential state characterized by "the perception of deeper meaning, the feeling of being moved, and the motivation to elaborate on thoughts and feelings inspired by the experience" (Oliver & Bartsch, 2010, p. 76). Last, media can facilitate social learning by modeling effective allyship and coping communication in movies and serial dramas depicting such moments between characters.

Coping with stigma involves competent interactions between stigmatized individuals and their allies. However, effective support interactions are not automatic, easy, or straightforward. People may experience paradoxical tensions when they seek or provide support to cope with a stigmatized identity (Crowley et al., 2023). For example, fear of stigmatization may lead the marked individuals to engage in certain strategies that elicit less supportive responses and more social rejection. Similarly, family members may encourage someone living with mental illness to seek professional help yet worry about implying that the person is incompetent or not normal. Communication training can address each step in a supportive interaction, including disclosing mental illnesses, communicating expectations for the desired amount and type of support, and providing support while protecting the identity needs of people experiencing stigma.

Conclusion

This chapter reviewed theories and research addressing the dynamic and complex intersections between communication, stigma, and mental illness. We encourage scholars to investigate stigma as a dynamic and emergent process, examine communication used to resist mental illness stigma at the personal level, and develop a more nuanced understanding of stigma coping and its effects on multiple dimensions of health and well-being. As our understanding of these processes and their intersections improves, we will have a better chance of creating interventions that eliminate stigma.

References

Afifi, T. D., Basinger, E. D., & Kam, J. A. (2020). The extended theoretical model of communal coping: Understanding the properties and functionality of communal coping. *Journal of Communication, 70*(3), 424–446. https://doi.org/10.1093/joc/jqaa006

American Psychiatric Association. (n.d.). *What is mental illness?* https://www.psychiatry.org/patients-families/what-is-mental-illness.

American Psychological Association. (2023). *Inclusive language guide* (2nd ed.). https://www.apa.org/about/apa/equity-diversity-inclusion/language-guidelines.pdf

Angermeyer, M. C., & Matschinger, H. (2003). The stigma of mental illness: Effects of labelling on public attitudes towards people with mental disorder. *Acta Psychiatrica Scandinavica, 108*(4), 304–309. https://doi.org/10.1034/j.1600-0447.2003.00150.x

Ashmore, R. D., & Del Boca, E. K. (1981). Conceptual approaches to stereotypes and stereotyping. In D. L. Hamilton (Ed.), *Cognitive processes in stereotyping and intergroup behavior* (pp. 1–35). Erlbaum.

Associated Press. (2016). *The associated press stylebook 2016*. Basic Books.

Baldwin, M. L., & Marcus, S. C. (2006). Perceived and measured stigma among workers with serious mental illness. *Psychiatric Services, 57*(3), 388–392. https://doi.org/10.1176/appi.ps.57.3.388

Bandura, A. (2001). Social cognitive theory of mass communication. *Media Psychology, 3*(3), 265–299. https://doi.org/10.1207/S1532785XMEP0303_03

Bhugra, D., Pathare, S., Gosavi, C., Ventriglio, A., Torales, J., Castaldelli-Maia, J., Tolentino, E. J., & Ng, R. (2016). Mental illness and the right to vote: A review of legislation across the world. *International Review of Psychiatry, 28*(4), 395–399. https://doi.org/10.1080/09540261.2016.1211096

Birch, S., Lavender, T., & Cupitt, C. (2005). The physical healthcare experiences of women with mental health problems: Status versus stigma. *Journal of Mental Health, 14*(1), 61–72. https://doi.org/10.1080/09638230500048032

Boysen, G. A., Isaacs, R. A., Tretter, L., & Markowski, S. (2020). Evidence for blatant dehumanization of mental illness and its relation to stigma. *The Journal of Social Psychology, 160*(3), 346–356. https://doi.org/10.1080/00224545.2019.1671301

Brody, G. H., Yu, T., Chen, E., Miller, G. E., Kogan, S. M., & Beach, S. R. (2013). Is resilience only skin deep? Rural African Americans' socioeconomic status- related risk and competence in preadolescence and psychological adjustment and allostatic load at age 19. *Psychological Science, 24*(7), 1285–1293. https://doi.org/10.1177/0956797612471954

Centers for Disease Control and Prevention. (2022). *Remove stigma: Talk with your patients about substance use disorder.* https://www.cdc.gov/opioids/addiction-medicine/conversation-starters/remove-stigma.html

Centers for Disease Control and Prevention. (2023). *Health equity guiding principles for inclusive communication.* https://www.cdc.gov/healthcommunication/Health_Equity.html

Chen, E., Brody, G. H., & Miller, G. E. (2022). What are the health consequences of upward mobility? *Annual Review of Psychology, 73*, 599–628. https://doi.org/10.1146/annurev-psych-033020-122814

Clarke, D. E., Dusome, D., & Hughes, L. (2007). Emergency department from the mental health client's perspective. *International Journal of Mental Health Nursing, 16*(2), 126–131. https://doi.org/10.1111/j.1447-0349.2007.00455.x

Corrigan, P., Michaels, P. J., & Morris, S. (2015). Do the effects of antistigma programs persist over time? Findings from a meta-analysis. *Psychiatric Services, 66*(5), 543–546. https://doi.org/10.1176/appi.ps.201400291

Corrigan, P. W. (2007). How clinical diagnosis might exacerbate the stigma of mental illness. *Social Work, 52*(1), 31–39. https://doi.org/10.1093/sw/52.1.31

Corrigan, P. W. (2018). *The stigma effect: Unintended consequences of mental health campaigns*. Columbia University Press.

Corrigan, P. W., Morris, S. B., Michaels, P. J., Rafacz, J. D., & Rüsch, N. (2012). Challenging the public stigma of mental illness: A meta-analysis of outcome studies. *Psychiatric Services, 63*(10), 963–973. https://doi.org/10.1176/appi.ps.201100529

Corrigan, P. W., Watson, A. C., Gracia, G., Slopen, N., Rasinski, K., & Hall, L. L. (2005). Newspaper stories as measures of structural stigma. *Psychiatric Services, 56*(5), 551–556. https://doi.org/10.1176/appi.ps.56.5.551

Crowley, J. L., High, A. C., Kotowski, M. R., & McCarty, D. N. (2023). Conflicting goals when seeking support for mental health concerns: Testing a stigma support activation model. *Communication Research*. Advance online publication. https://doi.org/10.1177/00936502231213129

Curtis, M. G., Kogan, S., Mitchell, J. W., & Stephenson, R. (2022). Dyadic effects of enacted stigma, internalized homophobia, and communal coping on depressive symptoms among cisgender sexual minority male couples. *Family Process, 61*(4), 1541–1558. https://doi.org/10.1111/famp.12746

Davoudpour, S. (2023). Superficial allies: The role of legal inclusion and social obedience in stigma processes. *Sociological Research Online, 29*(1), 101–119. https://doi.org/10.1177/13607804231156296

DeTurk, S. (2011). Allies in action: The communicative experiences of people who challenge social injustice on behalf of others. *Communication Quarterly, 59*(5), 569–590. https://doi.org/10.1080/01463373.2011.614209

Dickerson, F. B., Sommerville, J., Origoni, A. E., Ringel, N. B., & Parente, F. (2002). Experiences of stigma among outpatients with schizophrenia. *Schizophrenia Bulletin, 28*(1), 143–155. https://doi.org/10.1093/oxfordjournals.schbul.a006917

Dillard, J. P. (2014). Language, style, and persuasion. In T. Holtgraves (Ed.), *The Oxford handbook of language and social psychology* (pp. 177–187). Oxford University Press.

Dobson, K. S., & Rose, S. (2022). "Myths and facts" campaigns are at best ineffective and may increase mental illness stigma. *Stigma and Health*, *7*(1), 27–34. https://doi.org/10.1037/sah0000323

Donohue, D., & Swords, L. (2022). The portrayal of mental illness in popular children's programs on Netflix: A content and thematic analysis. *Psychology of Popular Media*, *13*(1), 102–110. https://dx.doi.org/10.1037/ppm0000445

Donovan, E. E., Thompson, C. M., LeFebvre, L., & Tollison, A. C. (2017). Emerging adult confidants' judgments of parental openness: Disclosure quality and post-disclosure relational closeness. *Communication Monographs*, *84*(2), 179–199. https://doi.org/10.1080/03637751.2015.1119867

Dunn, D. S., & Andrews, E. E. (2015). Person-first and identity-first language: Developing psychologists' cultural competence using disability language. *American Psychologist*, *70*(3), 255–264. https://doi.org/10.1037/a0038636

Durkheim, E. (1982). *The rules of sociological method and selected texts on sociology and its method.* Macmillan.

Earnshaw, V. A., Watson, R. J., Eaton, L. A., Brousseau, N. M., Laurenceau, J. P., & Fox, A. B. (2022). Integrating time into stigma and health research. *Nature Reviews Psychology*, *1*(4), 236–247. https://doi.org/10.1038/s44159-022-00034-2

Eden, A. L., Johnson, B. K., Reinecke, L., & Grady, S. M. (2020). Media for coping during COVID-19 social distancing: Stress, anxiety, and psychological well-being. *Frontiers in Psychology*, *11*, 577639. https://doi.org/10.3389/fpsyg.2020.577639

Favret, A. C. (2006). Archaeological investigations of unmarked graves at Eastern State Hospital Lexington, Fayette County, Kentucky. Kentucky Archaeological Survey. KAS Report No. 119. Kentucky. https://citeseerx.ist.psu.edu/document?repid=rep1&type=pdf&doi=19281939a36065b84777965127efaf44898dd10d

Ferrari, M., McIlwaine, S., Jordan, G., Shah, J., Lal, S., & Iyer, S. (2019). Gaming against stigma: An analysis of mental illness messages in video games. *JMIR Mental Health*, *6*(5), e12418. https://doi.org/10.2196/12418

Fischer, B. A. (2012). Maltreatment of people with serious mental illness in the early 20th century: A focus on Nazi Germany and eugenics in America. *The Journal of Nervous and Mental Disease*, *200*(12), 1096–1100. https://doi.org/10.1097/NMD.0b013e318275d391

Fox, A. B., Earnshaw, V. A., Taverna, E. C., & Vogt, D. (2018). Conceptualizing and measuring mental illness stigma: The mental illness stigma framework and critical review of measures. *Stigma and Health*, *3*(4), 348–376. https://doi.org/10.1037/sah0000104

Gary, F. A. (2005). Stigma: Barrier to mental health care among ethnic minorities. *Issues in Mental Health Nursing*, *26*(10), 979–999. https://doi.org/10.1080/01612840500280638

Gerbner, G. (1995). Casting and fate: Women and minorities on television drama, game shows, and news. In E. Hollander, D. Van der Linden, & P. Rutten (Eds.), *Communication, culture, community* (pp. 125–135). Bohn Stafleu van Loghum.

Goffman, E. (1963). *Stigma: Notes on the management of spoiled identity.* Prentice-Hall.

Goulden, R., Corker, E., Evans-Lacko, S., Rose, D., Thornicroft, G., & Henderson, C. (2011). Newspaper coverage of mental illness in the UK, 1992-2008. *BMC Public Health*, *11*, 1–8. https://doi.org/10.1186/1471-2458-11-796

Greene, K. (2009). An integrated model of health disclosure decision making. In T. D. Afifi & W. A. Afifi (Eds.), *Uncertainty and information regulation in interpersonal contexts: Theories and applications* (pp. 226–253). Routledge.

Griffiths, K. M., Carron-Arthur, B., Parsons, A., & Reid, R. (2014). Effectiveness of programs for reducing the stigma associated with mental disorders. A meta-analysis of randomized controlled trials. *World Psychiatry*, *13*(2), 161–175. https://doi.org/10.1002/wps.20129

Haslam, N. (2006). Dehumanization: An integrative review. *Personality and Social Psychology Review*, *10*(3), 252–264. https://doi.org/10.1207/s15327957pspr1003_4

Hatzenbuehler, M. L. (2016). Structural stigma: Research evidence and implications for psychological science. *American Psychologist*, *71*(8), 742–751. https://doi.org/10.1037/amp0000068

Hatzenbuehler, M. L., & Link, B. G. (2014). Introduction to the special issue on structural stigma and health. *Social Science & Medicine*, *103*, 1–6. https://doi.org/10.1016/j.socscimed.2013.12.017

Hecht, M., Kloß, A., & Bartsch, A. (2022). Stopping the stigma. How empathy and reflectiveness can help reduce mental health stigma. *Media Psychology*, *25*(3), 367–386. https://doi.org/10.1080/15213269.2021.1963991

Hildersley, R., Potts, L., Anderson, C., & Henderson, C. (2020). Improvement for most, but not all: Changes in newspaper coverage of mental illness from 2008 to 2019 in England. *Epidemiology and Psychiatric Sciences*, *29*(e177), 1–10. https://doi.org/10.1017/S204579602000089X

Jackson, R. G., Huskins, K., Skelton, S. M., & Thorius, K. A. K. (2020). *Allyship & accomplice: Two sides of the same coin.* Midwest & Plains Equity Assistance Center. https://greatlakesequity.org/sites/default/files/202003022136_newsletter.pdf

Jacobs, S., & Quinn, J. (2022). Cultural reproduction of mental illness stigma and stereotypes. *Social Science & Medicine*, *292*, 114552. https://doi.org/10.1016/j.socscimed.2021.114552

Jensen, P. R. (2018). Undignified dignity: Using humor to manage the stigma of mental illness and homelessness. *Communication Quarterly*, *66*(1), 20–37. https://doi.org/10.1080/01463373.2017.1325384

Jeong, M., & Bae, R. E. (2018). The effect of campaign-generated interpersonal communication on campaign-targeted health outcomes: A meta-analysis. *Health Communication, 33*(8), 988–1003. https://doi.org/10.1080/10410236.2017.1331184
Johnson, I. R., Pietri, E. S., Fullilove, F., & Mowrer, S. (2019). Exploring identity-safety cues and allyship among black women students in STEM environments. *Psychology of Women Quarterly, 43*(2), 131–150. https://doi.org/10.1177/0361684319830926
Jones, E. E., Farina, A., Hastorf, A. H., Markus, H., Miller, D. T., & Scott, R. A. (1984). *Social stigma: The psychology of marked relationships.* W. H. Freeman and Company.
Jones, K. P., King, E. B., Peddie, C. I., Gilrane, V. L., & Gray, A. L. (2016). Not so subtle: A meta-analytic investigation of the correlates of subtle and overt discrimination. *Journal of Management, 42*(6), 1588–1613. https://doi.org/10.1177/0149206313506466
Kam, J. A., Cornejo, M., Mendez Murillo, R., & Afifi, T. D. (2022). Communicating allyship according to college students with deferred action for childhood arrivals. *Journal of Social and Personal Relationships, 39*(6), 1623–1647. https://doi.org/10.1177/02654075211061715
Katz, E., & Lazarsfeld, P. F. (1955). *Personal influence: The part played by people in the flow of mass communications.* Free Press.
Keyes, C. L. M. (2002). The mental health continuum: From languishing to flourishing in life. *Journal of Health and Social Behavior, 43*(2), 207–222. https://doi.org/10.2307/3090197
Kleck, R. (1968). Physical stigma and nonverbal cues emitted in face-to-face interaction. *Human Relations, 21*(1), 19–28. https://doi.org/10.1177/001872676802100102
Klin, A., & Lemish, D. (2008). Mental disorders stigma in the media: Review of studies on production, content, and influences. *Journal of Health Communication, 13*(5), 434–449. https://doi.org/10.1080/10810730802198813
Ledford, V., Lim, J. R., Namkoong, K., Chen, J., & Qin, Y. (2022). The influence of stigmatizing messages on danger appraisal: Examining the model of stigma communication for opioid-related stigma, policy support, and related outcomes. *Health Communication, 37*(14), 1765–1777. https://doi.org/10.1080/10410236.2021.1920710
Link, B., Castille, D., & Stuber, J. (2008). Stigma and coercion in the context of outpatient treatment for people with mental illnesses. *Social Science & Medicine, 67*(3), 409–419. https://doi.org/10.1016/j.socscimed.2008.03.015
Link, B. G., Cullen, F. T., Struening, E., Shrout, P. E., & Dohrenwend, B. P. (1989). A modified labeling theory approach to mental disorders: An empirical assessment. *American Sociological Review, 54*(3), 400–423. https://doi.org/10.2307/2095613
Link, B. G., Mirotznik, J., & Cullen, F. T. (1991). The effectiveness of stigma coping orientations: Can negative consequences of mental illness labeling be avoided? *Journal of Health and Social Behavior, 32*(3), 302–320. https://doi.org/10.2307/2136810
Link, B. G., & Phelan, J. C. (2001). Conceptualizing stigma. *Annual Review of Sociology, 27*(1), 363–385. https://doi.org/10.1146/annurev.soc.27.1.363
Link, B. G., & Phelan, J. C. (2013). Labeling and stigma. In C. S. Aneshensel, J. C. Phelan, & A. Bierman (Eds.), *Handbook of the sociology of mental health* (pp. 521–539). Springer.
Link, B. G., Phelan, J. C., & Sullivan, G. (2018). Mental and physical health consequences of the stigma associated with mental illnesses. In B. Majro, J. F. Dovidio, & B. G. Link (Eds.), *The Oxford handbook of stigma, discrimination, and health* (pp. 525–541). Oxford University Press.
Livingston, J. D., & Boyd, J. E. (2010). Correlates and consequences of internalized stigma for people living with mental illness: A systematic review and meta-analysis. *Social Science & Medicine, 71*(12), 2150–2161. https://doi.org/10.1016/j.socscimed.2010.09.030
Lyons, R. F., Mickelson, K. D., Sullivan, M. J., & Coyne, J. C. (1998). Coping as a communal process. *Journal of Social and Personal Relationships, 15*(5), 579–605. https://doi.org/10.1177/0265407598155001
Mahomed, F. (2020). Addressing the problem of severe underinvestment in mental health and well-being from a human rights perspective. *Health and Human Rights, 22*(1), 35–50. https://www.jstor.org/stable/26923472
Mehta, S. I., & Farina, A. (1988). Associative stigma: Perceptions of the difficulties of college-aged children of stigmatized fathers. *Journal of Social and Clinical Psychology, 7*(2–3), 192–202. https://doi.org/10.1521/jscp.1988.7.2-3.192
Meisenbach, R. J. (2010). Stigma management communication: A theory and agenda for applied research on how individuals manage moments of stigmatized identity. *Journal of Applied Communication Research, 38*(3), 268–292. https://doi.org/10.1080/00909882.2010.490841
Meisenbach, R. J., & Hutchins, D. (2020). Stigma communication and power: Managing inclusion and exclusion in the workplace. In M. L. Doerfel & J. L. Gibbs (Eds.), *Organizing inclusion* (pp. 25–42). Routledge.
Miller, G. H., Marquez-Velarde, G., Williams, A. A., & Keith, V. M. (2021). Discrimination and black social media use: Sites of oppression and expression. *Sociology of Race and Ethnicity, 7*(2), 247–263. https://doi.org/10.1177/2332649220948179
Myrick, J. G., & Chen, J. (2022). Schadenfreude after watching the news: How audiences respond to media coverage of partisans disclosing illnesses. *Journalism & Mass Communication Quarterly, 99*(1), 135–155. https://doi.org/10.1177/10776990211008534

Nabi, R. L., Pérez, T. D., & Prestin, A. (2017). Guilty pleasure no more: The relative importance of media use for coping with stress. *Journal of Media Psychology, 29*, 126–136. https://doi.org/10.1027/1864-1105/a000223

National Alliance on Mental Illness. (2023). *Understanding your diagnosis*. https://www.nami.org/Your-Journey/Individuals-with-Mental-Illness/Understanding-Your-Diagnosis

National Institutes of Health. (2023). *Writing respectfully: Person-first and identity-first language*. https://www.nih.gov/about-nih/what-we-do/science-health-public-trust/perspectives/writing-respectfully-person-first-identity-first-language

Ng, S. H. (2007). Language-based discrimination: Blatant and subtle forms. *Journal of Language and Social Psychology, 26*(2), 106–122. https://doi.org/10.1177/0261927X07300074

O'Connor, C., Brassil, M., O'Sullivan, S., Seery, C., & Nearchou, F. (2022). How does diagnostic labelling affect social responses to people with mental illness? A systematic review of experimental studies using vignette-based designs. *Journal of Mental Health, 31*(1), 115–130. https://doi.org/10.1080/09638237.2021.1922653

Oexle, N., & Corrigan, P. W. (2018). Understanding mental illness stigma toward persons with multiple stigmatized conditions: Implications of intersectionality theory. *Psychiatric Services, 69*(5), 587–589. https://doi.org/10.1176/appi.ps.201700312

Oliver, M. B., & Bartsch, A. (2010). Appreciation as audience response: Exploring entertainment gratifications beyond hedonism. *Human Communication Research, 36*(1), 53–81. https://doi.org/10.1111/j.1468-2958.2009.01368.x

Olstead, R. (2002). Contesting the text: Canadian media depictions of the conflation of mental illness and criminality. *Sociology of Health & Illness, 24*, 621–643. https://doi.org/10.1111/1467-9566.00311

Perry, B. L., & Pescosolido, B. A. (2015). Social network activation: The role of health discussion partners in recovery from mental illness. *Social Science & Medicine, 125*, 116–128. https://doi.org/10.1016/j.socscimed.2013.12.033

Pescosolido, B. A., & Martin, J. K. (2015). The stigma complex. *Annual Review of Sociology, 41*, 87–116. https://doi.org/10.1146/annurev-soc-071312-145702

Pescosolido, B. A., Martin, J. K., Lang, A., & Olafsdottir, S. (2008). Rethinking theoretical approaches to stigma: A framework integrating normative influences on stigma (FINIS). *Social Science & Medicine, 67*(3), 431–440. https://doi.org/10.1016/j.socscimed.2008.03.018

Pietri, E. S., Johnson, I. R., & Ozgumus, E. (2018). One size may not fit all: Exploring how the intersection of race and gender and stigma consciousness predict effective identity-safe cues for Black women. *Journal of Experimental Social Psychology, 74*, 291–306. https://doi.org/10.1016/j.jesp.2017.06.021

Ranjit, Y. S., Das, M., & Meisenbach, R. (2022). COVID-19 courtesy stigma among healthcare providers in India: A study of stigma management communication and its impact. *Health Communication, 38*(13), 2833–2842. https://doi.org/10.1080/10410236.2022.2122279

Recovery Research Institute. (2023). *Addictionary*. https://www.recoveryanswers.org/addiction-ary

Riles, J. M., Miller, B., Funk, M., & Morrow, E. (2021). The modern character of mental health stigma: A 30-year examination of popular film. *Communication Studies, 72*(4), 668–683. https://doi.org/10.1080/10510974.2021.1953098

Ross, A. M., Morgan, A. J., Jorm, A. F., & Reavley, N. J. (2019). A systematic review of the impact of media reports of severe mental illness on stigma and discrimination, and interventions that aim to mitigate any adverse impact. *Social Psychiatry and Psychiatric Epidemiology, 54*, 11–31. https://doi.org/10.1007/s00127-018-1608-9

Ross, A. M., Morgan, A. J., Wake, A., Jorm, A. F., & Reavley, N. J. (2022). Key stakeholders' recommendations for improving Australian news media reporting of people with severe mental illness, violence and crime. *Advances in Mental Health, 20*(3), 253–265. https://doi.org/10.1080/18387357.2021.1942101

Rüsch, N., Angermeyer, M. C., & Corrigan, P. W. (2005). Mental illness stigma: Concepts, consequences, and initiatives to reduce stigma. *European Psychiatry, 20*(8), 529–539. https://doi.org/10.1016/j.eurpsy.2005.04.004

Samoilenko, S. A. (2016). Character assassination. In C. Carroll (Ed.), *The encyclopedia of corporate reputation* (pp. 115–118). Sage.

Smith, R. A. (2007). Language of the lost: An explication of stigma communication. *Communication Theory, 17*, 462–485. https://doi.org/10.1111/j.1468-2885.2007.00307.x

Smith, R. A. (2012a). An experimental test of stigma communication content with a hypothetical infectious disease alert. *Communication Monographs, 79*(4), 522–538. https://doi.org/10.1080/03637751.2012.723811

Smith, R. A. (2012b). Segmenting an audience into the own, the wise, and normals: A latent class analysis of stigma-related categories. *Communication Research Reports, 29*(4), 257–265. https://doi.org/10.1080/08824096.2012.704599

Smith, R. A. (2014). Testing the model of stigma communication with a factorial experiment in an interpersonal context. *Communication Studies, 65*(2), 154–173. https://doi.org/10.1080/10510974.2013.851095

Smith, R. A., & Bishop, R. E. (2019). Insights into stigma management communication theory: Considering stigmatization as interpersonal influence. *Journal of Applied Communication Research, 47*(5), 571–590. https://doi.org/10.1080/00909882.2019.1675894

Smith, R. A., & Hipper, T. J. (2010). Label management: Investigating how confidants encourage the use of communication strategies to avoid stigmatization. *Health Communication, 25*(5), 410–422. https://doi.org/10.1080/10410236.2010.483335

Smith, R. A., Sillars, A., Chesnut, R. P., & Zhu, X. (2018). Investigating married adults' communal coping with genetic health risk and perceived discrimination. *Communication Monographs*, *85*(2), 181–202. https://doi.org/10.1080/03637751.2017.1404618

Smith, R. A., Zhu, X., & Fink, E. L. (2019). Understanding the effects of stigma messages: Danger appraisal and message judgments. *Health Communication*, *34*(4), 424–436. https://doi.org/10.1080/10410236.2017.1405487

Smith, R. A., Zhu, X., & Quesnell, M. N. (2016). Stigma and health/risk communication. In J. Nussbaum (Ed.), *Oxford research encyclopedia of communication: Health and risk message design and processing* (pp. 1–33). Oxford University Press. https://doi.org/10.1093/acrefore/9780190228613.013.96

Smith-Frigerio, S. (2018). Intersectionality of race, class and gender: The complex representation of bipolar disorder on Fox Network's empire. *Howard Journal of Communications*, *29*(4), 387–402. https://doi.org/10.1080/10646175.2017.1407720

Southwell, B. G., & Yzer, M. C. (2007). The roles of interpersonal communication in mass media campaigns. *Annals of the International Communication Association*, *31*(1), 420–462. https://doi.org/10.1080/23808985.2007.11679072

Taniguchi-Dorios, E., Voorhees, H. L., & Donovan, E. (2023). Mental illness disclosure from confidants' perspective within romantic relationships: Validation and extension of the disclosure quality model. *Communication Monographs*, *90*(1), 112–135. https://doi.org/10.1080/03637751.2022.2125995

Thoits, P. A. (2011). Mechanisms linking social ties and support to physical and mental health. *Journal of Health and Social Behavior*, *52*(2), 145–161. https://doi.org/10.1177/0022146510395592

Thompson, T. L., & Seibold, D. R. (1978). Stigma management in normal-stigmatized interactions: Test of the disclosure hypothesis and a model of stigma acceptance. *Human Communication Research*, *4*(3), 231–242. https://doi.org/10.1111/j.1468-2958.1978.tb00612.x

Thornicroft, G., Sunkel, C., Aliev, A. A., Baker, S., Brohan, E., El Chammay, R., Davies, K., Demissie, M., Duncan, J., Fekadu, W., Gronholm, P. C., Guerrero, Z., Gurung, D., Habtamu, K., Hanlon, C., Heim, E., Henderson, C., Hijazi, Z., Hoffman, C., . . . Winkler, P. (2022). The lancet commission on ending stigma and discrimination in mental health. *The Lancet*, *400*(10361), 1438–1480. https://doi.org/10.1016/S0140-6736(22)01470-2

Tomiyama, A. J. (2014). Weight stigma is stressful. A review of evidence for the cyclic obesity/weight-based stigma model. *Appetite*, *82*, 8–15. https://doi.org/10.1016/j.appet.2014.06.108

Vayreda, A., & Antaki, C. (2009). Social support and unsolicited advice in a bipolar disorder online forum. *Qualitative Health Research*, *19*(7), 931–942. https://doi.org/10.1177/1049732309338952

Wahl, O. F. (2003). News media portrayal of mental illness: Implications for public policy. *American Behavioral Scientist*, *46*(12), 1594–1600. https://doi.org/10.1177/0002764203254615

Walter, G. (2000). The psychiatric patient in American cartoons, 1941–1990. *Humor*, *13*(1), 7–17. https://doi.org/10.1515/humr.2000.13.1.7

Williams, K. D. (2001). *Ostracism: The power of silence*. Guilford Press.

Wilson, C., Nairn, R., Coverdale, J., & Panapa, A. (2000). How mental illness is portrayed in children's television: A prospective study. *British Journal of Psychiatry*, *176*(5), 440–443. https://doi.org/10.1192/bjp.176.5.440

Wilson, S. R., Hintz, E. A., MacDermid Wadsworth, S. M., Topp, D. B., Southwell, K. H., & Spoont, M. (2021). Female US military veterans'(non) disclosure of mental health issues with family and friends: Privacy rules and boundary management. *Health Communication*, *36*(4), 412–423. https://doi.org/10.1080/10410236.2019.1693128

Wolenski, R., & Pettit, J. W. (2023). *Social media usage is associated with lower knowledge about anxiety and indiscriminate use of anxiety coping strategies*. Psychology of Popular Media. Advance online publication. https://doi.org/10.1037/ppm0000456

Wolfers, L. N., & Schneider, F. M. (2021). Using media for coping: A scoping review. *Communication Research*, *48*(8), 1210–1234. https://doi.org/10.1177/0093650220939778

World Health Organization. (2021). *Comprehensive mental health action plan 2013–2030*. https://www.who.int/publications/i/item/9789240031029

Yanos, P. T., DeLuca, J. S., Salyers, M. P., Fischer, M. W., Song, J., & Caro, J. (2020). Cross-sectional and prospective correlates of associative stigma among mental health service providers. *Psychiatric Rehabilitation Journal*, *43*(2), 85–90. https://doi.org/10.1037/prj0000378

Yin, M., Li, Z., & Zhou, C. (2020). Experience of stigma among family members of people with severe mental illness: A qualitative systematic review. *International Journal of Mental Health Nursing*, *29*(2), 141–160. https://doi.org/10.1111/inm.12668

Zhu, X. (2023). Mapping linguistic shifts during psychological coping with the COVID-19 pandemic. *Journal of Language and Social Psychology*, *42*(2), 203–216. https://doi.org/10.1177/0261927X221116335

Zhu, X., & Smith, R. (2016). Advancing research on the spread of stigmatizing beliefs with insights from rumor transmission. *American Behavioral Scientist*, *60*(11), 1342–1361. https://doi.org/10.1177/0002764216657382

Zhu, X., & Smith, R. A. (2021). Stigma, communication and health. In T. L. Thompson & N. G. Harrington (Eds.), *The Routledge handbook of health communication* (3rd ed., pp. 77–90). Routledge.

21

Reducing Mental Health Stigma Through School-Based Interventions: Assessing the Evidence and Translating It into Practice

Ashley Johnston[1], Supriya Misra[2], Rachel Banawa[1], John Anagnost[1], and Daniel Eisenberg[1]

[1] University of California Los Angeles
[2] San Francisco State University

Improving knowledge and attitudes related to mental health is important for increasing help seeking and creating a more supportive social environment for people experiencing mental health challenges (Shahwan et al., 2020). The roots of attitudes are developed in childhood, making schools an important setting for building a positive perception of mental health for children to carry through adulthood (Wahl et al., 2011). Schools can reach most of each child and youth cohort, and many already have a curriculum that addresses health and well-being issues.

There is considerable evidence that school-based interventions can be effective for improving knowledge and attitudes toward mental health and mental illness. A meta-analysis of 21 randomized clinical trial (RCT) evaluations of 20 unique school-based interventions concluded that moderate evidence exists for improving literacy and stigma attitudes and beliefs at posttest, with less evidence available to assess long-term sustainability (Ma et al., 2023). Another review used pooled data from pretest–posttest studies to examine behavioral intent of 21 contact-based school-based education interventions, finding that 18 studies showed nearly a threefold increase in the odds of a student scoring an A on the 11-item Social Acceptance scale at posttest compared with pretest (Koller & Stuart, 2016). Lastly, a review of seven studies (pretest–posttests and quasi-experimental designs) on school-based schizophrenia stigma interventions found that school-based interventions generally reduce stigma at posttest (Flanigan & Climie, 2020).

Although many interventions appear to be effective, the evidence has key limitations and weaknesses. Many studies do not measure outcomes beyond an immediate postintervention assessment, and those that do often find diminished effects over time. For instance, Mellor's (2014) analysis of 17 RCTs concluded that few studies demonstrated a positive impact on stigma or knowledge outcomes at a follow-up assessment. Moreover, many evaluation studies are vulnerable to selection and attrition bias (Mellor, 2014). Similarly, Schachter et al. (2008) purport poor reporting quality, mixed or null findings, and considerable heterogeneity across intervention content as critical barriers to the evidence for school-based interventions.

Ideally, schools throughout the United States and the world could easily identify which programs are most likely to be effective for improving knowledge and attitudes among their students. This would require making sense of the strengths and limitations of the continually evolving evidence

The Handbook of Mental Health Communication, First Edition.
Edited by Marco C. Yzer and Jason T. Siegel.

base, which is scattered across many sources. Currently, no single source summarizes and updates the evidence in a readily accessible format for schools and organizations that support schools.

To address this gap, we have begun to develop a repository of evidence on the effectiveness of school-based interventions that address mental health knowledge and attitudes. This chapter introduces this repository. A primary purpose of the repository is to assist school communities in identifying the most effective and promising interventions. Another purpose is to highlight for the research field the most important gaps that need to be addressed to provide even more useful evidence for school communities.

The remainder of this chapter is organized as follows. First, we provide an overview of how the repository was developed and organized, including the key criteria by which each intervention and evaluation study is assessed. Next, we briefly summarize the characteristics and findings of the evaluation studies as a whole. We then describe several examples of school-based programs that have been evaluated to illustrate in more detail some of the strengths and weaknesses in the evidence. Finally, we conclude with a brief discussion of next steps for improving and sharing evidence in this area.

Introduction to the Repository

The purpose of an evidence repository—also known as a registry or clearinghouse—is to "aggregate, standardize, review, and rate the evidence base of interventions" and thus provide input into decision-making by community and organization leaders (Neuhoff et al., 2015, p. 11). A repository can guide decisions about which interventions to implement, highlight strengths and limitations in the evidence, and motivate researchers and evaluators to address gaps with new studies and methods.

Although there are many repositories of evidence in a variety of areas related to youth well-being, such as the Blueprints Programs for Healthy Youth Development, no comprehensive repository critically assesses and summarizes evidence specifically for school-based mental health interventions. However, several sources are helpful for building such a repository, such as systematic reviews and meta-analyses of school-based evaluation studies (Ma et al., 2023; Mellor, 2014). A repository with a specific focus on school-based interventions has the potential to highlight the full variety of evidence in this area, whereas a broader registry such as Blueprints has strict methodological requirements that limit attention to only programs with the highest levels of evidence (Blueprints, 2003). A more narrowly focused repository can also be designed for the specific audience of schools and their partner organizations.

We have begun to develop a repository on school-based interventions addressing mental health. As a first step, we have compiled a database more specifically focused on interventions aimed at improving knowledge and attitudes related to mental health in schools. This includes interventions that explicitly address various aspects of mental health stigma as well as others that more generally address knowledge and attitudes related to mental health.

Our vision for the repository is to build a database of evidence and surround it with an active network of experts and partners who are engaging with the content. This network will help overcome the challenge that many repositories are underused due to a lack of visibility and support (Neuhoff et al., 2015). We anticipate that users of the repository will be able to engage with experts, peer organizations, and communities to better use the information in the database. This network will ideally include national and regional organizations that focus on student well-being and success (e.g., Jed Foundation, Steve Fund, American College Health Association) as well as leaders and practitioners from institutions that have experience implementing programs in the database. Also, users will be able to provide continuous feedback about what is helpful in the repository and what might be missing or in need of improvement. The repository is presently in development, and a description of our vision can be found at Healthy Minds Network (https://healthymindsnetwork.org/best-practices-repository; Lipson & Eisenberg, 2023).

To identify evaluations and programs for the repository, we searched databases such as Google Scholar, PubMed, and EBSCO using search terms including *schools, students, mental health, stigma, programs, interventions, knowledge,* and *attitudes.* We limited the search to English language studies. Our criteria for inclusion in the database are simply that a study must report outcomes from an evaluation of a school-based program or intervention addressing attitudes or knowledge related to mental health. In potentially relevant articles that we identified, we also reviewed the reference list for other studies that fit our criteria. As of August 2023, we have identified 111 evaluation studies meeting our criteria, corresponding to 84 school-based interventions across 24 countries.

For each eligible evaluation study, we have extracted meta-data with the aim of summarizing the quality and relevance of the evidence: internal validity, external validity, effect magnitude, and implementation readiness. Collectively, these elements represent some of the most important factors that school leaders will want to consider when choosing which intervention strategies to adopt. Whereas many previous repositories have focused on internal validity and effect magnitudes, external validity and implementation readiness are less commonly considered explicitly.

Internal validity refers to the accuracy and credibility of the estimated effects of the intervention for the population and setting in which it was tested. Key aspects of internal validity include overall study design, timing of assessments (baseline, posttest, follow-up), sample size, study power, participant attrition, outcome measures (e.g., type and validity), and differences between groups at baseline and how covariates are controlled (Chambless & Hollon, 2012). Although we have not yet settled on a specific formula, we anticipate summarizing internal validity through scores that represent a sum of ratings of each previously noted subcomponent.

External validity is more speculative to assess but is important to highlight so school communities can consider whether and how each piece of evidence pertains to their own population and setting. External validity cannot be summarized with a numerical rating, in part because the external validity of any given study will vary for each community considering the relevance of that study (depending on how similar the setting and population of the study are to their own). Thus, our plan is to summarize external validity in a more descriptive, qualitative manner by highlighting features such as the diversity of the sample in terms of demographic and socioeconomic characteristics, the geographical location of the study, and the results of any subgroup or modifier analyses that examine how intervention effects might vary across groups. Under external validity, we will also consider the number of schools and students in the study and how schools and students were recruited (e.g., a convenience sample versus a more representative or random sample).

In our categorization scheme, effect magnitude refers to the size of the estimated effects and also their statistical significance. In other words, this category represents whether the estimated impacts are large (or medium or small) and whether we can be confident that those estimates are real (and not due to statistical chance). We summarize effect sizes with standard measures such as Cohen's d, Cohen's f, and partial eta squared. Statistical significance is summarized by p values and confidence intervals. For studies that do not report these statistics, we calculate them using the data provided whenever possible. If the intervention produced positive effects, we document whether the effect is sustained, improved, or diminished at follow-up, when follow-up estimates are available.

Implementation readiness is the final category that we summarize for each program in the repository. This feature is sometimes ignored in other repositories, although there are notable exceptions such as Blueprints, which limits its scope only to programs that are readily available for dissemination and implementation. As in the case of external validity, implementation readiness is difficult to represent with a numerical score or grade, so instead we summarize it with qualitative information. We focus on factors such as the availability of guides, manuals, and organizations to assist a school or community with implementation, as well as the cost required for implementation. Additionally, we consider the time and personnel an intervention requires and the expectations for educators and other school personnel. For instance, is it an extra activity outside of regular class time, and are teachers expected to complete training before implementation?

Overall Findings: Summary of Programs and Evidence in Repository

We summarize key characteristics of the interventions and corresponding evaluations in the repository in Table 21.1. There are more evaluations than interventions because many interventions have been evaluated in multiple studies; for example, it is common for interventions to be tested first in smaller pilot studies and then later in larger evaluations. As shown in the table, the interventions and

Table 21.1 Summary of Interventions and Evaluations in the Repository (as of August 2023)

Number of interventions	84
Number of evaluation studies	111
Countries of evaluation studies	
Australia	11
Cambodia	1
Canada	10
Czech Republic	1
Egypt	1
England	12
Germany	2
Greece	3
Hong Kong	3
Italy	1
Japan	3
Malaysia	1
New Zealand	1
Nigeria	1
Norway	1
Pakistan	1
Portugal	3
Russia	2
Singapore	2
Spain	2
Taiwan	1
Turkey	4
United States	43
Vietnam	1
Education level	
Higher education/postsecondary	35
High school	58
Middle school	7
Elementary school	7
More than one of these levels	4
Study design	
Randomized controlled trial (RCT)	42
Quasi-experimental	22
Pretest–posttest	35
Other design (e.g., posttest only, pretest and follow-up)	12
Number of studies with a follow-up	
Studies with at least one follow-up	48
Studies with no follow-up	63
Intervention type	
Education	51
Contact	7
Education and contact	48
Education versus contact	5
Outcomes measured	
Mental health knowledge or literacy	64
Stigmatizing attitudes	93
Behavioral intention	29
Behavioral (actual)	9
Validity and reliability of measures	
Report valid or reliable measures	39
Report some measures are valid or reliable	19
Report only Cronbach's alpha	33
Report no information	16
Report not using valid or reliable measures	4

Table 21.1 (Continued)

Power analysis	
Conducted a power analysis	19
Report sufficient power	13 of 19
Implementation readiness	
Interventions readily available	22 of 84
Interventions partially available	12 of 84
Unknown or not reported	50 of 84
Positive findings at posttest	
Mental health knowledge or literacy	58 of 64
Stigmatizing attitudes	80 of 93
Behavioral intention	23 of 29
Behavioral (actual)	7 of 9
Positive findings for studies with a follow-up	
Mental health knowledge or literacy	22 of 26
Stigmatizing attitudes	27 of 34
Behavioral intention	13 of 15

evaluations have been implemented in many different countries throughout the world and across all grade levels, from elementary to higher education.

The majority of evaluations include a control group, with 42 RCTs and 22 quasi-experimental designs. The latter refers to prospective studies that compare outcomes for schools and students experiencing the intervention versus a nonrandomized control or comparison group, ideally selected for its similarity to the intervention group. Of all studies, 48 (43%) include at least one follow-up assessment. Overall, follow-up assessments range from one week posttest to three years, with six-month follow-ups being the most common, comprising 27% of studies with a follow-up.

We categorized interventions using the common nomenclature of ***education, contact***, and ***education and contact*** (Taniyama, 2016); this refers to whether the intervention is primarily designed to provide information, social contact with persons with a mental health condition, or both. Most studies focused on one of these categories, but a small number compared education with contact. There is considerable variability of content across interventions with ***education*** typically comprising role-playing, distribution of informational booklets, or an interactive lecture on a variety of topics such as identifying and debunking common myths about mental illness or identifying warning signs of mental illness and steps to seek assistance. Variations of ***contact*** include a live discussion with a person with lived experience of mental illness, viewing videos or documentaries of someone directly or indirectly discussing their experience with mental illness, or playing a video game imbued with concepts of mental illness.

The most common types of outcome measures are stigmatizing attitudes (93 studies) and mental health knowledge or literacy (64 studies). Many studies examine both of these outcomes. Stigmatizing attitudes encompass several measures of stigma, such as social distance, attitudes toward a specific mental illness, attitudes related to seeking or receiving treatment, stereotypes, self-stigma, and affect (emotional responses such as anger or fear). Fewer studies measure behavioral intentions (e.g., willingness or intention to seek help for oneself or provide support for others; 29 studies), and even fewer measure actual behavioral change (9 studies), and those that do vary in their approach. Among measures of actual behavioral change, examples include measures that assess whether or not a participant spoke to someone, sought treatment for a mental health concern, or engaged in positive actions such as befriending someone with a mental illness (Ahmad et al., 2020; Beaudry et al., 2019; Murman et al., 2014).

With respect to implementation readiness, we classify an intervention as readily available if it has all materials (e.g., written documents, videos) and guides or manuals publicly available. We classify an intervention as partially available if some but not all key materials and guides are available. Unknown or not reported refers to programs developed only for evaluation purposes, or a search for the intervention yields no information.

In classifying findings in Table 21.1, we define positive findings as showing statistically significant improvement on at least a few items of a single measure or positive findings on one of two measured dimensions. For example, several studies measure stigma using social distance and attitudes; if one of the two measures is significant, we report that study as yielding positive findings. Using this approach, the clear majority of studies have positive findings for each category of outcome, at both posttest and follow-up (for studies with a follow-up), as shown in the table. A key caveat, of course, is that this definition of positive findings does not account for limitations in the study design or for the risk of false positives when testing multiple related outcomes. In future iterations of the repository, our rating system noted earlier will score the quality of study design.

Findings for studies with a follow-up showed medium to large effect sizes on knowledge outcomes and small effects on attitude outcomes. This is consistent with literature demonstrating that attitude changes often happen gradually over weeks and sometimes years (Briñol et al., 2015). Thus, observing small effects on attitudes is not surprising. Moreover, small effects can still be considered a success in the context of relatively inexpensive school-based interventions that reach a large number of young people (Corrigan et al., 2012).

Examples of Interventions and Evaluation Studies

This section highlights examples of programs with promising efficacy for improving knowledge and attitudes toward mental health. We illustrate interventions from a variety of settings and modes of delivery. Though we strive for breadth, the programs highlighted here are not intended to be fully representative of all studies nor to be necessarily considered the best of all interventions.

The Mental Health & High School Curriculum Guide

The Mental Health & High School Curriculum Guide (also called the Guide) was developed in collaboration between mental health experts, educators, and the Canadian Mental Health Association (CMHA), a national mental health nongovernmental organization. It is designed to improve mental health literacy, increase understanding of mental illness, reduce the associated stigma, and promote students' help-seeking behaviors. It contains six distinct modules delivered over six hours of classroom time.

1. Stigma of mental illness
2. Understanding mental health and mental illness
3. Information on specific mental illnesses
4. Experiences of mental illness
5. Seeking help and finding support
6. The importance of positive mental health

Adapted from Milin et al. (2016).

The Guide has demonstrated efficacy in improving knowledge and attitudes across various evaluation studies and yielded some positive findings for cultural relevance. It has been evaluated using a variety of study designs and validated measures and has yielded consistently positive findings in a Western context. In addition, the intervention is freely and readily available. TeenMentalHealth.org (2023) actively supports the intervention by providing free access to lesson plans and teaching resources. Lesson plans include detailed instructions for each module, including an overview, learning objectives, major concepts, activities, and required materials. Teacher resources include suggested information to enhance understanding of the material, instructions for collecting and preparing materials, and pre-and post-quizzes to evaluate the efficacy of the intervention.

A secondary cross-sectional analysis conducted among Grade 9 students (n = 409) across four school boards in Durham, Canada, examined mental health literacy under the enhanced definition encompassing stigma reduction (McLuckie et al., 2014). The validity of the measuring instrument is not reported; however, internal consistency is acceptable (McLuckie et al., 2014). The chance for type I error was reduced by applying Bonferroni correction. Analysis showed significant improvements from baseline to posttest and baseline to two-month follow-up for knowledge and attitudes (McLuckie et al., 2014). By follow-up, knowledge had diminished from a large to medium effect size while attitudes sustained a small effect size (McLuckie et al., 2014).

Similar results were observed in a pretest–posttest with a two-month follow-up (Kutcher et al., 2015). This study was conducted among Grades 11 and 12 students across three schools ($n = 114$) in Toronto, Canada, using matched data (Kutcher et al., 2015). The intervention's efficacy on mental health knowledge and stigmatizing attitudes was assessed using scales with confirmed face validity (Kutcher et al., 2015). The chance for type I error was reduced by applying Bonferroni correction (Kutcher et al., 2015). Analysis showed a significant large effect of the intervention from baseline to posttest for knowledge and a significant medium effect for attitudes (Kutcher et al., 2015). Effects for knowledge were sustained at the two-month follow-up, albeit slightly diminished, and attitudes diminished, yielding a small effect size (Kutcher et al., 2015).

The intervention was also evaluated using an RCT of Grades 11 and 12 students across 25 schools in Ottawa, Canada (Milin et al., 2016). This study was sufficiently powered, the potential for type I error was reduced using Bonferroni correction, and measures were developed by the paper's authors and mental health and education experts (Milin et al., 2016). Knowledge and attitudes were assessed, yielding significant small effect sizes at the two-week posttest (Milin et al., 2016).

The Guide's cross-cultural relevance was tested in two studies in Southeast Asia: a controlled quasi-experimental design among 2,539 students in Grades 8 and 9 across 10 schools in Danang, Vietnam, and an RCT with 275 students from Grades 7, 8, 10, and 11 in one school in Phom Penh, Cambodia. Like previous scholars, the intervention assessed knowledge and attitudes with culturally adapted measures (Nguyen et al., 2020). Within-group results for the Cambodian study showed significant and small improvements in knowledge and stigma among intervention participants, with significant group effects found for both outcomes (Nguyen et al., 2020). Similarly, participants in the Vietnamese study showed significant but much smaller changes in both outcomes compared with the Cambodian study (Nguyen et al., 2020). Together, results were mixed; attitudes yielded a large effect size within the Cambodian study, contrary to the previously reported studies, which reported small to slightly medium effects for attitudes. At the same time, the Vietnamese study yielded much lower effects on attitude compared with the Cambodian study and all the previously reported studies (Nguyen et al., 2020).

Collectively, these studies suggest that the Guide is effective for improving knowledge and attitudes with promising findings for efficacy across cultural contexts (see Table 21.2).

Ending the Silence

Ending the Silence (ETS) is a program that aims to provide mental health education for young people to improve their understanding and acceptance of mental health conditions. The standard program is 50 minutes and traditionally delivered in person, but more recently it has been adapted for online instruction. Two trained facilitators deliver the program, which includes a PowerPoint presentation, a contact component, and an educational video followed by a group discussion. The PowerPoint presentation addresses facts about youth mental illness, warning signs of mental health conditions, and actions to take in response to warning signs, and discusses the acceptance of mental health conditions and urges stigma reduction. The contact component is delivered by a young adult who discusses their experience with a mental health condition. Lastly, the video, which is made by youth, encourages acceptance and support for peers with mental illness.

Description referenced from Deluca et al. (2021) and Wahl et al. (2019).

Ending the Silence (see Table 21.3) began in 2006 in DuPage, Illinois, and is a mental health stigma reduction and health promotion program developed by the National Alliance on Mental Illness (NAMI; DeLuca et al., 2021; Taniyama, 2016). Researchers at NAMI have estimated that as of 2012,

Table 21.2 The Curriculum Guide: Findings

References	*Outcomes*	*Reported findings*	*Effect size*
McLuckie et al. (2014)	Knowledge	Baseline to posttest: $p<0.001$ Baseline to two-month follow-up: $p<0.001$	Reported Cohen's *d* Baseline to posttest: $d = 0.90$ Baseline to two-month follow-up: $d = 0.73$
	Attitudes	Baseline to posttest: $p<0.001$ Baseline to two-month follow-up: $p<0.007$	Baseline to posttest: $d = 0.25$ Baseline to two-month follow-up: $d = 0.18$
Kutcher et al. (2015)	Knowledge	Baseline to posttest: $p<0.001$ Baseline to two-month follow-up: $p<0.001$	Reported Cohen's *d* Baseline to posttest: $d = 1.11$ Baseline to two-month follow-up: $d = 0.91$
	Attitudes	Baseline to posttest: $p<0.001$ Baseline to two-month follow-up: $p<0.001$	Baseline to posttest: $d = 0.66$ Baseline to two-month follow-up: $d = 0.52$
Milin et al. (2016)	Knowledge	$F_{1,495.33} = 25.78$, $p<0.001$, $B = 0.67$, 95% CI = 0.41–0.93	Conversion to Cohen's *d* Cohen's $d = 0.305$
	Positive attitudes	$F_{1,488.95} = 11.33$, $B = 0.51$, $p<0.01$, 95% CI = 0.21–0.81	Cohen's $d = 0.18$
Nguyen et al. (2020)	Vietnam	Baseline to posttest:	Conversion to Cohen's *d* Baseline to posttest: group effects
	Knowledge	$F_{(1,2536)} = 6.98$, $R^2<0.01$, $p<0.001$	Cohen's $d = 0.107$
	Attitudes	$F_{(1,2536)} = 12.72$, $R^2<0.01$, $p<0.001$	Cohen's $d = 0.144$
	Cambodia	Baseline to posttest:	Baseline to posttest:
	Knowledge	$F_{(1,272)} = 23.09$, $R^2 = 0.08$, $p<0.001$	Cohen's $d = 0.583$
	Attitudes	$F_{(1,272)} = 41.53$, $R^2 = 0.13$, $p<0.001$	Cohen's $d = 0.781$

approximately 750 presentations across California have reached an estimated 23,818 students and more than 1,000 presentations in the United States have reached an estimated 35,000 students (Taniyama, 2016). The intervention has shown consistently small effects on stigma measures across various study designs, and it is easily implemented. Designed for middle and high school students, NAMI provides the intervention at no fee, and its website includes step-by-step instructions for implementing the program, student testimonials, and resources (NAMI, 2023).

Our review includes four evaluations of ETS: two pretest–posttests, one without a follow-up and one with a six-week follow-up, a quasi-experimental study with a four- to six-week follow-up, and a cluster RCT with a four-week and eight-week follow-up (DeLuca et al., 2021; Taniyama, 2016; Wahl et al., 2019; Wong et al., 2016).

ETS was evaluated using a pretest–posttest design across three high schools (n = 250) in Northern California, using measures adapted from previous studies without reported reliability and validity (Wong et al., 2016). Stigma is the primary outcome, assessed on knowledge about mental illness, stigmatizing attitudes, emotional responses to students with a mental health problem at school, help seeking, and support-giving intentions (Wong et al., 2016). All outcomes showed significant findings except help seeking and support-giving intentions, but more data were needed to calculate effect sizes (Wong et al., 2016).

Comparable results were observed in another pretest–posttest design with a six-week follow-up across three high schools in California (n = 142; Taniyama, 2016). Outcomes included stigmatizing attitudes, knowledge of mental illness, and positive personal beliefs about those with mental illness.

Table 21.3 Ending the Silence: Findings

References	*Outcomes*	*Reported findings*	*Effect size*
Wong et al. (2016)	Emotional responses to students with a mental health problem at school	7 of 7 items significant ($p<0.001$ to $p<0.05$)	Not reported and not enough data reported to calculate Cohen's *d*
	Stigmatizing attitudes	5 of 8 items significant $p<0.010$	
	Knowledge about mental illness	4 of 5 items significant $p<0.001$	
	Help-seeking intentions and support giving	Not significant	
Taniyama (2016)	Stigma (r-AQ scale)	Baseline to posttest $t(137) = -1.93$, $p = 0.056$ Baseline to follow-up $t(140) = -2.60$, $p = 0.011$	Calculated Cohen's *d* Baseline to posttest: $d = 0.14$ Baseline to follow-up: $d = 0.20$
	Knowledge	Baseline to posttest $t(137) = 10.33$, $p<0.0001$ Baseline to follow-up $t(140) = 5.18$, $p<0.001$	Baseline to posttest: $d = 0.78$ Baseline to follow-up: $d = 0.43$
	Personal beliefs	Baseline to posttest $t(135) = -3.69$, $p<0.0001$ Baseline to follow-up $t(139) = 4.18$, $p<0.001$	Baseline to post-test: $d = 0.33$ Baseline to follow-up: $d = 0.06$
Wahl et al. (2019)	One instrument to measure all outcomes: Mental health knowledge, stigma, and help seeking	Baseline to posttest $p<0.010$ Baseline to four- to six-week follow-up $p<0.010$	Reported Cohen's *d* Baseline to posttest $d = 1.30$ Baseline to four- to six-week follow-up $d = 0.78$
DeLuca et al. (2021)	Stereotypes	$F_{3, 481.12} = 3.55$, $p = 0.014$	Reported Cohen's *d* $d = 0.44$
	Stigma-related mental health knowledge	$F_{3, 495.13} = 3.10$, $p = 0.026$	$d = 0.24$
	Disclosure of expectations: anticipated risk	$F_{3, 481.51} = 4.68$, $p = 0.003$	$d = 0.21$

Valid and reliable measures were used only to assess stigmatizing attitudes, and internal consistency was reported for all three measures (0.36–0.67; Taniyama, 2016). All outcomes were significant from baseline to posttest and baseline to follow-up, with effect sizes ranging from small to large (Taniyama, 2016).

ETS was evaluated using a quasi-experimental design across five states in the United States (Arizona, California, Florida, Illinois, and Texas) at 10 schools consisting of 60 classes (n = 932). Teachers assigned classes to the ETS or non-ETS groups based on schedule needs and limitations (Wahl et al., 2019). The study assessed knowledge, attitudes, and help seeking using highly reliable and moderately consistent measures. Results showed a significant interaction effect between time points ($p<0.010$), with the ETS group showing changes and scores with the non-ETS condition remaining essentially unchanged (Wahl et al., 2019). A large and significant effect from baseline to posttest was observed, which diminished from posttest to follow-up, yielding modestly large improvements (Wahl et al., 2019). However, mean changes were smaller for individual attitude questions than for the knowledge question, suggesting improvements in attitudes were smaller than knowledge (Wahl et al., 2019).

Most recently, ETS was assessed in a cluster RCT from one school in New York (n = 206) in Grades 9–12 across 14 classes (DeLuca et al., 2021). Primary outcomes include stigma-related mental health knowledge, attitudes, stereotypes, and intention to seek help (DeLuca et al., 2021). Secondary outcomes include anticipated stigma from others, self-stigma for seeking mental health treatment, and disclosure expectations (DeLuca et al., 2021). Disclosure expectations examine worries about confidentiality about mental health services and include anticipated risks (DES-AR) and anticipated benefits (DES-AB; DeLuca et al., 2021). The study was underpowered, and post hoc Bonferroni corrections were applied due to multiple comparisons (DeLuca et al., 2021). Results showed that small, significant effects were sustained at the eight-week follow-up on three of the 11 outcomes: stereotypes, stigma-related mental health knowledge, and the DES-AR (DeLuca et al., 2021).

Antistigma Program in Greece

This intervention is run by the University Mental Health Research Institute in Athens, Greece. It is delivered over two hours by two professionals of the program: an educational psychologist and a psychiatrist. The program actively engages students while aiming to reduce stigma and discrimination around mental illness using the example of schizophrenia. The intervention has two components. In the first part, students make notes on a card of a word, emotion, and color they think about when they hear the term *mental illness*. A discussion follows with students expressing their beliefs and feelings about schizophrenia and persons with schizophrenia. Stereotypes and myths emerge from this discussion and are written on the blackboard. Using scientific information and age-appropriate language, teachers dispel each one. Next, program administrators elaborate on the symptoms of schizophrenia and its available treatments. Narratives from persons living with mental illness about their experience are then read to students by program administrators. Subsequently, students actively engage by role-playing as the patient. In the second part of the program, students read narratives about being rejected due to schizophrenia, followed by another structured discussion. Program administrators then discuss alternate ways students can talk about persons with schizophrenia, ending with the motto, "Speak the language that respects, not the language that hurts." The program closes by having students collaborate on a drawing to express their feelings and thoughts about the program.

(Description referenced from Economou et al., 2012, 2014)

Another intervention from Athens, Greece, shows efficacy in improving knowledge and attitudes related to mental health across two evaluations (Economou et al., 2012, 2014; see Table 21.4). Both evaluations utilized rigorous designs, had low participating attrition rates, almost equivalent gender ratios (females comprised 51.4% and 53.1%, respectively), and consistent findings (Economou et al., 2012, 2014). The main drawback of the intervention is the absence of information regarding implementation readiness.

The intervention was first assessed using a cluster RCT with a 12-month follow-up among students aged 13–15 across 11 public schools (n = 616; Economou et al., 2012). Classes were randomized to either the intervention or control condition (a talk about nutrition and healthy living; Economou et al., 2012). A 94.16% response rate (n = 580) was reported, and attrition was primarily due to student's absence on the day of the intervention (Economou et al., 2012). Outcomes assessed include beliefs and attitudes, and stigma measured using social distance (Economou et al., 2012). The scale has been adapted from the Alberta Pilot Site Questionnaire Toolkit and has moderate internal consistency (Economou et al., 2012). At posttest, the intervention condition showed significant improvements on 9 of 10 belief and attitude items and all seven stigma (social distance) items, translating to small to medium Cohen's d effect sizes (Economou et al., 2012). Findings at the 12-month follow-up showed diminished effects from posttest but still significant from baseline on 7 of 10 items for beliefs and attitudes, indicating a sustained effect (Economou et al., 2012). However, a Bonferroni correction on social distance showed no significant effect of the intervention from baseline to 12-month follow-up, indicating that any improvements the intervention had on reducing social distance were erased by one year postintervention (Economou et al., 2012).

Table 21.4 Antistigma Program from Greece: Findings

References	*Outcomes*	*Reported findings*	*Effect size*
Economou et al. (2012)	Baseline to 12-month follow-up: Beliefs and attitudes items A person with schizophrenia:	Baseline mean, standard deviation (SD), and 12-month follow-up mean and SD All measures $p<0.010$	Calculated Cohen's d
	1. Suffers from split or multiple personalities	1. 2.97 (0.69) to 2.50 (0.91)	1. $d = 0.50$
	2. Tends to be mentally retarded or of lower intelligence	2. 2.40 (0.83) to 2.18 (0.83)	2. $d = 0.26$
	3. Can be seen talking to themself or shouting in the streets	3. 3.27 (0.69) to 3.40 (0.81)	3. $d = 0.31$
	4. Is dangerous to the public	4. 2.61 (0.82) to 2.05 (0.85)	4. $d = 0.67$
	5. Is a public nuisance due to panhandling, poor hygiene, or odd behavior	5. 2.36 (0.90) to 2.37 (0.93)	5. $d = 0.39$
	6. Can work at regular jobs	6. 1.70 (0.78) to 1.94 (0.86)	6. $d = 0.29$
	7. Can be creative	7. 2.85 (0.72) to 3.45 (0.73)	7. $d = 0.29$
Economou et al. (2014)	(Findings for the intervention group) Beliefs and attitude composite score	Baseline mean = 22.92 (4.20) Posttest mean = 16.81 (4.75) $p<0.001$	Calculated Cohen's d $d = 1.36$
	Social distance composite score	Baseline mean = 21.77 (5.83) Posttest mean = 18.76 (6.11) $p<0.001$	$d = 0.50$

A second cluster RCT was conducted among students aged 13–15 with a two-week posttest across 20 schools (n = 1081; Economou et al., 2014). The randomization protocol is consistent with the 2012 study, except the control condition received a discussion on immunization; the same outcomes and measures were also used (Economou et al., 2014). Two-week posttest results showed significant reductions on beliefs and attitudes and social distance, translating to large and medium effect sizes, respectively (Economou et al., 2014).

Eliminating the Stigma of Differences

Eliminating the Stigma of Differences (ESD) is a three-hour curriculum delivered by teachers over one week and combines an educational component, group discussion, and homework exercises. Teachers receive a video outlining the program's purpose and information to help guide delivery. In-class and homework exercises and paper materials to display in the classroom are also provided to teachers. ESD is delivered in three modules. Module 1 encompasses a basis for judging others to be different; definitions, causes, and consequences of stigma; a definition, description, causes, and treatments of mental illness; barriers to help seeking; how stigma applies to mental illness; and a contact component where two young adults with mental illness speak about the onset of their illness, course of symptoms, hospitalizations, and treatments, feelings about the illness, coping strategies, and impact the illness has on social relationships, school, and work. Modules 2 and 3 introduce mental health disorders: attention deficit hyperactivity disorder (ADHD), anxiety disorders, depression, schizophrenia, and bipolar disorders; describe each disorder; and discuss causes and treatment. Suicide is also discussed as part of module 2.

Description referenced from Link et al. (2020) and Painter et al. (2017).

Table 21.5 Eliminating the Stigma of Differences: Findings

Reference	*Significant related outcomes*	*Findings*
Painter et al. (2017)	Knowledge and attitudes	Curriculum plus contact: $p<0.010$, 95% CI = 3.60–3.72
	Behavioral intention: stigma awareness and action	Curriculum condition: $p<0.010$, 95% CI = 0.14–0.18 Curriculum + contact condition: $p<0.001$, 95% CI = 0.16–0.22
	Social distance: more acceptable forms	Curriculum condition: $p<0.050$ Curriculum + contact condition: $p<0.050$
Link et al. (2020)	Knowledge and positive attitudes	Two-year follow-up $d = 0.35$, $p<0.001$
	Social distance	$d = 0.16$, $p<0.050$
	Treatment seeking for high-risk students	OR = 3.90, $p<0.050$ Converted to Cohen's $d = 0.75$

ESD has shown promising results from a single longitudinal RCT (2011–2015) reported on by two teams of scholars: Link et al. (2020) and Painter et al. (2017). We have chosen to highlight this program based on its longitudinal nature, which demonstrated sustained effects two years postintervention (see Table 21.5). In addition, ESD is short (three hours over one week), and specialized training is not required (Link et al., 2020; Painter et al., 2017).

This longitudinal RCT comprised middle school students from 19 classes across 14 schools ($n = 751$) in one Texas school district (Link et al., 2020; Painter et al., 2017). Conditions included an ESD condition, a contact condition, a printed materials condition, and a no-intervention control group; schools were randomized to receive all three interventions, two, one, or no intervention (Link et al., 2020; Painter et al., 2017). The study was conducted in two phases. Phase 1 included a baseline and posttest, reported on by Painter et al. (2017), and Phases 1 and 2 are reported on by Link et al. (2020); the latter includes follow-up assessments at 6, 12, 18, and 24 months postintervention. Measures have established psychometric properties for this sample population and a few newly developed items specific to this intervention (Painter et al., 2017). Both studies assessed the intervention on knowledge and attitudes, actual behavior and behavioral intentions, and help seeking (Link et al., 2020; Painter et al., 2017). Painter et al. (2017) also include an analysis of beliefs, social distance, and help-seeking recommendations using vignette characters. Link et al. (2020) represent one of the few studies that include actual behavioral-seeking measures. Behavior was measured by asking, "Whether youth had taken medicine for a mental health problem or talked to a therapist or counselor about a mental health problem"; responses were binary yes or no (Link et al., 2020, p. 4). Subsequently, students completed the National Institute of Mental Health Diagnostic Schedule for Children (DSIC), Version IV, which identifies students at high risk of needing professional mental health treatment, and were compared across conditions (Link et al., 2020).

Results at posttest showed that knowledge and attitudes were only significant for the curriculum + contact condition (Painter et al., 2017). One of two items was significant for behavioral intention, one of two items for the social distance measures, and six of eight items were significant at posttest for the curriculum contact group (Painter et al., 2017). Moreover, the curriculum + contact condition and the curriculum-only condition did not significantly differ, implying that the effect of adding the contact to the curriculum was negligible (Painter et al., 2017). This is consistent with Link et al. (2020), who found no effect of the contact intervention.

Findings from the Phase 2 report on the curriculum-only group show that participants sustained a small, significant increase in knowledge and positive attitudes and a small, significant effect in reducing one's desire for social distance across the two-year follow-up period compared to the nonintervention groups (Link et al., 2020). Moreover, these effects were sustained when covariates (sex, age, social desirability, race/ethnicity, parental educational attainment, and primary language spoken at home) were controlled (Link et al., 2020). Regarding actual behavioral outcomes, the analysis showed that high-risk students in the curriculum group were significantly more likely to seek treatment than their counterparts in the other conditions (Link et al., 2020). The intervention had no effect on treatment seeking for low-risk students (Link et al., 2020).

Next Steps for Improving Evidence and Practice

Our review of school-based interventions to address mental health knowledge and attitudes revealed a number of strengths and limitations in the evidence. Moreover, in building a repository of evidence to help guide school and community leaders, we are particularly interested in how this evidence can best translate to practice. Here, we highlight a few areas in which future evaluations and research would ideally focus attention.

First, we were not able to identify a clear pattern regarding which types of interventions are most effective. This indicates a need to classify and study intervention types in a more nuanced way than broad classifications such as *contact* and *education*. For example, we suspect that the most effective interventions benefited from the highest quality training and other implementation strategies, but there is no way to assess this hypothesis with currently available data. The skills of teachers and others who deliver interventions are undoubtedly important; teacher depression literacy has been found to be significantly associated with student depression literacy (p = 0.035, 95% CI [0.044, 0.355]; Miller et al., 2019).

Another approach may involve assessing the underlying mechanisms that are theorized to produce behavioral change to shed light on why some interventions are effective while others are not. For example, some interventions are founded on the theory of planned behavior, which predicts one's intention to engage in a particular behavior. In our context, a change in one's perception of mental illness and persons it affects. It can predict and explain health behaviors such as smoking, drinking, and substance use (LaMorte, 2022). It comprises three components, which work together to yield behavioral change: (a) behavioral beliefs (beliefs about the likely consequences of the behavior); (b) normative beliefs (beliefs about the normative expectations of others); and (c) control beliefs (beliefs about the presence of factors that may facilitate or impede performance of the behavior) (Bosnjak et al., 2020, p. 353).

Recent studies outside of mental health have examined how variables affect these foundational considerations such as the importance of group identification on one's attitudes toward binge drinking and assessing behavioral change by framing it as the development of a new habit (Bosnjak et al., 2020, p. 353).

Relatedly, a study (Ferchaud et al., 2020) in our collection used transportation theory and identification to evaluate how playing a video game with a main character affected by psychosis could reduce stigma. Transportation theory has demonstrated efficacy in changing attitudes and posits that when one disengages from reality and absorbs oneself in a story, their intentions change as a result of the story (Ferchaud et al., 2020). Identification is an "imaginative process wherein an individual takes on the thoughts and perspectives of media characters" (Ferchaud et al., 2020, p. 3). Results indicated that playing the game increased transportation, which then increased identification; subsequently, identification decreased the desire for social distance (Ferchaud et al., 2020).

Future research and evaluations should prioritize identifying these core components, or active ingredients, that are essential for the effectiveness of the intervention. This type of research facilitates the adaptation of interventions to diverse settings and populations by highlighting which components must remain in place and which are potentially modifiable without sacrificing effectiveness. Also, this research will allow for modifications of interventions that maximize efficiency, which is important in the context of schools with limited time and attention to implement new programs.

Another priority for future work is incorporating actual behavioral measures into analysis rather than using behavioral intention as a proxy for change. Few studies to date use actual behavioral measures, which means that it is still unclear whether and how school-based interventions are changing these important outcomes. Measuring actual behavioral change requires reframing questions from intention to action oriented. For example, actual behavior for help seeking may be measured by asking whether one has spoken to or sought out mental health professionals or a school counselor or whether one has engaged in supportive or distancing behavior with someone experiencing mental health challenges (Lindow et al., 2020; Link et al., 2020; Schilling et al., 2016). Although changes in attitudes and knowledge might have value in their own right, the ultimate goal of most interventions is to change behaviors, too, but the latter is rarely measured in evaluations.

Statistical power is another challenge for many studies in this area. This partially reflects the challenge that school-based interventions are typically delivered at a group level—a classroom, grade, or entire school. Group-level interventions require clustered study designs in which high statistical power might necessitate a large number of groups or clusters. However, alternative methods exist to enhance power, such as "increasing sample homogeneity, using instructional manipulation checks, or controlling for relevant covariates" (Sommet et al., 2022, p. 27). However, these options can impede generalizability or create spurious suppression effects (Sommet et al., 2022). Another potentially more feasible approach is using measures that have demonstrated reliability. For example, Heo et al. (2015) demonstrated that by increasing Cronbach's alpha from the minimum acceptable level of 0.70 to a high value of 0.90, power to detect an interaction in a mixed design can increase from approximately 0.40 to almost 0.90 (Sommet et al., 2022, p. 28). Thus, future research should attempt to assess and maximize study power. Scholars can employ alternative measures to increase study power if the suggested sample size is unattainable.

Another important gap is the lack of information and support regarding how to implement many of the interventions that have promising evidence of effectiveness. Ideally, all interventions with strong evidence of effectiveness would have purveyor organizations that help schools and communities with the process of implementing the intervention. There would also ideally be intervention manuals and guidance on how to ensure fidelity to the model. However, our review identified programs, such as the one from Greece, that appear to exist only in research studies and are not available for implementation.

Our hope is that the repository of evidence that we are building will help focus attention on these and other emerging gaps. We envision a virtuous cycle in which schools and communities using the repository will give feedback about what is missing, which will spur new research, which in turn will provide more relevant guidance to practice. As evidence and practice both improve in this area, young people will emerge from schooling with greater knowledge and more positive attitudes related to mental health, and this in turn will contribute to healthier and more supportive communities for people experiencing mental health conditions.

References

Ahmad, S. I., Leventhal, B. L., Nielsen, B. N., & Hinshaw, S. P. (2020). Reducing mental-illness stigma via high school clubs: A matched-pair, cluster-randomized trial. *Stigma and Health*, 5(2), 230–239. https://doi.org/10.1037/sah0000193

Beaudry, M. B., Swartz, K., Miller, L., Schweizer, B., Glazer, K., & Wilcox, H. (2019). Effectiveness of the adolescent depression awareness program (ADAP) on depression literacy and mental health treatment. *Journal of School Health*, *89*(3), 165–172. https://doi.org/10.1111/josh.12725

Blueprints. (2003). *Blue Prints Certification*. Blue Prints. https://www.blueprintsprograms.org/blueprints-certification

Bosnjak, M., Ajzen, I., & Schmidt, P. (2020). The theory of planned behavior: Selected recent advances and applications. *Europe's Journal of Psychology*, *16*(3), 352–356. https://doi.org/10.5964/ejop.v16i3.3107

Briñol, P., Rucker, D. D., & Petty, R. E. (2015). Naïve theories about persuasion: Implications for information processing and consumer attitude change. *International Journal of Advertising*, *34*(1), 85–106. https://doi.org/10.1080/02650487.2014.997080

Chambless, D. L., & Hollon, S. D. (2012). Treatment validity for intervention studies. In H. Cooper, P. M. Camic, D. L. Long, A. T. Panter, D. Rindskopf, & K. J. Sher (Eds.), *APA handbook of research methods in psychology. Research designs: Quantitative, qualitative, neuropsychological, and biological* (Vol. 2, pp. 529–552). American Psychological Association. https://doi.org/10.1037/13620-028

Corrigan, P. W., Morris, S. B., Michaels, P. J., Rafacz, J. D., & Rüsch, N. (2012). Challenging the public stigma of mental illness: A meta-analysis of outcome studies. *Psychiatric Services, 63*(10), 963–973. https://doi.org/10.1176/appi.ps.201100529

DeLuca, J. S., Tang, J., Zoubaa, S., Dial, B., & Yanos, P. T. (2021). Reducing stigma in high school students: A cluster randomized controlled trial of the National Alliance on Mental Illness' ending the silence intervention. *Stigma and Health, 6*(2), 228–242. https://doi.org/10.1037/sah0000235

Economou, M., Louki, E., Peppou, L. E., Gramandani, C., Yotis, L., & Stefanis, C. N. (2012). Fighting psychiatric stigma in the classroom: The impact of an educational intervention on secondary school students' attitudes to schizophrenia. *International Journal of Social Psychiatry, 58*(5), 544–551. https://doi.org/10.1177/0020764011413678

Economou, M., Peppou, L. E., Geroulanou, K., Louki, E., Tsaliagkou, I., Kolostoumpis, D., & Stefanis, C. N. (2014). The influence of an anti-stigma intervention on adolescents' attitudes to schizophrenia: a mixed methodology approach. *Child and Adolescent Mental Health, 19*(1), 16–23. https://doi.org/10.1111/j.1475-3588.2012.00669.x

Ferchaud, A., Seibert, J., Sellers, N., & Escobar Salazar, N. (2020). Reducing mental health stigma through identification with video game avatars with mental illness. *Frontiers in Psychology, 11*, 2240. https://doi.org/10.3389/fpsyg.2020.0224

Flanigan, L. K., & Climie, E. A. (2020). A review of school-based interventions to reduce stigma towards schizophrenia. *Psychiatric Quarterly, 91*(4), 983–1002. https://doi.org/10.1007/s11126-020-09765-y

Heo, M., Kim, N., & Faith, M. S. (2015). Statistical power as a function of Cronbach alpha of instrument questionnaire items. *BMC Medical Research Methodology, 15*(1), 86. https://doi.org/10.1186/s12874-015-0070-6

Koller, M., & Stuart, H. (2016). Reducing stigma in high school youth. *Acta Psychiatrica Scandinavica, 134*, 63–70. https://doi.org/10.1111/acps.12613

Kutcher, S., Wei, Y., & Morgan, C. (2015). Successful application of a Canadian mental health curriculum resource by usual classroom teachers in significantly and sustainably improving student mental health literacy. *The Canadian Journal of Psychiatry, 60*(12), 580–586. https://doi.org/10.1177/070674371506001209

LaMorte, W. (2022). *The theory of planned behavior*. Boston University School of Public Health. https://sphweb.bumc.bu.edu/otlt/mph-modules/sb/behavioralchangetheories/BehavioralChangeTheories3.html

Lindow, J. C., Hughes, J. L., South, C., Minhajuddin, A., Gutierrez, L., Bannister, E., Trivedi, M. H., & Byerly, M. J. (2020). The youth aware of mental health intervention: Impact on help seeking, mental health knowledge, and stigma in U.S. adolescents. *Journal of Adolescent Health, 67*(1), 101–107. https://doi.org/10.1016/j.jadohealth.2020.01.006

Link, B. G., DuPont-Reyes, M. J., Barkin, K., Villatoro, A. P., Phelan, J. C., & Painter, K. (2020). A school-based intervention for mental illness stigma: A cluster randomized trial. *Pediatrics, 145*(6), e20190780. https://doi.org/10.1542/peds.2019-0780

Lipson, S., & Eisenberg, D. (2023, September, 08). *Best practices repository*. The healthy minds network. https://healthymindsnetwork.org/best-practices-repository

Ma, K. K. Y., Anderson, J. K., & Burn, A. (2023). Review: School-based interventions to improve mental health literacy and reduce mental health stigma—A systematic review. *Child and Adolescent Mental Health, 28*(2), 230–240. https://doi.org/10.1111/camh.12543

McLuckie, A., Kutcher, S., Wei, Y., & Weaver, C. (2014). Sustained improvements in students' mental health literacy with use of a mental health curriculum in Canadian schools. *BMC Psychiatry, 14*(1), 379. https://doi.org/10.1186/s12888-014-0379-4

Mellor, C. (2014). School-based interventions targeting stigma of mental illness: Systematic review. *The Psychiatric Bulletin, 38*(4), 164–171. https://doi.org/10.1192/pb.bp.112.041723

Milin, R., Kutcher, S., Lewis, S. P., Walker, S., Wei, Y., Ferrill, N., & Armstrong, M. A. (2016). Impact of a mental health curriculum on knowledge and stigma among high school students: A randomized controlled trial. *Journal of the American Academy of Child & Adolescent Psychiatry, 55*(5), 383–391.e1. https://doi.org/10.1016/j.jaac.2016.02.018

Miller, L., Musci, R., D'Agati, D., Alfes, C., Beaudry, M. B., Swartz, K., & Wilcox, H. (2019). Teacher mental health literacy is associated with student literacy in the adolescent depression awareness program. *School Mental Health, 11*(2), 357–363. https://doi.org/10.1007/s12310-018-9281-4

Murman, N. M., Buckingham, K. C. E., Fontilea, P., Villanueva, R., Leventhal, B., & Hinshaw, S. P. (2014). Let's erase the stigma (LETS): A quasi-experimental evaluation of adolescent-led school groups intended to reduce mental illness stigma. *Child & Youth Care Forum, 43*(5), 621–637. https://doi.org/10.1007/s10566-014-9257-y

NAMI. (2023). NAMI ending the silence. https://ets.nami.org

Neuhoff, A., Axworthy, S., Glazer, S., & Berfond D. (2015). *The what works marketplace: Helping leaders use evidence to make smarter choices*. The Bridgespan Group. https://www.bridgespan.org/getmedia/248532cb-8ae1-4560-908e-79f044c630d1/the-what-works-marketplace.pdf

Nguyen, A. J., Dang, H.-M., Bui, D., Phoeun, B., & Weiss, B. (2020). Experimental evaluation of a school-based mental health literacy program in two southeast Asian nations. *School Mental Health, 12*(4), 716–731. https://doi.org/10.1007/s12310-020-09379-6

Painter, K., Phelan, J. C., DuPont-Reyes, M. J., Barkin, K. F., Villatoro, A. P., & Link, B. G. (2017). Evaluation of antistigma interventions with sixth-grade students: A school-based field experiment. *Psychiatric Services, 68*(4), 345–352. https://doi.org/10.1176/appi.ps.201600052

Schachter, H. M., Girardi, A., Ly, M., Lacroix, D., Lumb, A. B., Van Berkom, J., & Gill, R. (2008). Effects of school-based interventions on mental health stigmatization: A systematic review. *Child and Adolescent Psychiatry and Mental Health*, *2*(1), 18. https://doi.org/10.1186/1753-2000-2-18

Schilling, E. A., Aseltine, R. H., & James, A. (2016). The SOS suicide prevention program: Further evidence of efficacy and effectiveness. *Prevention Science*, *17*(2), 157–166. https://doi.org/10.1007/s11121-015-0594-3

Shahwan, S., Lau, J. H., Goh, C. M. J., Ong, W. J., Tan, G. T. H., Kwok, K. W., Samari, E., Lee, Y. Y., Teh, W. L., Seet, V., Chang, S., Chong, S. A., & Subramaniam, M. (2020). The potential impact of an anti-stigma intervention on mental health help-seeking attitudes among university students. *BMC Psychiatry*, *20*(1), 562. https://doi.org/10.1186/s12888-020-02960-y

Sommet, N., Weissman, D. L., Cheutin, N., & Elliot, A. (2022). How many participants do I need to test an interaction? Conducting an appropriate power analysis and achieving sufficient power to detect an interaction. *Open Science Framework*. https://doi.org/10.31219/osf.io/xhe3u

Taniyama, S. L. (2016). *An evaluation of the effectiveness of the National Alliance of Mental Illness's ending the silence program*. [Master's Thesis, California Polytechnic State University]. https://doi.org/10.15368/theses.2016.34

Teenmentalhealth.org. (2023). *Mental health and high school curriculum guide* (Version 3). Teen mental health. https://mentalhealthliteracy.org/product/mental-health-high-school- curriculum/

Wahl, O., Rothman, J., Brister, T., & Thompson, C. (2019). Changing student attitudes about mental health conditions: NAMI ending the silence. *Stigma and Health*, *4*(2), 188–195. https://doi.org/10.1037/sah0000135

Wahl, O. F., Susin, J., Kaplan, L., Lax, A., & Zatina, D. (2011). Changing knowledge and attitudes with a middle school mental health education curriculum. *Stigma Research and Action*, *1*(1), 44–53. https://doi.org/10.5463/sra.v1i1.17

Wong, E. C., Collins, R. L., Cerully, J. L., Roth, E., Marks, J., & Yu, J. (2016). Effects of stigma and discrimination reduction trainings conducted under the California mental health services authority: An evaluation of the National Alliance on Mental Illness adult programs. *Rand Health Quarterly*, *5*(4), 9. https://doi.org/10.7249/RR1240

22

Application of Weiner's Attribution-Emotion-Action Model to Increase Support to People With Depression

Tara Muschetto and Jason T. Siegel
Claremont Graduate University

Depression is a pervasive mental illness that affects approximately 280 million people worldwide (World Health Organization [WHO], 2023), and symptoms can have major social consequences for those affected. Interpersonal theories of depression (e.g., Coyne, 1976; Erlbaum Hillsdale et al., 1992) posit that individuals with the illness behave in ways that elicit social rejection, such as engaging in excessive reassurance seeking. Further, depressive symptoms are negatively associated with the quality and quantity of social interactions (Elmer & Stadtfeld, 2020), and affected individuals tend to report lower perceived social support relative to healthy individuals (Visentini et al., 2018).

Attempts to increase social support to individuals with depression can mitigate the myriad interpersonal consequences the illness presents. Perceived social support is associated with reduced symptom severity and duration (Wang et al., 2018), as well as lower likelihood of attempting suicide (Kleiman & Liu, 2013). Attribution theory (Weiner, 1980a) has guided numerous research efforts examining ways to increase support for individuals with depression.

There has been extraordinary work on ways to increase social support (e.g., Angermeyer et al., 2011; Corrigan, 2000; Liu et al., 1992; Rippere, 1977; Tullett & Plaks, 2016), much of which has inspired and heavily guided the research reported in this chapter. However, this chapter focuses on our research lab's application of Weiner's attribution theory to the depression domain (depressionlab.org). The central objective of the chapter is to synthesize findings from 26 of our attribution studies on depression to derive actionable insights on how attribution theory can best be applied to mental health communication. The chapter begins with an overview of attribution theory, then proceeds to a discussion of attribution dimensions (i.e., controllability, stability) and related appraisals (i.e., deservingness), including how each has been investigated in the context of depression and their applications to campaign settings. The chapter concludes with a summary of attribution theory-related implications for mental health communication.

Attribution Theory Overview

Attribution theory is a social psychological theory of motivation. The theory was formalized by with Fritz Heider's (1958) publication of *The Psychology of Interpersonal Relations* and has since been highly influential across a range of disciplines. Heider regarded humans as intuitive psychologists motivated

The Handbook of Mental Health Communication, First Edition.
Edited by Marco C. Yzer and Jason T. Siegel.

to understand their social world by drawing inferences about their own and others' behavior. According to Heider, the causes of one's behavior or predicament could be attributed to factors within (e.g., ability) or outside of (e.g., task difficulty) a person. These ideas were the theoretical foundation upon which subsequent iterations of attribution theory were developed (e.g., Kelley, 1967).

Earlier attribution theories focused on antecedents (e.g., Jones & Davis, 1965), whereas the most contemporary theory reformulation (Weiner, 1980a) concerns attributions' consequences. Weiner's attribution-emotion-action (AEA) model was developed based on Heider's (1958) theorizing, scholarship on achievement motivation (Weiner, 1974; Weiner et al., 1971), and studies of helping behavior (e.g., Barnes et al., 1979; Berkowitz, 1969; Ickes & Kidd, 1976; Schopler & Matthews, 1965). Building upon this range of scholarship, Weiner (1980a) introduced a classification system of three causal dimensions: locus, controllability, and stability. Locus is the location of a cause (internal-external), controllability refers to the degree of volitional control (controllable-uncontrollable), and stability deals with the duration of a cause (stable-unstable). Of these dimensions, locus has received limited attention, whereas controllability and stability have been identified as most relevant to understanding human motivation (Corrigan, 2000). As such, this chapter focuses exclusively on the latter two dimensions and their applications to mental health communication.

Each causal dimension is theorized to produce discrete emotional responses (Weiner, 1985). The affective consequence of attributions is central to Weiner's theory, which posits that attributions influence emotions, and these affective responses in turn drive action (Weiner, 1980a). The model also has been called the attribution-affect-action (AAA) model (Schmidt & Weiner, 1988; Weiner, 2018), but we maintain AEA for consistency (and because AAA reminds us of needing roadside assistance). The following sections discuss controllability and related responsibility judgments, deservingness (another appraisal related to controllability and responsibility), and stability. Each section includes a review of our empirical studies on depression and the AEA model and highlights how attribution messages have been tested experimentally in applied settings.

Controllability Dimension

Most empirical work on attribution theory has concentrated on perceived controllability, which is particularly relevant in the help-giving context (see Rudolph et al., 2004 for review). According to the theory (Weiner, 1980a, 1980b), the decision to offer aid is partially based on whether the cause is perceived as controllable, resulting in emotional responses that influence the decision to help. Uncontrollable causes give rise to sympathy and, by extension, help giving, whereas controllable causes produce anger and consequently inhibit aid.

Weiner (1980a) tested the effect of controllability using a scenario from Piliavin et al. (1969) involving a confederate who fell in the subway. The reason for the fall was manipulated by depicting the fallen person with a cane (illness, uncontrollable) or with a bottle and smelling of alcohol (drunkenness, controllable). Drunkenness was perceived as more controllable than sickness, and emotional reactions toward the ill person were more positive (e.g., sympathy, concern), whereas responses to the drunk person were more negative (e.g., anger, disgust). Sympathy was positively associated, and anger/disgust was negatively associated, with the likelihood of helping.

Although the basic tenets of the AEA model have remained largely unchanged, specificity has been added and clarifications have been made. Brickman et al. (1982) further specified controllability by differentiating between whether people are perceived as responsible for causing (i.e., onset controllability) and/or solving (i.e., offset controllability) their problems. For example, people could perceive someone as not responsible for becoming depressed but responsible for remaining depressed. Differentiating between onset and offset controllability marks an important advancement of attribution theory. As later discussed, we make this distinction explicitly at times (e.g., Ruybal & Siegel, 2021) but not others (Muschetto & Siegel, 2024), depending on the context.

Another advancement concerns the association between controllability and responsibility. Weiner (1995) noted, "I tended not to make a distinction between causal controllability and responsibility, considering them as synonyms. But now I believe that I erred in my conceptual analysis: Causal controllability is not to be equated with responsibility" (p. 8). Weiner further described that controllability refers to whether "characteristics of the cause" (e.g., a lack of effort) are "subject to volitional alteration" (p. 8). Responsibility is a judgment regarding whether the person should have acted differently. Even though controllability attributions often lead to judgments of responsibility, mitigating factors can weaken the influence of controllability on responsibility (Weiner, 1995). Many studies, including ours, do not always make this distinction, though considering controllability and responsibility as separate constructs has proven fruitful (Dolphin & Hennessy, 2014; Yao & Siegel, 2024).

Decades of studies have supported Weiner's (1980a, 1980b) proposal that controllable causes, and thus persons responsible for their plight, elicit less sympathy, more anger, and subsequently less help (see Rudolph et al., 2004 for a meta-analysis; see Muschetto & Siegel, 2021 for a bibliometric review). This model has successfully explained topics as diverse as unvaccinated individuals who spread COVID-19 (Claudy et al., 2022), sexual assault (Sperry & Siegel, 2013), driver aggression (Wickens et al., 2011), and schizophrenia (Angermeyer et al., 2015). Moreover, the model has received support across populations of various ages (e.g., adolescents; Corrigan et al., 2007) and diverse backgrounds with studies conducted in China (Zhang et al., 2013), Kuwait (Badahdah & Alkhder, 2006), and Germany (Greitemeyer & Rudolph, 2003).

Perceived Controllability or Responsibility and Reactions Toward Individuals with Depression

We have conducted numerous correlational and experimental studies to assess the controllability or responsibility component of the AEA model in the realm of depression with the long-term goal of crafting messages that increase support for people with depression (e.g., Siegel et al., 2012). Our experimental studies have focused on onset controllability, offset controllability, and responsibility explicitly. In line with many attribution studies, the method commonly used in our experiments involved comparing two opposing conditions (e.g., controllable versus uncontrollable or responsible versus not responsible).

One set of vignettes used in our experiments involved randomly assigning participants to read about a woman with postpartum depression (PPD). In one condition, she could have prevented the illness but did not. In the other condition, the woman was described as not at fault for developing the illness (i.e., onset controllability; Ruybal & Siegel, 2021). Respondents who read about a woman who was not at fault for developing PPD reported a greater willingness to provide support through increased sympathy and reduced anger.

A different experiment examining onset controllability revealed a similar pattern of results (Muschetto & Siegel, 2019). This experiment explicitly told participants that the subject of the vignette (a loved one or a close other) was (or was not) responsible for becoming depressed (e.g., becoming depressed was something within/beyond their control). Findings revealed an indirect effect of controllability on willingness to provide social support (WPSS) and desire for social distance through sympathy and anger among close others and acquaintances.

Another set of experiments focused on offset controllability. These studies involved randomly assigning respondents to consider a loved one with depression who did (or did not) take their prescribed medication. Whether tested in the realm of PPD (Ruybal & Siegel, 2017) or major depressive disorder (MDD; Yao & Siegel, 2024), respondents who read about a loved one who took their medication reported greater willingness to help through increased sympathy and/or reduced anger compared to those who read about a loved one who *did not* take their medication. Ruybal and Siegel (2017, Study 2) also found an effect of the controllability manipulation on social support outcome expectations (SSOEs; the belief that providing support would be beneficial) through increased sympathy.

The same pattern of results was indicated in a study focused explicitly on responsibility. Respondents were asked to think of someone they knew with depression and read a scenario where the person's symptoms improved after taking medication, but the person then stopped the medication despite this improvement (Muschetto & Siegel, 2024). Unlike the manipulation used by Ruybal and Siegel (2017), all scenarios involved the person stopping their medication. Responsibility varied based on whether the doctor strongly did (high responsibility) or did not (low responsibility) emphasize the importance of continuing the medication. This responsibility manipulation significantly influenced WPSS and willingness to provide general support (WPGS) through anger and sympathy in the expected directions.

In sum, people who read vignettes that described depression as onset uncontrollable (versus controllable; Muschetto & Siegel, 2019; Ruybal & Siegel, 2021), offset uncontrollable (versus controllable; Ruybal & Siegel, 2017; Yao & Siegel, 2024), or for which the affected person was not responsible (versus responsible; Muschetto & Siegel, 2024) reported increased willingness to provide support through emotional responses. These studies offer stalwart support for Weiner's AEA model within the realm of depression. As discussed next, however, comparing opposing conditions (controllable versus uncontrollable) may not be as useful when implemented as part of a campaign.

Perceived Controllability as a Campaign Approach

Campaigns have been developed, both formally and informally, based on the idea that reducing the culpability of depression can be advantageous for affected individuals. For example, the National Alliance on Mental Illness (NAMI, 2006) sponsored a campaign that stated, "You would not say 'get over it, it's just cancer.' So why would you say that about depression?" Such a message can be expected to lead to favorable responses based on attribution theory and prior research. Recent studies, however, have revealed cause for a more cautious outlook.

Ruybal and Siegel (2017, Study 3) provided initial support for messages designed to minimize responsibility. The authors randomly assigned respondents to view one of three print depression public service announcements (DPSAs) or a control. Each DPSA included an image from a PPD news article (Fischinger & Corbis, 2013) that portrayed a woman holding her infant, looking sad and exhausted. All three DPSAs blamed PPD on factors associated with the illness rather than the mother (e.g., shifting hormone levels and the need to feed the baby every three hours). Results indicated an indirect effect of the DPSAs on WPSS and SSOEs through anger but not sympathy. A limitation of this study was the use of a no-message control group as the sole comparison. Although the DPSAs reduced anger, which was associated with increased WPSS, this effect may have been driven by the image or demand characteristics rather than the actual message. The shortcomings of this approach became fully realized in our later studies.

Subsequent experiments overcame the limitations of a no-message control by randomly assigning respondents to view a message that encouraged them to offer support to people with depression or an identical message that only differed by the inclusion of attribution-specific information (Muschetto & Siegel, 2024; Ruybal & Siegel, 2021). For example, all respondents in Ruybal and Siegel's study received the following standard message:

> Are you concerned your loved one may have postpartum depression? Postpartum depression is more than just sadness. It is a mental illness that affects how your loved one thinks, feels, and acts. Please consider reaching out to your loved one with postpartum depression. For more information, call 1–800-PPD-MOMS or visit www.postpartum.net.

In the experimental group, respondents also read two additional sentences: "Uncontrollable changes in hormones after pregnancy can cause postpartum depression. Your loved one is not responsible for developing depression" before the sentence "Please consider reaching out to your loved one with postpartum depression." Unexpectedly, results showed that information on responsibility did not lead to differences in emotional responses, SSOEs, or WPSS.

Muschetto and Siegel (2024) conducted a similar experiment to Ruybal and Siegel (2021), albeit focused on MDD, comparing vignettes that did or did not include messages about responsibility attributions. Like Ruybal and Siegel's (2021) findings, information about general responsibility (i.e., "Your loved one is not responsible for their illness. It is not their fault they have depression") did not significantly influence emotional responses or willingness to help (though there was an effect of an *undeservingness* message, which will be discussed shortly).

These null results should not be interpreted as a theoretical shortcoming of the AEA model. As described, several experiments whereby respondents were asked to consider close others either as responsible or not responsible for their depression indirectly influenced willingness to help through affective changes. Using opposing conditions in these studies maximized the variance of perceived responsibility between the two experimental groups. In the previously discussed campaign studies, however, respondents in the experimental group viewed a message about depression that emphasized how people with depression are not responsible, whereas those in the comparison group received a depression message that was identical except it did not include information about responsibility. Therefore, the potentially influenced responsibility beliefs of the experimental condition respondents were compared to the comparison group respondents' existing beliefs about depression and responsibility. Between group variance in responsibility was minimized to the degree that respondents already believed people with depression are not responsible.

In support of existing responsibility beliefs possibly minimizing between group differences, Muschetto and Siegel (2019) asked respondents about their perception of people's responsibility for depression on a 7-point scale (1 = *Not at all*, 7 = *Very much*). The mean score was 2.48 ($SD = 1.25$). Similarly, Marshburn and Siegel (2025) asked graduate students the extent to which they agreed with the statement, "People with depression are not at fault for what they are experiencing," and the mean on a 7-point scale was 6.10 ($SD = 1.33$). If people already perceive others with depression as not responsible for their ailment, a campaign promoting such a message would be limited in its ability to influence those beliefs further.

To be sure, people already holding favorable attributions does not necessarily indicate that an attribution campaign would be futile. Priming can influence behavior without changing beliefs (Fishbein & Yzer, 2003). Therefore, messages can prime existing beliefs, making them more salient (e.g., Ajzen, 1991; Cialdini et al., 1990) and accessible (Fazio, 2014). In turn, these beliefs would have greater influence on behavior than they would have otherwise. We are unsure why making responsibility attributions salient did not lead to significant differences, but messages focused on effort, a precursor of responsibility, were successful.

Effort (A Form of Offset Controllability)

Effort is considered a form of offset controllability as it represents the extent to which a person is trying to overcome their situation (e.g., Brickman et al., 1982). The role of effort has long been noted in attribution research. For example, Heider (1958) theorized that "can" (ability) and "try" (effort) are key determinants of action. Before the development of the AEA model, attribution research was concentrated in the achievement domain, where effort and ability played a critical role in determining outcomes and evaluations (e.g., reward versus punishment). Success can be attributed to high ability or high effort, and failure can be attributed to low ability or low effort (Weiner, 1972). Overcoming low ability through expended effort is commended, while failing (despite high ability) due to lack of effort is considered immoral (Weiner & Kukla, 1970).

Studies on the effect of ability and effort became less common following debates in the achievement domain over the consequences of ascribing the cause of success and failure to such attributions (Brown & Weiner, 1984; Weiner, 1994). Some scholars preferred ascriptions of success to high ability and failure to low effort (Covington & Omelich, 1979), whereas others favored the reverse (success ascribed to high effort and failure to low ability; Weiner & Kukla, 1970). Although investigations of the influence of effort beyond the achievement domain, particularly on helping behavior, are limited, Weiner et al. (1988) posited that requests for help following failure to expend effort would elicit anger and inhibit help giving.

Achievement-related studies support the relationships among effort attributions, affective reactions, and helping responses. For example, Karasawa (1991) experimentally varied the reason for falling behind in school (sick versus effort versus no effort) and found that students who expended effort were perceived as less responsible for falling behind and elicited less anger and more sympathy. Further, respondents were more likely to help and less likely to criticize students who expended effort relative to those who gave no effort (see Bennett & Flores, 1998, for similar results). Although limited in number, studies conducted outside the achievement domain also indicate that attributing a person's situation to lack of effort generally inhibits help giving through reduced sympathy and increased anger (e.g., Jones & Ruthig, 2015; Reynolds et al., 2023).

Effort and Reactions to Individuals With Depression

Although not focused on depression, these prior works suggest that reactions toward individuals with the illness would be more favorable if those affected are perceived as having expended effort to recover. Ruybal and Siegel (2021, Study 1) tested this possibility in the depression realm by randomly assigning respondents to think of a loved one with PPD who did or did not expend effort to overcome their illness. Onset controllability and stability attributions also were assessed, though the pertinent findings in this context relate to the effect of effort. Findings revealed that perceiving a loved one as expending effort to overcome her depression, relative to no effort, led to more sympathy and less anger, both of which were associated with greater WPSS and WPGS.

Effort as a Campaign Approach

The previous study highlighted the potential value of focusing on effort as another attribution component. In a campaign setting, however, the critical question is whether adding information about the effort affected individuals make to overcome PPD will be more effective than when such information is omitted.

Ruybal and Siegel (2021, Study 2) investigated this possibility. The authors manipulated several variables (i.e., effort, stability, responsibility) in a factorial design, though results associated with effort are most relevant to the present context. All DPSAs in the study included the standard opening (i.e., "Are you concerned your loved one may have postpartum depression?") and ending message (i.e., "Please consider reaching out to your loved one with postpartum depression"). The following text was presented in the effort condition: "She is making an effort to get better. Although it might not always seem like it, she is trying her best to overcome her depression." The mere addition of these 25 words caused more sympathy toward a loved one with PPD, which was associated with greater WPSS. These findings revealed the potential value of effort as an attribution component and its utility in a campaign message.

The success of the effort message is particularly noteworthy given that a pilot study indicated people already believed others with PPD are likely putting forth effort. Respondents were asked how much effort they thought their loved one would expend to overcome PPD if they experienced the illness (1 = *No effort at all*) to (7 = *A lot of effort*), and the mean score was 5.85 (*SD* = 1.02), indicating limited room for upward movement. Still, adding two sentences about expended effort indirectly increased WPSS through emotions. This finding further leads us to believe that attribution campaigns can be successful by making attributions salient and that belief changes may not be necessary (Fishbein & Yzer, 2003).

Given the success of the effort attribution, which is a form of offset controllability, it is unclear why messages explicitly focused on responsibility were not successful (e.g., Muschetto & Siegel, 2024), particularly given the tight association between controllability and responsibility (Weiner, 1995). The effort attribution likely reduced perceptions of responsibility, yet the direct responsibility messages were unsuccessful. Until the null effect of direct responsibility manipulations can be explained, focusing on constructs associated with responsibility rather than responsibility itself may be prudent. One such construct is deservingness, which is an appraisal closely linked to responsibility with the potential to improve favorable responses toward people with depression.

Deservingness

Deservingness refers to the relationship between the valence of actions and outcomes (Feather, 1996). Deservingness judgments, like responsibility, produce discrete emotions (Feather, 2006); most relevant to the current context are undeserved negative outcomes (e.g., depression), which give rise to sympathy. Deservingness theory suggests that deservingness and responsibility are inherently linked, as "a person cannot be judged to deserve an outcome for which he or she is not responsible" (Feather, 1999, p. 92). Studies have yielded empirical support for the relationship between deservingness and responsibility, as well as affective responses. For example, perceived responsibility for a negative event (e.g., domestic violence, plagiarism, shoplifting) predicted the deservingness of penalty and, by extension, lower levels of sympathy (Feather, 1996). Perceived responsibility for aggressive behavior has also been found to be inversely related to the deservingness of help (Feather & Johnstone, 2001). Although responsibility is often used as a proxy for deservingness (e.g., Bringham et al., 1997; Feather et al., 2011), scholars have cautioned against equating the two constructs.

Deservingness Judgments and Reactions to Individuals With Depression

Researchers have attempted to increase support for people with depression by highlighting how the illness is undeserved. Muschetto and Siegel (2024) examined deservingness as an antecedent of emotions (sympathy, anger) and subsequent helping judgments. Their correlational study revealed that deservingness was positively associated with responsibility and anger, and negatively related to sympathy and willingness to help. Muschetto and Siegel (Study 1) also included measures of responsibility and deservingness as predictors in the same model and found that only responsibility significantly predicted emotional responses. However, deservingness attributions were worth further investigation, given the associations with emotional responses and willingness to help.

A follow-up experiment manipulated deservingness using vignettes (deserved versus undeserved) and found that deservingness directly predicted sympathy and anger. People experienced more sympathy and less anger when others were perceived as undeserving rather than deserving of their depression. Higher levels of sympathy also predicted greater willingness to help. Overall, deservingness, though not part of attribution theory, is an important appraisal that influences emotional responses and subsequent helping judgment.

Deservingness as a Campaign Approach

Building upon the studies described, Muschetto and Siegel (2024; Study 3) tested the effect of communicating that no one deserves to be depressed. However, pilot studies indicated most respondents already perceived depression as undeserved ($M = 1.85$, $SD = 1.48$; 7-point scale), making it difficult to reduce deservingness perceptions further (as discussed shortly, the same pattern emerged regarding the stability attributions of PPD). Deservingness, as a campaign strategy, would be successful to the extent that priming these attributions would be influential. Therefore, we tested whether making deservingness attributions salient could have a positive impact on emotional responses and help giving (see Ruybal & Siegel, 2021, for the success of effort attributions despite the common consensus that people with PPD exert effort to recover).

The study included DPSA manipulations of responsibility and deservingness. The responsibility manipulation discussed earlier did not significantly influence sympathy, anger, or WPSS. The standard text across all messages and the only text in the control condition read:

> Are you concerned that your loved one might have depression? Depression is more than just sadness. It is a mental illness that affects how people think, act, and feel. Please consider reaching out to your loved one with depression. For more information: Call 1-800-622-HELP or text 435748 (HELP4U).

In addition to this standard message, used as the basis in many of our studies, respondents randomly assigned to the undeserving condition viewed the following text: "No one deserves to feel this kind of sadness. No one deserves to have depression." The difference between the control and undeserving DPSAs was two sentences comprising 15 words. Results revealed that adding those 15 words had a statistically significant influence. Emphasizing that others do not deserve to feel depressed increased sympathy (but did not reduce anger), which was associated with a greater willingness to help a close other with depression. These findings provide further evidence of the utility of deservingness as a campaign approach, though this appraisal has been relatively understudied.

Responsibility as a Central Pillar

Our research has taught us much about attribution theory and its nuances. Considering the totality of work, we realize that responsibility can be considered a central pillar of a linear path. Onset and offset controllability are critical variables on one side of the pillar. Controllability attributions and possible mitigators (e.g., self-blame) lead to judgments of responsibility. Responsibility is in the center. Responsibility and the resulting outcome also generate appraisals of deservingness (i.e., the punishment must fit the crime; Weiner, 2006).

Every step of the linear path has received experimental support for its inclusion in the AEA model when tested within the realm of depression using bipolar approaches (e.g., responsible versus not responsible). Potential helpers are more likely to offer assistance through increased sympathy or reduced anger when depression is perceived as onset uncontrollable rather than controllable, when the person experiencing depression expends effort rather than no effort (offset controllable), when they are judged as not responsible rather than responsible, and when depression is perceived as undeserved rather than deserved.

When these components (i.e., onset controllability, effort [offset controllability], responsibility, deservingness) are tested using a more conservative approach that does not include an opposing condition, success is less consistent. Messages that emphasize the effort put forth to overcome depression or the undeservingness of the illness increased willingness to help through increased sympathy or reduced anger. In contrast, messages about general responsibility and onset controllability did not have a significant effect. Although responsibility is the central component of attribution theory, campaigns that make salient the effort people expend to overcome depression, and the undeservingness of the illness, lead to positive outcomes that are not achieved when responsibility, at a more global level, is the focus. These findings highlight the nuances of responsibility-based campaigns and the considerations required to develop a successful approach.

Additional Considerations for Responsibility-Based Campaign Development

Some attribution studies on the specific aspects of responsibility have yielded unexpected findings that warrant further attention. First, campaign developers must be careful not to assume people from different cultures will perceive the same event as controllable or uncontrollable. Siegel et al. (2012) surveyed Spanish-dominant Hispanics on their agreement with reasons as to why a loved one became and remained depressed (e.g., a lack of willpower and motivation). Beliefs that someone became or remained depressed for reasons such as a lack of willpower were associated with increased rather than decreased sympathy, the opposite finding from non-Hispanics. The authors reasoned that Spanish-dominant Hispanic respondents likely perceived a lack of motivation and willpower as uncontrollable rather than controllable, thus eliciting more sympathy. This finding indicates that perceived causality can differ across cultures, an important consideration from a mental health communication standpoint (Barksdale et al., 2025; Marciano et al., 2025).

Consideration of the intended audience is also imperative (e.g., parents or close others). Yao and Siegel (2024) conducted a series of studies in China and found an unexpected positive association between controllability and sympathy among parents who were asked to consider their child experiencing depression. This finding was not evident among respondents who considered a non-child close other with depression. Follow-up studies revealed that parents experienced self-blame when their child's depression was perceived as controllable. Self-blame mediated the relationship between controllability and responsibility among parents but not those considering a non-child close other. Additional studies indicated that this association was not specific to parents but anyone who felt responsible for the person with controllable depression. These data highlight the importance of considering the communication target and possible unintended outcomes of attribution messages (e.g., self-blame among parents). The findings also echo Weiner's (1995) position that controllability and responsibility are not interchangeable under certain circumstances.

Stability Dimension

The stability dimension has received much less research attention than perceived controllability. Stability refers to the temporal duration of a cause, including reversibility and changeability (Weiner, 1985). Weiner's work on perceived stability and helping behavior originated in the achievement domain (e.g., Weiner, 1979; Weiner et al., 1971; also see Barnes et al., 1979), where it was theorized that ability and task difficulty are stable, and effort and luck are unstable. Weiner et al. (1971) proposed that stability attributions would primarily cause expectation shifts. Stability was not associated with affect initially (Weiner et al., 1971), but a path between the two constructs was later added.

Achievement studies indicated that respondents reported different emotional responses depending on whether success was due to stable or unstable effort (Weiner et al., 1979). Regarding helping behavior, Weiner et al. (1982) noted that stability influences the magnitude of experienced emotions rather than the direction, but they also noted that "most experiences of anger are associated with unstable causes" (p. 232). Ickes and Kidd (1976) reasoned that someone with unstable needs is in a less dire situation than someone with stable needs. Likewise, Weiner (1985) proposed that pity and help are most likely when causes are perceived as stable and uncontrollable (versus unstable and controllable) because the person in need is less able to help themselves. As Weiner (1985, p. 563) noted, "affects such as pity are exacerbated when the cause of the negative state is stable rather than unstable (e.g., we tend to pity the blind more than we pity those with temporary eye problems)."

Early research supported these propositions and found that stable needs led to more help giving than unstable needs (e.g., Barnes et al., 1979). However, later studies, particularly those in applied settings, revealed another pattern of results. For example, care staff who perceived patients' challenging behavior as stable tended to be less willing to help and less likely to believe their help would improve the patient's behavior (Willner & Smith, 2008). These inconsistent findings, in contrast to the robust effect of controllability, may explain why stability received limited attention in the literature relative to controllability. Stability was not included in Weiner's (2018) description of attribution theory and helping behavior, nor in a meta-analysis of attributions and help-giving (Rudolph et al., 2004).

Perceived Stability and Reactions Toward Individuals With Depression

Debates surrounding the biogenetic approach piqued our initial interest in perceived stability. Biogenetic approaches conceptualize depression as a biological disorder to minimize blame placed on affected individuals (e.g., Han & Chen, 2014; Lebowitz & Ahn, 2014). Although such an approach may reduce perceptions of blame, it also could give the impression that depression is permanent. As noted, some attribution literature indicated that increased perceptions of permanence led to more helping behavior (e.g., Barnes et al., 1979), whereas other studies indicated otherwise (e.g., Willner & Smith, 2008). Because campaigns often take a biogenetic approach, investigations on the effect of stability on reactions toward individuals with depression were warranted.

Our initial attempt investigated the inconsistent associations between perceived stability and affective reactions. We noticed the relationship between the potential helper and the person in need was varied throughout the literature. For example, Meyer and Mulherin (1980) asked respondents to consider acquaintances. Han and Chen (2014) asked about individuals with depression. Willner and Smith (2008) and Mackay and Barrowclough (2005) inquired about responses to patients. We considered whether the interpersonal relationship between a potential helper and a person in need could account for the mixed results in prior research because the duration of depression likely would have differential effects for close others and strangers (Muschetto & Siegel, 2019).

We manipulated interpersonal relationship, stability, and controllability attributions to explore this possibility (Muschetto & Siegel, 2019, Study 2). Regarding stability and interpersonal relationship, findings revealed that perceiving depression as permanent was associated with less WPSS and greater desire for social distance through reduced sympathy and increased anger. However, this finding was evident only among those who considered a close other, not an acquaintance. Yao and Siegel (2021) replicated this finding in China, though the effect of stability was through sympathy and not anger. Ruybal and Siegel (2019) examined the perceived stability of PPD and found a similar pattern of results. Perceiving a loved one's PPD as permanent rather than temporary reduced WPSS, relational closeness, and SSOEs through reduced sympathy, but not anger.

These findings prompted an investigation to determine the rationale behind the negative effect of perceived stability (Muschetto & Siegel, 2023). Two complementary explanations were investigated: the negative personal impact (NPI) of having a loved one with depression (e.g., Bodenmann & Randall, 2013) and psychological contract breach (PCB; Rousseau, 1989). A series of studies using the experimental-causal-chain design (Spencer et al., 2005) were conducted to examine the effect of perceived stability on NPI, PCB, and the ensuing affective and helping responses. Findings revealed that respondents who perceived a loved one's depression as permanent (versus temporary) felt their lives would be more negatively affected and believed their loved ones would be less able to fulfill relational obligations. These beliefs were associated with more anger (NPI, PCB) and less sympathy (PCB), which were related to less willingness to help. Qualitative responses further indicated that respondents believed they would feel distress from worrying about their loved ones and assuming additional responsibilities. Respondents also reported that their loved one's depression would be contagious and change the dynamic of their relationship.

NPI and PCB were manipulated experimentally in a follow-up study. Findings showed that perceiving one's life to be negatively affected by a loved one's depression led to more anger but not less sympathy, which was associated with less WPSS/WPGS. The PCB manipulation did not have a significant indirect effect on willingness to help through sympathy or anger. Together, these results suggest that perceived stability leads to less favorable responses because relational partners perceive their lives will also be negatively affected by their loved one's depression.

Stability and Outcome Expectations

Stability attributions initially were theorized to be associated with expectation shifts, not emotional responses (Weiner et al., 1971). Accordingly, we have tested SSOEs as a mediator between perceptions of temporality and willingness to provide support. Initially, Siegel et al. (2012) investigated the association between SSOEs and help giving and found that SSOEs were predictive of willingness to provide support over and above sympathy and anger. This finding emerged in both Spanish-dominant Hispanic and non-Hispanic samples. Likewise, Ruybal and Siegel (2017, 2019) found an association between SSOEs and willingness to provide support to people with PPD. These studies demonstrate the crucial role of SSOEs in determining helping judgments. The studies described next further underscore the influence of perceived stability on SSOEs.

Muschetto and Siegel (2020) randomly assigned respondents to think of a loved one with either temporary or permanent depression. Participants in the temporary condition had greater SSOEs and less anger, which were associated with greater WPSS/WPGS. Ruybal and Siegel (2021) replicated these findings and found that presenting PPD as temporary (versus permanent) increased WPSS through increased SSOEs; anger and sympathy also served as mediators. These studies highlight the influence of stability attributions on both affect and expectations.

Stability as a Campaign Approach

Two experiments indicated that campaigns focused on the temporary nature of depression have the potential to influence favorable outcomes. In the studies to be described, all respondents viewed a DPSA encouraging them to extend support to others with depression. The difference between the conditions is whether extra sentences about the temporary nature of depression were included. One experiment focused on MDD (Muschetto & Siegel, 2020), and the other experiment focused on PPD (Ruybal & Siegel, 2021).

Our first experiment focused on MDD. Unlike the basement effect that was present with perceptions of undeservingness, prior studies indicated that people tend to perceive MDD as temporary, but there was still room for further influence. For example, Muschetto and Siegel (2019) found a mean depression stability score of 3.20 (*SD* = 0.94; 1 = *Temporary*, 7 = *Permanent*). Similarly, Marshburn and Siegel (2024) surveyed graduate students on their level of agreement with a statement about the temporary nature of depression, and the mean score was 5.30 (*SD* = 1.86; 1 = *Strongly Disagree*, 7 = *Strongly Agree*).

Muschetto and Siegel (2020) compared two DPSAs that differed only by three sentences composed of 26 words. All respondents received a standard message about depression. Those in the experimental condition received this additional text: "Your loved one's depression can be temporary. They do not have to live with depression forever. Your loved one can feel better and overcome their depression." The additional 26 words focused on temporality resulted in significant differences in WPSS/WPGS through SSOEs, but not emotions, though anger was negatively associated with SSOEs.

In a conceptual replication, Ruybal and Siegel (2021) investigated the effect of a PPD stability DPSA. A pilot study indicated that most respondents already perceived PPD as temporary (*M* = 2.33; *SD* = 1.13; 1 = *Temporary*, 7 = *Permanent*). Unlike the stability attributions of MDD described earlier, this finding represents another situation where messages may not change attributions because of basement effects but can still have the potential to influence affect by priming existing stability attributions.

All respondents received the standard message, and those in the stability condition read two extra sentences: "Postpartum depression can be temporary and treatable. Your loved one does not have to live with depression forever." Even though most respondents already believed PPD was temporary, the addition of these two sentences increased SSOEs, which was associated with greater WPSS/WPGS. The temporary message, however, did not significantly influence emotions.

These two experiments used different scripts and targeted different types of depression but exhibited the same pattern of results. Adding two or three sentences about the temporary nature of depression to DPSAs positively influenced willingness to provide support through SSOEs (but not affect). Notably, as described earlier, when studies compared temporary and permanent depression, there was a significant indirect effect on WPSS/WPGS through both affect and SSOEs. However, this more conservative assessment (i.e., the presence or absence of information that makes the temporary nature of depression salient) revealed only an indirect effect of stability through SSOEs. Campaigns focused on the temporary nature of depression may have appeared unsuccessful if SSOEs were not included. Weiner et al.'s (1971) initial theorizing about stability attributions primarily causing expectation shifts appears to have been on target. Regardless of the mechanism, these studies indicate that adding two sentences about the temporary nature of depression to DPSAs can indirectly increase the amount of support people with depression receive.

Implications for Mental Health Communication

Stability, Effort, and Deservingness Have High Potential

The most critical implication for mental health communication is that messages that make salient the temporary nature of depression, the effort put forth by people with depression, and how people are undeserving of depression have strong potential to indirectly increase social support for people with the illness. Messages that highlighted the temporary nature of depression increased willingness to provide support through SSOEs in two different studies. Effort and undeservingness messages indirectly influenced help giving through affect in one study each. Additional replications are warranted, but the potential of these approaches is highly promising, particularly given that the only difference between the experimental and comparison DPSAs was two or three sentences. Increasing social support for people with depression can have life-saving implications, and these studies offer a potential guide for doing so.

Messages focused broadly on onset controllability and responsibility, however, did not appear to have the same potential as effort, deservingness, and stability. Although responsibility should be considered the central pillar of attribution efforts, and messages focused on effort and deservingness also likely influence responsibility, two different experiments indicated that focusing on responsibility explicitly does not influence affective responses to people with depression. From a theoretical standpoint, and when tested using opposing conditions, responsibility attributions worked as Weiner (1980a) suggested. However, two different experiments lead us to believe that depression campaigns focused only on responsibility may not be the best use of resources—at least not in cultures where people with the illness are not perceived as responsible. The effects of perceived responsibility in campaigns, however, still warrant further investigation, as different messaging approaches may be more successful.

Bipolar Comparisons Are Likely Necessary But Not Sufficient

The use of bipolar conditions (e.g., controllable versus uncontrollable) was a helpful methodological tool for theory development and investigating the generalizability of the AEA model (Weiner, 1980) to the depression domain. However, we have learned that more is needed for predicting campaign success. Many of our attribution experiments on controllability or responsibility compared emotional responses toward someone either responsible or not responsible for their depression. We found indirect effects of controllability or responsibility on willingness to help through emotional responses in studies of PPD (Ruybal & Siegel, 2017) and MDD (Muschetto & Siegel, 2019), as well as in the United States (Ruybal & Siegel, 2021) and China (Yao & Siegel, 2021). However, these effects were not significant when we compared MDD (Muschetto & Siegel, 2024) and PPD (Ruybal & Siegel, 2021) DPSAs that either did or did not include text focused exclusively on responsibility attributions.

We also conducted scores of experiments that randomly assigned respondents to consider a loved one with temporary or permanent depression. We found indirect effects on willingness to provide support through emotional responses and SSOEs in experiments with PPD (Ruybal & Siegel, 2019) and MDD (Muschetto & Siegel, 2019), as well as in the United States (Muschetto & Siegel, 2020) and China (Yao & Siegel, 2021). When we compared MDD (Muschetto & Siegel, 2020) and PPD (Ruybal & Siegel, 2021) DPSAs that either did or did not include text focused on stability, we found significant effects but only through SSOEs. Differences identified by comparing opposing attributions may be a necessary first step, but it cannot be the only approach.

Changing Attributions or Making Them Salient

People generally believe others with PPD put forth effort to recover and that PPD can be temporary (Ruybal & Siegel, 2021). People also believe those experiencing depression do not deserve to be depressed (Muschetto & Siegel, 2024). At first glance, creating campaign messages focused on these topics may appear futile. However, this thinking assumes that the only goal of such campaigns is to change attributions. Such an assumption would be limiting as campaigns also can prime attributions, making them more salient. As noted earlier, beliefs (Ajzen, 1991), norms (Cialdini et al., 1990), and attitudes (Crano & Prislin, 1995) are more predictive of behavior when they are salient, and changing them may not be necessary (Fishbein & Yzer, 2003).

Even if mental health messages do not change the attributions, they have the capacity to increase the salience of different attributions and, by extension, influence emotional responses and helping judgments. Our deservingness study highlighted this possibility (Muschetto & Siegel, 2024). Two pilot studies were unsuccessful because people already believed that depression was not deserved and perceptions of deservingness could not be influenced further. However, respondents reported greater willingness to provide support through more favorable affect after viewing a DPSA that highlighted how no one deserves to feel depressed (versus the comparison DPSA).

Some attributions have the potential to be influenced in a more favorable direction (e.g., the temporary nature of MDD); however, favorable attributions (e.g., the temporary nature of PDD) should not be ignored, as making those beliefs salient can have a positive influence. Moreover, the previously mentioned studies were conducted in cultural contexts where existing attributions were largely favorable. The success of these approaches may be vastly amplified if implemented in a culture where attributions are less favorable and could be further influenced.

The Specificity of Attributions

Researchers are also advised to consider nuanced differences between seemingly similar attributions. Yao and Siegel (2024) measured controllability with items that asked whether depression is controllable, preventable, and beyond the person's power. Responsibility was measured with items about responsibility, blame, and fault. The difference between these two constructs is seemingly so minor that they may only be recognized by academics with too much time on their hands. However, the correlation between these two measures was $r = 0.43$ (Study 2) among respondents who considered a non-child close other with depression and $r = 0.23$ among those who considered their child with depression. Moreover, findings revealed that responsibility, but not controllability, was significantly correlated with sympathy.

A similar argument can be made for responsibility and deservingness (e.g., Muschetto & Siegel, 2024). The responsibility measure was identical to Yao and Siegel (2024), and the deservingness measure included items about whether depression was deserved, fair, and justified. The correlation between the two constructs was $r = 0.29$. Moreover, the deservingness message ("No one deserves to feel this kind of sadness. No one deserves to have depression") indirectly influenced WPSS/WPGS through increased sympathy, but the responsibility message ("Your loved one is not responsible for their illness. It is not their fault they have depression") had no such influence. Altogether, these data indicate that nuances that appear superficial or purely academic can significantly influence outcomes.

Consider the Totality of Attributions

Communications designed to change beliefs must not make one attribution more favorable while unintentionally making another less favorable. This possibility is best illustrated by biogenetic explanations used to reduce the stigmatization of people with depression (e.g., Han & Chen, 2014). As explained by Deacon and Baird (2009), attributing depression to "a chemical imbalance in the brain involving the neurotransmitter serotonin" compared to a combination of "biological, environmental, and psychological factors" (p. 421) resulted in reduced responsibility but increased stability attributions (see Haslam & Kvaale, 2015 for similar theorizing with general mental illness). Scholars have argued against this approach (e.g., Angermeyer et al., 2015; Dumas-Mallet & Gonon, 2020; Yao et al., 2021), and mental health communication researchers must be cautious about the second-order consequences of changing certain attributions.

Consider the Target of the Messages

Attributions may lead to varying outcomes depending on the target of a DPSA. For example, perceived stability had differential effects based on whether the person in need was a close other or an acquaintance with depression (Muschetto & Siegel, 2019; Ruybal & Siegel, 2021; Yao & Siegel, 2021). Yao and Siegel (2024, Studies 1 and 4) also found a negative association between controllability and sympathy among Chinese respondents who thought of a non-child close other with depression but a positive association when respondents thought of their own child with depression. This finding was partially due to self-blame experienced when potential helpers felt responsible for the person with controllable depression. These data convey that attribution messages can lead to different outcomes based on interpersonal relationships, and extensive pilot tests are required before implementation.

Consider Nontargets of the Messages

Public communication about mental health requires more than good intentions, as too many well-intended efforts have led to iatrogenic effects. Communications that are intended to educate the general population will also be seen by people with depression. Numerous scholars have echoed this concern (Chambers et al., 2005; Corrigan, 2016; Niederkrotenthaler et al., 2014; Siegel et al., 2017). As Klimes-Dougan and colleagues described (2016, p. 6), "because PSA [public service announcement] exposure may not be limited to the target population, it is also critical to determine the efficacy and safety for other potentially vulnerable populations who may incidentally view PSAs." Highlighting the need for caution, Siegel et al. (2019) exposed people with and without depressive symptomatology to two DPSAs intended to increase social support for people with depression. Nearly 25% of respondents with depressive symptomatology put forth responses coded as indicating that at least one of the two DPSAs resulted in negative affect; 1.5% of viewers without heightened depressive symptomatology were coded as such.

Conclusion

This research program began with the goal of using Weiner's AEA model (1980a) to guide the development of messages to increase support for people with depression. Our journey has involved numerous missteps, misreadings, and mistakes. We have learned much about appreciating theoretical nuances, the importance of replication, and methodological rigor. We also learned that Weiner's AEA model is more sophisticated, accurate, and useful than anticipated. This research program also allowed us to uncover critical pathways for creating messages to increase the likelihood that people with depression are met with sympathy and receive ongoing support (i.e., attributions of effort, deservingness, and stability). We sincerely hope the lessons learned and the findings uncovered lead others to continue this research stream and develop it further. We also hope this scholarship can help campaign creators develop messages that improve and potentially save the lives of people experiencing depression.

References

Ajzen, I. (1991). The theory of planned behavior. *Organizational Behavior and Human Decision Processes, 50*(2), 179–211. https://doi.org/10.1016/0749-5978(91)90020-T

Angermeyer, M. C., Daubmann, A., Wegscheider, K., Mnich, E., Schomerus, G., & Knesebeck, O. V. D. (2015). The relationship between biogenetic attributions and desire for social distance from persons with schizophrenia and major depression revisited. *Epidemiology and Psychiatric Sciences, 24*(4), 335–341. https://doi.org/10.1017/S2045796014000262

Angermeyer, M. C., Holzinger, A., Carta, M. G., & Schomerus, G. (2011). Biogenetic explanations and public acceptance of mental illness: Systematic review of population studies. *British Journal of Psychiatry, 199*(5), 367–372. https://doi.org/10.1192/bjp.bp.110.085563

Badahdah, A. M., & Alkhder, O. H. (2006). Helping a friend with AIDS: A test of Weiner's attributional theory in Kuwait. *Illness, Crisis, & Loss, 14*(1), 43–54. https://doi.org/10.1177/105413730601400103

Barksdale, C. L., Lawnhorn, C., Alvidrez, & Schwartz, K. (2025). Considerations for optimizing mental health communication to advance mental health equity. In M. C. Yzer & J. T. Siegel (Eds.), *Handbook of mental health communication*. Wiley.

Barnes, R. D., Ickes, W., & Kidd, R. F. (1979). Effects of the perceived intentionality and stability of another's dependency on helping behavior. *Personality and Social Psychology Bulletin, 5*(3), 367–372. https://doi.org/10.1177/014616727900500320

Bennett, T. R., & Flores, M. S. (1998). Help giving in achievement contexts: A developmental and cultural analysis of the effects of children's attributions and affects on their willingness to help. *Journal of Educational Psychology, 90*(4), 659–669. https://doi.org/10.1037/0022-0663.90.4.659

Berkowitz, L. (1969). Resistance to improper dependency relationships. *Journal of Experimental Social Psychology, 5*(3), 283–294. https://doi.org/10.1016/0022-1031(69)90054-7

Bodenmann, G., & Randall, A. K. (2013). Close relationships in psychiatric disorders. *Current Opinion in Psychiatry, 26*(5), 464–467. https://doi.org/10.1097/YCO.0b013e3283642de7

Brickman, P., Rabinowitz, V. C., Karuza, J., Coates, D., Cohn, E., & Kidder, L. (1982). Models of helping and coping. *American Psychologist, 37*(4), 368–384. https://doi.org/10.1037/0003-066X.37.4.368

Bringham, N. L., Kelso, K. A., Jackson, M. A., & Smith, R. H. (1997). The roles of invidious comparisons and deservingness in sympathy and schadenfreude. *Basic and Applied Social Psychology, 19*(3), 363–380. https://doi.org/10.1207/s15324834basp1903_6

Brown, J., & Weiner, B. (1984). Affective consequences of ability versus effort ascriptions: Controversies, resolutions, and quandaries. *Journal of Educational Psychology, 76*(1), 146–158. https://doi.org/10.1037/0022-0663.76.1.146

Chambers, D. A., Pearson, J. L., Lubell, K., Brandon, S., O'Brien, K., & Zinn, J. (2005). The science of public messages for suicide prevention: A workshop summary. *Suicide and Life-Threatening Behavior, 35*, 134–145. https://doi.org/10.1521/suli.35.2.134.62871

Cialdini, R. B., Reno, R. R., & Kallgren, C. A. (1990). A focused theory of normative conduct: Recycling the concept of norms to reduce littering in public places. *Journal of Personality and Social Psychology, 58*(6), 1015–1026. https://doi.org/10.1037/0022-3514.58.6.1015

Claudy, M. C., Vijayakumar, S., & Campbell, N. (2022). Reckless spreader or blameless victim? How vaccination status affects responses to COVID-19 patients. *Social Science & Medicine, 305*, 1–8. https://doi.org/10.1016/j.socscimed.2022.115089

Corrigan, P. W. (2000). Mental health stigma and social attribution: Implications for research methods and attitude change. *Clinical Psychology: Science and Practice*, *7*(1), 48–67. https://doi.org/10.1019/clipsy.7.1.48
Corrigan, P. W. (2016). Lessons learned from unintended consequences about erasing the stigma of mental illness. *World Psychiatry*, *15*, 67–73. https://doi.org/10.1002/wps.20295
Corrigan, P. W., Watson, A. C., Otey, E., Westbrook, A. L., Gardner, A. L., Lamb, T. A., & Fenton, W. S. (2007). How do children stigmatize people with mental illness? *Journal of Applied Social Psychology*, *37*(7), 1405–1417. https://doi.org/10.1111/j.1559-1816.2007.00218.x
Covington, M. V., & Omelich, C. L. (1979). Are causal attributions causal? *Journal of Personality & Social Psychology*, *37*, 1487–1504. https://doi.org/10.1037/0022-3514.37.9.1487
Coyne, J. C. (1976). Depression and the response of others. *Journal of Abnormal Psychology*, *85*(2), 186–193. https://doi.org/10.1037/0021-843X.85.2.186
Crano, W. D., & Prislin, R. (1995). Components of vested interest and attitude-behavior consistency. *Basic and Applied Social Psychology*, *17*(1–2), 1–21. https://doi/org/10.1080/01973533.1995.9646129
Deacon, B. J., & Baird, G. L. (2009). The chemical imbalance explanation of depression: Reducing blame at what cost? *Journal of Social and Clinical Psychology*, *28*(4), 415–435. https://doi.org/10.1521/jscp.2009.28.4.415
Dolphin, L., & Hennessy, E. (2014). Adolescents' perceptions of peers with depression: An attributional analysis. *Psychiatry Research*, *218*(3), 295–302. https://doi.org/10.1016/j.psychres.2014.04.051
Dumas-Mallet, E., & Gonon, F. (2020). Messaging in biological psychiatry: Misrepresentations, their causes, and potential consequences. *Harvard Review of Psychiatry*, *28*(6), 395–403. https://doi.org/10.1097/HRP.0000000000000276
Elmer, T., & Stadtfeld, C. (2020). Depressive symptoms are associated with social isolation in face-to-face interaction networks. *Scientific Reports*, *10*(1). https://doi.org/10.1038/s41598-020-58297-9
Erlbaum Hillsdale, N. J., Joiner, T. E., Alfano, M. S., & Metalsky, G. I. (1992). When depression breeds contempt: Reassurance seeking, self-esteem, and rejection of depressed college students by their roommates. *Journal of Abnormal Psychology*, *101*(1), 165–173. https://doi.org/10.1037/0021-843X.101.1.165
Fazio, R. H. (2014). On the power and functionality of attitudes: The role of attitude accessibility. In A. R. Pratkanis, S. J. Breckler, & A. G. Greenwald (Eds.), *Attitude structure and function* (pp. 153–179). Taylor & Francis.
Feather, N. T. (1996). Reactions to penalties for an offense in relation to authoritarianism, values, perceived responsibility, perceived seriousness, and deservingness. *Journal of Personality and Social Psychology*, *71*(3), 57–587. https://doi.org/10.1037/0022-3514.71.3.571
Feather, N. T. (1999). Judgments of deservingness: Studies in the psychology of justice and achievement. *Personality and Social Psychology Review*, *3*(2), 86–107. https://doi.org/10.1207/s15327957pspr0302_1
Feather, N. T. (2006). Deservingness and emotions: Applying the structural model of deservingness to the analysis of affective reactions to outcomes. *European Review of Social Psychology*, *17*(1), 38–73. https://doi.org/10.1080/10463280600662321
Feather, N. T., & Johnstone, C. (2001). Social norms, entitlement, and deservingness: Differential reactions to aggressive behavior of schizophrenic and personality disorder patients. *Personality & Social Psychology Bulletin*, *27*(6), 755–767. https://doi.org/10.1177/0146167201276010
Feather, N. T., McKee, I. R., & Bekker, N. (2011). Deservingness and emotions: Testing a structural model that relates discrete emotions to the perceived deservingness of positive or negative outcomes. *Motivation and Emotion*, *35*(1), 1–13. https://doi.org/10.1007/s11031-011-9202-4
Fischinger, M. (Photographer), & Corbis. (2013). [Photograph]. Retrieved July 31, 2024, from www.dailymail.co.uk/health/article-2451174/Many-newmothers- developing-depression-feel-pressureright.html
Fishbein, M., & Yzer, M. C. (2003). Using theory to design effective health behavior interventions. *Communication Theory*, *13*(2), 164–183. https://doi.org/10.1111/j.1468-2885.2003.tb00287.x
Greitemeyer, T., & Rudolph, U. (2003). Help giving and aggression from an attributional perspective: Why and when we help or retaliate. *Journal of Applied Social Psychology*, *33*(5), 1069–1087. https://doi.org/10.1111/j.1559-1816.2003.tb01939.x
Han, D. Y., & Chen, S. H. (2014). Reducing the stigma of depression through neurobiology-based psychoeducation: A randomized controlled trial. *Psychiatry and Clinical Neurosciences*, *68*(9), 666–673. https://doi.org/10.1111/pcn.12174
Haslam, N., & Kvaale, E. P. (2015). Biogenetic explanations of mental disorder: The mixed-blessings model. *Current Directions in Psychological Science*, *24*(5), 399–404. https://doi.org/10.1177/0963721415588082
Heider, F. (1958). *The psychology of interpersonal relations*. Wiley.
Ickes, W., & Kidd, R. (1976). An attributional analysis of helping behavior. In J. Harvey, W. Ickes, & R. Kidd (Eds.), *New directions in attribution research* (Vol. 1, pp. 311–334). Erlbaum.
Jones, E. E., & Davis, K. E. (1965). From acts to dispositions: The attribution process in person perception. In L. Berkowitz (Ed.), *Advances in experimental social psychology* (pp. 219–266). Elsevier. https://doi.org/10.1016/S0065-2601(08)60107-0
Jones, K. M., & Ruthig, J. C. (2015). The impact of positive thinking, gender, and empathy on social attributions for cancer outcomes. *Current Psychology*, *34*(4), 762–771. https://doi.org/10.1007/s12144-014-9288-4
Karasawa, K. (1991). The effects of onset and offset responsibility on affects and helping judgments. *Journal of Applied Social Psychology*, *21*(6), 482–499. https://doi.org/10.1111/j.1559-1816.1991.tb00532.x
Kelley, H. H. (1967). Attribution theory in social psychology. *Nebraska Symposium on Motivation*, *15*, 192–238.

Kleiman, E. M., & Liu, R. T. (2013). Social support as a protective factor in suicide: Findings from two nationally representative samples. *Journal of Affective Disorders*, *150*(2), 540–545. https://doi.org/10.1016/j.jad.2013.01.033

Klimes-Dougan, B., Wright, N., & Klingbeil, D. A. (2016). Suicide prevention public service announcements impact help-seeking attitudes: The message makes a difference. *Frontiers in Psychiatry*, *7*, 1–8. https://doi.org/10.3389/fpsyt.2016.00124

Lebowitz, M. S., & Ahn, W. K. (2014). Effects of biological explanations for mental disorders on clinicians' empathy. *Proceedings of the National Academy of Sciences*, *111*(50), 17786–17790. https://doi.org/10.1073/pnas.1414058111

Liu, J. H., Karasawa, K., & Weiner, B. (1992). Inferences about the causes of positive and negative emotions. *Personality and Social Psychology Bulletin*, *18*(5), 603–615. https://doi.org/10.1177/0146167292185011

Mackay, N., & Barrowclough, C. (2005). Accident and emergency staff's perceptions of deliberate self-harm: Attributions, emotions and willingness to help. *British Journal of Psychology*, *44*(2), 255–267. https://doi.org/10.1348/014466505x29620

Marciano, L., Kikut-Stein, A., & Viswanath, K. (2025). Communication, equity, and mental well-being: The road ahead. In M. C. Yzer & J. T. Siegel (Eds.), *Handbook of mental health communication*. Wiley.

Marshburn, A., & Siegel, J. T. (2025). Depression, mental health culture, and graduate students: A low-cost, poster-based intervention using attribution messages. *Journal of American College Health*, 1–10. Advance online publication. https://doi.org/10.1080/07448481.2024.2446441

Meyer, J. P., & Mulherin, A. (1980). From attribution to helping: An analysis of the mediating effects of affect and expectancy. *Journal of Personality & Social Psychology*, *39*, 201–210. https://psycnet.apa.org/doi/10.1037/0022-3514.39.2.201

Muschetto, T., & Siegel, J. T. (2019). Attribution theory and support for individuals with depression: The impact of controllability, stability, and interpersonal relationship. *Stigma and Health*, *4*(2), 126–135. https://doi.org/10.1037/sah0000131

Muschetto, T., & Siegel, J. T. (2020). Use of attribution vignettes and public service announcements to influence perceived stability of depression: The impact on affect, outcome expectations, and helping judgments. *Stigma and Health*, *5*(1), 69–78. https://doi.org/10.1037/sah0000174

Muschetto, T., & Siegel, J. T. (2021). Bibliometric review of attribution theory: Document cocitation analysis. *Motivation Science*, *7*(4), 439–450. https://doi.org/10.1037/mot0000253

Muschetto, T., & Siegel, J. T. (2023). Perceived stability of depressive symptomology and willingness to help relational partners: An attributional perspective. *Current Psychology*, *42*, 14076–14091. https://doi.org/10.1007/s12144-022-02708-9

Muschetto, T., & Siegel, J. T. (2024). *Reactions to others with depression: An investigation of responsibility and deservingness judgments* [Manuscript under review]. Division of Behavioral & Organizational Sciences, Claremont Graduate University.

National Alliance on Mental Illness. (2006, September 14). *Diverse new coalition launches education campaign to counter misconceptions about depression* [Press release]. https://www.nami.org/Press-Media/Press-Releases/2006/Diverse-New-Coalition-Launches-Education-Campaign

Niederkrotenthaler, T., Reidenberg, D. J., Till, B., & Gould, M. S. (2014). Increasing help-seeking and referrals for individuals at risk for suicide by decreasing stigma: The role of mass media. *American Journal of Preventive Medicine*, *47*, S235–S243. https://doi.org/10.1016/j.amepre.2014.06.010

Piliavin, I. M., Rodin, J., & Piliavin, J. A. (1969). Good samaritanism: An underground phenomenon? *Journal of Personality and Social Psychology*, *13*(4), 289–299. https://doi.org/10.1037/h0028433

Reynolds, R. M., Holmstrom, A. J., Shebib, S. J., Clare, D. D., Edwards, A. A. H., Mazur, A. P., Poland, T. L., Summers, M. E., Royer, H. R., & Zhang, L. (2023). The impact of effort attributions on the quality of esteem support messages produced. *Communication Studies, 1–20.* https://doi.org/10.1080/10510974.2023.2290297

Rippere, V. (1977). Some cognitive dimensions of antidepressive behaviour. *Behaviour Research and Therapy*, *15*(1), 57–63. https://doi.org/10.1016/0005-7967(77)90088-2

Rousseau, D. M. (1989). Psychological and implied contracts in organizations. *Employee Responsibilities and Rights Journal*, *2*(2), 121–139. https://doi.org/10.1007/BF01384942

Rudolph, U., Roesch, S., Greitemeyer, T., & Weiner, B. (2004). A meta-analytic review of help giving and aggression from an attributional perspective: Contributions to a general theory of motivation. *Cognition and Emotion*, *18*(6), 815–848. https://doi.org/10.1080/02699930341000248

Ruybal, A. L., & Siegel, J. T. (2017). Increasing social support for women with postpartum depression: An application of attribution theory. *Stigma and Health*, *2*(2), 137–156. https://doi.org/10.1037/sah0000047

Ruybal, A. L., & Siegel, J. T. (2019). Attribution theory and reducing stigma toward women with postpartum depression: Examining the role of perceptions of stability. *Stigma and Health*, *4*(3), 320–329. https://doi.org/10.1037/sah0000146

Ruybal, A. L., & Siegel, J. T. (2021). Increasing social support for women with postpartum depression through attribution theory guided vignettes and video messages: The understudied role of effort. *Journal of Experimental Social Psychology*, *97*(1), 1–22. https://doi.org/10.1016/j.jesp.2021.104197

Schmidt, G., & Weiner, B. (1988). An attribution-affect-action theory of behavior: Replications of judgments of help-giving. *Personality and Social Psychology Bulletin, 14*(3), 610–621. https://doi.org/10.1177/0146167288143021

Schopler, J., & Matthews, M. W. (1965). The influence of the perceived causal locus of partner's dependence on the use of interpersonal power. *Journal of Personality and Social Psychology, 2*(4), 609–612. https://doi.org/10.1037/h0022488

Siegel, J. T., Alvaro, E. M., Crano, W. D., Lienemann, B. A., Hohman, Z. P., & O'Brien, E. (2012). Increasing social support for depressed individuals: A cross-cultural assessment of an affect-expectancy approach. *Journal of Health Communication, 17*(6), 713–732. https://doi.org/10.1080/10810730.2011.635775

Siegel, J. T., Flores-Medel, E., Martinez, D. A., & Berger, D. E. (2019). Can mental health anti-stigma messages have untoward effects on some people with depression? An exploratory study. *Journal of Health Communication, 24*(11), 821–828. https://doi.org/10.1080/10810730.2019.1672838

Siegel, J. T., Lienemann, B. A., & Rosenberg, B. D. (2017). Resistance, reactance, and misinterpretation: Highlighting the challenge of persuading people with depression to seek help. *Social and Personality Psychology Compass, 11*, e12322. https://doi.org/10.1111/spc3.12322

Spencer, S. J., Zanna, M. P., & Fong, G. T. (2005). Establishing a causal chain: Why experiments are often more effective than mediational analyses in examining psychological processes. *Journal of Personality and Social Psychology, 89*(6), 845–851. https://doi.org/10.1037/0022-3514.89.6.845

Sperry, K., & Siegel, J. T. (2013). Victim responsibility, credibility, and verdict in a simulated rape case: Application of Weiner's attribution model. *Legal and Criminological Psychology, 18*(1), 16–29. https://doi.org/10.1111/j.2044-8333.2011/02022.x

Tullett, A. M., & Plaks, J. E. (2016). Testing the link between empathy and lay theories of happiness. *Personality and Social Psychology Bulletin, 42*(11), 1505–1521. https://doi.org/10.1177/0146167216665092

Visentini, C., Cassidy, M., Bird, V. J., & Priebe, S. (2018). Social networks of patients with chronic depression: A systematic review. *Journal of Affective Disorders, 241*, 571–578. https://doi.org/10.1016/j.jad.2018.08.022

Wang, J., Mann, F., Lloyd-Evans, B., Ma, R., & Johnson, S. (2018). Associations between loneliness and perceived social support and outcomes of mental health problems: A systematic review. *BMC Psychiatry, 18*, 1–16. https://doi.org/10.1186/s12888-018-1736-5

Weiner, B. (1972). Attribution theory, achievement motivation, and the educational process. *Review of Educational Research, 42*(2), 203–215. https://doi.org/10.3102/00346543042002203

Weiner, B. (1974). Motivation psychology and educational research. *Educational Psychologist, 11*(2), 96–101. https://doi.org/10.1080/00461527409529130

Weiner, B. (1979). A theory of motivation for some classroom experiences. *Journal of Educational Psychology, 71*(1), 3–25. https://doi.org/10.1037/0022-0663.71.1.3

Weiner, B. (1980a). A cognitive (attribution)–Emotion–Action model of motivated behavior: An analysis of judgments of help-giving. *Journal of Personality and Social Psychology, 39*(2), 186–200. https://doi.org/10.1037/0022-3514.39.2.186

Weiner, B. (1980b). May I borrow your class notes? An attributional analysis of judgments of help giving in an achievement-related context. *Journal of Education Psychology, 72*(5), 676–681. https://doi.org/10.1037/0022-0663.72.5.676

Weiner, B. (1985). An attributional theory of achievement motivation and emotion. *Psychological Review, 92*(4), 548–573. https://doi.org/10.1037/0033-295X.92.4.548

Weiner, B. (1994). Integrating social and personal theories of achievement striving. *Review of Educational Research, 64*(4), 557–573. https://doi.org/10.3102/00346543064004557

Weiner, B. (1995). *Judgements of responsibility: A foundation for a theory of social conduct.* Guilford Press.

Weiner, B. (2006). *Social motivation, justice, and the moral emotions: An attributional approach.* Lawrence Erlbaum Associates.

Weiner, B. (2018). The legacy of an attribution approach to motivation and emotion: A no-crisis zone. *Motivation Science, 4*(1), 4–14. https://doi.org/10.1037/mot0000082

Weiner, B., Frieze, I., Kukla, A., Reed, L., Rest, S., & Rosenbaum, R. M. (1971). Perceiving the causes of success and failure. In E. E. Jones, D. E. Kanouse, H. H. Kelley, R. E. Nisbett, S. Valins, & B. Weiner (Eds.), *Attribution: Perceiving the causes of behavior* (pp. 95–120)). General Learning Press.

Weiner, B., Graham, S., & Chandler, C. (1982). Pity, anger, and guilt: An attributional analysis. *Personality and Social Psychology Bulletin, 8*(2), 226–232. https://doi.org/10.1177/0146167282082007

Weiner, B., & Kukla, A. (1970). An attributional analysis of achievement motivation. *Journal of Personality and Social Psychology, 15*(1), 1–20. https://doi.org/10.1037/h0029211

Weiner, B., Perry, R. P., & Magnusson, J. (1988). An attributional analysis of reactions to stigmas. *Journal of Personality and Social Psychology, 55*, 738–748. https://doi.org/10.1037/0022-3514.55.5.738

Weiner, B., Russell, D., & Lerman, D. (1979). The cognition-emotion process in achievement-related contexts. *Journal of Personality and Social Psychology, 37*(7), 1211–1220. https://doi.org/10.1037/0022-3514.37.7.1211

Wickens, C. M., Wiesenthal, D. L., Flora, D. B., & Flett, G. L. (2011). Understanding driver anger and aggression: Attributional theory in the driving environment. *Journal of Experimental Psychology: Applied, 17*(4), 354–370. https://doi.org/10.1037/a0025815

Willner, P., & Smith, M. (2008). Can attribution theory explain carers' propensity to help men with intellectual disabilities who display inappropriate sexual behaviour? *Journal of Intellectual Disability Research*, *52*, 79–88. https://doi.org/10.1111/j.1365-2788.2007.00989.x

World Health Organization. (2023, March 31). *Depressive disorder (depression)*. https://www.who.int/news-room/fact-sheets/detail/depression

Yao, E., & Siegel, J. T. (2021). Examining the role of interpersonal relationship on attribution, emotion, and depression support provision: Experimental evidence from the People's Republic of China. *Motivation Science*, *7*(1), 46–55. http://dx.doi.org/10.1037/mot0000180

Yao, E., & Siegel, J. T. (2024). Weiner's attribution-emotion-action model: Uncovering the mediating role of self-blame and the moderating effect of the helper's responsibility for the help recipient's behavior. *Personality and Social Psychology Bulletin*. https://doi.org/10.1177/01461672241238132

Yao, E., Wang, C., & Sun, M. (2021). An empirical examination of the biogenetic approach in schizophrenia stigma reduction through an attribution lens. *International Journal of Social Psychiatry*, *67*(3), 227–231. https://doi.org/10.1177/0020764020944202

Zhang, A., Rivkin, I., & An, N. (2013). Responsibility judgments and responses to people living with AIDS in China: Testing an attributional perspective. *Journal of Applied Social Psychology*, *43*(5), 1029–1039. https://doi.org/10.1111/jasp.12066

23

The Benefits and Unintended Consequences of Anti-Stigma Campaigns

Miranda Twiss, Nataliya Turchmanovych-Hienkel, and Patrick Corrigan
Illinois Institute of Technology

Stigma is a pernicious force exacerbating the already poor outcomes of many marginalized demographics, including low-income populations, racial and sexual minorities, and people with mental illness (PWMI). These communities have campaigned to reduce stigma and its negative consequences. Mental health stigma, especially, has seen increased advocacy in recent decades. However, stigma around mental illness is a complex construct, and many advocates do not fully understand its scope before rushing into their activism, leading to unintended consequences from anti-stigma campaigns, which can harm the very community they are attempting to uplift. This chapter begins with a review of the components and manifestations of mental health stigma and the agendas of anti-stigma efforts before diving into four common approaches to stigma change, specifically examining their efficacy and unintentional harms.

Overview of Stigma

Stigma consists of three main components: stereotypes, prejudice, and discrimination. Stereotypes are ingrained beliefs that set the stigmatized group apart from the so-called normal majority, such as the idea that PWMI are violent. Most people are aware of stereotypes (Corrigan et al., 2011), as they are ingrained by cultural representations from childhood and hard to avoid. Prejudice occurs when stereotypes create negative emotions and judgments about the stigmatized group, like feeling fearful of someone with mental illness due to believing they are violent. Discrimination is the behavioral result of prejudice, usually punitive and causing loss of rightful opportunity, such as refusing to employ someone with a mental health diagnosis due to being afraid of them.

Various forms of stigma exist, including public stigma (stigmatizing attitudes and behaviors from others), self-stigma (internalized prejudices directed at oneself), label avoidance (delaying, avoiding, or terminating treatment to evade a stigmatizing diagnosis), perceived stigma (the belief that others will judge you based on certain traits), courtesy or associative stigma (being judged due to proximity to a stigmatized identity, like family members of individuals with mental illness), structural stigma (bias embedded in systems or policies), and practitioner stigma (biases from health care workers affecting their treatment provision).

The Handbook of Mental Health Communication, First Edition.
Edited by Marco C. Yzer and Jason T. Siegel.

Goals of Stigma Change

Many individuals strive to eliminate mental illness stigma but with varying ideologies. Three agendas for stigma change have emerged: the services agenda, the rights agenda, and the self-worth agenda (Corrigan & Al-Khouja, 2018). The services agenda focuses on combating label avoidance to enhance treatment engagement. The rights agenda mirrors civil rights efforts, countering public stigma to reduce discrimination and enhance access to rightful opportunities. The self-worth agenda targets self-stigma to boost self-esteem, replacing shame with empowerment and self-determination.

While these perspectives share the goal of reducing stigma harm, they are often in competition for limited resources. The agendas can also clash conceptually. For instance, a rights agenda campaign may promote normalcy messaging, suggesting that those with mental illness are no different from others. Paradoxically, this may harm the self-worth agenda, intensifying self-stigma and leading individuals to hide or downplay their symptoms to fit the so-called normalcy ascribed to them. Such closeting can negatively affect self-esteem and relationships (Newheiser & Barreto, 2014; Wegner & Smart, 2000). Promoting normalcy may likewise undermine the services agenda by suggesting symptoms are common and therefore do not warrant special treatment. Portraying experiences as normal might foster the cycle of avoidance, where individuals with mental illness, especially adolescents, widen their concept of normal to encompass their experiences instead of seeking necessary treatment (Biddle & Gowen, 2009).

Approaches to Stigma Change

Anti-stigma efforts employ four primary approaches. The first approach, changing words, seeks to replace stigmatizing labels with more respectful terms. However, language is neither the root cause nor the most harmful manifestation of stigma, and attempting to censor words may create a rebound effect. The second approach is protest, wherein instances of stigma are publicly called out and remonstrated. This approach has successfully influenced media representation and policy changes, but can also alienate those outside the movement and trigger psychological reactance, intensifying the stigmatizing behavior. The third strategy, education, combats stereotypes with factual information about mental illness. Education has improved mental health literacy and led to earlier interventions, but often falls short of reducing bias in adults, and certain messages can exacerbate self-stigma. The fourth strategy, contact, involves facilitating personal interactions between the public and those in recovery from mental illness. This approach utilizes personal experiences to challenge negative expectations about individuals with mental illness, and has demonstrated larger and more enduring stigma change—although certain aspects of contact must be in place for efficacy. The positive and negative outcomes of these four strategies are explored in greater detail in the rest of this chapter.

Changing Words

People often think of stigma as the words used to express it, including the standard names for stigmatized characteristics as well as slurs (e.g., the N-word for Black people, the F-word for the lesbian, gay, bisexual, transgender, and queer/questioning [LGBTQ] community, or *psycho* and *schizo* for PWMI). Consequently, some people advocate reducing stigma by changing words. For example, changing ***Black*** to ***African American*** attempted to replace dehumanizing language with culturally meaningful language emphasizing both African ancestry and American identity, while mirroring the labels for less stigmatized racial groups, such as Asian Americans, to evoke the same respect and social category (Smith, 1992). Changing labels to reduce stigma also occurs with certain medical conditions. *Leprosy*, for example—a condition so stigmatized that it is a biblical symbol of outcasts—has been replaced with ***Hansen's disease*** in some regions. Mental health diagnoses have seen similar changes, such as ***mental retardation*** becoming ***intellectual disability*** or ***Alzheimer's disease*** replacing ***dementia***. Renaming schizophrenia has been endorsed by over 75 psychopathology experts due to its high stigma (Maruta et al., 2014), and some East Asian countries like China and Japan have already changed their diagnostic labels. This could target the service agenda by reducing label avoidance with a less stigmatizing diagnosis.

Central to language-focused anti-stigma efforts is the question of who leads the movement. Are changes being advocated for by doctors, who want medical terminology to better represent epidemiology, or by members of the community? Diagnostic relabeling carries professional legitimacy but centers stigma changes within the medical perspective instead of lived experience. Mental health practitioners are highly stigmatizing (Schulze, 2007), and many psychiatrists do not endorse recovery as a legitimate model for serious disorders like schizophrenia (Torrey, 2011), highlighting the disconnect between medical legitimacy and lack of stigma. Advocates speaking on behalf of a group also frequently miss the mark. For instance, ***Latinx*** was introduced as a gender-inclusive alternative to ***Latino/Latina*** but is largely disconnected from the Hispanic community: Less than 25% of American Hispanics are aware of the term, and only 3% use it themselves (Noe-Bustamante et al., 2020).

Ideally, the decision on appropriate terminology should rest with the people being described. Within stigmatized groups, people often have conflicting preferences for how they want to be referred. For example, some mental health advocates have moved away from the term ***patient*** to alternatives including ***consumer, customer***, or ***client***. One study found that ***client*** was most preferred across four mental health sites, followed by ***patient*** (Mueser et al., 1996). A later survey found that ***patient*** was most widely preferred, apparently due to participants' dislike of the other terms' emphasis on market relationships (Deber et al., 2005). Most language questions lack easily accessible statistics on group preference, but even with research there is not always a clear answer because each group is not a monolith. Even if a majority consensus exists, personal preferences matter.

Benefits

Japan's renaming of schizophrenia has been used to examine the impact of language. Providers who used the new term were more likely to inform patients of their diagnosis (Sato, 2006) and had better knowledge of psychosocial interventions (Sartorius et al., 2014). Among the public, awareness of the new label correlated with a reduced desire for social distance (Takahashi et al., 2009), although the direction of this relationship remains uncertain. People may use so-called correct language out of professionalism or social pressure, but even insincere respect influences the transmission of stigmatizing attitudes because different language elicits different responses. For example, describing criminality and schizophrenia with person-first language (i.e., ***person convicted of crime***, not ***convicted criminal***; ***person with schizophrenia***, not ***schizophrenic***) evoked more positive reactions (Denver et al., 2017; Penn & Nowlin-Drummond, 2001).

Using appropriate and well-understood labels can also reduce stigma by contextualizing unusual behavior. The discounting principle (Kelley, 1971) posits that people will discount one explanation if another is available. Therefore, individuals with mental illness may face less judgment for their actions if others have a diagnostic explanation. For example, students exhibited more positive attitudes toward social challenges or inappropriate communication when a peer was labeled as autistic compared with being presented as neurotypical (Brosnan & Mills, 2016; Matthews et al., 2015).

Unintended Consequences

Reducing stigma to language oversimplifies the issue, implying it is easier to address than it is. This misinterpretation of respectful language as actual respect has caused some professionals to argue that anti-stigma programs are outdated (Rosenberg, 2013), contributing to fluctuating support for stigma research over the past decade from funding organizations like the National Institute of Mental Health. Changing words also allows for ***slacktivism***—symbolic gestures of allyship that feel good but lack meaningful impact—such as liking and sharing social media posts; little effort is required, and little impact is realized. It can also enable individuals to maintain their biases while appearing politically correct, similar to the phenomenon of ***modern racism*** that emerged when traditional racism became socially unacceptable. Modern racism encompasses three elements: (a) emotional hostility toward Black individuals; (b) resistance to their political demands; and (c) the belief that racism no longer exists (McConahay, 1986). Similarly, changing words around mental illness can lead people to mistakenly believe that the problem of mental health stigma is resolved, justifying their reluctance to support further advocacy while retaining emotional hostility and prejudice.

The language focus serves as a political distraction from more effective stigma change. Like funding, the public's cognitive capacity is limited, and censoring words takes up mental energy that would be better spent working through the actual bias. For example, so-called politically correct terms such as *urban*, *inner city*, or *poor* have cropped up as euphemisms for Black populations expressing the same prejudiced sentiments. Even the relatively progressive President Joe Biden once remarked that "poor kids are just as bright and just as talented as White kids" (*The New York Times*, 2019): A perfect example of what happens when language is changed without addressing the underlying association. Being inundated with politically correct language obscures the real problem and desensitizes to other anti-stigma efforts.

The focus on changing words is also a misrepresentation of causality between stigma and language. The label for a stigmatized characteristic may develop a negative connotation, but it does not create prejudice that did not previously exist. Changing language may confuse people briefly, but stigma will eventually become associated with the new term as well. For example, Brazil made the official change from *lepra* (leprosy) to *Hanseniase* (Hansen's disease) in 1975, almost 50 years ago. Over time, the same stigmatizing language surrounding lepra became associated with Hanseniase as well (Oliveira et al., 2003). A study conducted 30 years after lepra was outlawed found that the introduction of Hanseniase had done little to reduce stigma (Femina et al., 2007).

Language-centered efforts can lead to direct harm when advocates act as word police, scolding those who use outdated terms. These rebukes are often aimed at potential allies, making them feel alienated and discouraging further engagement (Corrigan, 2019). Word policing creates barriers to entry for both advocacy and treatment, potentially driving individuals away from support groups or social justice involvement due to being admonished for using the "wrong" words when they try to participate. Moreover, asking people to suppress the old term can backfire and actually increase its salience, known as the rebound effect in social psychology. Attempting not to think about something causes people to put active effort into avoiding it, increasing attention to the subject at the same rate as actively thinking about it (Wegner et al., 1990). Similarly, telling people not to use certain words could wind up increasing the likelihood that those words will pop into their heads.

Protest

Protest publicly denounces injustices and their perpetrators, usually through collective action. It is often used to combat stigmatizing media portrayal of mental illness. For instance, Burger King's 2010 advertisement "The King's Gone Crazy," which involved a cartoon burger in a psych ward being called "crazy" and "insane," was removed after protests from mental health groups (Watson et al., 2014). StigmaBusters, an online National Alliance on Mental Illness (NAMI) group that organizes writing campaigns in response to offensive media, similarly targeted ABC's TV show *Wonderland* for negative portrayals of characters with mental illness. The show was canceled in 2000 after just two episodes due to protest pressure on corporate advertisers (Corrigan, 2004).

Protests employ different mediums, including social media campaigns, marches, legal action, boycotts, and petitions. Medium choice depends on the target; businesses may react to boycotts and negative reviews, while governments respond to representative outreach and campaign donations. With *Wonderland*, TV executives were not bothered by audience reaction because any engagement increases visibility, but involving ABC's sponsors created the necessary financial incentives. It's important to understand that protests may not solely target the object of rebuke; reaching third-party witnesses or like-minded entities, such as the viewers or other showrunners, can be of equal or higher priority.

Protest messaging often focuses on reducing negative attitudes without promoting positive, evidence-based alternatives. Protests frequently employ reactive language and negative emotions like anger and shame. These emotions can motivate participants: Anger may cultivate a desire to punish offenders (Landmann & Rohmann, 2020), and collective action is predicted by anticipated shame if the transgression goes unaddressed (Shepherd et al., 2013). However, this approach can backfire on the object of the protest. Shame, in particular, can solidify or increase stigma, with the shamed entity blaming their ostracization on the outgroup (Jasper, 2014).

Distinguishing between different types of shame is important. Reintegrative shaming (Braithwaite et al., 1999) conveys that an action was wrong but allows the individual to repair harm and reintegrate into the community. Stigmatizing shame, on the other hand, labels the person themselves as bad, advocating their exclusion from society. Brené Brown's *TED Talk* (2012) has popularized this distinction by using *shame* for stigmatizing shame ("I am bad") and *guilt* for reintegrative shaming ("I did something bad"). Guilt, or reintegrative shame, encourages change and offers redemption, while shame, or stigmatizing shame, demotivates change by suggesting the offender can never be morally good again. A protest that employs outrage, anger, and stigmatizing shame can be potent for participants and observers but is likely to cement or even increase stigmatizing attitudes for the object of the protest.

Benefits

Anti-stigma protests evoke righteous anger among participants, which research has identified as a healthy response to stigma inversely linked to depression (Stevenson et al., 1997) and a protective factor against internalized stigma (Steinberg, 2021). Anger also correlates with engaging in collective and affirming responses to stigma (Wright, 1997), making protest an empowering experience that encourages PWMI to reject stigmatizing messages and respond with action rather than helplessness.

Protests may reduce perceived stigma by displaying support for PWMI, akin to LGBTQ Pride marches increasing the visibility of acceptance. Protest also may impact public stigma by spreading awareness of stigma harm, facilitating discussions around mental health, and improving media representation of mental illness. Successful campaigns can even impact structural stigma; for instance, the right to community placement came from a successful legal protest by two women who remained institutionalized despite being able to live in the community (Corrigan, 2018). Similarly, the Americans with Disabilities Act (ADA), which grants civil rights protections for people with disabilities, was catalyzed by the Capitol Crawl protest in 1990 (Davis, 2016), when activists left wheelchairs and mobility aids behind to climb up the 82 Capitol Building steps, demonstrating the need for accessibility features such as ramps.

Unintended Consequences

Protest has significant drawbacks as a tool for reducing stigma. The same emotions that empower participants and replace self-stigma with anger can be off-putting to outsiders. Whereas feeling outraged is associated with motivation and can cause someone to take action, being shamed is more likely to produce avoidance (Schmader & Lickel, 2006). That shame mostly falls into the category of stigmatizing shame, not reintegrative shame (or guilt), because protests are punitive and often advocate for boycotts or other parallels of shunning. As a result, the people who are being chastised are not motivated to engage in the protest, instead building up resentment and even starting to consider themselves as the victims—which will only increase their bias against the group in question (Jasper, 2014).

Alternatively, someone who encounters the chastising message might change their behavior according to social desirability rather than actual understanding and agreement. When someone's motivations are not addressed—even if they eliminate the socially unacceptable behavior—stigma will continue to be expressed in subtler, more politically correct terms. Using protest to reduce the most egregious expressions of bias is still a move in the right direction but may result in a modern version of stigma that is harder to identify and address (Barreto & Ellemers, 2005).

One major issue with protests is psychological reactance, a phenomenon in which people are motivated to do the opposite of what they are told in order to resolve the threat to their autonomy (Brehm & Brehm, 2013). The theory is framed in terms of freedom and control: When told what to do, people reject the external control by engaging in behavioral freedom that was restricted (Brehm, 1989). With anti-stigma protests, that means that the audience may react to the protest by doubling down on their stigmatizing behavior. This "do not tell me what to do" attitude is especially prevalent in Western, individualist cultures, where the eliminated option is seen as more desirable because individual freedom is more highly valued (Graupmann et al., 2012).

As with changing language, protests may also suffer from a rebound effect. Protests over a problematic stereotype of mental illness are asking the audience to suppress that stereotype, which can have the opposite effect and instead increase the salience of the stereotype (Wegner et al., 1987). For example, being told not to think of PWMI as dangerous could strengthen the association due to the heightened attention toward suppressing it.

Education

Education seeks to provide factual, evidence-based information about mental illness to dispel the stigmatizing myths and common misperceptions. For example, education interventions might provide information about the role of genetics in the development of mental illness to counter the myth that people are responsible for their symptoms. This information can be delivered through a variety of mediums, including public service announcements (PSAs), books, flyers, movies, videos, and other audio and visual aids. Educational campaigns are particularly popular for social justice issues because they are easy to develop and disseminate to a wide audience.

The efficacy of PSAs can be assessed in terms of penetration (how much of the targeted population observed and remembered the PSA) and impact (the degree to which the message prompted change in those who saw it; Corrigan & Shapiro, 2010). The greatest benefit of media-based campaigns is the scope of their ability to reach people, with the broadest penetration among television and online anti-stigma campaigns. PSAs that are distributed on the Web are heavily reliant on those websites having high numbers of visitors that would be exposed to the PSAs, because without traffic the PSAs may not penetrate a wide audience. Impact, however, is better achieved by the in vivo approach, occurring when the targeted group is able to interact with individuals in recovery (Corrigan et al., 2007), discussed further in the section on contact.

Public service campaigns are prominent examples of the social marketing and education used in anti-stigma reduction strategies. For instance, in 2004 the Substance Abuse and Mental Health Administration (SAMHSA) launched the Campaign for Mental Health Recovery, a multiyear public service effort to promote social inclusion and support (Power, 2010). The campaign, which encouraged young adults to support friends living with mental health problems, was launched through webpages, television, radio, and print and distributed to over 28,000 media outlets nationwide. It included several anti-stigma PSAs, which would need to be observable by the public to sufficiently penetrate and impact the population. One such PSA, the "Elimination of Barriers Initiative" (EBI), was sent to 627 television organizations, 62% of broadcast outlets, and 225 cable systems (Bell et al., 2005). Notably, receiving the PSA did not mean that it would be aired; only 20% of receiving stations pledged to air the EBI content at least once. Airtime for PSAs is often limited since they are competing with coverage of other prominent current issues, such as immigration, abortion rights, or climate. PSAs are often broadcast during off hours (e.g., between 2 and 4 a.m.) when fewer people are watching television, and are pulled from air rather quickly due to many actors' contracts stipulating a time frame for the video's broadcast, usually one year. Distributors would need to pay residuals to actors in order to show the PSA beyond the contracted time limit, but funding is often unavailable or prioritized elsewhere.

Benefits

Education around mental illness promotes mental health literacy, an important goal for the services agenda of getting people into treatment. Knowledge is especially impactful at the beginning of someone's journey with mental health when they might be unaware that their symptoms have a diagnosis and can be treated. Helping PWMI label strange experiences can be a source of relief, providing an answer to the question of "What is happening to me?" Education programs also enhance psychiatric literacy of students and practitioners of mental health disciplines, who become informed about evidence-based practices, as well as service gatekeepers such as primary care physicians or nurse practitioners, who become trained on early identification.

Education is especially effective at reducing stigma among adolescents, whose beliefs and attitudes are less ingrained and therefore more variable in degree of stigma (Corrigan et al., 2012). Research has found that increased knowledge of mental health resulted in decreased stigma among teenage students (Simmons et al., 2017). Education also improves mental health knowledge in adults; for example, population understanding of depression and schizophrenia as brain disorders increased from 55% to 75% between 1990 and 2006 (Schomerus et al., 2011). Unfortunately, knowledge does not seem to reduce stigma in adults as it does for youth: Stigma actually worsened among adult respondents in the same time span that understanding improved, with acceptance of a coworker with schizophrenia falling from 50% to 30% (Schomerus et al., 2011).

Unintended Consequences

PSAs have been shown to boomerang. For example, one study examined reactions to a printed depression advertisement prompting viewers to seek support for their depressive symptoms. However, participants with greater depressive symptoms often interpret the world through a negativity bias, and results found that viewing the advertisement actually increased self-stigma and decreased help-seeking intention (Lienemann et al., 2013). Another article described a similar disparity between the reactions of individuals with and without heightened depressive symptoms in response to an anti-stigma PSA targeted at the general public: Around one in five respondents with heightened depression reported negative affect caused by the PSA, compared with less than 2% of respondents without heightened symptomatology (Siegel et al., 2019). The PSA in question focused on the importance of supporting a friend with mental health challenges, which the authors posited may have caused severely depressed viewers to instead reflect on their lack of support. The authors suggested that such unintended consequences are likely to occur if the unique mindsets of people with high symptomatology are not specifically accounted for.

Another example of broadcasted mental health campaigns with mixed results is direct-to-consumer advertising (DTCA). DTCA refers to marketing strategies that bypass a provider's promotion of a product and drive product sales directly from the customer's side. Unfortunately, these advertisements can become problematic. DTCA for prescription medications exploded after the U.S. Food and Drug Administration (FDA) lifted its restrictions in 1985, triggering some unintended effects on public stigma. For example, viewers of an advertisement for an antidepressant medication called Cymbalta were less likely to endorse recovery or self-determination (Corrigan et al., 2014). However, for people with lived experience of mental health challenges, the Cymbalta advertisement seemed to cause less blame and more support of empowerment. Like PSAs, the positive and negative impacts of DTCAs show up differently for the general population compared with PWMI. Although both of these examples were intended to improve stigma, each accidentally worsened it for either the public or the patients.

Some government-funded education programs were intended to pursue public health goals but did not achieve the desired outcomes and, in some instances, contributed to unintended negative outcomes. An example of this is the Drug Abuse Resistance Education (DARE) program, which was intended to dissuade youth from engaging in substance use and was implemented in 75% of US school districts and 43 countries around the world. Research conducted on this program revealed that the program either had no measurable impact on participant attitudes and behaviors or, interestingly, had the opposite of the intended result, with children who completed the DARE program being more likely to use hallucinogenic drugs during follow-up (Evans & Bosworth, 1998).

In 1990, the National Institute of Mental Health launched the Decade of the Brain in an effort to bring modern psychiatry into the age of neuroscience. It sought to ground the understanding of diagnosis and treatment in bench science. Mental illness became branded as a brain disorder. A meta-analysis of several studies found that this medicalization of mental illness consistently had a harmful impact on stigma (Kvaale et al., 2013). Although it is true that individuals blame people with serious mental illness less after learning about the genetic origins of some disorders, they are also more likely to believe that the person will not be able to recover, which increases stigma (Read et al., 2006). Beliefs that undermine recovery can lead to employers not hiring PWMI, landlords not wanting to rent to them, and primary care physicians potentially offering substandard care. Other educational approaches, such as framing mental illness like any other illness, have similarly shown few benefits and instead were associated with greater perceptions of dangerousness and unpredictability (Corrigan, 2018; Read et al., 2006).

Contact

The final approach to stigma reduction aims to facilitate interpersonal contact between the public and people in recovery from mental illness. Knowing someone in a stigmatized group is often associated with lower levels of stigma toward that group. For example, a study of homophobia in the 1990s (Herek & Capitanio, 1996) found that heterosexual respondents reporting interpersonal contact with gay or lesbian individuals exhibited more positive attitudes toward homosexuality than those without contact—and, notably, increasing from *none* to *some* gay acquaintances at a one-year follow up was correlated with decreases in stigma/homophobia. The impact of contact on stigmatizing attitudes was stronger for respondents who had a higher number of gay acquaintances, closer relationships with those acquaintances, and direct knowledge of the acquaintance's homosexuality through their self-disclosure (as opposed to via third party). Contact strategies for mental health stigma are based on the same principle: Personal experience with an individual with a stigmatized attribute reduces stigma against that group.

Contact can take place in vivo or through video-based media. A meta-analysis found that video-mediated contact leads to less stigma and more affirming attitudes but that face-to-face contact is more effective (Corrigan et al., 2012). Person-to-person contact presents more obstacles and slower dissemination than digital media, so public service campaigns rely heavily on e-media, which may be misguided given its lower efficacy at diminishing stigma.

Allport (1954) identified four elements of effective intergroup contact:

1 Equal status between groups: PWMI and the public interact as peers, in contrast with the power dynamics of doctor–patient or supervisor–employee relationships.
2 Common goals: The groups collaborate on shared objectives like puzzles or community projects, with meaningful tasks being more impactful.
3 No competition: The interaction is not competitive in any direction; for example, participants do not challenge the rights of individuals with mental illness, who seek full belonging without hostile messages about bigoted "normals."
4 Authoritative sanction for the contact: The contact is endorsed by management of an organization or a respected community member, for example, a rabbi prominently introduces someone with mental illness as a fellow human with an important message for the congregation.

Impactful contact requires effective messaging from the individual with lived experience, which comprises three components: (1) on-the-way-down story; (2) on-the-way-up rejoinder; and (3) change moral (Corrigan, 2018). On-the-way-down stories focus on an individual's personal experiences with mental illness that are foreign to the audience, including symptoms, diagnostic labels, medications, psychiatric care, and hospitalizations. Because mental illness is often invisible, the audience may not believe that a speaker who presents well truly qualifies as a person with a serious mental illness, so these compelling details of their story prove their status. Once the contact has established legitimacy, they address stigma with an on-the-way-up rejoinder, the story of *despite*: Despite symptoms and disabilities, the individual has accomplished a great deal (e.g., gainful employment, independent apartment lease), highlighting that individuals with mental illness aspire and achieve just like everyone else. An effective message concludes with a three-part change moral, a plea for the audience to recognize that (a) the speaker's story is representative of others with mental illness and not an exception; (b) despite recovery, prejudice and discrimination continue to impact the speaker and can be as harmful as the illness itself; and (c) mental illness stigma is a societal injustice like racism or sexism, and needs to be replaced with affirming attitudes and equal treatment.

Benefits

Contact shows great promise as a stigma reduction tool. A recent meta-analysis by Maunder and White (2019) sought to investigate the effectiveness of intergroup contact as a strategy for reducing mental health stigma and found that at three different time points (immediately after the intervention, short-term, and medium-term) the effect of contact was significant, with small to medium effect size at all three time points. A review summarizing 79 studies found that adults who participated in contact exhibited improvements in stigmatizing attitudes and behavioral intentions two to three times greater than adults who participated in education alone (Corrigan et al., 2012). Additionally, a subsequent analysis indicated that the benefits of contact were maintained better over time than those of education alone (Corrigan et al., 2015). This shows that contact is more effective at reducing stigma short-term as well as long-term.

Contact can also improve the impact of education interventions. Research on training health practitioners found that health education and experience decreased stigma for students who previously had a friend with mental illness but exacerbated stigma among students without contact (Sadow et al., 2002). Accordingly, incorporating contact into education interventions improves stigma reduction (Corrigan et al., 2007). Direct contact allows the public to check for itself the humanity of someone living with mental illness, adding personal meaning to any information on paper.

Best practices for stigma-reducing contact have been outlined in a set of guidelines called strategic stigma change (SSC). Effective person-to-person contact should always be led by a person with lived experience. SSC delineates five additional practices, abbreviated to the acronym TLC4: targeted, local, credible, continuous contact leading to change.

1. Targeted: Contact interventions target key influential groups (e.g., employers, community leaders, health care providers, legislators, and media outlets), leveraging existing opportunities like staff meetings or medical rounds.
2. Local: Contact programs consider local influences (both geographic and sociopolitical) on target group interests (e.g., neighborhood variations, socioeconomic status, ethnicity, and religion).
3. Credible: The contact person establishes credibility with the target group through three factors: shared characteristics (e.g., ethnicity or socioeconomic status); similar roles (e.g., health care provider); and being in the process of recovery (e.g., employment, independence, quality of life; Corrigan, 2018).
4. Continuous: One-time contact has some effect, but lasting change requires ongoing interaction. Multiple contacts, with variations in peer and target partners, messages, venues, and opportunities, are more effective in reducing stigma.
5. Contact leading to change: Contact programs lead toward clear and actionable goals for behavioral change in the audience, such as a group of employers interviewing, offering positions to, and providing reasonable accommodations for employees with mental illness.

Specific programs have been designed to incorporate TLC4 principles. For example, the US Department of Veterans Affairs (VA) used TLC4 principles through its website www.maketheconnection.net (MTC), where veterans and their families can learn from peers' stories about behavioral health challenges experienced by ex-military and evidence-based interventions for recovery with the services agenda goal of increasing veterans' engagement in VA behavioral health services. Consequently, all stories end with a similar moral that veterans with mental illness challenges recover when they engage in evidence-based interventions. Stories are targeted through different drop-down menus that direct site visitors to report previous service branch (e.g., army, navy, marines, reserves), gender, era (e.g., WWII through Korean War, Vietnam War, post–Vietnam War era, Desert Storm era), and combat experience in order to tailor the experience to each site visitor.

Unintended Consequences

The impact of contact is dependent on the degree to which the individual fits various stereotypes of PWMI; the interaction essentially provides a chance to test those stereotypes for accuracy. Although contact is most effective with someone in recovery, involving only people who are symptom-free may create unrealistic expectations of PWMI or increase public stigma by implying that people with current symptoms are somehow less than (Corrigan, 2018). Alternatively, individuals that highly disconfirm prevalent stereotypes may not be believed as representative of the larger population with mental illness, regarded instead as special exceptions to the pertinacious prejudice against the group. At the other extreme, having contact with individuals who behave in ways consistent with stereotypes about their group, such as people who are actively psychotic or homeless, may actually reinforce the stigmatizing attitudes that the public holds (Reinke et al., 2004).

Another downside to contact is that it places the burden of stigma change on the stigmatized group, requiring them to be vulnerable to people who are prejudiced against them in order to disprove their expectations. Moreover, because mental illness is often invisible, contact requires disclosure, which can improve self-stigma but may expose the individual to negative consequences or loss of rightful opportunities. Perceptions of disclosure seem to vary by culture; one study on sociocultural factors and mental illness disclosure found that collectivist cultures like China were more likely to recommend limiting disclosure (An & McDermott, 2014) due to negative community reactions and associative stigma.

Conclusion

Stigma around mental illness can have devastating impacts, so it is not surprising that many advocates dive headfirst into anti-stigma campaigns. Unfortunately, these well-intended efforts often backfire. The four common approaches to stigma change each have their own aspects of efficacy and pitfalls that must be taken into account to prevent unintentional harm.

Changing words misconstrues the root of stigmatizing beliefs, and this strategy can easily distract and take resources from more impactful anti-stigma work. When engaging with language, advocates should be careful of the rebound effect and aware of the endurance of stigmatizing beliefs, regardless of terminology.

Protests have an important role in addressing specific injustices but can easily provoke psychological reactance and alienate the public. Participants in collective action should be aware of the differential response they are likely to evoke in their protest target and outside observers. Demonstrations that might cultivate sympathy and outrage in allies could result in the object of the protest doubling down on the behavior to protect their sense of freedom and blaming the marginalized group for the negative consequences the protest brings about.

Education strategies have the benefit of increasing mental health literacy and can reduce stigma in children and adolescents whose beliefs are still developing. However, learning about mental illness has repeatedly failed to reduce stigma in adults and may even reinforce their bias despite increasing their understanding. Advocates of education campaigns should also be careful of how the presented information could be interpreted by people with more severe mental illness, as PSAs are not often tested for adverse impacts on those specific populations.

Contact with someone in recovery is especially effective at impacting mental health stigma by providing interpersonal experiences that conflict with the previously held bias. Still, facilitators of contact interventions should ensure that the necessary ingredients are in place so that the interaction does not reinforce stereotypes and so that the individual is interpreted as representative of the broader group of PWMI.

It is crucial to take the time to clarify the goal of any advocacy and identify the possible harms before jumping into action. The competing agendas of stigma change and the diverse impacts of a given strategy must be carefully weighed to minimize unintended consequences, even if they cannot be totally eliminated. For example, consulting people with lived experience of mental illness or testing impact in focus groups can help optimize a strategy before it is implemented on a larger scale. These accidental harms do not make anti-stigma campaigns any less important, but they do necessitate that caution is exercised to reduce negative impacts on persons with mental illness and on the public's attitudes.

References

Allport, G. W. (1954). *The nature of prejudice*. Addison-Wesley.

An, Z., & McDermott, V. M. (2014). The effects of sociocultural factors and perceptions of mental illness on indirect disclosure preferences. *Communication Research Reports, 31*(3), 281–291. https://doi.org/10.1080/08824096.2014.924338

Barreto, M., & Ellemers, N. (2005). The burden of benevolent sexism: How it contributes to the maintenance of gender inequalities. *European Journal of Social Psychology, 35*(5), 633–642. https://doi.org/10.1002/ejsp.270

Bell, J., Colangelo, A., & Pillen, M. (2005). *Final report of the evaluation of the elimination of barriers initiative*. James Bell Associates.

Biddle, L., & Gowen, L. K. (2009). Stigma and the cycle of avoidance: Why young people fail to seek help for their mental distress. *Focal Point: Research, Policy, and Practice in Children's Mental Health, 23*(1), 26–28. http://archives.pdx.edu/ds/psu/15837

Braithwaite, J., Braithwaite, V., & Ahmed, E. (1999). Reintegrative shaming. In S. Henry & M. Lanier (Eds.), *The Essential Criminology Reader* (pp. 286–295). Taylor & Francis.

Brehm, J. W. (1989). *Psychological reactance: Theory and applications. ACR North American Advances.*

Brehm, S. S., & Brehm, J. W. (2013). *Psychological reactance: A theory of freedom and control*. Academic Press.

Brosnan, M., & Mills, E. (2016). The effect of diagnostic labels on the affective responses of college students towards peers with 'Asperger's Syndrome' and 'Autism Spectrum Disorder'. *Autism, 20*(4), 388–394. https://doi.org/10.1177/1362361315586721

Brown, B. (2012, March). *Listening to Shame* [Video]. TED Conferences. https://www.ted.com/talks/brene_brown_listening_to_shame?language=en

Corrigan, P., Michaels, P. J., & Morris, S. (2015). Do the effects of antistigma programs persist over time? Findings from a meta-analysis. *Psychiatric Services, 66*(5), 543–546. https://doi.org/10.1176/appi.ps.201400291

Corrigan, P. W. (2004). Target-specific stigma change: A strategy for impacting mental illness stigma. *Psychiatric Rehabilitation Journal, 28*(2), 113–121. https://doi.org/10.2975/28.2004.113.121

Corrigan, P. W. (2018). *The stigma effect: Unintended consequences of mental health campaigns*. Columbia University Press. https://doi.org/10.7312/corr18356

Corrigan, P. W. (2019). Beware the word police. *Psychiatric Services, 70*(3), 234–236. https://doi.org/10.1176/appi.ps.201800369

Corrigan, P. W., & Al-Khouja, M. A. (2018). Three agendas for changing the public stigma of mental illness. *Psychiatric Rehabilitation Journal, 41*(1), 1–7. https://doi.org/10.1037/prj0000277

Corrigan, P. W., Kosyluk, K. A., Konadu Fokuo, J., & Park, J. H. (2014). How does direct to consumer advertising affect the stigma of mental illness? *Community Mental Health Journal, 50*, 792–799. https://doi.org/10.1007/s10597-014-9698-7

Corrigan, P. W., Larson, J., Sells, M., Niessen, N., & Watson, A. C. (2007). Will filmed presentations of education and contact diminish mental illness stigma? *Community Mental Health Journal, 43*, 171–181. https://doi.org/10.1007/s10597-006-9061-8

Corrigan, P. W., Morris, S. B., Michaels, P. J., Rafacz, J. D., & Rüsch, N. (2012). Challenging the public stigma of mental illness: A meta-analysis of outcome studies. *Psychiatric Services, 63*(10), 963–973. https://doi.org/10.1176/appi.ps.201100529

Corrigan, P. W., Rafacz, J., & Rüsch, N. (2011). Examining a progressive model of self-stigma and its impact on people with serious mental illness. *Psychiatry Research, 189*(3), 339–343. https://doi.org/10.1016/j.psychres.2011.05.024

Corrigan, P. W., & Shapiro, J. R. (2010). Measuring the impact of programs that challenge the public stigma of mental illness. *Clinical Psychology Review, 30*(8), 907–922. https://doi.org/10.1016/j.cpr.2010.06.004

Davis, L. J. (2016). *Enabling acts: The hidden story of how the Americans with Disabilities Act gave the largest US minority its rights*. Beacon Press.

Deber, R. B., Kraetschmer, N., Urowitz, S., & Sharpe, N. (2005). Patient, consumer, client, or customer: What do people want to be called? *Health Expectations, 8*(4), 345–351. https://doi.org/10.1111/j.1369-7625.2005.00352.x

Denver, M., Pickett, J. T., & Bushway, S. D. (2017). The language of stigmatization and the mark of violence: Experimental evidence on the social construction and use of criminal record stigma. *Criminology, 55*(3), 664–690. https://doi.org/10.1111/1745-9125.12145

Evans, A., & Bosworth, K. (1998). *Building effective drug education programs*. Phi Delta Kappa International.

Femina, L. L., Soler, A. C. P., Nardi, S. M. T., Del, V., & Paschoal, A. (2007). Lepra para hanseníase: A visão do portador sobre a mudança de terminologia. *Hansenologia Internationalis: Hanseníase e Outras Doenças Infecciosas*, *32*(1), 37–48. https://doi.org/10.47878/hi.2007.v32.35192

Graupmann, V., Jonas, E., Meier, E., Hawelka, S., & Aichhorn, M. (2012). Reactance, the self, and its group: When threats to freedom come from the ingroup versus the outgroup. *European Journal of Social Psychology*, *42*(2), 164–173. https://doi.org/10.1002/ejsp.857

Herek, G. M., & Capitanio, J. P. (1996). "Some of my best friends": Intergroup contact, concealable stigma, and heterosexuals' attitudes toward gay men and lesbians. *Personality and Social Psychology Bulletin*, *22*(4), 412–424. https://doi.org/10.1177/0146167296224007

Jasper, J. M. (2014). Constructing indignation: Anger dynamics in protest movements. *Emotion Review*, *6*(3), 208–213. https://doi.org/10.1177/1754073914522863

Kelley, H. H. (1971). *Attribution in social interaction*. General Learning Press.

Kvaale, E. P., Haslam, N., & Gottdiener, W. H. (2013). The 'side effects' of medicalization: A meta-analytic review of how biogenetic explanations affect stigma. *Clinical Psychology Review*, *33*(6), 782–794. https://doi.org/10.1016/j.cpr.2013.06.002

Landmann, H., & Rohmann, A. (2020). Being moved by protest: Collective efficacy beliefs and injustice appraisals enhance collective action intentions for forest protection via positive and negative emotions. *Journal of Environmental Psychology*, *71*, 101491. https://doi.org/10.1016/j.jenvp.2020.101491

Lienemann, B. A., Siegel, J. T., & Crano, W. D. (2013). Persuading people with depression to seek help: Respect the boomerang. *Health Communication*, *28*(7), 718–728. https://doi.org/10.1080/10410236.2012.712091

Maruta, T., Volpe, U., Gaebel, W., Matsumoto, C., & Iimori, M. (2014). Should schizophrenia still be named so? *Schizophrenia Research*, *152*(1), 305–306. https://doi.org/10.1016/j.schres.2013.11.005

Matthews, N. L., Ly, A. R., & Goldberg, W. A. (2015). College students' perceptions of peers with autism spectrum disorder. *Journal of Autism and Developmental Disorders*, *45*(1), 90–99. https://doi.org/10.1007/s10803-014-2195-6

Maunder, R. D., & White, F. A. (2019). Intergroup contact and mental health stigma: A comparative effectiveness meta-analysis. *Clinical Psychology Review*, *72*, 101749. https://doi.org/10.1016/j.cpr.2019.101749

McConahay, J. B. (1986). Modern racism, ambivalence, and the modern racism scale. In J. F. Dovidio & S. L. Gaertner (Eds.), *Prejudice, discrimination, and racism* (pp. 91–125). Academic Press.

Mueser, K. T., Glynn, S. M., Corrigan, P. W., & Baber, W. (1996). What's in a name? The preferences of participants in mental health services. *Psychiatric Services*, *47*, 760–761. https://doi.org/10.1007/s11606-022-07813-w

Newheiser, A. K., & Barreto, M. (2014). Hidden costs of hiding stigma: Ironic interpersonal consequences of concealing a stigmatized identity in social interactions. *Journal of Experimental Social Psychology*, *52*, 58–70. https://doi.org/10.1016/j.jesp.2014.01.002

Noe-Bustamante, L., Mora, L., & Lopez, M. H. (2020). *About one-in-four US Hispanics have heard of Latinx, but just 3% use it* (Vol. *11*). *Pew Research Center*. https://www.pewresearch.org/hispanic/2020/08/11/about-one-in-four-u-s-hispanics-have-heard-of-latinx-but-just-3-use-it

Oliveira, M. L., Mendes, C. M., Tardin, R. T., Cunha, M. D., & Arruda, A. (2003). Social representation of Hansen's disease thirty years after the term "'leprosy"' was replaced in Brazil. *História, Ciências, Saúde-Manguinhos*, *10*(S1), 41–48. https://doi.org/10.1590/s0104-59702003000400003

Penn, D. L., & Nowlin-Drummond, A. (2001). Politically correct labels and schizophrenia: A rose by any other name? *Schizophrenia Bulletin*, *27*(2), 197–203. https://doi.org/10.1093/oxfordjournals.schbul.a006866

Power, A. K. (2010). Transforming the nation's health: Next steps in mental health promotion. *American Journal of Public Health*, *100*(12), 2343–2346. https://doi.org/10.2105/AJPH.2010.192138

Read, J., Haslam, N., Sayce, L., & Davies, E. (2006). Prejudice and schizophrenia: A review of the 'mental illness is an illness like any other' approach. *Acta Psychiatrica Scandinavica*, *114*(5), 303–318. https://doi.org/10.1111/j.1600-0447.2006.00824.x

Reinke, R. R., Corrigan, P. W., Leonhard, C., Lundin, R. K., & Kubiak, M. A. (2004). Examining two aspects of contact on the stigma of mental illness. *Journal of Social and Clinical Psychology*, *23*(3), 377–389. https://doi.org/10.1521/jscp.23.3.377.35457

Rosenberg, L. (2013). *Is mental health stigma overrated?* National Council for Behavioral Health.

Sadow, D., Ryder, M., & Webster, D. (2002). Is education of health professionals encouraging stigma towards the mentally ill? *Journal of Mental Health*, *11*(6), 657–665. https://doi.org/10.1080/09638230021000058210

Sartorius, N., Chiu, H., Heok, K. E., Lee, M. S., Ouyang, W. C., Sato, M., Yang, Y. K., & Yu, X. (2014). Name change for schizophrenia. *Schizophrenia Bulletin*, *40*(2), 255–258. https://doi.org/10.1093/schbul/sbt231

Sato, M. (2006). Renaming schizophrenia: A Japanese perspective. *World Psychiatry*, *5*(1), 53–55. https://doi.org/10.1017/S2045796018000598

Schmader, T., & Lickel, B. (2006). The approach and avoidance function of guilt and shame emotions: Comparing reactions to self-caused and other-caused wrongdoing. *Motivation and Emotion*, *30*(1), 42–55. https://doi.org/10.1007/s11031-006-9006-0

Schomerus, G., Lucht, M., Holzinger, A., Matschinger, H., Carta, M. G., & Angermeyer, M. C. (2011). The stigma of alcohol dependence compared with other mental disorders: A review of population studies. *Alcohol and Alcoholism*, 46(2), 105–112. https://doi.org/10.1093/alcalc/agq089

Schulze, B. (2007). Stigma and mental health professionals: A review of the evidence on an intricate relationship. *International Review of Psychiatry*, 19(2), 137–155. https://doi.org/10.1080/09540260701278929

Shepherd, L., Spears, R., & Manstead, A. S. (2013). "This will bring shame on our nation": The role of anticipated group-based emotions on collective action. *Journal of Experimental Social Psychology*, 49(1), 42–57. https://doi.org/10.1016/j.jesp.2012.07.011

Siegel, J. T., Flores-Mendel, F., Martinez, D. A., & Berger, D. E. (2019). Can mental health anti-stigma messages have untoward effects on some people with depression?: An exploratory study. *Journal of Health Communication*, 24(11), 821–828. https://doi.org/10.1080/10810730.2019.1672838

Simmons, L., Jones, T., & Bradley, E. (2017). Reducing mental health stigma: The relationship between knowledge and attitude change. *European Journal of Mental Health*, 12(1), 25–40. https://doi.org/10.5708/EJMH.12.2017.1.2

Smith, T. W. (1992). Changing racial labels: From "colored" to "negro" to "Black" to "African American". *Public Opinion Quarterly*, 56(4), 496–514. https://doi.org/10.1086/269339

Steinberg, L. (2021). *Emotional Responses to Contemporary Media Representations of Disability as a Predictor of Internalized Stigma among Physically Disabled Adults* (Publication No. 28867480) [Doctoral dissertation, Alliant International University]. ProQuest Dissertations & Theses Global.

Stevenson, H. C., Reed, J., Bodison, P., & Bishop, A. (1997). Racism stress management: Racial socialization beliefs and the experience of depression and anger in African American youth. *Youth & Society*, 29(2), 197–222. https://doi.org/10.1177/0044118X97029002003

Takahashi, H., Ideno, T., Okubo, S., Matsui, H., Takemura, K., Matsuura, M., Kato, M., & Okubo, Y. (2009). Impact of changing the Japanese term for "schizophrenia" for reasons of stereotypical beliefs of schizophrenia in Japanese youth. *Schizophrenia Research*, 112(1–3), 149–152. https://doi.org/10.1016/j.schres.2009.03.037

The New York Times. (2019, August 9). '*Poor Kids*' *Just as Bright as White Kids, Biden Says* [Video]. https://www.nytimes.com/2019/08/09/us/politics/joe-biden-poor-kids.html

Torrey, E. F. (2011). Stigma and violence: Isn't it time to connect the dots? *Schizophrenia Bulletin*, 37(5), 892–896. https://doi.org/10.1093/schbul/sbr057

Watson, A. C., Corrigan, P., & Kosyluk, K. (2014). Challenging stigma. In E. Byrne & A. Rosen (Eds.), *Early intervention in psychiatry: EI of nearly everything for better mental health* (pp. 358–371). Wiley Blackwell.

Wegner, D. M., Schneider, D. J., Carter, S. R., & White, T. L. (1987). Paradoxical effects of thought suppression. *Journal of Personality and Social Psychology*, 53(1), 5–13. https://doi.org/10.1037/0022-3514.53.1.5

Wegner, D. M., Shortt, J. W., Blake, A. W., & Page, M. S. (1990). The suppression of exciting thoughts. *Journal of Personality and Social Psychology*, 58(3), 409–418. https://doi.org/10.1037/0022-3514.58.3.409

Wegner, D. M., & Smart, L. (2000). The hidden costs of hidden stigma. In T. F. Heatherton, R. E. Kleck, M. R. Hebl & J. G. Hull (Eds.), *The social psychology of stigma* (pp. 220–242). Guilford Press.

Wright, S. C. (1997). Ambiguity, social influence, and collective action: Generating collective protest in response to tokenism. *Personality and Social Psychology Bulletin*, 23(12), 1277–1290. https://doi.org/10.1177/01461672972312005

Part VI

Promising Strategies

24

Minimizing Reactance to Increase Help Seeking for Depression

Christopher M. Falco[1] and Benjamin D. Rosenberg[2]
[1] Claremont Graduate University
[2] Dominican University of California

Depression afflicts over 320 million people worldwide and is considered the leading cause of disability globally (World Health Organization, 2017); further, the prevalence of depression sharply increased during the COVID-19 pandemic (Ettman et al., 2020). Thankfully, myriad treatments (e.g., psychotherapy; Barth et al., 2013) are effective in reducing depressive symptomatology, and greater perceived social support is predictive of quicker recovery (Wang et al., 2018). However, in stark contrast to many conditions for which more severe symptoms predict help seeking (e.g., influenza-like illness; Peppa et al., 2017), people become less likely to seek help from both professional and nonprofessional sources as depressive symptomatology heightens (Siegel et al., 2015; Yamaguchi et al., 2023; Yzer et al., 2022) due in part to characteristics of depression itself (Lienemann et al., 2013; Siegel et al., 2017).

Convincing people with depression to seek help is a notable challenge (Siegel et al., 2017; Yzer & Siegel, 2025). While some persuasive messages designed to increase help seeking are successful, others backfire, resulting in lowered help-seeking likelihood (Lienemann et al., 2013). Psychological factors significantly contribute to this issue (Siegel et al., 2017), including the negative bias and cognitive distortions characteristic of depression (Beck, 1967). A complementary but relatively understudied explanation for the failure of campaigns to persuade people with depression to seek help is psychological reactance theory (PRT; Brehm, 1966; Brehm & Brehm, 1981), which offers an account of how people respond to perceived threats to their autonomy.

According to PRT (Brehm, 1966), when people perceive their freedom as being threatened, a motivational state—psychological reactance—can be aroused, which motivates them to restore their freedom. Reactance can arise in many circumstances, including when people view or hear persuasive messages (Brehm, 1966; Dillard & Shen, 2005). Messages that display persuasive intent can be perceived as freedom threatening and thus lead to diminished compliance as a form of freedom restoration (for a meta-analysis, see Rains, 2013). Reactance reduces the effectiveness of persuasive messages across many contexts, including in attempting to convince those with depression to seek help for their condition (Lienemann & Siegel, 2016).

It is crucial to design persuasive messages that minimize reactance to increase the positive effects of messages and avoid backfires that undermine help seeking (Lienemann & Siegel, 2016; Siegel et al., 2017). In the hopes of stimulating future research on this topic, we review PRT (Brehm, 1966) and Beck's (1967) cognitive theory of depression (CTD). Then, we discuss tactics used to minimize reactance that we believe are especially promising for the current context while considering the relation between reactance and the cognitive patterns typical of people with depression (Beck, 1967) that cause them to respond differently to persuasive messages than people without depression (Siegel et al., 2017).

The Handbook of Mental Health Communication, First Edition.
Edited by Marco C. Yzer and Jason T. Siegel.

Psychological Reactance Theory

PRT (Brehm, 1966; Brehm & Brehm, 1981; for a review, see Rosenberg & Siegel, 2018) rests upon the premise that people have free behaviors—actions, thoughts, or feelings that they perceive to have the freedom and ability to enact or experience—and their ability to engage in these free behaviors is highly valued. According to PRT, if people's ability to engage in a free behavior is eliminated or threatened, an unpleasant motivational state called reactance is often aroused that spurs them to restore that freedom. Reactance is typified by an amalgam of anger and negative cognitions (Dillard & Shen, 2005).

Freedom restoration often manifests behaviorally; people may restore their freedom by engaging in a threatened behavior or attempting to regain an eliminated behavior (Brehm, 1966). Beyond behavioral consequences, reactance arousal causes attitudinal shifts such as increases in the attractiveness of threatened behaviors (Brehm et al., 1966) and derogation of sources of freedom threats (Worchel & Brehm, 1971). As an illustration of freedom restoration, the more people felt forced to wear masks during the height of the COVID-19 pandemic, the less likely they were to do so (Taylor & Asmundson, 2021).

Reactance arousal and magnitude depend on many factors (Brehm, 1966). Reactance should be most robust when: (a) the free behavior is highly important; (b) there are few or no alternative free behaviors; (c) a large number of free behaviors are threatened or eliminated; (d) when threatened, the threat is severe; (e) future threats or eliminations are implied; (f) the threat or elimination is illegitimate; (g) the threat or elimination is unjustified; and/or (h) the freedom is eliminated rather than threatened (Brehm, 1966; Brehm & Brehm, 1981). However, if a free behavior is genuinely lost, reactance should dissipate and result in helplessness (Wortman & Brehm, 1975). Individual characteristics and conditions may also affect reactance arousal, such as uncertainty (Rosenberg & Siegel, 2023), trait reactance (i.e., the disposition to become reactant; Shoham et al., 2004), reactance itself (Siegel & Rosenberg, 2024), and most pertinently, depressive symptomatology (Lienemann & Siegel, 2016).

To the detriment of pro-health persuasive attempts (e.g., efforts to reduce smoking; So, 2022), people often perceive them as freedom threats (Dillard & Shen, 2005). Thus, the messages arouse reactance, which diminishes the effectiveness of persuasive messages—even leading to boomerang effects (i.e., message backfiring; Quick & Stephenson, 2007). However, it is possible to minimize reactance toward persuasive messages with many tactics, such as using language that is minimally controlling (Staunton et al., 2022).

From a PRT standpoint (Brehm, 1966), people with depression are likely to become reactant toward messages attempting to persuade them to seek help. If people with depression perceive such messages as freedom threatening and consider the decision of whether to seek help as an important free behavior, reactance is likely to result (Lienemann & Siegel, 2016). To the extent that messages are incongruent with their beliefs about the effectiveness of help seeking and their attitudes toward help seeking—both of which tend to be less favorable than those of people without depression (Siegel et al., 2015)—reactance should be greater due to interfering with both their freedom of behavior and freedom of thought. Beyond the possibility that encouraging someone to seek help could cause reactance due to the topic and persuasive nature of the message, the prospect of circumstances in which the directives of others may restrict their freedoms (e.g., therapy or inpatient treatment; Addis & Mahalik, 2003) should cause further resistance. Complementing the insights provided by PRT (Brehm, 1966), there is theoretical rationale that suggests depression itself leads to heightened reactance toward persuasive help-seeking messages (Lienemann et al., 2013; Siegel et al., 2017).

Beck's Cognitive Theory of Depression

CTD (Beck, 1963, 1967; Beck et al., 1979) holds that individuals with depression think and process information differently than those without, especially in the case of self-relevant information (Wisco, 2009). This framework (Beck, 1967) states that depression is typified by three major components: the cognitive triad, the depressogenic schema, and cognitive distortions. The cognitive triad consists of enduring negative views of oneself, one's experiences, and one's expectations of the future. The depressogenic schema directs those with depression to attend more to negative information.

Cognitive distortions, which tend to arise involuntarily, entail misinterpreting information or making invalid inferences in a manner that supports the overall negative bias. For example, magnification refers to inflating the extremity of an adverse event, making it seem more consequential than it may actually be (Beck et al., 1979). These three components (i.e., the cognitive triad, the depressogenic schema, and cognitive distortions) are thought to become progressively more negative as depression heightens, resulting in a further departure from objectivity.

Such negative biases are evident in the help-seeking context; more severe depressive symptomatology is associated with less favorable attitudes toward seeking help, less positive outcome expectations of seeking help, and lower intentions to seek help (e.g., Siegel et al., 2015). The ideal target of a persuasive message would understand the content of the message perfectly and hold either relatively positive attitudes toward help seeking or less favorable attitudes that are weak. However, people with depression are the opposite: They are likely to attend to negative information, misinterpret information negatively, and hold strong, less favorable attitudes toward help seeking (Lienemann et al., 2013; Siegel et al., 2017). This cognitive profile presents difficulties in persuading people with depression to seek help, even without considering how reactance relates to the condition and topic (Lienemann & Siegel, 2016).

Reactance and Persuading People with Depression to Seek Help

Grounded in the implications of both PRT (Brehm, 1966) and CTD (Beck, 1967), researchers have posited that help-seeking messages may result in especially heightened reactance among people with depression due to characteristics of depression itself (Lienemann & Siegel, 2016). In two studies, Lienemann and Siegel (2016) exposed participants to advertisements, including two that encouraged those with depression to seek help. Findings showed that reactance mediated the relationship between higher depressive symptomatology and less favorable help-seeking inclinations. In addition, results revealed that depression itself predicted reactance toward help-seeking messages over and above trait reactance. Further, the use of a reactance minimization tactic was ineffective among those with high levels of depressive symptomatology, contrary to consistent findings in other contexts (e.g., discouraging binge drinking; Dillard & Shen, 2005).

Lienemann and Siegel (2016) theorized that this pattern of results occurred for four main reasons. First, those with depression likely regard the choice to seek help as an important free behavior, making suggestions to seek help likely to arouse reactance and reduce help-seeking likelihood—even among those who are already unlikely to do so. Second, messages advocating for help seeking may be incongruent with the less favorable beliefs and attitudes of people with depression toward help seeking compared with those without (Siegel et al., 2015), threatening their freedom of belief. Third, cognitive biases inherent in depression (Beck, 1967) may cause people with heightened depressive symptomatology to overly attend to negative information, such as apparent threats to their freedom. Fourth, cognitive distortions could lead to heightened reactance; for instance, people with depression may magnify any apparent threat to freedom. In support of Lienemann and Siegel's (2016) ideas, higher depressive symptomatology is associated with both higher levels of trait reactance (Hong & Faedda, 1996) and irritability (Balbuena et al., 2016).

Put simply, persuading people with depression to seek help presents a perfect storm for increased reactance and, as a result, decreased message effectiveness—or even iatrogenic effects. This is not to say that every help-seeking message will induce reactance. Rather, help-seeking messages have a high potential to arouse reactance; when aroused, reactance poses a considerable issue for the success of campaigns and the well-being of people experiencing depression. Given the significance of this issue, the current chapter discusses reactance minimization tactics that we believe may both increase the effectiveness of messages and reduce the risk of backfires, such as further inhibited help seeking. However, a few caveats are necessary to keep in mind. The techniques discussed are meant to complement the content of a message; even the strongest reactance minimization tactics are unlikely to succeed with poorly planned content. Although there is theoretical and empirical backing for each tactic, many have not yet been tested on those with depression. These tactics' effectiveness is likely to depend on people's levels of depressive symptomatology—as symptomatology heightens, success becomes less likely regardless of approach. While the techniques we propose should lessen the arousal of reactance, there is still the chance that a tactic might result in further help-seeking inhibition due to the consequences of unexpected cognitive distortions. Regardless, we are optimistic that with careful study, these strategies may be used to minimize reactance and increase help seeking for depression.

Low-Controlling Language

A well-intentioned message designer might assume that saying targets *must* engage in a healthy behavior would be more effective than saying they *have the choice* to do so. Although this sort of language has its strengths (e.g., clarity; Staunton et al., 2022), it can also be detrimental, as phrasing that implies or asserts that people do not have autonomy can be perceived as freedom threatening (e.g., Dillard & Shen, 2005). In reactance parlance, such phrasing is called high-controlling language (HCL; Staunton et al., 2022). Messages that use HCL are likely to be perceived as threatening and high in persuasive intent, leading to greater reactance than those that employ low-controlling language (LCL), which uses suggestions, remains polite, emphasizes recipients' autonomy, and errs on the side of implicitness.

LCL often results in lower reactance through reduced perceptions of freedom threat compared with HCL in myriad contexts (for a meta-analysis, see Rains, 2013). For example, LCL used in an antismoking advertisement attributed to parents resulted in lower intentions to use cannabis among adolescents than an HCL advertisement (Crano et al., 2017). Owing to how reliably HCL arouses reactance, manipulating controlling language is a common paradigm used to conduct basic research on PRT (e.g., Dillard & Shen, 2005).

Considerations for Depression

Based on such consistent results in favor of LCL (Rains, 2013), it could be reasonably predicted that using LCL would minimize reactance among those with depression when persuading them to seek help. However, these language manipulations may not have as pronounced an impact on this population due to the cognitive aspects of depression (Beck, 1967). Lienemann and Siegel (2016) found that manipulating the controlling nature of language in persuasive messages was not effective in minimizing reactance among people with high levels of depressive symptomatology. These researchers theorized that cognitive distortions responsible for increasing reactance to help-seeking messages rendered HCL and LCL messages equally reactance inducing. For example, any freedom threats the message posed may have been magnified, while the positive characteristics of LCL may have been minimized (Beck, 1967).

Nevertheless, it may be the case that those with lower levels of depressive symptomatology who do still meet diagnostic criteria benefit from LCL, as their cognitions are skewed less severely (Beck, 1967). Supporting this idea, an LCL message resulted in less reactance than an HCL message among those just shy of a clinical cutoff for depression (Lienemann & Siegel, 2016). Further, it is noteworthy that LCL did not produce worse outcomes than HCL among those with heightened depressive symptomatology.

Future Directions for Low-Controlling Language

Among those with high levels of depressive symptomatology, LCL may not minimize reactance (Lienemann & Siegel, 2016), though people with mild depression may benefit from its use. There is currently little reason to suspect that HCL should be used instead of LCL in help-seeking messages, as evidence suggests that, at worst, they are equivalent in the arousal of reactance. We recommend, pending further study, that message designers exercise caution and use LCL in help-seeking messages, such as *please consider* and *it is your choice*.

In addition, it is notable that Lienemann and Siegel (2016) focused on the autonomy-supportive aspect of LCL, which emphasizes freedom of choice. It may be worth examining how other elements of LCL may affect the arousal of reactance in this context; for example, language that is minimally dogmatic may be effective in mitigating reactance toward help-seeking messages, as has been found in other contexts (e.g., binge drinking reduction; Bensley & Wu, 1991). Though here we emphasize the benefits of LCL, there are benefits of HCL—namely, clarity and efficiency (Staunton et al., 2022). Help-seeking messages may be able to capitalize upon those benefits and instead use other tactics to minimize reactance (e.g., mistargeting, discussed later; Siegel et al., 2015); however, this approach carries more risk.

Restoration Postscripts

A restoration postscript is a message provided after the actual persuasive content has been communicated, emphasizing that recipients can choose whether to comply with the request (Miller et al., 2007). For example, a postscript used in a prior study included: "You know what is best for yourself. . . The choice is yours. You're free to decide for yourself" (Miller et al., 2007, p. 240). By making it clear and salient that recipients are free to choose their course of action, postscripts are thought to decrease perceived threat to freedom and provide an opportunity to restore freedom, thereby reducing reactance.

In line with these predictions, postscripts have reduced perceptions of freedom threats (Miller et al., 2007), reduced reactance (Richards et al., 2022), and increased desired behavioral intentions (Reynolds-Tylus et al., 2022). Despite this supportive evidence, the success of postscripts may depend on factors that merit further investigation. Adding postscripts to messages that use LCL may have no effect (Bessarabova et al., 2017) or inhibit persuasion (Bessarabova et al., 2013). Further, the relationship between restoration postscripts and reduced perceptions of freedom threat may be dose-dependent, with insufficiently detailed postscripts resulting in null findings (Quick et al., 2015).

Considerations for Depression

If people with heightened depressive symptomatology are prone to reactance (Lienemann & Siegel, 2016), it may be easier to reduce reactance than prevent its arousal. Given restoration postscripts are intended to minimize reactance (Miller et al., 2007), this tactic may be especially appropriate for use in help-seeking messages. Following a message urging people with depression to seek help, a postscript could include content such as, "After considering these options, the choice is ultimately yours."

However, cognitive distortions (Beck, 1967) may arise in response to the emphasis that restoration postscripts place on people's freedom of choice. Arbitrary inference (Beck et al., 1979), making a conclusion in the absence of supporting evidence or the presence of contrary evidence, could be especially problematic. This distortion could lead people with depression to conclude that if they had the freedom to choose whether to seek help and did not do so, they may be too weak to seek help. People may fall prey to this distortion even if the message convinced them of the benefits of help seeking. Although postscripts may potentially spark negative cognitions, a subtle reminder of autonomy may avoid backfiring, just as LCL did not backfire in prior studies (Lienemann & Siegel, 2016).

Future Directions for Restoration Postscripts

Using restoration postscripts (Miller et al., 2007) to reduce reactance after exposure to help-seeking messages among those with heightened depressive symptomatology is a promising avenue for research. Given that the effects of postscripts may be dependent upon the use of controlling language (e.g., Bessarabova et al., 2013), studies that examine postscripts in this context may benefit from the concurrent manipulation of postscripts and controlling language to determine whether these effects generalize to help-seeking messages targeting people with depression. Researchers should also consider that the success of postscripts may depend on their length, as some have hypothesized that short postscripts may not be sufficient to reduce reactance (Quick et al., 2015). When considering postscript length, literature on the *but you are free* compliance technique (Guéguen & Pascual, 2000) could be informative. Adding short phrases like *but you are free to refuse* to the end of requests may increase compliance by reducing reactance (Carpenter & Pascual, 2016). A postscript that may toe the line between freedom restoration and inadvertently causing arbitrary inference could include content to the effect of, "While we recommend that you talk to a mental health professional if you feel depressed, you are free to decide what is best for yourself. It is entirely your decision, and you may do as you wish."

Providing Compliance Options

Another method of minimizing reactance is simply offering more than one way that recipients can comply with a persuasive message. For example, when advocating for people to engage in cancer-preventive behaviors, requesting they either use sunscreen or wear protective clothing rather than asking them to do both (Shen, 2015). The more restrictive a threat or elimination, the greater the magnitude of reactance (Brehm, 1966); by "loosening these constraints" (Heilman & Garner, 1975, p. 912), reactance should be diminished. Offering multiple methods of compliance achieves this aim, yet the options offered remain in service of inducing compliance with the general goal of a message.

Although providing compliance options has been less frequently examined than other methods of minimizing reactance in response to persuasive communication (e.g., LCL; Rains, 2013), findings are thus far encouraging. Early research (Heilman & Garner, 1975) found that when only one method of compliance was available, messages that threatened punishment for noncompliance resulted in lower compliance rates than messages that promised rewards. In contrast, when participants could choose from four methods of compliance, this difference was nonsignificant. More recent evidence also suggests that this tactic is effective: Offering two options of compliance with a persuasive message advocating for cancer-preventive behaviors led to lower state reactance than offering just one (Shen, 2015). However, a possible downside of this approach is that recipients could perceive a message as mandating compliance with every option. If so, the threat to freedom would likely be perceived as greater than if one method of compliance had been offered (e.g., Reynolds-Tylus et al., 2019).

Considerations for Depression

This tactic may be particularly suitable for the current context, as there are many ways people with depression can seek help, such as meeting with health professionals (of which there are many kinds) or asking for social support. Further, people may prefer certain sources from which they could seek help (Nolan & O'Connor, 2019). By listing more than one source that recipients could seek help from, there is also a greater chance that their preferred source would be presented in the message, a potential benefit of the approach. Although the effectiveness of this tactic in help-seeking messages has been seldom investigated, we expect that the number of compliance options presented and help-seeking inclinations likely exhibit a curvilinear relationship due to choice overload (Iyengar & Lepper, 2000). As the number of options increases, help-seeking inclinations may initially become more favorable due to minimized reactance and then reach a point where additional options are detrimental.

Future Directions for Providing Compliance Options

From a PRT perspective (Brehm, 1966), offering compliance options in help-seeking messages should minimize reactance and thus be helpful (e.g., Shen, 2015). However, if too many options are provided, motivation to seek help may decrease despite minimized reactance (Iyengar & Lepper, 2000). There is also the chance that offering compliance options may heighten reactance; if recipients interpret the message as indicating that complying with each option is necessary, reactance may heighten (e.g., Reynolds-Tylus et al., 2019).

These concerns notwithstanding, a minimal manipulation of compliance options could be effective—perhaps offering two sources of help instead of one. Similarly subtle manipulations have effectively minimized reactance in the past (e.g., Shen, 2015). Given these findings, we believe that research on incorporating compliance options into help-seeking messages is merited. Researchers may benefit from carefully varying the options listed to look for minimal manipulations that mitigate reactance and a point at which doing so may be counterproductive. It may also be worthwhile to examine how the match between recipients' preferences and the help-seeking sources presented affects reactance. One possibility for leveraging options for compliance in help-seeking messages could be a portion that reads, "There is more than one type of person who can give you support. Mental health professionals and loved ones can all be there for you. Please consider speaking with one of them."

Source Characteristics

Much research indicates that reactance can result in derogation of the source of persuasive messages—that is, the source of the freedom threat (e.g., Miller et al., 2007). Just as reactance may affect perceptions of source characteristics, so can source characteristics affect reactance arousal. Sources perceived as authoritative, expert, or having power over the recipient can result in greater reactance arousal because they are likely to be perceived as freedom threatening (Brehm, 1966; Brehm & Brehm, 1981). For example, pro-health messages attributed to doctors may, at times, lead to less favorable evaluations of messages than those attributed to peers (Crano et al., 2007).

The effectiveness of peer sources in minimizing reactance may also be due in part to similarity. High source similarity minimizes the arousal of reactance and can increase desired persuasive outcomes (Song et al., 2018), sometimes even nullifying the detrimental effects of threatening messages (Silvia, 2005). Likewise, manipulating the group status of a source (i.e., making a source more like message recipients in terms of group membership) may minimize reactance (Song et al., 2018) in a manner consistent with social identity theory literature (for a review, see Hogg & Smith, 2007).

Considerations for Depression

Source characteristics may be critical to consider when attempting to persuade people with depression, as some literature suggests that source characteristics are more influential in changing the attitudes of those with higher depression than those without (Neimeyer et al., 1990). This may be due to a heightened motivation to reduce uncertainty about social information (Weary et al., 1993). Further, those with depression may generally judge message sources less positively than those without.

By offering information that is self-relevant to those with depression, the source of such information could become self-relevant as well and may thus trigger cognitive distortions. This should be especially problematic when those sources are seen as freedom threatening; people with depression could magnify (Beck, 1967) a power differential, which would likely lead to heightened reactance. Another possibility is that the cognitive distortion of selective abstraction (i.e., latching onto a minor detail and interpreting an entire event based on the detail; Beck et al., 1979) may result in dissimilar sources being deemed as not understanding of the message recipients' experiences, leading people experiencing depression to view messages as illegitimate freedom threats. In addition, negative mood often skews judgments in a valence-congruent manner (Forgas, 1995), so those with depression should be expected to judge sources more negatively from an affective perspective as well. Indeed, greater depressive symptomatology is associated with lower trust in governmental sources that offer information regarding COVID-19 (Wilkinson et al., 2022).

Future Directions for Source Characteristics

As source characteristics may particularly influence people with depression (Neimeyer et al., 1990) and people with depression are likely to judge sources less positively given their persistent negative cognitions (Beck, 1967) and mood (Forgas, 1995), further research is needed to determine which source characteristics are most effective in minimizing reactance toward help-seeking messages as well as which are most detrimental. The two source characteristics outlined above—authority and similarity—would be a reasonable place to begin these investigations.

However, manipulating source characteristics in actual campaigns may pose a challenge, as governmental agencies and nonprofits tend to organize and fund such endeavors and are likely to be perceived as authoritative, expert, or holding power over the recipients. To sidestep this issue, it may be practical to use spokespeople who are known to have experienced depression, as doing so would heighten similarity to intended recipients in both an identity- and message-relevant manner. Until further research is conducted on this topic, we recommend that researchers studying other methods of minimizing reactance bear in mind that authoritative or expert sources may, at times, heighten reactance toward messages, whereas sources similar to recipients may minimize its arousal.

Mistargeting

Another method of minimizing reactance is mistargeted communication, which refers to purposefully directing a persuasive message to someone or some group other than the true targets (Siegel et al., 2015). By doing so, persuasive intent can be masked, thereby increasing the effectiveness of a message. For example, a mistargeted message used to increase help seeking among people with depression led with, "Do you know someone who fights depression?" (Siegel et al., 2015, p. 2).

Early researchers noted, "It is widely believed that a communication, if inadvertently overheard, is more likely to be effective in changing the opinion of the listener than if it had been deliberately addressed to him" (Walster & Festinger, 1962, p. 395). In a formative study, participants were led to believe that they were overhearing someone attempting to persuade another person that the link between smoking and lung cancer was not evidenced by research (Walster & Festinger, 1962). Of participants who were smokers, those who did not believe that the people speaking were aware of them listening exhibited greater agreement with the persuasive communication than those who did believe that the individuals were aware of them listening. Both smokers and nonsmokers rated the speaker as having greater honesty and sincerity in the overheard condition compared to the regular condition.

This research inspired the technique of mistargeting (Crano et al., 2007; Siegel et al., 2015), which uses the overheard communication technique within a persuasive message. Although a paucity of research has directly tested the idea, mistargeting holds promise as a reactance minimization technique (Miller et al., 2007; Staunton et al., 2022). The rationale for overheard communication and mistargeting effectiveness is entirely compatible with PRT (Brehm, 1966): If targets are unaware someone is attempting to persuade them, they should be unaware that their freedom is being threatened.

Considerations for Depression

As noted, a significant trigger of cognitive distortions in those with depression is self-relevant information (Wisco, 2009). Therefore, lowering the self-relevance of messages by using mistargeting may be especially effective when persuading those with depression to seek help (Siegel et al., 2019). Siegel et al. (2015) phrased messages so that their apparent intent was to persuade recipients to recommend help seeking to others who have depression rather than persuading people with depression to seek help. These mistargeted messages increased help-seeking intentions, attitudes, and outcome expectations in those with heightened depressive symptomatology compared with a direct message (for similar findings, see Siegel & Marshburn, 2025). As an illustration, one mistargeted message included: "Do you know someone who is feeling distressed? Feeling hopeless? They might be depressed" (Siegel et al., 2015, p. 12). Further, if cognitive distortions lead to heightened reactance (Lienemann & Siegel, 2016), minimizing self-relevant information by using mistargeting could reduce the arousal of the very cognitive distortions that intensify reactance in tandem with the benefit of lowering perceptions of persuasive intent.

Future Directions for Mistargeting

As mistargeted communication can increase help-seeking inclinations among those with heightened depressive symptomatology (Siegel et al., 2015; Siegel & Marshburn, 2025), lower self-relevance, and likely minimizes reactance, we believe that this technique merits both immediate implementation and further study. Beyond facilitating persuasion, mistargeted messages and overheard communication can result in more favorable source (Walster & Festinger, 1962) and message evaluations as well (Crano et al., 2007)—all of which align with reactance literature. Beyond using the approach and further testing its efficacy, we recommend investigating whether minimized reactance mediates the positive persuasive effects of mistargeting.

Narratives

Another persuasive strategy that minimizes self-relevance is using narrative-form messages (for a review, see Hinyard & Kreuter, 2007), or messages conveyed in a story with a beginning, middle, and end, whether fictional or factual. At times, narratives can be more effective than non-narrative messages. In comparing an educational program about teenage pregnancy to a dramatic television program in which an adolescent couple became pregnant, female viewers exposed to the narrative reported greater safe-sex intentions than those exposed to the nonnarrative message due in part to the narrative cloaking persuasive intent and thus mitigating reactance (Moyer-Gusé & Nabi, 2010). In addition to mitigating reactance by lowering perceived persuasive intent, the persuasive effects of narratives may be mediated by empathy and identification (Shen, 2011; Shen et al., 2017).

Empathy, in part, consists of cognitive and affective components—people experiencing empathy take on the thoughts and/or emotions of the object of empathy yet can still differentiate between their own experiences and those of the object of empathy (Eisenberg, 1989). Empathizing with characters in narratives can lead to diminished reactance, consequently increasing the effectiveness of persuasive messages (e.g., Shen, 2011). The influence of narrative messages may also be mediated by identification, which refers to a similar cognitive–affective process in which a narrative consumer takes on the perspective of a character, including their goals, with concurrent loss of self-awareness (Cohen, 2001). As with empathy, identification likely leads to minimized reactance, followed by more desirable persuasive outcomes (Shen et al., 2017).

Considerations for Depression

Narrative communication is promising for use in the current context because it works through perspective-taking processes that lower not only perceived threat and minimize reactance (e.g., Shen et al., 2017) but also possibly self-relevance and thus the risk of cognitive distortions arising (for similar theorizing, see Siegel et al., 2019). Although direct examinations of this idea using samples of people with depression are rare, narrative communication may increase help-seeking behaviors among this population (Dixon De Silva, 2021).

Despite the promise of using narratives to increase help seeking among people with depression, there are also reasons for caution to consider. Depressive symptomatology exhibits complex relationships with both affective and cognitive empathy (Tully et al., 2016). Among people with high emotion dysregulation, moderate-to-high affective empathy is associated with more significant depressive symptomatology; conversely, both high and low cognitive empathy are predictive of heightened symptomatology. Depressive symptomatology is negatively correlated with the tendency to identify with characters (O'Connor et al., 2002), another concern given the importance of identification in narrative communication. In brief, not everyone with depression may reap the full benefits of narrative communication.

Among those who experience high levels of empathy and identification, narratives should have the most significant effect; however, this effect could be counterproductive depending on the content of the narrative. Suppose people with depression perceive a character with whom they empathize or identify as displaying negative affect and an unwillingness to seek help. In that case, they may experience more significant negative affect and a decreased willingness to seek help. This would be especially concerning if such perceptions spark or coincide with emotional reasoning. This cognitive distortion entails believing something is the case because one feels it is the case (DeRubeis et al., 2010). If a message recipient perceives a character as hopeless about help seeking, they may feel the same and believe that it is futile.

Future Directions for Narratives

At present, limited research has examined the effect of narrative help-seeking messages among people with depression (Dixon De Silva, 2021). We recommend that researchers study both the utility of narratives in increasing help seeking for depression and how minimized reactance may drive this effect. However, researchers investigating narrative communication should bear in mind that its strengths (i.e., empathy and identification) could pose problems if not handled with care. Specifically, researchers who attempt to use narratives to increase help seeking should consider that including characters who exhibit negative affect or seem unwilling to seek help by the end of the narrative could be detrimental among people with depression.

Inducing Reactance to Motivate Help Seeking

As reactance motivates people to restore or reassert their freedom (Brehm, 1966), we have primarily discussed how to avoid or reduce reactance so that messages attempting to convince people with depression to seek help may be optimized (e.g., Lienemann & Siegel, 2016). Counterintuitively, reactance arousal could be leveraged to promote a desired behavior—so long as reactance is directed toward the correct behavior and source (e.g., Quick et al., 2009).

Florida's Truth campaign portrayed tobacco companies and media depictions of tobacco as manipulative (i.e., freedom threatening) and resulted in lowered smoking among adolescents (Sly et al., 2001). Similarly, Quick et al. (2009) found that trait reactance predicted anger (evidenced as a component of reactance; Dillard & Shen, 2005) toward secondhand smoke exposure, which in turn was associated positively with attitudes toward clean air policies. Together, these findings indicate that messages may be used to induce reactance toward an undesirable behavior to increase engagement in a desired behavior.

Considerations for Depression

Inducing reactance to take advantage of its motivational properties may be especially appropriate in the help-seeking context. Those with depression seem predisposed to reactance (Hong & Faedda, 1996; Lienemann & Siegel, 2016); leveraging its arousal may be easier than attempting to avoid or reduce the state. However, a significant challenge would be selecting the source of the threat to freedom.

One possibility is that by framing depression as a threat to the freedom of those with depression to seek help or not, they could become reactant toward depression itself and, attempting to restore their freedom, seek help as a result. In a way, depression does threaten people's freedom of belief and choice when it comes to help seeking due to its cognitive characteristics (Siegel et al., 2015). If attempted, framing depression as a freedom threat must be done with caution. If people perceive depression as too threatening or believe that depression has already won by being able to influence their thoughts and feelings, help-seeking likelihood may fall (Brehm & Brehm, 1981; Wortman & Brehm, 1975). If researchers take this approach, they should deliberately communicate that while depression threatens people's freedom, it does not entirely determine their behavior.

Future Directions for Inducing Reactance

Considering that those with depression may be prone to reactance (Hong & Faedda, 1996; Lienemann & Siegel, 2016), we believe it would be worthwhile to attempt inducing reactance to increase the motivation to engage in help-seeking behaviors. To do so, researchers should consider using the exact opposite of the tactics we have thus far advocated for (e.g., using HCL instead of LCL; Staunton et al., 2022) to arouse the state.

As noted, a possible source of a freedom threat to help seeking that could be used in messages is depression itself. Theoretically, if those with depression become reactant toward depression due to it infringing upon their freedom to choose whether to seek help, they should become more likely to seek help. We suggest that it would be useful to determine if messages that frame depression as a freedom threat could increase help-seeking inclinations in a manner mediated by reactance. In doing so, testing the boundaries of this potential effect would be necessary; that is, examining at what point emphasizing the threatening nature of depression may decrease people's motivation to seek help (Wortman & Brehm, 1975).

A persuasive message attempting to induce reactance could describe how depression influences people's decision-making about whether to seek help (e.g., making them think more negatively about the outcomes of seeking help than those without depression; Siegel et al., 2015). For example, a message could contain content along the lines of the following: “Depression is not just feeling sad. At times, it can influence how we think and make decisions. If you feel hopeless about seeking support, that might be depression thinking for you and limiting your freedom. However, it does not decide what you do. You have the ability to make your own decisions.”

Interactions

Up to this point, we have primarily discussed reactance mitigation strategies in isolation. However, simultaneously used tactics often interact (e.g., Miller et al., 2007). As reactance is challenging to minimize among those with depression (Lienemann & Siegel, 2016), it may be beneficial to examine how the concurrent use of multiple reactance minimization tactics could result in maximally favorable outcomes. A single help-seeking message could incorporate LCL (Staunton et al., 2022), mistargeting (Siegel et al., 2015), and a restoration postscript (Miller et al., 2007) all at once. Such a message could be apparently directed at the loved ones of those with depression, espouse the benefits of help seeking using soft phrases such as *please consider* and avoiding absolutes, then recommend help seeking followed by a reminder that whether to seek help is the choice of the individual. Determining which tactics combine effectively would require thorough study; some tactics might not interact in the desired manner (e.g., Bessarabova et al., 2013), and at some point, adding more tactics into the mix may yield diminishing returns. Nevertheless, if the aim is to increase help seeking by minimizing reactance to the greatest extent possible, implementing more than one technique may be necessary.

Conclusion

Persuading people with depression to seek help is extremely difficult due to the cognitive patterns characteristic of depression (Siegel et al., 2017) and reactance (Brehm, 1966), the motivation to restore threatened or eliminated freedom. Reactance can be aroused due to simply perceiving a persuasive attempt, potentially leading message recipients to engage in the opposite of the advocated behavior. In the context of persuading people with depression to seek help, simply trying to convince them to seek help may make them less likely to do so. While research has seldom examined how to minimize reactance to increase the effectiveness of help-seeking messages directed toward people with depression, findings thus far indicate that doing so is challenging (Lienemann & Siegel, 2016).

To offer avenues for future research to address this critical issue, we have reviewed reactance minimization strategies that we believe are promising for use in help-seeking messages, as well as the degree to which we caution their use given the cognitive aspects of depression (Beck, 1967): LCL (Staunton et al., 2022), restoration postscripts (Miller et al., 2007), providing compliance options (Shen, 2015), considering source characteristics (Song et al., 2018), mistargeting (Siegel et al., 2015), and narratives (Moyer-Gusé & Nabi, 2010). We additionally discussed the possibility of inducing reactance to motivate help seeking. However, our list is not exhaustive; other techniques, such as inoculating against reactance (e.g., Richards & Banas, 2015), may be effective. Overall, we hope this chapter points to potential lines of research on how to minimize reactance in response to help-seeking messages among those with depression; in minimizing reactance, help seeking may increase.

References

Addis, M. E., & Mahalik, J. R. (2003). Men, masculinity, and the contexts of help seeking. *American Psychologist, 58*(1), 5–14. https://doi-org.ccl.idm.oclc.org/10.1037/0003-066X.58.1.5

Balbuena, L., Bowen, R., Baetz, M., & Marwaha, S. (2016). Mood instability and irritability as core symptoms of major depression: An exploration using Rasch analysis. *Frontiers in Psychiatry, 7*, 214927. https://doi.org/10.3389/fpsyt.2016.00174

Barth, J., Munder, T., Gerger, H., Nüesch, E., Trelle, S., Znoj, H., Jüni, P., & Cuijpers, P. (2013). Comparative efficacy of seven psychotherapeutic interventions for patients with depression: A network meta-analysis. *PLoS Medicine, 10*(5), e1001454. https://doi.org/10.1371/journal.pmed.1001454

Beck, A. T. (1963). Thinking and depression: I. Idiosyncratic content and cognitive distortions. *Archives of General Psychiatry, 9*(4), 324–333. https://doi.org/10.1001/archpsyc.1963.01720160014002

Beck, A. T. (1967). *Depression: Clinical, experimental, and theoretical aspects.* Hoeber.

Beck, A. T., Rush, A. J., Shaw, B. F., & Emery, D. (1979). *Cognitive therapy of depression.* Guilford Press.

Bensley, L. S., & Wu, R. (1991). The role of psychological reactance in drinking following alcohol prevention messages. *Journal of Applied Social Psychology, 21*(13), 1111–1124. https://doi-org.ccl.idm.oclc.org/10.1111/j.1559-1816.1991.tb00461.x

Bessarabova, E., Fink, E. L., & Turner, M. (2013). Reactance, restoration, and cognitive structure: Comparative statics. *Human Communication Research, 39*(3), 339–364. https://doi-org.ccl.idm.oclc.org/10.1111/hcre.12007

Bessarabova, E., Miller, C. H., & Russell, J. (2017). A further exploration of the effects of restoration postscripts on reactance. *Western Journal of Communication, 81*(3), 385–403. https://doi-org.ccl.idm.oclc.org/10.1080/10570314.2016.1254815

Brehm, J. W. (1966). *A theory of psychological reactance.* Academic Press.

Brehm, J. W., Stires, L. K., Sensenig, J., & Shaban, J. (1966). The attractiveness of an eliminated choice alternative. *Journal of Experimental Social Psychology, 2*(3), 301–313. https://doi.org/10.1016/0022-1031(66)90086-2

Brehm, S. S., & Brehm, J. W. (1981). *Psychological reactance: A theory of freedom and control.* Academic Press.

Carpenter, C. J., & Pascual, A. (2016). Testing the reactance vs. the reciprocity of politeness explanations for the effectiveness of the "but you are free" compliance-gaining technique. *Social Influence, 11*(2), 101–110. https://doi-org.ccl.idm.oclc.org/10.1080/15534510.2016.1156569

Cohen, J. (2001). Defining identification: A theoretical look at the identification of audiences with media characters. *Mass Communication & Society, 4*(3), 245–264. https://doi-org.ccl.idm.oclc.org/10.1207/S15327825MCS0403_01

Crano, W. D., Alvaro, E. M., Tan, C. N., & Siegel, J. T. (2017). Social mediation of persuasive media in adolescent substance prevention. *Psychology of Addictive Behaviors, 31*(4), 479–487. https://doi-org.ccl.idm.oclc.org/10.1037/adb0000265

Crano, W. D., Siegel, J. T., Alvaro, E. M., & Patel, N. M. (2007). Overcoming adolescents' resistance to anti-inhalant appeals. *Psychology of Addictive Behaviors, 21*(4), 516–524. https://doi-org.ccl.idm.oclc.org/10.1037/0893-164X.21.4.516

DeRubeis, R. J., Webb, C. A., Tang, T. Z., & Beck, A. T. (2010). Cognitive therapy. In K. S. Dobson (Ed.), *Handbook of cognitive-behavioral therapies* (pp. 277–316). Guilford Press.

Dillard, J. P., & Shen, L. (2005). On the nature of reactance and its role in persuasive health communication. *Communication Monographs, 72*(2), 144–168. https://doi.org/10.1080/03637750500111815

Dixon De Silva, L. E. (2021). Entertainment education for depression in Latin adults: Testing mediators and moderators of a culture-centric narrative intervention to promote help-seeking behavior [Doctoral dissertation, University of California, Los Angeles]. Proquest Dissertations Publishing. https://www-proquest-com.ccl.idm.oclc.org/docview/2567952026

Eisenberg, N. (1989). Empathy and sympathy. In W. Damon (Ed.), *Child development today and tomorrow* (pp. 137–154). Jossey-Bass/Wiley.

Ettman, C. K., Abdalla, S. M., Cohen, G. H., Sampson, L., Vivier, P. M., & Galea, S. (2020). Prevalence of depression symptoms in US adults before and during the COVID-19 pandemic. *JAMA Network Open, 3*(9), e2019686. https://doi.org/10.1001jamanetworkopen.2020.19686

Forgas, J. P. (1995). Mood and judgment: The affect infusion model (AIM). *Psychological Bulletin, 117*(1), 39–66. https://doi.org/10.1037/0033-2909.117.1.39

Guéguen, N., & Pascual, A. (2000). Evocation of freedom and compliance: The "but you are free of. . ." technique. *Current Research in Social Psychology, 5*(18), 264–270.

Heilman, M. E., & Garner, K. A. (1975). Counteracting the boomerang: The effects of choice on compliance to threats and promises. *Journal of Personality and Social Psychology, 31*(5), 911–917. https://doi.org/10.1037/h0076788

Hinyard, L. J., & Kreuter, M. W. (2007). Using narrative communication as a tool for health behavior change: A conceptual, theoretical, and empirical overview. *Health Education & Behavior, 34*(5), 777–792. https://doi.org/10.1177/10901981062919

Hogg, M. A., & Smith, J. R. (2007). Attitudes in social context: A social identity perspective. *European Review of Social Psychology, 18*(1), 89–131. https://doi.org/10.1080/10463280701592070

Hong, S. M., & Faedda, S. (1996). Refinement of the Hong psychological reactance scale. *Educational and Psychological Measurement, 56*(1), 173–182. https://doi.org/10.1177/001316449605600101

Iyengar, S. S., & Lepper, M. R. (2000). When choice is demotivating: Can one desire too much of a good thing? *Journal of Personality and Social Psychology, 79*(6), 995–1006. https://doi.org/10.1037/0022-3514.79.6.995

Lienemann, B. A., & Siegel, J. T. (2016). State psychological reactance to depression public service announcements among people with varying levels of depressive symptomatology. *Health Communication, 31*(1), 102–116. https://doi.org/10.1080/10410236.2014.940668

Lienemann, B. A., Siegel, J. T., & Crano, W. D. (2013). Persuading people with depression to seek help: Respect the boomerang. *Health Communication, 28*(7), 718–728. https://doi.org/10.1080/10410236.2012.712091

Miller, C. H., Lane, L. T., Deatrick, L. M., Young, A. M., & Potts, K. A. (2007). Psychological reactance and promotional health messages: The effects of controlling language, lexical concreteness, and the restoration of freedom. *Human Communication Research, 33*(2), 219–240. https://doi.org/10.1111/j.1468-2958.2007.00297.x

Moyer-Gusé, E., & Nabi, R. L. (2010). Explaining the effects of narrative in an entertainment television program: Overcoming resistance to persuasion. *Human Communication Research, 36*(1), 26–52. https://doi.org/10.1111/j.1468-2958.2009.01367.x

Neimeyer, G. J., Metzler, A. E., & Dongarra, T. (1990). Changing attitudes regarding the effectiveness of cognitive restructuring for treating depression. *Social Behavior and Personality: An International Journal, 18*(2), 181–188. https://doi.org/10.2224/sbp.1990.18.2.181

Nolan, A., & O'Connor, C. (2019). The effect of causal attributions for depression on help- seeking and treatment preferences. *Journal of Affective Disorders, 257*, 477–485. https://doi.org/10.1016/j.jad.2019.07.017

O'Connor, L. E., Berry, J. W., Weiss, J., & Gilbert, P. (2002). Guilt, fear, submission, and empathy in depression. *Journal of Affective Disorders, 71*(1–3), 19–27. https://doi.org/10.1016/S0165-0327(01)00408-6

Peppa, M., John Edmunds, W., & Funk, S. (2017). Disease severity determines health-seeking behaviour amongst individuals with influenza-like illness in an internet-based cohort. *BMC Infectious Diseases, 17*(1), 1–13. https://doi.org/10.1186/s12879-017-2337-5

Quick, B. L., Bates, B. R., & Quinlan, M. R. (2009). The utility of anger in promoting clean indoor air policies. *Health Communication, 24*(6), 548–561. https://doi.org/10.1080/10410230903104939

Quick, B. L., Kam, J. A., Morgan, S. E., Montero Liberona, C. A., & Smith, R. A. (2015). Prospect theory, discrete emotions, and freedom threats: An extension of psychological reactance theory. *Journal of Communication, 65*(1), 40–61. https://doi.org/10.1111/jcom.12134

Quick, B. L., & Stephenson, M. T. (2007). Further evidence that psychological reactance can be modeled as a combination of anger and negative cognitions. *Communication Research, 34*(3), 255–276. https://doi.org/10.1177/0093650207300427

Rains, S. A. (2013). The nature of psychological reactance revisited: A meta-analytic review. *Human Communication Research, 39*(1), 47–73. https://doi.org/10.1111/j.1468-2958.2012.01443.x

Reynolds-Tylus, T., Martinez Gonzalez, A., & Quick, B. L. (2019). The role of choice clustering and descriptive norms in attenuating psychological reactance to water and energy conservation messages. *Environmental Communication, 13*(7), 847–863. https://doi.org/10.1080/17524032.2018.1461672

Reynolds-Tylus, T., Smith, K. E., & Moore, M. E. (2022). Reducing psychological reactance to bystander intervention messages: Comparing preemptive and postscript mitigation strategies. *Communication Research Reports, 39*(5), 259–265. https://doi.org/10.1080/08824096.2022.2130227

Richards, A. S., & Banas, J. A. (2015). Inoculating against reactance to persuasive health messages. *Health Communication, 30*(5), 451–460. https://doi-org.ccl.idm.oclc.org/10.1080/10410236.2013.867005

Richards, A. S., Bessarabova, E., Banas, J. A., & Bernard, D. R. (2022). Reducing psychological reactance to health promotion messages: Comparing preemptive and postscript mitigation strategies. *Health Communication, 37*(3), 366–374. https://doi.org/10.1080/10410236.2020.1839203

Rosenberg, B. D., & Siegel, J. T. (2018). A 50-year review of psychological reactance theory: Do not read this article. *Motivation Science, 4*(4), 281–300. https://doi.org/10.1037/mot0000091

Rosenberg, B. D., & Siegel, J. T. (2023). Threatening uncertainty and psychological reactance: Are freedom threats always noxious? *Current Psychology, 42*(5), 3968–3977. https://doi-org.ccl.idm.oclc.org/10.1007/s12144-021-01640-8

Shen, L. (2011). The effectiveness of empathy- versus fear-arousing antismoking PSAs. *Health Communication, 26*(5), 404–415. https://doi.org/10.1080/10410236.2011.552480

Shen, L. (2015). Antecedents to psychological reactance: The impact of threat, message frame, and choice. *Health Communication, 30*(10), 975–985. https://doi.org/10.1080/10410236.2014.910882

Shen, L., Seung, S., Andersen, K. K., & McNeal, D. (2017). The psychological mechanisms of persuasive impact from narrative communication. *Studies in Communication Sciences, 17*(2), 165–181. https://doi.org/10.24434/j.scoms.2017.02.003

Shoham, V., Trost, S. E., & Rohrbaugh, M. J. (2004). From state to trait and back again: Reactance theory goes clinical. In R. A. Wright, J. Greenberg, & S. S. Brehm (Eds.), *Motivational analyses of social behavior: Building on Jack Brehm's contributions to psychology* (pp. 167–185). Lawrence Erlbaum Associates Publishers.

Siegel, J. T., Flores-Medel, E., Martinez, D. A., & Berger, D. E. (2019). Can mental health anti- stigma messages have untoward effects on some people with depression? An exploratory study. *Journal of Health Communication, 24*(11), 821–828. https://doi-org.ccl.idm.oclc.org/10.1080/10810730.2019.1672838

Siegel, J. T., Lienemann, B. A., & Rosenberg, B. D. (2017). Resistance, reactance, and misinterpretation: Highlighting the challenge of persuading people with depression to seek help. *Social and Personality Psychology Compass, 11*(6), e12322. https://doi.org/10.1111/spc3.12322

Siegel, J. T., Lienemann, B. A., & Tan, C. N. (2015). Influencing help-seeking among people with elevated depressive symptomatology: Mistargeting as a persuasive technique. *Clinical Psychological Science, 3*(2), 242–255. https://doi.org/10.1177/2167702614542846

Siegel, J. T. & Marshburn, A. (2025). Increasing help-seeking for, and reducing the stigmatization of, people experiencing depression: A dual-DV (dependent variable) assessment of the overheard communication approach. *Manuscript under review.*

Siegel, J. T., & Rosenberg, B. D. (2024). When reactance begets more reactance: The reactive spiral. *Motivation Science.* Advance online publication. https://doi.org/10.1037/mot0000363

Silvia, P. J. (2005). Deflecting reactance: The role of similarity in increasing compliance and reducing resistance. *Basic and Applied Social Psychology, 27*(3), 277–284. https://doi.org/10.1207/s15324834basp2703_9

Sly, D. F., Hopkins, R. S., Trapido, E., & Ray, S. (2001). Influence of a counteradvertising media campaign on initiation of smoking: The Florida "truth" campaign. *American Journal of Public Health, 91*(2), 233–238. https://doi.org/10.2105/ajph.91.2.233

So, J. (2022). Counterproductive effects of overfamiliar antitobacco messages on smoking cessation intentions via message fatigue and resistance to persuasion. *Psychology of Addictive Behaviors, 36*(8), 931–941. https://doi.org/10.1037/adb0000776

Song, H., McComas, K. A., & Schuler, K. L. (2018). Source effects on psychological reactance to regulatory policies: The role of trust and similarity. *Science Communication, 40*(5), 591–620. https://doi.org/10.1177/1075547018791293

Staunton, T. V., Alvaro, E. M., & Rosenberg, B. D. (2022). A case for directives: Strategies for enhancing clarity while mitigating reactance. *Current Psychology, 41*(2), 611–621. https://doi-org.ccl.idm.oclc.org/10.1007/s12144-019-00588-0

Taylor, S., & Asmundson, G. J. (2021). Negative attitudes about facemasks during the COVID-19 pandemic: The dual importance of perceived ineffectiveness and psychological reactance. *PLoS One, 16*(2), e0246317.

Tully, E. C., Ames, A. M., Garcia, S. E., & Donohue, M. R. (2016). Quadratic associations between empathy and depression as moderated by emotion dysregulation. *The Journal of Psychology, 150*(1), 15–35. https://doi-org.ccl.idm.oclc.org/10.1080/00223980.2014.992382

Walster, E., & Festinger, L. (1962). The effectiveness of "overheard" persuasive communications. *Journal of Abnormal and Social Psychology, 65*(6), 395–402. https://doi-org.ccl.idm.oclc.org/10.1037/h0041172

Wang, J., Mann, F., Lloyd-Evans, B., Ma, R., & Johnson, S. (2018). Associations between loneliness and perceived social support and outcomes of mental health problems: A systematic review. *BMC Psychiatry, 18*, 1–16. https://doi-org.ccl.idm.oclc.org/10.1186/s12888-018-1736-5

Weary, G., Marsh, K. L., Gleicher, F., & Edwards, J. A. (1993). Depression, control motivation, and the processing of information about others. In G. Weary, F. Gleicher, & K. L. Marsh (Eds.), *Control motivation and social cognition* (pp. 255–287). Springer-Verlag. https://doi-org.ccl.idm.oclc.org/10.1007/978-1-4613-8309-3_10

Wilkinson, T. J., Lightfoot, C. J., Palmer, J., & Smith, A. C. (2022). Navigating the COVID-19 infodemic in those living with kidney disease: Access and trust in health information sources and the association with anxiety and depression. *Current Medical Research and Opinion, 38*(1), 35–42. https://doi-org.ccl.idm.oclc.org/10.1080/03007995.2021.1984221

Wisco, B. E. (2009). Depressive cognition: Self-reference and depth of processing. *Clinical Psychology Review, 29*(4), 382–392. https://doi.org/10.1016/j.cpr.2009.03.003

Worchel, S., & Brehm, J. W. (1971). Direct and implied social restoration of freedom. *Journal of Personality and Social Psychology, 18*(3), 294–304. https://doi-org.ccl.idm.oclc.org/10.1037/h0031000

World Health Organization. (2017). *Depression and other common mental disorders: Global health estimates.* https://apps.who.int/iris/bitstream/handle/10665/254610/WHO-MSD-MER-2017.2-eng.pdf

Wortman, C. B., & Brehm, J. W. (1975). Responses to uncontrollable outcomes: An integration of reactance theory and the learned helplessness model. In L. Berkowitz (Ed.), *Advances in experimental social psychology* (Vol. 8, pp. 277–336). Academic Press.

Yamaguchi, S., Ando, S., Miyashita, M., Usami, S., Yamasaki, S., Endo, K., DeVylder, J., Stanyon, D., Baba, K., Nakajima, N., Niimura, J., Nakanishi, M., Hiraiwa-Hasegawa, M., Kasai, K., & Nishida, A. (2023). Longitudinal relationships between help-seeking intentions and depressive symptoms in adolescents. *Journal of Adolescent Health, 73*(6), 1061–1067. https://doi.org/10.1016/j.jadohealth.2023.06.033

Yzer, M., Kinzer, H., & Malone, M. (2022). A reasoned action approach to depression help- seeking messaging for college students: Implications of cognitive biases in depression. *Health Communication, 37*(14), 1731–1739. https://doi-org.ccl.idm.oclc.org/10.1080/10410236.2021.1917744

Yzer, M., & Siegel, J. T. (2025). Cognitive biases in depression: Implications for help-seeking messaging. In G. J. de Bruijn & H. Vandebosch (Eds.), *Handbook on health, media, and communication* (pp. 391–410). De Gruyter Mouton. https://doi.org/10.1515/9783110775426-021

25

Suicide Prevention Media Campaigns: An Application of the Papageno Effect

Thomas Niederkrotenthaler[1], Stefanie Kirchner[1], Benedikt Till[1], Angela Nicholas[2], Maria Ftanou[2], and Jane Pirkis[2]

[1] Medical University of Vienna
[2] University of Melbourne

Suicide prevention media campaigns are often recommended in the suite of interventions that might be used to bring down suicide rates. They are featured in some form in many national suicide prevention strategies (Schlichthorst et al., 2022) and have the imprimatur of the World Health Organization (World Health Organization, 2018, 2021).

Like other communication campaigns, suicide prevention media campaigns are “purposive attempts to inform or influence behaviors in large audiences within a specified time period using an organized set of communication activities and featuring an array of mediated messages in multiple channels generally to produce noncommercial benefits to individuals and society” (Atkin & Rice, 2013, p. 3). In the case of suicide prevention campaigns, there are two main types of mediated messages: (a) ones that target the general population and are designed to raise awareness of suicide (e.g., by presenting rates of suicide, highlighting risk factors and warning signs, and/or providing advice about reaching out to someone who might be at risk); and (b) ones that target suicidal individuals and are designed to encourage help seeking (Pirkis et al., 2016). Often these messages are encapsulated in brief community services announcements (CSAs) that take the form of short videos delivered via a variety of channels (e.g., on television, in cinemas, via social media). These CSAs are often the core element of any campaign.

This chapter is concerned with suicide prevention campaigns that are designed to encourage help seeking. In particular, it deals with one of the key theoretical underpinnings of these sorts of campaigns, namely, the *Papageno effect* (Niederkrotenthaler et al., 2010a, 2010b). The Papageno effect has been demonstrated in the context of other media presentations of recovery from suicidal crises where the main purpose is to inform or entertain, rather that to directly encourage help-seeking. This chapter considers the Papageno effect in the context of suicide prevention media campaigns, generally mentioning other forms of media presentation for scene-setting purposes only. The scope of the chapter is summarized in Figure 25.1. Readers who are interested in learning more about suicide prevention media campaigns in general or about broader applications of the Papageno effect might wish to read the following references: Torok et al. (2017), Pirkis et al. (2019), Niederkrotenthaler and Till (2019), and Niederkrotenthaler et al. (2022).

The Handbook of Mental Health Communication, First Edition.
Edited by Marco C. Yzer and Jason T. Siegel.

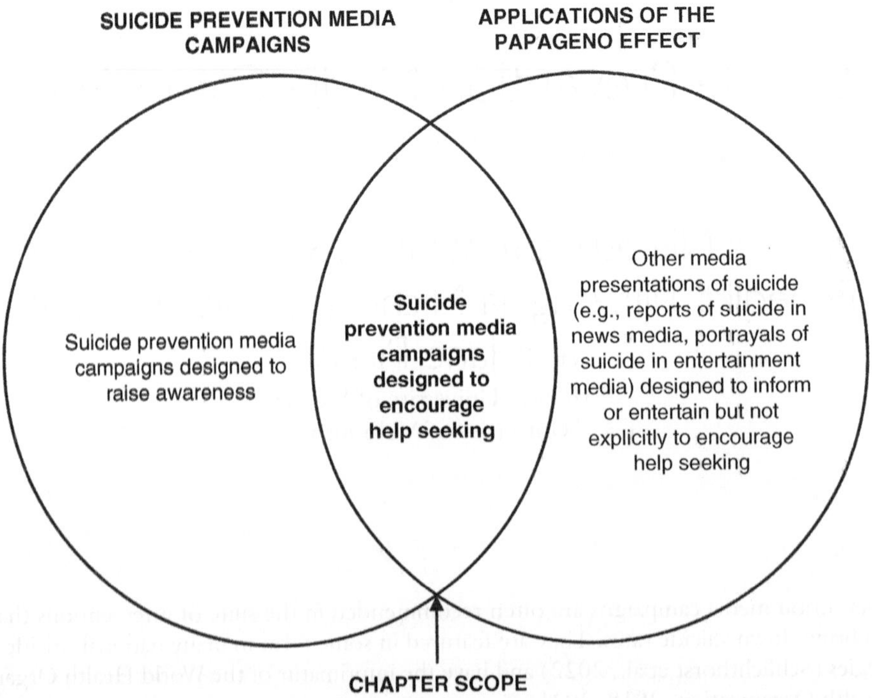

Figure 25.1 Chapter scope.

Before Papageno: The Werther Effect

Before discussing the Papageno effect in detail, it is worth taking a step back to mention the *Werther effect.* In suicide prevention, the Werther effect describes the phenomenon whereby media coverage of suicide deaths has the potential to induce imitative suicides. There is compelling evidence for the Werther effect from more than 150 studies that have explored the impact of suicide media coverage in many different countries (Niederkrotenthaler et al., 2020; Pirkis & Blood, 2001; Pirkis et al., 2018; Sisask & Varnik, 2012). The Werther effect takes its name from Goethe's 1774 novel, *The Sorrows of Young Werther*, which ends with the protagonist taking his own life. Following the release of the novel, there were a number of suicides by young males who appeared to have been influenced by the book. Some were dressed like Werther, some were found with the novel at the scene of their death, and most used the same method as Werther. Decades later, Phillips (1974) coined the term Werther effect when he observed an increase in suicides in the United States in the months in which major newspapers ran a front-page story and no equivalent increase in the months when no such stories were published. Since then, the Werther effect has been observed in studies conducted in diverse cultural contexts (Niederkrotenthaler et al., 2020; Pirkis & Blood, 2001; Pirkis et al., 2018; Sisask & Varnik, 2012). Many of these studies have considered the impact of news reports of suicide, but some have also examined the influence of depictions of suicide in the entertainment media. These studies have consistently demonstrated that certain portrayals of suicide (e.g., sensationalist, prominent or repeated stories, stories involving celebrity suicides) are associated with increases in suicide rates. Concerns about the Werther effect have led to guidelines for media professionals being developed in many countries (Pirkis et al., 2006).

The Papageno Effect

For many years, research relating to suicide and the media tended to focus on the negative Werther-type media impacts. As time went on, however, consideration was given to whether some types of media content might have positive effects. The first major study in this area was conducted in 2010 in

Austria. Niederkrotenthaler et al. (2010b) classified approximately 500 suicide-related newspaper articles into various classes and assessed the association between these different classes and suicide. The aim of this study was to better understand which media items were associated with increases in suicides subsequently. In this study, the authors replicated findings about the Werther effect. But, to their surprise, they also found that a specific class of article, namely, those featuring individuals who had suicidal thoughts but managed to cope with them, were associated with *decreases* in suicides. Niederkrotenthaler et al. (2010b) coined the term the Papageno effect to describe this phenomenon. The name refers to a character in Mozart's opera *The Magic Flute* who prepares to end his own life but ultimately overcomes his suicidal crisis, changing his mind when three boys encourage him to take an alternative course of action. Considering this, Niederkrotenthaler et al. (2010b) thought that the best possible outcome a media report about suicide prevention could have would be to remind audiences of alternatives to suicide when they were in difficult life situations and having suicidal thoughts. Other studies of news media similarly suggested that fewer suicides occurred following stories about suicidal ideation, including stories about recovery from suicidal crises (Pirkis et al., 2006; Sinyor et al., 2021).

Niederkrotenthaler et al. (2014) argued that media narratives that convey messages of hope and recovery from a suicidal crisis can expand the outlook of individuals experiencing suicidal thoughts, highlighting alternative approaches to dealing with difficult circumstances other than resorting to suicide.

Proposed Mechanisms for the Papageno Effect

So far, the psychological mechanisms behind both the Werther and Papageno effects are not fully understood (Niederkrotenthaler & Stack, 2017; Niederkrotenthaler & Till, 2019), though some have been proposed. It is often assumed in suicide research literature that people considering suicide fluctuate between life-sustaining and death-oriented impulses and that media messages on suicide that are observed while in this state may influence the outcome of this inner conflict (Shneidman, 1995).

Another concept that has often been referred to in the literature when explaining these effects is Bandura's (1977) *social learning theory*. The central tenet of this theory is that behavior is learned through the observation and imitation of others (Bandura, 1977). Media portrayals of other peoples' behavior can therefore enhance individual learning processes, which promote and stimulate the respective observed behavior. In the case of media portrayals of suicide, a person experiencing suicidal thoughts might observe suicidal behaviors (in case of the Werther effect) or coping or help-seeking behaviors (in case of the Papageno effect; Niederkrotenthaler & Till, 2019). Therefore, the resulting imitation could have positive or negative outcomes.

Some authors also refer to *social identification processes* when explaining Werther and Papageno effects (Arendt et al., 2016; Braun et al., 2023; Kirchner et al., 2022; Stack, 1992). Research has shown accordingly that audiences who identify with the protagonists featured in a story of hope and recovery benefit most strongly from watching or reading the story, in terms of a reduction in their suicidal thoughts (Braun et al., 2023, Kirchner et al., 2022). In relation to media and social identification, it is important that, when trying to change behavior, individuals exposed to media messages see the person delivering that message as part of their in-group, who then model the positive behavior (Harwood, 2020). In this case, to elicit a Papageno effect, it seems that the message needs to be delivered by an individual with personal experience of suicidal ideation or suicidal behavior (Niederkrotenthaler et al., 2022). In most studies on the Papageno effect, exposure to educative news articles on suicide prevention without a personal narrative on overcoming a suicidal crisis did not reduce suicide risk (Niederkrotenthaler & Till, 2020b; Till et al., 2021).

Papageno-Type Messaging in Suicide Prevention Media Campaigns

Recently, consideration has been given to whether Papageno-type messaging in suicide prevention media campaigns might have a positive impact by demonstrating that it is possible for people to get through suicidal crises. There are numerous examples of campaigns with Papageno-type messaging, many of which either preceded the notion of the Papageno effect or were created without specific reference to it. This suggests that practice in this area may well have advanced without the theory to underpin it but that once the theory was articulated it supported the direction that the field was already taking.

Ftanou et al. (2017) conducted an Internet search for short, English-language CSAs that had been screened as the core element of a suicide prevention media campaign prior to 2014 and identified a number that had Papageno-type messages. Examples of these include:

- *Human Race* (implemented by Lifeline in Australia in 2007): This CSA featured a young male jumping over hurdles in a race, with each hurdle representing a life stressor. It concluded with the message that participating (in life) is what is important and, "Without you there is no race."
- *Choose Life* (implemented by the Scottish Association for Mental Health in Scotland in 2010): This CSA featured a young male with suicidal thoughts and feelings getting to work and struggling to get through his day. His peers actively included him in social activities and asked him about how he was feeling. The CSA urged viewers to talk about suicide.
- *Talk About It* (implemented by Embrace Life Council in Canada in 2012): This CSA features a teenage boy and his girlfriend having a fight. After the disagreement, he wanders off looking upset and calls his friends for help. The CSA stressed the importance of talking about suicide.
- *Ask for Help* (implemented by the Trevor Project in the United States in 2013): This CSA featured a number of young people from different cultural backgrounds talking about their life struggles, asking for help from a variety of sources (e.g., a teacher, an aunt, the Trevor Project), and experiencing the benefits of receiving support.

Evaluations of Papageno-Type Suicide Prevention Media Campaigns

Increasingly, Papageno-type suicide prevention media campaigns—or core elements of them—are being evaluated. In one example, Too et al. (2020) evaluated the *Pause. Call. Be heard* campaign that was run by Lifeline, Australia's largest crisis line. The campaign was delivered via animated billboards at railway stations in response to concern about railway suicides. It imparted a message of hope and recovery, indicating that calling Lifeline was a positive course of action. In addition, it actively encouraged people who might be feeling vulnerable to stop and breathe along with a moving image. The evaluation showed that the campaign had a wide reach, with 25% of rail commuters at the relevant stations noticing the campaign, and the majority of these engaging with it and indicating that it influenced their likelihood of seeking help. There was also a significant increase in calls to Lifeline during the campaign period and a nonsignificant decrease in suicidal behaviors at the stations where *Pause. Call. Be heard* had been promoted.

Niederkrotenthaler et al. (2021b) conducted another study that demonstrated the impact of Papageno-type messages, this time delivered in a campaign not originally designed as a campaign. They investigated the impact of the song "1-800-273-8255" by US hip-hop star Logic, which promoted the number of the National Suicide Prevention Lifeline in the United States and told the story of a person in a suicidal crisis who calls the Lifeline and finds help. The results of the study showed that during days of high public attention on the song, there was an increase in calls to the Lifeline of approximately 7% (corresponding to 10,000 additional calls) and a decrease in suicides of 5.5% (i.e., 250 fewer suicides) in the United States.

The studies by Too et al. (2020) and Niederkrotenthaler et al. (2021b) are examples of evaluations of purpose-designed or serendipitous campaigns with Papageno-type content conducted in the real world. Although their findings were positive, their designs had distinct limitations. The former involved a post-test design only. The latter employed a much stronger design (an ecological time-series analysis), but even this did not allow definitive conclusions to be drawn about any causal relationship between the exposure and the outcome because it was not possible to control for important confounding factors. For this reason, the real-world evaluations of suicide prevention media campaigns are increasingly being complemented with randomized controlled trials of core elements of them, conducted in laboratory settings.

These randomized controlled trials of suicide prevention media campaign content have been conducted alongside other trials of stories of hope and recovery delivered via news media (Arendt et al., 2016; Niederkrotenthaler et al., 2021a; Niederkrotenthaler & Till, 2020b) or entertainment media (Till et al., 2015; Ungar et al., 2017). The campaign-related trials have evaluated Papageno-type content delivered in a variety of ways. For example, Till et al. (2017) explored the impact on users of educative suicide prevention websites that included stories of hope and recovery immediately after surfing these websites and one week later. They found a sustained decrease in suicidal ideation among users with comparatively higher suicidal ideation at baseline (i.e., suicidal ideation scores above the median of the sample) and a sustained increase in suicide prevention–related knowledge in the entire sample.

King et al. (2018) evaluated a documentary called *Man Up*, which was the centerpiece of an Australian campaign addressing the relationship between masculinity and suicide that also included a widespread digital strategy. The documentary, which ran over three one-hour episodes, featured many suicide prevention experts and laypeople, including a number of men who had experienced a suicidal crisis and come through it. Several of these individuals were now trying to help others. King et al. (2018) found that participants who watched *Man Up* demonstrated significant increases in their likelihood of seeking help if they were facing emotional difficulties, whereas there was no change for participants in the control group.

Other studies have examined the impact of much shorter videos that are more akin to the CSAs that might typically sit at the heart of a media campaign. Braun et al. (2023) investigated the impact of a five-minute suicide prevention video that was produced by students within a school project in Austria, testing its effects in a sample of adolescents. The video followed an adolescent boy who was struggling but ultimately began to come through an episode of suicidal thinking. The participants in the trial who viewed the intervention video experienced a decrease in suicidal ideation whereas those in the control group did not. The impact was particularly evident for those who reported comparatively higher identification with the protagonist. Furthermore, there was an increase in help-seeking intentions and a reduction of favorable attitudes toward suicide. Both effects were found not just immediately after the intervention but also four weeks later.

Ftanou et al. (2021) conducted a similar study to Braun et al. (2023), except they tested three different intervention videos, each of which was only about 30 seconds in duration. All three videos targeted young people and had Papageno-type messages: "Find what works for you," "Talk to someone," and "Life can get better." Ftanou et al. (2021) did not find any impact of any of the videos on attitudes toward the preventability of suicide.

Other randomized controlled trials have examined the impacts of suicide prevention media campaign materials for specific target audiences. Kirchner et al. (2022) tested the impact on lesbian, gay, bisexual, transgender, and queer/questioning (LGBTQ+) young people of videos made for the *It Gets Better* project. These videos featured the personal narratives of LGBTQ+ young people coming out. One featured a male and was seven minutes long, and the other featured a female and lasted for three minutes. The protagonists in each video described the difficulties they experienced when coming out, including struggles with suicidal ideation. Participants in the intervention group watched one of these two videos. Kirchner et al. (2022) found no overall effect of the videos on suicidal ideation. However, they did find an increase in help-seeking intentions.

Niederkrotenthaler and Till (2020a) explicitly looked at the impacts of campaign materials for a clinical sample. More specifically, they explored the effect of a short video that featured an interview with a young woman about overcoming her depression and suicidal ideation in a sample of young adults with current depressive symptoms and suicidal thoughts. After watching their allocated video, those in the intervention group experienced reductions in their depressed mood, whereas those in the control group did not.

Summarizing the Evidence

Two systematic reviews relating to suicide prevention media campaigns (Pirkis et al., 2019; Torok et al., 2017) and one meta-analysis relating to the Papageno effect (Niederkrotenthaler et al., 2022) have synthesized findings from the kinds of aforementioned studies mentioned. These reviews provide an indicative picture of where the evidence base is, although they have some limitations. The two systematic reviews cover studies of all suicide prevention media campaigns, not just those with Papageno-type messages, and the meta-analysis covers studies of the Papageno effect in general, not just its specific application to suicide prevention media campaigns. In addition, some further studies have been conducted since these reviews were published. Nonetheless, their conclusions are worth considering.

Together, Pirkis et al. (2019), Torok et al. (2017), and Niederkrotenthaler et al. (2022) suggest that media campaigns with Papageno-type messages show promise but that their effectiveness depends on the kinds of outcomes that are observed in evaluations. In general, the narratives relating to hope and recovery appear to have some impact on distal outcomes, with some (though not all) studies showing that these could improve understanding of suicide, increase the likelihood of help seeking, and decrease suicidal ideation. There is less evidence of these sorts of narratives being able to shift more proximal outcomes relating to behaviors (e.g., actual help seeking, reductions in suicidal acts). It is worth noting here that there is no evidence of these narratives having a negative, Werther-type impact.

It is worth considering the likely reasons for this picture. One possibility is that Papageno-type media campaigns genuinely do not have the ability to change behavior. This seems unlikely. We know from elsewhere (e.g., other communication campaigns, the broader advertising industry) that the media can exert a very persuasive influence on behavior. We also know that some of the more distal outcomes are likely to lead to some of the proximal ones in the longer term, although we should be careful here. For example, although suicidal ideation is a relevant outcome, it is obviously not the case that everyone who has suicidal thoughts will die by suicide (McHugh et al., 2019).

Another possibility is that not all Papageno-type messages are the same and that some will be more persuasive than others. Although the Papageno effect is based on messages of hope and recovery, there are different ways of crafting and delivering this message. Karras et al. (2022) interviewed 33 veterans about why campaigns designed to encourage help seeking may sometimes miss the mark. The study's participants indicated that messages that were not sufficiently tailored to the audience and were delivered by people with whom the audience did not resonate were likely to fail.

Finally, the way the evaluations of Papageno-type media campaigns have been conducted may have a bearing on the findings. As noted, these evaluations tend to either involve real-world examinations of whole campaigns or randomized controlled trials of core elements of campaigns. Both types of evaluation generally involve fairly short follow-up periods and/or have relatively small sample sizes, which limits the likelihood of behavioral outcomes being observed. The real-world evaluations have relatively weak study designs which mean they cannot fully control for confounders, limiting causal inferences. The randomized controlled trials have stronger study designs but the components of campaigns that they test tend to be very brief, making it difficult for them to demonstrate effectiveness. It is noticeable that some of the randomized controlled trials that have found campaign material to be effective have tended to involve longer exposures (e.g., to a three-hour documentary in the *Man Up* trial). We would argue that a different approach is needed that combines the benefits of the real-world evaluations (i.e., exposure to whole campaigns outside of a laboratory setting) with the benefits of randomized controlled trials (i.e., methodological rigor which allows conclusions about causality to be drawn). There are examples of large-scale randomized controlled trials of complex interventions elsewhere in suicide prevention (e.g., Wasserman et al., 2015), but they are lacking in the area of suicide prevention media research.

Conclusions

The suicide prevention community has made substantial progress in exploring the potential of suicide prevention media campaigns to have a positive impact. There is now a strong theoretical basis for campaigns that are designed to encourage those who are in a suicidal state to take alternative courses of action, in the form of the Papageno effect. There is also mounting evidence that these campaigns can be effective, although we need to drill down into the nuances of Papageno-type messages to determine whether some work better than others, whether their impact depends on the audience and the outcome under consideration, and whether a threshold level of exposure is required. We also need to become more ambitious in our evaluation efforts, testing the impacts of whole campaigns in well-designed trials. Identifying the elements and conditions that make Papageno-type suicide prevention media campaigns most effective will allow them to achieve their full potential. Until this research is expanded upon, existing evidence for the Papageno effect suggests that those attempting to craft suicide prevention media messages would do well to consider the inclusion of narratives of hope and recovery. These messages are likely to be best communicated by a person with lived experience of suicidal crisis and recovery to whom the audience can relate. Therefore, the characteristics and experiences of the target audience for such messages should be given thorough consideration and the language, content, and protagonist of the narrative matched well to that audience.

References

Arendt, F., Till, B., & Niederkrotenthaler, T. (2016). Effects of suicide awareness material on implicit suicide cognition: A laboratory experiment. *Health Communication*, *31*(6), 718–726. https://doi.org/10.1080/10410236.2014.993495

Atkin, C., & Rice, R. (2013). Theory and principles of public communication campaigns. In R. Rice & C. Atkin (Eds.), *Public communication campaigns* (4th ed., pp. 3–19). Sage.

Bandura, A. (1977). *Social learning theory*. Prentice-Hall.

Braun, M., Till, B., Pirkis, J., & Niederkrotenthaler, T. (2023). Effects of suicide prevention videos developed by and targeting adolescents: A randomized controlled trial. *European Child and Adolescent Psychiatry*, *32*(5), 847–857. https://doi.org/10.1007/s00787-021-01911-6

Ftanou, M., Cox, G., Nicholas, A., Spittal, M. J., Machlin, A., Robinson, J., & Pirkis, J. (2017). Suicide prevention public service announcements (PSAs): Examples from around the world. *Health Communication*, *32*(4), 493–501. https://doi.org/10.1080/10410236.2016.1140269

Ftanou, M., Ross, A., Machlin, A., Spittal, M. J., King, K., Nicholas, A., Hocking, J., Robinson, J., Reavley, N., & Pirkis, J. (2021). Public service announcements to change attitudes about youth suicide: A randomized controlled trial. *Archives of Suicide Research*, *25*(4), 829–844. https://doi.org/10.1080/13811118.2020.1765929

Harwood, J. (2020). Social identity theory. In J. Van den Bulck, D. Ewoldsen, M.-L. Mares, & E. Scharer (Eds.), *The international encyclopedia of media psychology*. John Wiley & Sons Inc. https://doi.org/10.1002/9781119011071.iemp0153

Karras, E., Levandowski, B., & McCarten, J. (2022). An exploration of barriers to suicide prevention messaging with US veterans. *Crisis*, *43*(1), 28–34. https://doi.org/10.1027/0227-5910/a000756

King, K., Schlichthorst, M., Spittal, M., Phelps, A., & Pirkis, J. (2018). Can a documentary increase help-seeking intentions in men? A randomised controlled trial. *Journal of Epidemiology and Community Health*, *72*(1), 92–96. https://doi.org/10.1136/jech-2017-209502

Kirchner, S., Till, B., Ploderl, M., & Niederkrotenthaler, T. (2022). Effects of "It Gets Better" suicide prevention videos on youth identifying as lesbian, gay, bisexual, transgender, queer, or other sexual or gender minorities: A randomized controlled trial. *LGBT Health*, *9*(6), 436–446. https://doi.org/10.1089/lgbt.2021.0383

McHugh, C., Corderoy, A., Ryan, C., Hickie, I., & Large, M. (2019). Association between suicidal ideation and suicide: Meta-analyses of odds ratios, sensitivity, specificity and positive predictive value. *BJPsych Open*, *5*(2), e18. https://doi.org/10.1192/bjo.2018.88

Niederkrotenthaler, T., Braun, M., Pirkis, J., Till, B., Stack, S., Sinyor, M., Tran, U. S., Voracek, M., Cheng, Q. J., Arendt, F., Scherr, S., Yip, P. S. F., & Spittal, M. J. (2020). Association between suicide reporting in the media and suicide: Systematic review and meta-analysis. *British Medical Journal*, *368*, m575. https://doi.org/10.1136/bmj.m575

Niederkrotenthaler, T., Kirchner, S., Till, B., Sinyor, M., Tran, U. S., Pirkis, J., & Spittal, M. (2021a). Systematic review and meta-analyses of suicidal outcomes following fictional portrayals of suicide and suicide attempt in entertainment media. *eClinicalMedicine*, *36*, 100922. https://doi.org/10.1016/j.eclinm.2021.100922

Niederkrotenthaler, T., Reidenberg, D. J., Till, B., & Gould, M. S. (2014). Increasing help-seeking and referrals for individuals at risk for suicide by decreasing stigma: The role of mass media. *American Journal of Preventive Medicine*, *47*(3 Suppl 2), S235–S243. https://doi.org/10.1016/j.amepre.2014.06.010

Niederkrotenthaler, T., & Stack, S. (2017). *Media and suicide: International perspectives on research, theory, and policy* (1st ed.). Routledge. https://doi-org.ccl.idm.oclc.org/10.4324/9781351295246

Niederkrotenthaler, T., & Till, B. (2019). Suicide and the media: From Werther to Papageno effects – A selective literature review. *Suicidologi*, *2*, 1–12. https://doi.org/10.5617/suicidologi.7398

Niederkrotenthaler, T., & Till, B. (2020a). Effects of awareness material featuring individuals with experience of depression and suicidal thoughts on an audience with depressive symptoms: Randomized controlled trial. *Journal of Behavior Therapy and Experimental Psychiatry*, *66*, 101515. https://doi.org/10.1016/j.jbtep.2019.101515

Niederkrotenthaler, T., & Till, B. (2020b). Effects of suicide awareness materials on individuals with recent suicidal ideation or attempt: Online randomised controlled trial. *British Journal of Psychiatry*, *217*(6), 693–700. https://doi.org/10.1192/bjp.2019.259

Niederkrotenthaler, T., Till, B., Kirchner, S., Sinyor, M., Braun, M., Pirkis, J., Tran, U. S., Voracek, M., Arendt, F., Ftanou, M., Kovacs, R., King, K., Schlichthorst, M., Stack, S., & Spittal, M. J. (2022). Effects of media stories of hope and recovery on suicidal ideation and help-seeking attitudes and intentions: Systematic review and meta-analysis. *The Lancet Public Health*, *7*(2), e156–e168. https://doi.org/10.1016/s2468-2667(21)00274-7

Niederkrotenthaler, T., Tran, U. S., Gould, M., Sinyor, M., Sumner, S., Strauss, M., Voracek, M., Till, B., Murphy, S., Gonzalez, F., Spittal, M., & Draper, J. (2021b). Association of Logic's hip hop song "1-800-273-8255" with Lifeline calls and suicides in the United States: Interrupted time series analysis. *British Medical Journal*, *375*, e067726. https://doi.org/10.1136/bmj-2021-067726

Niederkrotenthaler, T., Voracek, M., Herberth, A., Till, B., Strauss, M., Etzersdorfer, E., Eisenwort, B., & Sonneck, G. (2010a). Media and suicide: Papageno v Werther effect. *British Medical Journal*, *341*, c5841, Article c5841. https://doi.org/10.1136/bmj.c5841

Niederkrotenthaler, T., Voracek, M., Herberth, A., Till, B., Strauss, M., Etzersdorfer, E., Eisenwort, B., & Sonneck, G. (2010b). Role of media reports in completed and prevented suicide: Werther v. Papageno effects. *British Journal of Psychiatry*, *197*(3), 234–243. https://doi.org/10.1192/bjp.bp.109.074633

Phillips, D. (1974). The influence of suggestion on suicide: Substantive and theoretical implications of the Werther effect. *American Sociological Review*, *39*(3), 340–354. https://doi.org/10.2307/2094294

Pirkis, J., & Blood, R. W. (2001). Suicide and the media. Part I: Reportage in nonfictional media. *Crisis*, *22*(4), 146–154. https://doi.org/10.1027//0227-5910.22.4.146

Pirkis, J., Blood, R. W., Beautrais, A., Burgess, P., & Skehan, J. (2006). Media guidelines on the reporting of suicide. *Crisis*, *27*(2), 82–87. https://doi.org/10.1027/0227-5910.27.2.82

Pirkis, J., Blood, R. W., Sutherland, G., & Currier, D. (2018). *Suicide and the news and information media: A critical review*. Everymind.

Pirkis, J., Rossetto, A., Nicholas, A., & Ftanou, M. (2016). Advancing knowledge about suicide prevention media campaigns. *Crisis*, *37*(5), 319–322. https://doi.org/10.1027/0227-5910/a000441

Pirkis, J., Rossetto, A., Nicholas, A., Ftanou, M., Robinson, J., & Reavley, N. (2019). Suicide prevention media campaigns: A systematic literature review. *Health Communication*, *34*(4), 402–414. https://doi.org/10.1080/10410236.2017.1405484

Schlichthorst, M., Reifels, L., Spittal, M., Clapperton, A., Scurrah, K., Kolves, K., Platt, S., Pirkis, J., & Krysinska, K. (2022). Evaluating the effectiveness of components of national suicide prevention strategies. *Crisis*, *44*(4), 318–328. https://doi.org/10.1027/0227-5910/a000887

Shneidman, E. S. (1995). *Suicide as psychache: A clinical approach to self-destructive behavior*. Aronson.

Sinyor, M., Kiss, A., Williams, M., Zaheer, R., Pirkis, J., Heisel, M., Schaffer, A., Redelmeier, D., Cheung, A. H., & Niederkrotenthaler, T. (2021). Changes in suicide reporting quality and deaths in Ontario following publication of national media guidelines. *Crisis*, *42*(5), 378–385. https://doi.org/10.1027/0227-5910/a000737

Sisask, M., & Varnik, A. (2012). Media roles in suicide prevention: A systematic review. *International Journal of Environmental Research and Public Health*, *9*(1), 123–138. https://doi.org/10.3390/ijerph9010123

Stack, S. (1992). Social correlates of suicide by age. Media impacts. In A. A. Leenaars (Ed.), *Life span perspectives of suicide: Time lines in the suicidal process* (pp. 187–214). Plenum Publishing.

Till, B., Strauss, M., Sonneck, G., & Niederkrotenthaler, T. (2015). Determining the effects of films with suicidal content: A laboratory experiment. *British Journal of Psychiatry*, *207*(1), 72–78. https://doi.org/10.1192/bjp.bp.114.152827

Till, B., Tran, U., Voracek, M., & Niederkrotenthaler, T. (2017). Beneficial and harmful effects of educative suicide prevention websites: Randomised controlled trial exploring Papageno v. Werther effects. *British Journal of Psychiatry*, *211*(2), 109–115. https://doi.org/10.1192/bjp.bp.115.177394

Till, B., Tran, U. S., & Niederkrotenthaler, T. (2021). The Impact of educative news articles about suicide prevention: A randomized controlled trial. *Health Communication*, *36*(14), 2022–2029. https://doi.org/10.1080/10410236.2020.1813953

Too, L. S., Ross, A., Pirkis, J., Reavley, N., & Reifels, L. (2020). The impact of the "Pause. Call. Be Heard" campaign on help-seeking and suicidal behaviors within rail environment in Victoria, Australia. *Suicide & Life-Threatening Behavior*, *50*(2), 490–501. https://doi.org/10.1111/sltb.12604

Torok, M., Calear, A., Shand, F., & Christensen, H. (2017). A Systematic review of mass media campaigns for suicide prevention: Understanding their efficacy and the mechanisms needed for successful behavioral and literacy change. *Suicide & Life-Threatening Behavior*, *47*(6), 672–687. https://doi.org/10.1111/sltb.12324

Ungar, T., Norman, C. D., & Knaak, S. (2017). Think you can shrink? A proof-of-concept study for men's health education through edutainment. *Journal of Technology in Behavioral Science*, *2*(2), 71–76. https://doi.org/10.1007/s41347-016-0009-8

Wasserman, D., Hoven, C., Wasserman, C., Wall, M., Eisenberg, R., Hadlaczky, G., Kelleher, I., Sarchiapone, M., Apter, A., Balazs, J., Bobes, J., Brunner, R., Corcoran, P., Cosman, D., Guillemin, F., Haring, C., Iosue, M., Kaess, M., Kahn, J. P., ... Carli, V. (2015). School-based suicide prevention programmes: The SEYLE cluster-randomised, controlled trial. *Lancet*, *385*(9977), 1536–1544. https://doi.org/10.1016/s0140-6736(14)61213-7

World Health Organization. (2018). *National suicide prevention strategies: Progress, examples and indicators*. https://www.who.int/publications/i/item/national-suicide-prevention-strategies-progress-examples-and-indicators

World Health Organization. (2021). *LIVE LIFE: An implementation guide for suicide prevention in countries*. https://www.who.int/publications/i/item/9789240026629

26

Positive Emotion Infusions as a Means of Increasing Help Seeking Among People Experiencing Depression: Savoring, Elevation, and Gratitude

Tasha Straszewski and Jason T. Siegel
Claremont Graduate University

Depression is a leading cause of disability worldwide (World Health Organization, 2017), and approximately 22.5 million American adults experience a major depressive episode annually (Substance Abuse and Mental Health Services Administration, 2023). This debilitating mental illness impairs myriad aspects of a person's life. Depression negatively impacts work performance, and common correlates of depression, such as sleep disturbance and anxiety, amplify this relationship (Kessler et al., 2008). Depression is also associated with an increased risk for other diseases (e.g., Alzheimer's disease; Diniz et al., 2013) and, most critically, an increased risk of suicide (Centers for Disease Control and Prevention, 2023).

Several models explain the experience of someone experiencing depression (e.g., the metacognitive model; Huntley & Fisher, 2016; Wells et al., 2009). As described elsewhere in this handbook, depression is commonly characterized as an information-processing disorder (Bathina et al., 2021) whereby people experiencing depression process information with a negative bias (Hoerger et al., 2012). People experiencing depression possess negative self-schemas consisting of negative beliefs about themselves, their world, and their future (i.e., the cognitive triad; Beck, 1967). As Gotlib and Joorman (2010) describe, "Depression not only changes the way we feel, it also changes how we perceive ourselves and the world around us" (p. 286).

Fortunately, depression is treatable through various means, such as medication (Fournier et al., 2010) and various forms of psychotherapy (Barth et al., 2013). However, one-third of adults experiencing depression do not seek help (Hasin et al., 2018). The longer someone goes without treatment, the likelihood of recovery decreases while the likelihood of recurring episodes increases (Ghio et al., 2014).

Identifying ways to increase help seeking among people experiencing depression could save lives; however, there are several challenges (Yzer & Siegel, 2025). Unlike many other ailments where help seeking increases as symptoms worsen, there is a negative association between levels of depression and help-seeking attitudes and intentions (Siegel et al., 2015). Higher levels of depression are also associated with less favorable help seeking outcome expectations (Hollar & Siegel, 2020), which further increases the challenge of persuading people experiencing depression to seek help (e.g., Lienemann & Siegel, 2016). As noted by Siegel et al. (2017), the negative schema through which people experiencing depression process information is the same negative schema through which they process messages advocating help seeking.

The Handbook of Mental Health Communication, First Edition.
Edited by Marco C. Yzer and Jason T. Siegel.

Although some attempts to increase help seeking have been effective (Hollar & Siegel, 2024), others have backfired. Lienemann et al. (2013) found that a depression message intended to be helpful resulted in increased self-stigma among people experiencing depression. Lueck (2018) chronicled how a persuasive attempt caused less favorable attitudes for people with moderate depression. Even antistigma messages can harm people experiencing depression (Corrigan, 2018; Siegel et al., 2019).

As highlighted throughout this handbook, there is a critical need for novel means of increasing help seeking for depression. In the next few pages, we present a newly proposed approach for doing so: positive emotion infusions (PEIs). We begin by describing the impetus for the approach and then describe our team's experimental work assessing its utility. We then propose future steps for PEI scholarship, lessons learned from the prior studies, and implications for mental health communication.

Positive Emotion Infusions

In describing the experience of depression, Beck (2002) noted, "Even though situations may be favorable and indeed may temporarily reduce dysphoria and introduce some satisfaction, the overall set of futility persists" (p. 36). Although this overall prognosis is unfavorable, Siegel and Thomson (2017) focused on what they saw as a promising aspect of the description: it is possible to "temporarily reduce dysphoria and introduce some satisfaction" (p. 36). The notion that dysphoria could be temporarily reduced led Siegel and Thomson to consider an approach for increasing help seeking among people with depression. Siegel and Thomson reasoned that if there were means of causing a temporary reduction in dysphoria, it could lead the person experiencing depression to perceive help seeking more favorably, at least for a short period.

Siegel and Thomson (2017) did not see the short-lived aspect of the influence as necessarily problematic. Although long-term change is the goal of many persuasive attempts, guided by the IIFF (information, immediate and complete registration mechanism, focused engagement, and favorable activation) model (Siegel et al., 2010b), Siegel and Thomson (2017) proposed that long-term change was not necessarily needed. If an immediate mechanism for seeking help were provided at the same time the momentary change occured, the short-term nature of the change would not be a barrier. Even though the change in help-seeking perceptions would be short-lived, if the person experiencing depression used the immediate help-seeking mechanism to contact another person, it would "ideally set off a chain reaction that will proactively engage the person with depression after the PEI wears off" (Siegel & Thomson, 2017, p. 511). If an immediate mechanism for help seeking were not provided at the same time the change in help-seeking perceptions occurred, help-seeking perceptions would soon return to prior levels, and help seeking would be much less likely to happen.

Siegel and Thomson's (2017) first step was to figure out how to cause a temporary reduction in dysphoria among people experiencing depression. Guided by their recent work on positive emotions (Siegel et al., 2014; Thomson & Siegel, 2013; Thomson et al., 2014), they considered the possibility of temporarily reducing dysphoria by infusing people experiencing depression with a short burst of positive emotions. Although the focus is rarely specific to people experiencing depression, various streams of research support the idea that infusing people with positive emotions can favorably influence perceptions. For example, according to Fredrickson's (2001) broaden-and-build theory, positive emotions are adaptive. They can increase one's cognitive scope, broaden one's thought–action repertoire, and build one's personal resources (i.e., intellectual, social, psychological, and physical) through an upward spiral effect. People in a positive emotional state may be more open to new experiences (Fredrickson, 2001), experience greater cognitive flexibility (Isen & Daubman, 1984), engage in more creative problem-solving (Isen et al., 1987), and experience increased mood-congruent recall (Isen et al., 1978). Further, positive emotions can have an undoing effect on negative emotions (Fredrickson, 2001). Decades of research also support the general view that people in more favorable moods or emotional states generally make more favorable judgments (e.g., Izard, 1964); the judgment's target does not even need to be related to the cause of the emotion (Forgas, 1995; Lerner et al., 2015; Lerner & Keltner, 2000).

The totality of this literature led Siegel and Thomson (2017) to propose that if it were possible to infuse someone experiencing depression with a burst of positive emotions, it could possibly reduce dysphoria temporarily, causing a host of behaviors—including help seeking—to be perceived more favorably. They proposed the term *positive emotion infusion*, to refer "to the elicitation of a surge of positive emotions intended to catalyze a momentary change in the mindset of the recipient" (p. 510). This approach is in line with what Lerner et al. (2015) put forward as a "dual-emotion solution" (p. 812), whereby a new emotion is induced to counteract a current emotional state.

Based on extensive literature that notes differences among discrete positive emotions on numerous outcomes (e.g., Graham et al., 2019), Siegel and Thomson (2017) chose two discrete positive emotions for their initial test of the PEI approach: 1) *elevation* (i.e., the uplifted feeling associated with being a spectator of moral beauty; Algoe & Haidt, 2009); and 2) *gratitude* (Emmons & McCullough, 2003).

Siegel and Thomson (2017) first examined whether they could infuse people experiencing depression with elevation and gratitude through a story and an autobiographical recall task. In line with all the studies testing the PEI approach that we describe in this chapter, only respondents with at least mild depressive symptomatology were eligible for participation. Results indicated that both elevating tasks (i.e., elevation story and elevation autobiographical recall tasks) led to higher self-reported elevation than the control condition (Study 2a). The same pattern of results was evident with the gratitude tasks, as both the gratitude story and the autobiographical recall task led to higher self-reported gratitude compared with the control condition (Study 2b). In line with Beck's (2002) description of the possibility of dysphoria being temporarily reduced among people with depression, the results indicated it is possible to infuse people experiencing depressive symptomatology with a burst of positive emotion.

Siegel and Thomson (2017) then assessed whether these PEIs would increase help-seeking intentions among people with heightened depressive symptomatology. They used the same two elevation and gratitude manipulations (i.e., story and autobiographical recall tasks) from their first study, with help-seeking intentions as the dependent measure. Siegel and Thomson found that invoking feelings of elevation through a story led to increased help-seeking intentions from numerous sources (i.e., overall help-seeking intentions composite, close-others composite, romantic partner, mental health professional, and a website). In contrast, the elevation autobiographical recall task only increased help-seeking intentions from a romantic partner and a website. For gratitude, the story increased help-seeking intentions from a friend; the autobiographical recall condition increased help-seeking intentions only from a parent but reduced help-seeking intentions from a website.

These initial tests indicated that success through the PEI approach is possible (Siegel & Thomson, 2017). It is possible to infuse people experiencing depression with positive emotions, and it is possible to increase help-seeking intentions as a result. Given that prior attempts to increase help seeking have backfired (Siegel et al., 2017), the ability of the story-based elevation PEI to successfully increase help-seeking intentions—even without any mention of depression or help seeking—highlighted the potential of this approach. As the gratitude induction had less influence on help-seeking intentions, it appeared the specific discrete emotion being infused could dictate the utility of the PEI. Given the promising findings of the initial PEI studies, Straszewski and Siegel (2018) were motivated to explore the PEI approach further and turned to savoring.

Savoring as a PEI Approach for Increasing Help Seeking for Depression

Savoring is a process by which people attend to, appreciate, and prolong the enjoyment of positive experiences (Bryant & Veroff, 2007). Bryant and Veroff described four main savoring processes: basking, luxuriating, thanksgiving, and marveling. These processes differ in attentional focus (i.e., internally or externally focused) and whether they involve cognitive reflection or experiential absorption. Savoring processes are not restricted to the present moment, as one can also savor the past or savor something that has yet to happen (anticipatory savoring). To elicit the savoring processes, one can experience triggers or life events that produce appreciation without taking deliberate actions or engaging in cognitive and behavioral savoring strategies, which are consciously employed to increase one's appreciation of a positive experience (Bryant & Veroff, 2007). Cognitive savoring strategies include absorption, counting blessings, positive mental time travel, temporal awareness, and awareness that each moment is fleeting. People can also engage in behavioral strategies such as behavioral expression (e.g., smiling) and sharing good news with others. Cognitive and behavioral savoring strategies can be used alone or in combination.

In addition to increasing positive emotion (e.g., Borelli et al., 2015), happiness (e.g., Bryant et al., 2005), and relationship satisfaction (e.g., Borelli et al., 2015), among other psychological constructs (e.g., Borelli et al., 2019; see Bryant, 2021, for a review), researchers have used savoring to reduce depressive symptomatology. For example, in a one-week intervention, Smith and Hanni (2017) had older adults focus on a positive experience for five minutes at the start and end of each day. Following the intervention, participants reported using fewer dampening strategies compared with their baseline level of downregulating their positive emotions. Furthermore, those who completed the savoring exercises for at least six days saw improvements in resilience and a decrease in stress and depressive symptomatology. In another past-focused intervention, McMakin et al. (2011) had female university students with mild to moderate depressive symptomatology complete a 20-minute savoring task on three separate occasions for two weeks. Participants described a past positive experience, their role in the event, and the feelings they experienced. Those in the control condition wrote objectively about how they use their time. Savoring had a moderate effect on reducing depressive symptomatology and increasing positive emotions following each writing session compared with those in the control condition.

Inspired by the success of prior applications of savoring, particularly to people experiencing heightened depressive symptomatology (e.g., McMakin et al., 2011), Straszewski and Siegel (2018, 2020, 2021) examined whether leading people experiencing depression to savor a positive experience could favorably influence help-seeking inclinations. Across a series of studies, Straszewski and Siegel (2018, 2020, 2021) experimentally assessed savoring-based PEIs, tested savoring mediators, and developed different forms of implementation.

The Initial Savoring Studies

Following the studies previously discussed on the use of savoring to reduce depressive symptomatology (e.g., McMakin et al., 2011) and the prior PEI studies (Siegel & Thomson, 2017), Straszewski and Siegel (2018) tested savoring's ability to increase help-seeking intentions using writing tasks. Straszewski and Siegel drew inspiration from McMakin et al.'s (2011) adoption of Pennebaker's (1997) writing paradigm to create the task. Participants in the savoring condition were asked to think about a recent positive event. They were then instructed to recall details associated with the memory (e.g., emotions, sights, smells). They were instructed to replay the memory in their mind, and to think about various aspects of the event, including their role in making the event occur (see Straszewski & Siegel, 2018, for a complete description of the writing tasks).

Straszewski and Siegel (2018) conducted two initial studies using participants screened for experiencing at least mild depressive symptomatology. In the first study, participants (i.e., people with at least mild depressive symptomatology) who were randomly assigned to engage in the savoring writing task reported significantly more favorable help-seeking intentions than those randomly assigned to a comparison task. Even though the savoring writing task had nothing to do with depression or help seeking, engaging in the task increased intentions to seek help among people with depression.

The efficacy of the savoring-based PEI led Straszewski and Siegel (2018) to consider what variables, beyond positive emotions, might be responsible for the PEI's success. A perceived sense of control was considered as a second mediator. Savoring is one of the four factors of perceived control (i.e., savoring, obtaining, avoiding, and coping) that represents perceived control over positive emotions (Bryant & Veroff, 2007). Bryant (2003) reported an association between one's belief in their ability to savor the moment and beliefs about self-control, internal locus of control, and obtaining (i.e., perceived control over positive outcomes). Moreover, as described in the theory of planned behavior (Ajzen, 1985), the extent to which people think they can control their behaviors (i.e., perceived behavioral control) impacts both their intentions to engage in a behavior and the behavior directly. Accordingly, Straszewski and Siegel (2018) hypothesized that a sense of personal control would act as a complementary mediator to positive emotion through which intentions to seek help are influenced.

To allow for comparison with similar studies, Straszewski and Siegel (2018) measured positive emotion and control using a three-item measure of positive emotion, arousal, and personal control (Self-Assessment Manikin [SAM]; Bradley & Lang, 1994; as used in McMakin et al., 2011). They were not directly interested in arousal at that time, but it was included as it was part of the scale. A significant indirect effect of savoring on help-seeking intentions through positive emotion was indicated but not through arousal or personal control. Although the indirect effects of savoring on help seeking through arousal and personal control were not statistically significant, those who savored reported a greater sense of arousal than control participants.

Comparing High-Arousal Versus Low-Arousal Savoring

Following their initial applications of savoring to increase help-seeking intentions, Straszewski and Siegel (2020) sought to test if isolating the type of positive experience savored, namely an experience associated with high- versus low-arousal positive emotions, would lead to different effects on help-seeking intentions. As depressive symptomatology is associated with cortical underarousal (Jaworska et al., 2012) and low reactivity (see Bylsma et al., 2008, for a meta-analysis), Straszewski and Siegel speculated that people experiencing depression might benefit more from an induction of high-arousal positive emotion as opposed to low-arousal positive emotion. High-arousal positive emotions are associated with a heightened motivational state (Harmon-Jones et al., 2012), and heightened arousal can increase people's preferences for goal-relevant stimuli (Mather & Sutherland, 2011). Although people with heightened depressive symptomatology may struggle to seek help (e.g., Ghio et al., 2014), people experiencing depressive symptomatology typically want assistance (Farmer et al., 2012). Being in a high-arousal positive emotional state may motivate someone experiencing depression to take a step toward their goal of seeking help. As such, Straszewski and Siegel hypothesized that savoring a past positive experience associated with high-arousal positive emotion (i.e., excitement) would lead to greater help-seeking intentions compared with savoring a low-arousal (i.e., calm) positive experience.

Straszewski and Siegel (2020) conducted three studies to examine the effects of savoring high- versus low-arousal positive experiences on help-seeking intentions and made small modifications to their study procedure, discussed later. They first wanted to assess whether they could increase levels of arousal among people with heightened depressive symptomatology. In Study 1, Straszewski and Siegel randomly assigned participants to write about a time they felt excited, a time they felt calm, or what they did that day and the day before (i.e., the control condition). As hypothesized, those who savored a time when they felt excited reported greater arousal than those in the calm memory condition and the control condition. However, counter to Straszewski and Siegel's hypothesis, the calm memory condition was not associated with lower arousal levels than the control condition.

Before testing the writing tasks' effects on help-seeking intentions, Straszewski and Siegel (2020) wanted to ensure that the calm memory and control conditions, even if similar in arousal, would still differ on positive emotion. Even if the calm memory condition was not arousing, the goal was that it would still elicit positive emotion, whereas the control writing task would not. In Study 2, Straszewski and Siegel (2020) found that both savoring writing tasks were associated with significantly greater positive emotion than the control condition and were not significantly different from each other in positive emotion.

Straszewski and Siegel (2020) then tested the central hypotheses regarding the predicted effects of the high- and low-arousal writing tasks on help-seeking intentions. Study 3 results indicated that savoring an exciting memory, compared with the control writing task, was effective at increasing help-seeking intentions, while savoring a calm memory was not. When Straszewski and Siegel conducted an exploratory analysis focused exclusively on participants experiencing depression who also believed they might have been experiencing the disorder, the effect size of the relationship between savoring an exciting memory and help-seeking intentions more than doubled.

Testing Savoring in the Form of a Video

To utilize savoring in mass media communications to target help seeking on a larger scale, Straszewski and Siegel (2021) conducted an initial test of savoring in the form of a video. They first sought to identify the strongest form of savoring to test. Researchers have found that depressogenic schemas are more dysfunctional when information is greater in self-relevance (Beck et al., 1979). Therefore, Straszewski and Siegel (2021) hypothesized that savoring with less self-focus may lead to greater help-seeking intentions. They tested five savoring writing tasks that varied in self-focus and a neutral control writing task: vicarious savoring, self-distanced savoring, relational savoring, combination savoring, and personal savoring (see Straszewski, 2019, for the writing task instructions).

Straszewski and Siegel (2021) found no significant differences between the conditions on help-seeking intentions. However, among the planned comparisons, relational savoring had a stronger effect on help-seeking intentions than the combination savoring condition. Straszewski and Siegel (2021) conducted a series of unregistered, exploratory analyses to examine the results further. They decided to include only the participants who self-reported paying full attention during the study based on a question at the end of the survey. When only these participants were selected, relational savoring was associated with greater help-seeking intentions than the neutral control, but relational savoring did not differ from the combination condition. Although relational savoring was not significantly better or worse than vicarious, self-distanced, or personal savoring, Straszewski and Siegel selected relational savoring to test in a video, as it was the only condition that differed significantly from another savoring condition when the entire sample of eligible participants was used, and it also differed significantly from the control condition when using only participants who paid full attention (i.e., self-reported paying full attention to the study).

In Study 2, Straszewski and Siegel (2021) created a six-minute relational savoring public service announcement (S-PSA) that introduced savoring and guided participants through an exercise. Unlike the previously used savoring manipulations, which instructed participants to complete a writing task, the S-PSA asked participants to think about a positive experience they shared with someone they cared about and with whom they enjoyed spending time. Participants were then asked to think about their feelings associated with the experience. Providing empirical support for this processing method, thinking about a positive experience has been found to be more effective at increasing life satisfaction than writing or talking about it aloud (Lyubomirsky et al., 2006). As the effects of the savoring exercise were expected to be fleeting, Straszewski and Siegel included a help-seeking message immediately following the savoring exercise. This 30-second message at the end of the S-PSA provided participants with resources to access help. Straszewski and Siegel created a similar six-minute video that discussed the KonMari method of tidying up and reducing clutter to use as a comparison PSA. The control condition included only the 30-second help-seeking message. (See Straszewski, 2019, for the video transcripts). Straszewski and Siegel's results indicated that, contrary to their hypotheses, no significant differences existed among the conditions on help-seeking attitudes, intentions, or behavior.

The studies described in this chapter all focused on using positive emotions to create a fleeting window where dysphoria is reduced and help seeking is viewed in a different light. Although not every PEI experiment indicated success, the totality of the experimental studies indicated that it is possible to infuse people experiencing depression with positive emotions, and doing so can influence help-seeking intentions. The success of the PEI approach in favorably influencing help-seeking intentions among people experiencing depression is particularly important given the number of approaches that have struggled to influence this population (Siegel et al., 2017).

Methodologically Maximizing the Strength of PEIs

For those attempting to maximize the range of emotions that can be used for PEIs and looking to understand further why PEIs work the way they do, some steps can be taken to help maximize effectiveness. Throughout the range of experiments conducted, particularly the savoring studies, we learned a fair amount about minor and major adjustments that can be made to maximize the infusion's strength.

The (Non)specificity of PEI Instructions

Across the savoring studies, the greatest success was found when participants were asked to recall a general positive experience (Straszewski & Siegel, 2016, 2018) instead of a specific positive one (Straszewski & Siegel, 2020, 2021). It is possible that minimizing participants' freedom to select any past positive experience by asking them to select a specific experience to recall (Straszewski & Siegel, 2020, 2021) may have reduced savoring's effect among this population. It also may have reduced participants' autonomy, a fundamental psychological need, due to not having as much of a say in which positive experience they wanted to recall (Ryan & Deci, 2000). A more open-ended savoring manipulation will allow participants to select any positive experience that may have been uplifting. Some may select a shared experience, while others may select an individualized experience.

The Recency of the Positive Event

Straszewski and Siegel (2020, 2021) found a reduction in the effects of the savoring manipulation following modification of the instructions from having participants recall a positive experience that occurred recently as opposed to in the last week (Straszewski & Siegel, 2016, 2018). While they had hoped that opening the recall window would have provided participants with more memories to savor, this may have had the opposite effect. The "recent" part of the instruction may have been interpreted differently by different participants, so some may have recalled events that happened weeks or months ago, which would have allowed for greater rumination and dampening of the positive emotions associated with the experience by the time they were asked to savor it. In conjunction, the results of Straszewski and Siegel's (2016, 2018, 2020, 2021) studies trend toward savoring being most effective when participants have a more concrete task to complete, the task instructions are more general, and the recall time is within the last week.

Sample Screening

Small changes regarding which participants are included in analyses can greatly impact the outcomes. In the initial PEI studies (e.g., Siegel & Thomson, 2017), participants were included regardless of whether they perceived themselves to be depressed. However, in direct response to a reviewer request, Straszewski and Siegel (2021) limited participants to those who perceived themselves as experiencing depression, and the effect size doubled. Accordingly, we recommend limiting samples to individuals who perceive themselves as experiencing depression.

Besides this lesson learned during the PEI savoring studies, there are additional lessons from studies in other domains. We strongly recommend that studies seeking to increase help seeking among people with depression focus analyses explicitly on people experiencing depression and, ideally, those who have yet to seek help (e.g., Straszewski & Siegel, 2018). Regarding the recommendation to focus exclusively on people with depression, there are numerous examples of help-seeking messages working favorably on people without depression but backfiring on those experiencing the disorder (e.g., Lienemann et al., 2013; see Siegel et al., 2017 for a review).

We also recommend excluding people who have already sought help for their current bout of depression. If someone is already seeking help, it could be difficult to interpret their responses to a help-seeking intentions scale. Likewise, if a person is already receiving assistance, it would be challenging to determine how to interpret the person's decision not to seek help when provided with an immediate mechanism.

Future Directions

Beyond maximizing future replications of the studies already conducted, there are myriad next steps for the PEI approach (e.g., Siegel & Straszewski, 2019).

Exploration of Different Positive Emotions

As described earlier, Siegel and Thomson (2017) tested elevation- and gratitude-based inductions. They were able to induce both emotions among those experiencing depression. However, Siegel and Thomson found greater success in increasing help-seeking intentions using an elevation-based induction than a gratitude-based one. This set of studies indicates that the specific emotion can make a difference between the PEI failing or succeeding.

PEI research has only begun to explore the myriad of discrete positive emotions that can be used to maximize the PEI approach. Additional, theory-guided, studies are warranted to determine which specific positive emotions will lead to the greatest levels of success. For example, violation-elicited discrete emotions refer to a family of emotions that occur in response to unexpected and novel stimuli (i.e., amusement, awe, curiosity, and positive surprise; Graham et al., 2019). The unexpected nature of the positive stimuli might draw extra attention and greater levels of processing, thus making the PEI more effective.

It is also important to consider arousal level when considering which positive emotion to induce. Positive emotions scholarship is becoming increasingly aware of the differences between high-and low-arousal positive emotions (e.g., McManus et al., 2019, 2024). As described, Straszewski and Siegel (2020) showed that recalling an experience associated with a high-arousal positive emotion (i.e., excitement) led to increased help-seeking intentions. In contrast, the low-arousal positive emotion condition (i.e., calm) did not. As future studies examine how to maximize the PEI approach, the level of arousal associated with specific emotions likely plays a critical role.

The Explanatory Mechanisms

A greater understanding of the mediators that cause the effect and the moderators that maximize the effect are warranted. Straszewski and Siegel (2018) found that savoring influenced help-seeking intentions directly (Study 1) and indirectly through positive emotion (Study 2); it would be useful to explore what mediators specific to positive emotions are responsible for increased help seeking. Siegel and Thomson (2017) proposed that the PEIs may work because of the positive emotions increasing cognitive flexibility (Isen & Daubman, 1984), openness to new experiences (Fredrickson, 2001), mood-congruent recall (Isen et al., 1978), and—depending on the specific positive emotion—approach-oriented behaviors (Harmon-Jones et al., 2012). A complementary possibility is that specific discrete positive emotions could reduce perceptions of risks (Lerner & Keltner, 2001), thus increasing help seeking among people with depression and offering a useful starting point. Constructs that moderate the influence of the PEI would also ideally be explored. For example, due to experience with help seeking likely being associated with more crystalized beliefs about help seeking, PEIs might be most effective among those who have never sought help (Forgas, 1995).

Maximizing Theoretical Guidance

The exploration of different positive emotions that can be used for PEIs, and the considerations of explanatory mechanisms, will ideally continue to take advantage of the rich literature on emotion and cognition (e.g., Forgas, 1995; Lerner et al., 2015). The idea of momentarily infusing people experiencing depression with positive emotions while providing an immediate help-seeking mechanism has rarely been investigted. However, numerous frameworks have explored and explained qualities of emotions and affect, such as function, arousal, valence, and approach/avoidance (e.g., Harmon-Jones et al., 2012; Lench, 2018; Shiota et al., 2017). Some models have explored emotions' influence over judgment and cognition, the role of motivation, and when the influence of emotion is expected to be most potent (e.g., Bower, 1981; Bradley & Lang, 2007; Forgas, 1995; Lerner & Keltner, 2001; Nabi, 2003; Wyer & Carlston, 1979). As exploration of the PEI approach continues, future studies will ideally take advantage of the rich information about emotion, information processing, and action to maximize the likelihood of PEI success.

Testing the Complete Approach

A crucial next step is to ensure that offering an immediate help-seeking mechanism during the PEI will indeed increase help-seeking behavior. There is evidence of the strong impact that the immediate mechanism for action can have on interventions in other domains (Alvaro et al., 2011; Siegel et al., 2010a). However, we believe this needs to be explicitly tested in the realm of help seeking. Moreover, the approach rests on the assumption that if a person experiencing depression reaches out and makes first contact, further help seeking will continue for many. A study on medical trainees and physicians provides evidence of this possibility (Mortali & Moutier, 2018), but explicit assessment within the PEI approach is warranted.

Implementation

If an assessment of the complete PEI approach is successful, attention will ideally turn toward learning how to maximize intervention success. This will involve consideration of all aspects of the PEI, including delivery mode, environment, message appeal, and the help-seeking mechanism that will be most useful. Messages that appear on apps or social media are highly likely to succeed, as most will view these messages on their smartphones or personal computers, both of which could provide an immediate and complete help-seeking mechanism. For example, a link to a hotline could be provided if the PEI takes the form of a social media (e.g., TikTok) video. A school counselor could also deliver the PEI to one classroom at a time. If the counselor provides a written recall-based PEI to a classroom and then asks students to check a box and provide their email if they want mental health assistance, the counselor could then contact them regarding their mental health and provide help. Since all students would be doing the written recall task, the student would be able to check the box and ask for help without other students knowing, which may make help seeking more likely.

Implications for Mental Health Communication

The PEI approach is built on the idea that changes in help-seeking perceptions do not have to be permanent (Siegel & Thomson, 2017); instead, the goal is to create a temporary change in perceptions. Put differently, core beliefs do not have to be changed; the focus can be state-level changes (i.e., increased positive emotions). This could require a different messaging approach than would be needed otherwise. For example, attitudes do not have to be directly targeted in this context. Messages can be created with the goal of emotional and motivational changes such that attitudes toward help seeking become more favorable.

Highly relevant to mental health mass communication is, as just noted, whether a PEI is best delivered before a persuasive help-seeking PSA, such that the PEI will be used to maximize message acceptance of a help-seeking PSA that follows or if it should be part of the message itself (i.e., having the help-seeking message be the source of the infusion). Both approaches seem plausible, and both would ideally be explored. For example, a short news story that infuses positive emotion could come directly before a help-seeking PSA (e.g., Siegel & Straszewski, 2019). Alternatively, the PSA itself could tell a story about someone with depression helping others with depression, thus causing elevation while encouraging immediate help-seeking action on the viewer's part.

If the PEI comes before the help-seeking communication, one decision to be made is whether the PEI should focus on depression (e.g., help seeking) or be completely unrelated (see Lerner et al., 2015 for a discussion of incidental emotions). Throughout numerous PEI studies (e.g., Siegel & Thomson, 2017; Straszewski & Siegel, 2021), help-seeking intentions were moved even though the writing tasks had nothing to do with help seeking or depression. There might be advantages to not focusing on depression per se (e.g., reduced counterarguing) but instead providing an unrelated narrative to infuse positive emotion. If an unrelated narrative infuses positive emotion, the most helpful combination of PEI and providing a help-seeking mechanism must be considered. Survey participants might not be surprised to receive help-seeking questions after a video; however, in the field, there will have to be a transition from the unrelated PEI to the provision of the help-seeking mechanism. There must be a minimum amount of messaging around the provision of a help-seeking mechanism; there are likely ways this can be done to amplify, rather than harm, the PEI.

Along these lines, an additional implication of the PEI approach (i.e., the focus on short-term change in mindset and the need to deliver an immediate help-seeking mechanism) is that some modes of communication might not be viable. For example, it might be possible to deliver a PEI through a radio message, either such that it enhances acceptance of the help-seeking message that follows or such that it is part of the PSA; however, if the person is driving and cannot immediately seek help, the effect of the PEI will likely wear off before action can be taken. If the PEI were in the form of a mass media PSA, there would need to be a QR code that can be scanned to allow for immediate help seeking. The success of this approach might depend on the viewing context, as a person viewing the PSA on their own might not hesitate to scan the code, but this might not be the case for someone watching with others.

Conclusion

Increasing help seeking among people experiencing depression is challenging but critical. In this chapter, we reviewed research focusing on PEIs, with most of the work conducted in the savoring domain. We have conducted multiple studies to explore the potential utility of using PEIs to increase help seeking among people experiencing depression. Although success was not universal, numerous experiments using different methods, emotions, and outcomes indicate the potential success of PEIs. Numerous future directions are ripe for investigation, including examining the specific positive emotions to infuse, the explanatory mechanisms, and the different help-seeking mechanisms that could be provided. There have been many lessons learned that researchers may wish to consider in future work on PEIs, including the most effective methodological approaches for minimizing measurement errors, the importance of minimizing the cognitive demand associated with the PEI, the instructions associated with the greatest success, and how the recency of events being recalled could influence outcomes. Although there is much work to be done, the prior work underscores the potential for this approach to increase help seeking among people experiencing depression and, therefore, save lives.

References

Ajzen, I. (1985). From intentions to action: A theory of planned behavior. In J. Kuhl & J. Beckmann (Eds.), *Action-control: From cognition to behavior* (pp. 11–39). Springer-Verlag. http://dx.doi.org/10.1007/978-3-642-69746-3_2

Algoe, S. B., & Haidt, J. (2009). Witnessing excellence in action: The 'other-praising' emotions of elevation, gratitude, and admiration. *The Journal of Positive Psychology*, *4*(2), 105–127. https://doi.org/10.1080/17439760802650519

Alvaro, E. A., Siegel, J. T., & Jones, S. P. (2011). Increasing organ donor registration rates by providing an immediate and complete registration opportunity: An experimental assessment of the IIFF model. *Psychology, Health and Medicine*, *16*, 686–694. https://doi.org/10.1080/13548506.2011.564353

Barth, J., Munder, T., Gerger, H., Nüesch, E., Trelle, S., Znoj, H., Jüni, P., & Cuijpers, P. (2013). Comparative efficacy of seven psychotherapeutic interventions for patients with depression: A network meta-analysis. *PLoS Medicine*, *10*(5), 1–17. https://doi.org/10.1371/journal.pmed.1001454

Bathina, K. C., ten Thij, M., Lorenzo-Luaces, L., Rutter, L. A., & Bollen, J. (2021). Individuals with depression express more distorted thinking on social media. *Nature Human Behaviour*, *5*(4), 458–466. https://doi.org/10.1038/s41562-021-01050-7

Beck, A. T. (1967). *Depression: Clinical, experimental, and theoretical aspects*. Hoeber.

Beck, A. T. (2002). Cognitive models of depression. In R. L. Leahy & E. T. Dowd (Eds.), *Clinical advances in cognitive psychotherapy: Theory and application* (pp. 29–61). Springer Publishing Company.

Beck, A. T., Rush, A. J., Shaw, B. F., & Emery, G. (1979). *Cognitive therapy of depression*. Guilford Press.

Borelli, J. L., Bond, D. K., Fox, S., & Horn-Mallers, M. (2019). Relational savoring reduces physiological reactivity and enhances psychological agency in older adults. *Journal of Applied Gerontology*, *39*(3), 332–342. https://doi.org/10.1177/0733464819866972

Borelli, J. L., Rasmussen, H. F., Burkhart, M. L., & Sbarra, D. A. (2015). Relational savoring in long-distance romantic relationships. *Journal of Social and Personal Relationships*, *32*(8), 1083–1108. https://doi.org/10.1177/0265407514558960

Bower, G. H. (1981). Mood and memory. *American Psychologist*, *36*, 129–148. https://doi.org/10.1037//0003-066X.36.2.129

Bradley, M. M., & Lang, P. J. (1994). Measuring emotion: The self-assessment manikin and the semantic differential. *Journal of Behavior Therapy and Experimental Psychiatry*, *25*(1), 49–59. https://doi.org/10.1016/0005-7916(94)90063-9

Bradley, M. M., & Lang, P. J. (2007). Motivation and emotion. In J. T. Cacioppo, L. G. Tassinary, & G. Berntson (Eds.), *Handbook of psychophysiology* (2nd ed., pp. 581–607). Cambridge University Press.

Bryant, F. B. (2003). Savoring beliefs inventory (SBI): A scale for measuring beliefs about savoring. *Journal of Mental Health*, *12*, 175–196. https://doi.org/10.1080/0963823031000103489

Bryant, F. B. (2021). Current progress and future directions for theory and research on savoring. *Frontiers in Psychology*, *12*, 771698. https://doi.org/10.3389/fpsyg.2021.771698

Bryant, F. B., Smart, C. M., & King, S. P. (2005). Using the past to enhance the present: Boosting happiness through positive reminiscence. *Journal of Happiness Studies*, *6*, 227–260. http://dx.doi.org/10.1007/s10902-005-3889-4

Bryant, F. B., & Veroff, J. (2007). *Savoring: A new model of positive experience*. Erlbaum Associates.

Bylsma, L. M., Morris, B. H., & Rottenberg, J. (2008). A meta-analysis of emotional reactivity in major depressive disorder. *Clinical Psychology Review*, *28*(4), 676–691. https://doi.org/10.1016/j.cpr.2007.10.001

Centers for Disease Control and Prevention. (2023). *Suicide prevention: Risk and protective factors*. https://www.cdc.gov/suicide/factors/index.html

Corrigan, P. W. (2018). *The stigma effect: Unintended consequences of mental health campaigns*. Columbia University Press.

Diniz, B. S., Butters, M. A., Albert, S. M., Dew, M. A., & Reynolds, C. F. (2013). Late-life depression and risk of vascular dementia and Alzheimer's disease: Systematic review and meta-analysis of community-based cohort studies. *The British Journal of Psychiatry*, *202*(5), 329–335. https://doi.org/10.1192/bjp.bp.112.118307

Emmons, R. A., & McCullough, M. E. (2003). Counting blessings versus burdens: An experimental investigation of gratitude and subjective well-being in daily life. *Journal of Personality and Social Psychology*, *84*, 377–389. https://doi.org/10.1037/0022-3514.84.2.377

Farmer, C., Farrand, P., & O'Mahen, H. (2012). 'I am not a depressed person': How identity conflict affects help-seeking rates for major depressive disorder. *BMC Psychiatry*, *12*, 1–10. https://doi.org/10.1186/1471-244X-12-164

Forgas, J. P. (1995). Mood and judgment: The affect infusion model (AIM). *Psychological Bulletin*, *117*(1), 39–66. https://doi.org/10.1037/0033-2909.117.1.39

Fournier, J. C., DeRubeis, R. J., Hollon, S. D., Dimidjian, S., Amsterdam, J. D., Shelton, R. C., & Fawcett, J. (2010). Antidepressant drug effects and depression severity: A patient-level meta-analysis. *JAMA*, *303*(1), 47–53. https://doi.org/10.1001/jama.2009.1943

Fredrickson, B. L. (2001). The role of positive emotions in positive psychology: The broaden-and-build theory of positive emotions. *American Psychologist*, *56*(3), 218–226. https://doi.org/10.1037/0003-066X.56.3.218

Ghio, L., Gotelli, S., Marcenaro, M., Amore, M., & Natta, W. (2014). Duration of untreated illness and outcomes in unipolar depression: A systematic review and meta-analysis. *Journal of Affective Disorders*, *152–154*, 45–51. https://doi.org/10.1016/j.jad.2013.10.002

Gotlib, I. H., & Joormann, J. (2010). Cognition and depression: Current status and future directions. *Annual Review of Clinical Psychology*, *6*, 285–312. https://doi.org/10.1146/annurev.clinpsy.121208.131305

Graham, L. E., Thomson, A. L., Nakamura, J., Brandt, I. A., & Siegel, J. T. (2019). Finding a family: A categorization of enjoyable emotions. *The Journal of Positive Psychology*, *14*(2), 206–229. https://doi.org/10.1080/17439760.2017.1402074

Harmon-Jones, E., Price, T. F., & Gable, P. A. (2012). The influence of affective states on cognitive broadening/narrowing: Considering the importance of motivational intensity. *Social and Personality Psychology Compass*, *6*(4), 314–327. https://doi-org.org/10.1111/j.1751-9004.2012.00432.x

Hasin, D. S., Sarvet, A. L., Meyers, J. L., Saha, T. D., Ruan, W. J., Stohl, M., & Grant, B. F. (2018). Epidemiology of adult DSM-5 major depressive disorder and its specifiers in the United States. *JAMA Psychiatry*, *75*(4), 336–346. https://doi.org/10.1001/jamapsychiatry.2017.4602

Hoerger, M., Quirk, S. W., Chapman, B. P., & Duberstein, P. R. (2012). Affective forecasting and self-rated symptoms of depression, anxiety, and hypomania: Evidence for a dysphoric forecasting bias. *Cognition and Emotion*, *26*(6), 1098–1106. https://doi.org/10.1080/02699931.2011.631985

Hollar, S., & Siegel, J. T. (2024) Self-distancing as a persuasive amplifier for increasing help-seeking among people with depression. *Manuscript under review*.

Hollar, S. M., & Siegel, J. T. (2020). Self-distancing as a path to help-seeking for people with depression. *Social Science & Medicine*, *245*, 112700. https://doi.org/10.1016/j.socscimed.2019.112700

Huntley, C. D., & Fisher, P. L. (2016). Examining the role of positive and negative metacognitive beliefs in depression. *Scandinavian Journal of Psychology*, *57*(5), 446–452. https://doi.org/10.1111/sjop.12306

Isen, A. M., & Daubman, K. A. (1984). The influence of affect on categorization. *Journal of Personality and Social Psychology, 47*(6), 1206–1217. http://dx.doi.org/10.1037/0022-3514.47.6.1206

Isen, A. M., Daubman, K. A., & Nowicki, G. P. (1987). Positive affect facilitates creative problem solving. *Journal of Personality and Social Psychology, 52*(6), 1122–1131. http://dx.doi.org/10.1037/0022-3514.52.6.1122

Isen, A. M., Shalker, T. E., Clark, M., & Karp, L. (1978). Affect, accessibility of material in memory, and behavior: A cognitive loop? *Journal of Personality and Social Psychology, 36*(1), 1–12. https://doi.org/10.1037/0022-3514.36.1.1

Izard, C. E. (1964). The effects of role-played emotion on affective reactions, intellectual functioning and evaluative ratings of the actress. *Journal of Clinical Psychology, 20*, 444–446. https://doi.org/10.1002/1097-4679(196410)20:4<444::AID-JCLP2270200410>3.0.CO;2-5

Jaworska, N., Blier, P., Fusee, W., & Knott, V. (2012). Alpha power, alpha asymmetry and anterior cingulate cortex activity in depressed males and females. *Journal of Psychiatric Research, 46*(11), 1483–1491. https://doi.org/10.1016/j.jpsychires.2012.08.003

Kessler, R., White, L. A., Birnbaum, H., Qiu, Y., Kidolezi, Y., Mallett, D., & Swindle, R. (2008). Comparative and interactive effects of depression relative to other health problems on work performance in the workforce of a large employer. *Journal of Occupational and Environmental Medicine, 50*(7), 809–816. https://doi.org/10.1097/JOM.0b013e318169ccba

Lench, H. (2018). *The function of emotions: When and why emotions help us.* Springer. https://doi.org/10.1007/978-3-319-77619-4

Lerner, J. S., & Keltner, D. (2000). Beyond valence: Toward a model of emotion-specific influences on judgement and choice. *Cognition and Emotion, 14*, 473–493. https://doi.org/10.1080/026999300402763

Lerner, J. S., & Keltner, D. (2001). Fear, anger, and risk. *Journal of Personality and Social Psychology, 81*, 146–159. https://doi.org/10.1037/0022-3514.81.1.146

Lerner, J. S., Li, Y., Valdesolo, P., & Kassam, K. S. (2015). Emotion and decision making. *Annual Review of Psychology, 66*, 799–823. https://doi.org/10.1146/annurev-psych-010213-115043

Lienemann, B. A., & Siegel, J. T. (2016). State psychological reactance to depression public service announcements among people with varying levels of depressive symptomatology. *Health Communication, 31*(1), 102–116. https://doi.org/10.1080/10410236.2014.940668

Lienemann, B. A., Siegel, J. T., & Crano, W. D. (2013). Persuading people with depression to seek help: Respect the boomerang. *Health Communication, 28*(7), 718–728. https://doi.org/10.1080/10410236.2012.712091

Lueck, J. A. (2018). Respecting the 'stages' of depression: Considering depression severity and readiness to seek help. *Patient Education and Counseling, 101*(7), 1276–1282. https://doi.org/10.1016/j.pec.2018.02.007

Lyubomirsky, S., Sousa, L., & Dickerhoof, R. (2006). The costs and benefits of writing, talking, and thinking about triumphs and defeats. *Journal of Personality and Social Psychology, 90*(4), 692–708. https://doi.org/10.1037/0022-3514.90.4.692

Mather, M., & Sutherland, M. R. (2011). Arousal-biased competition in perception and memory. *Perspectives on Psychological Science, 6*(2), 114–133. https://doi.org/10.1177/1745691611400234

McMakin, D. L., Siegle, G. J., & Shirk, S. R. (2011). Positive affect stimulation and sustainment (PASS) module for depressed mood: A preliminary investigation of treatment-related effects. *Cognitive Therapy and Research, 35*, 217–226. https://doi.org/10.1007/s10608-010-9311-5

McManus, M., Siegel, J. T., & Nakamura, J. (2019). The predictive power of low-arousal positive affect. *Motivation and Emotion, 43*, 130–144. https://doi.org/10.1007/s11031-018-9719-x

McManus, M. D., Nakamura, J., & Siegel, J. T. (2024). Hiding in plain sight: The distinct importance of low-arousal positive affect. *Motivation and Emotion.* https://doi.org/10.1007/s11031-024-10062-5

Mortali, M., & Moutier, C. (2018). Facilitating help-seeking behavior among medical trainees and physicians using the interactive screening program. *Journal of Medical Regulation, 104*(2), 27–36. https://doi.org/10.30770/2572-1852-104.2.27

Nabi, R. L. (2003). Exploring the framing effects of emotion do discrete emotions differentially influence information accessibility, information seeking, and policy preference? *Communication Research, 30*(2), 224–247. https://doi.org/10.1177/0093650202250881

Pennebaker, J. W. (1997). Writing about emotional experiences as a therapeutic process. *Psychological Science, 8*(3), 162–166. https://doi.org/10.1111/j.1467-9280.1997.tb00403.x

Ryan, R. M., & Deci, E. L. (2000). Self-determination theory and the facilitation of intrinsic motivation, social development, and well-being. *American Psychologist, 55*(1), 68–78. s//dx.doi.org/10.1037/0003-066X.55.1.68

Shiota, M. N., Campos, B., Oveis, C., Hertenstein, M. J., Simon-Thomas, E., & Keltner, D. (2017). Beyond happiness: Building a science of discrete positive emotions. *American Psychologist, 72*(7), 617–643. https://doi.org/10.1037/a0040456

Siegel, J. T., Alvaro, E. A., Crano, W. D., Gonzalez, A., Tang, J., & Jones, S. P. (2010a). Passive-positive organ donor registration behavior: A mixed method assessment of the IIFF model. *Psychology, Health and Medicine, 15*, 198–209. https://doi.org/10.1080/13548501003623922

Siegel, J. T., Alvaro, E. A., & Hohman, Z. (2010b). A dawning recognition of factors for increasing donor registration: The IIFF model. In J. Siegel & E. Alvaro (Eds.), *Understanding organ donation: Applied behavioral science approaches* (pp. 313–330). Blackwell-Wiley.

Siegel, J. T., Flores-Medel, E., Martinez, D. A., & Berger, D. E. (2019). Can mental health anti-stigma messages have untoward effects on some people with depression? An exploratory study. *Journal of Health Communication, 24*(11), 821–828. https://doi.org/10.1080/10810730.2019.1672838

Siegel, J. T., Lienemann, B. A., & Rosenberg, B. D. (2017). Resistance, reactance, and misinterpretation: Highlighting the challenge of persuading people with depression to seek help. *Social and Personality Psychology Compass, 11*(6), e12322. https://doi.org/10.1111/spc3.12322

Siegel, J. T., Lienemann, B. A., & Tan, C. N. (2015). Influencing help-seeking among people with heightened depressive symptomatology: Mistargeting as a persuasive technique. *Clinical Psychological Science, 3*(2), 242–255. https://doi.org/10.1177/2167702614542846

Siegel, J. T. & Straszewski, T. (2019). *The influence of elevation on help-seeking intentions and PSA effectiveness* [Panel presentation]. Association for Psychological Science Annual Conference, Washington, D. C., United States.

Siegel, J. T., & Thomson, A. (2017). Positive emotion infusions of elevation and gratitude: Increasing help-seeking among people with elevated levels of depressive symptomatology. *The Journal of Positive Psychology, 12*(6), 509–524. https://doi.org/10.1080/17439760.2016.1221125

Siegel, J. T., Thomson, A. L., & Navarro, M. N. (2014). Experimentally distinguishing elevation from gratitude: Oh, the morality. *Journal of Positive Psychology, 9*(5), 414–427. https://doi.org/10.1080/17439760.2014.910825

Smith, J. L., & Hanni, A. A. (2017). Effects of a savoring intervention on resilience and well-being of older adults. *Journal of Applied Gerontology, 38*(1), 137–152. https://doi.org/10.1177/0733464817693375

Straszewski, T. (2019). *An extension of the savoring approach to increasing help-seeking for depression: Reducing self-focus through a writing task and savoring PSA* (Publication No. 27668287) [Doctoral dissertation, Claremont Graduate University]. ProQuest Dissertations Publishing. https://scholarship.claremont.edu/cgu_etd/328

Straszewski, T., & Siegel, J. T. (2016, May 31–June 3). *Not a cure but a catalyst: Using savoring to increase help-seeking intentions for depression* [Panel presentation]. Society for Prevention Research Annual Meeting, San Francisco, CA, United States. https://spr.confex.com/spr/spr2016/webprogram/Paper24882.html

Straszewski, T., & Siegel, J. T. (2018). Positive emotion infusions: Can savoring increase help-seeking intentions among people with depression? *Applied Psychology: Health and Well-Being, 10*(1), 171–190. https://doi.org/10.1111/aphw.12122

Straszewski, T., & Siegel, J. T. (2020). Differential effects of high- and low-arousal positive emotions on help-seeking for depression. *Applied Psychology: Health and Well-Being, 12*(3), 887–906. https://doi.org/10.1111/aphw.12214

Straszewski, T., & Siegel, J. T. (2021). From writing tasks to a public service announcement: Experimentally assessing savoring as a means of increasing help-seeking for depression. *Social Science & Medicine, 287*, 114362. https://doi.org/10.1016/j.socscimed.2021.114362

Substance Abuse and Mental Health Service Administration. (2023). *Key substance use and mental health indicators in the United States: Results from the 2022 national survey on drug use and health.* https://www.samhsa.gov/data/sites/default/files/reports/rpt42731/2022-nsduh-nnr.pdf

Thomson, A. L., Nakamura, J. N., Siegel, J. T., & Csikszentmihalyi, M. (2014). Elevation and mentoring: An experimental assessment of causal relations. *Journal of Positive Psychology, 9*, 402–413. https://doi.org/10.1080/17439760.2014.910824

Thomson, A. L., & Siegel, J. T. (2013). A moral act, elevation, and prosocial behavior: Moderators of morality. *Journal of Positive Psychology, 8*(1), 50–64. https://doi.org/10.1080/17439760.2012.754926

Wells, A., Fisher, P., Myers, S., Wheatley, J., Patel, T., & Brewin, C. R. (2009). Metacognitive therapy in recurrent and persistent depression: A multiple-baseline study of a new treatment. *Cognitive Therapy and Research, 33*(3), 291–300. https://doi.org/10.1007/s10608-007-9178-2

World Health Organization. (2017). *Depression and other common mental disorders: Global health estimates.* https://apps.who.int/iris/bitstream/handle/10665/254610/WHO-MSD-MER-2017.2-eng.pdf

Wyer, R. S., & Carlston, D. (1979). *Social cognition, inference, and attribution.* Erlbaum.

Yzer, M., & Siegel, J. T. (2025). Cognitive biases in depression: Implications for help-seeking messaging, Chapter 20. In G. De Bruijn & H. Vandebosch (Eds.), *Health, Media, and Communication* (pp. 391–410). Berlin, Boston: De Gruyter Mouton. https://doi.org/10.1515/9783110775426-021

27

A Research Protocol for Determining Depression Help-Seeking Message Content

Marco C. Yzer[1] and Xuan Zhu[2]
[1] University of Minnesota
[2] Mayo Clinic

Depression is a common mental disorder that affects large proportions of the global population (Lim et al., 2018; Xiong et al., 2021). Individuals with depression experience sustained negative mood, characterized by persistent negative views of oneself that cause biases in attention to, interpretation of, and memory for self-relevant information (e.g. Beck, 1967; Vos et al., 2025; Wisco, 2009). Left untreated, depression can significantly diminish a person's well-being and reduce their functioning. Unfortunately, however, whereas therapeutic and pharmaceutical treatment options exist for many (but certainly not all) who are afflicted with depression, a substantial proportion of the people who have depression do not seek help for their depression (Mekonen et al., 2021). To address this treatment gap, messaging campaigns have been used to encourage people with depression to seek professional help.

To inform the design of depression help-seeking messaging, two primary questions need to be addressed; questions about message *content* (what should the message say?) and about message *format* (how should the message say this?). Whereas there is much excellent work on message format questions (for review, see Nan et al., 2022; Yzer & Siegel, in press), there is much less guidance on message content deliberations. In this chapter, we therefore exclusively focus on message content, and more specifically on the question of how one can determine the appropriate content for a message that aims to encourage seeking help for depression. To answer this question, we present a research protocol for determining message content.

A Protocol for Determining Content for Depression Help-Seeking Messages

We define help-seeking message content as information about one or more variables that are expected to predict help-seeking. Thus, message content should be chosen based on knowledge of which variables predict help-seeking in the population that the message planner seeks to serve. The logic behind this idea is that messages that successfully improve factors that are strongly related to seeking help should be more effective in encouraging people to seek help than messages that improve factors that do not matter much for seeking help. For example, even if a message successfully persuades message recipients that they will gain support resources if they seek help for depression, that message would not move those message recipients to take action if for them expansion of support resources is not an important motivator for seeking help. Consistent with this, one objective of the message content

The Handbook of Mental Health Communication, First Edition.
Edited by Marco C. Yzer and Jason T. Siegel.

determination (or MCD) protocol is to conduct research to systematically identify the variables that predict help-seeking in the target population.

The MCD research protocol that we describe here attributes its origins to what has become known as the Hornik and Woolf approach, or in short, H&W. Hornik and Woolf (1999) argued that of the many advantages of research for the development of social marketing campaigns, the most important is the guidance it provides for the determination of what they called "message strategies." Message strategies, later referred to as "campaign themes" (e.g. Brennan et al., 2017; Hornik et al., 2019) or "message themes" (e.g. Rath et al., 2021; Yang et al., 2023), are "the essential belief(s) that a message will be designed to impart" (Hornik & Woolf, 1999, p. 35). These beliefs pertain to perceptions of the behavior that a message encourages.

The Hornik and Woolf approach focuses on how, once a set of beliefs is selected for further scrutiny, quantitative survey data regarding those beliefs as well as intention and behavior should be analyzed in order to identify beliefs that are promising candidates for message content. Hornik et al. (2019) explain that:

> the H&W approach requires that planners consider three key points: the proportion of people who do not endorse the belief at baseline (i.e. the number of people who are available for belief change), the strength of association between the potential targeted belief and the desired outcome (i.e. behavior or behavioral intention), and whether the belief could reasonably be affected by a communication campaign. (p. 60)

Whereas the Hornik and Woolf approach emphasizes analytical aspects of determining message content, the MCD protocol provides additional guidance on how to select beliefs or other variables that potentially explain help-seeking intention or behavior for further examination as candidates for message content. Specifically, the MCD protocol is a four-step research process. In step 1, the help-seeking behavior that a message aims to encourage is defined at a high level of specificity. In step 2, audience characteristics that will be used as stratification or moderator variables are chosen. For depression help-seeking messaging, the most relevant audience characteristic is depression severity. In step 3, a set of variables is selected for inclusion in a logic model that explains which variables the message planner thinks predict help-seeking in their target population. We recommend that variable selection is guided by behavioral theory and the empirical literature on predictors of help-seeking for depression. In step 4, similar to the Hornik and Woolf approach, survey data on the help-seeking predictor variables that were selected in step 3 are collected and analyzed to identify which of these variables should be considered as candidates for message content. In the next sections, we describe the four steps of the MCD protocol in more detail.

Step 1: Defining the Behavior

As the first step in research for health message design, the behavior that one wants to address in the audience needs to be defined (Hawkins & Dobes, 1977; Hornik et al., 2019). Our discussion thus far used the phrase "seeking help for depression" which works well for a general review, but is not sufficiently specific for MCD research and message design purposes. This is because the more specific a behavior is defined in questionnaires and presented in intervention messages, the more likely it is that research participants and message recipients interpret questions about the behavior and behavioral recommendations as intended. Behavioral definitions can be specified in terms of four components; an *action* (e.g. seeking), directed at a *target* (e.g. help from a health professional), performed in a certain *context* (e.g., for depression), and at a certain point in *time* (e.g. in the next 2 weeks; Fishbein & Ajzen, 2010). The more these components are specified, the clearer the behavioral definition. For example, a behavioral recommendation to "seek help for depression" has an action and a target component but leaves message recipients with ample room for interpretation because of the absence of context (e.g. help from whom?) and time (e.g. seek help immediately or at some later point in time?).

Variations in the specification of behavioral definitions have important implications. First, because messages address variables that predict the behavior and the variables that predict one behavior often are different for other behaviors, different messages are needed for each of these behaviors. For example, the variables that explain why people do or do not seek help for depression from friends and the variables that explain why people do or do not seek help for depression from a professional therapist may overlap to some extent but likely will also include uniquely different variables, in part because relationships with friends are different from relationships with health professionals.

Second, variations in how help-seeking was defined in research may result in the selection of different variables as candidates for message content. For example, Bohon et al. (2016), Zorrilla et al. (2019), and Yzer et al. (2022) examined help-seeking intentions in similar samples of US college students using similar attitude–perceived norms–perceived control prediction variables. Their definitions of help-seeking clearly differed, however: Bohon et al. defined the target behavior as "seeking mental health services," Zorrilla et al. as "seeking help from mental health professionals," and Yzer et al. as "making an appointment with a health professional on campus to discuss depressive symptoms if I were to experience depressive symptoms anytime in the next 2 months." These definitional differences may explain that in Bohon et al. (2016) intention was primarily a function of attitude, in Zorrilla et al. (2019) intention was a function of attitude, perceived norms, and perceived control, and in Yzer et al. (2022) intention was a function of attitude and perceived control.

Step 2: Choosing Audience Characteristics as Stratification Variables

Depression affects how people think and feel (Beck, 1967; Wisco, 2009). Increased depression is associated with increasingly persistent negative biases when people think about themselves (Beck & Bredemeier, 2016). For example, people with heightened depression symptoms have more negative views of their competence and of their future outcomes and are more likely to blame themselves for their own symptoms than people with lower depression symptoms (Wisco, 2009). Such negative biases extend to thinking about seeking help for one's own depression symptoms, which means that it should be expected that people with heightened depression will respond differently to messages about seeking help for depression than people with lower depression (Siegel et al., 2017; Yzer & Siegel, in press). Depression severity is therefore a particularly important audience characteristic to consider in depression help-seeking research.

Surprisingly, however, research on predictors of help-seeking for depression has not universally taken participants' depression levels into account. For example, in some studies depression levels were controlled in analyses and in other studies depression levels were overlooked entirely.[1] In contrast, much other research has been designed in recognition of the influence of depression on predictors of seeking help, either by purposively sampling participants with heightened depression or by stratifying analyses by depression levels. Let us describe several such studies with the objective of illustrating common approaches (rather than offer a comprehensive research synthesis).

Boerema et al. (2016) recruited 102 Dutch adults who were diagnosed with major depression. They found that the duration of depression symptoms and personal stigma (measured as participants' own attitude toward depression) explained whether participants had sought help for their depression in the 6 months prior to the study. Damghanian and Alijanzadeh (2018) recruited 1,011 Iranian adults who had heightened anxiety, depression, or both. Using a longitudinal design, they found that perceived control explained intention to seek mental health services from a professional and actual help-seeking assessed, impressively, 2 years later. Trusty and Swift (2023) recruited 253 US adults whose depression levels ranged from moderate to severe depression and who were not in psychotherapy. Using a longitudinal design, they found that increasing depression was associated with higher perceived effort of seeking psychotherapy, and that anticipated effort explained psychotherapy use as assessed 3 months later.

Schomerus et al. (2009) recruited 2,302 German adults, of whom 136 had heightened depression. Their analyses of the extent to which attitude, perceived norms, and perceived control explain intention to see a psychiatrist for their depression were stratified by depression. Schomerus et al. reported that in both the nondepressed group and depressed group attitude toward seeing a psychiatrist was the strongest predictor of intention but they did not report whether depressed participants had more negative attitudes and intention than nondepressed participants. Yzer et al. (2022)

measured depression in a convenience sample of 374 US college students and stratified analyses using depression scores. They found that beliefs about positive and negative outcomes of seeking help from university health services as well as attitude, perceived norms, perceived control, and intention were more negative for students with moderately to severely depressed students than for students with no or mild depression. Further, for moderately to severely depressed students, intention was primarily a function of perceived control, but intention was a function of attitude and perceived control for nondepressed students and primarily a function of attitude for mildly depressed students.

As a final example, Siegel et al. (2024) recruited a total of 2,189 US medical residents from a large hospital system. In three studies, they tested the effects of residents' depression severity on beliefs about positive outcomes of seeking help and on intention to seek help from seven different sources. In each of the three studies, they found that depression negatively affected the extent to which residents believed that seeking help has positive outcomes and that these outcome expectations in turn explained intention to seek help.

This brief review illustrates the point that it is critical to include depression severity as a moderator or stratification variable in research for MCD purposes. The example studies demonstrated that depression affects variables that predict help-seeking, which implies that people with heightened depression may need different messages to encourage them to seek help than people with relatively lower depression severity. The brief review also illustrated that a range of different variables have been found to predict help-seeking intentions and behavior. This leads to the question: What makes a variable useful as a basis for MCD research? We turn to that question next.

Step 3: Selecting Variables for a Logic Model of Seeking Help for Depression

The ultimate objective of the MCD protocol is to identify which variables among a set of variables most strongly relate to help-seeking in the population that the campaign targets, so that if a message positively changes these variables, help-seeking intentions and behaviors also improve. This initial pool of variables can be informed by a literature review of research on predictors of help-seeking, an assessment of variables that emerged from clinical experience, and a review of predictor variables that behavioral theories propose. We recommend that once a pool of variables has been achieved, the message planner creates a logic model that represents the relations between these variables that the message planner thinks predict help-seeking intentions and behavior in the intervention's population and context. This logic model should then be tested, because even if a strong theoretical argument exists for particular variables to predict help-seeking or even if particular variables have been shown to predict help-seeking in previous research or in clinical experience, there is no guarantee that these variables will also explain help-seeking in the population and context of the intervention for which MCD research is conducted.

We discussed sources that can be used to inform an initial pool of variables to include in a logic model of help-seeking for depression. But how can a message planner decide which variables should be included in a logic model of help-seeking? To answer this question, consider that the logic of MCD is based on three principles: (a) messages can contribute to behavior change by *changing* variables that predict that behavior, (b) determining message content requires research to assess which variables best explain the behavior, and (c) a variable is useful as a message content candidate if it offers clear ideas about what that content should be. Consistent with these, we put forward two criteria for assessing a variable's usefulness for inclusion in a help-seeking logic model for MCD purposes: The *malleability* criterion and the *precision* criterion.

The Malleability Criterion

The malleability criterion asks: Can the variable be changed by message recipients? The content of messages that encourage help-seeking should reflect factors that the message recipient in principle can change, even if that is challenging, and not factors that clearly are beyond the control of the message recipient. To use an example from Hornik and Woolf (1999) about messages that encourage youth to quit smoking; even if parental education is found to strongly influence whether youth will smoke, parental educational level is not a very useful factor to address in messages directed at youth as youth cannot change their parents' education.

A wide array of variables across many levels (e.g. individual, interpersonal, community, and environmental) have been found to be associated with help-seeking for depression. Each of these variables can offer important insights into help-seeking processes, yet many are not useful for message content candidates because they are not malleable by message recipients. For example, in a sample of 1,122 Swiss adolescents and adults who reported mental health problems, Michel et al. (2018) found that help-seeking from a health professional was a function of psychosocial functioning, age, having a partner, and having had past treatment. In a sample of 672 Chinese adults with elevated depression, Fang et al. (2019) found that age, education level, and living in urban areas were positively related to seeking help. Whereas these findings are helpful for understanding who seeks help, none of these variables are malleable by individuals and these variables are therefore not useful for targeting as message content.

In Boerema et al. (2016), the duration of depression symptoms and personal stigma explained whether Dutch participants with depression had sought help. Duration of symptoms clearly does not pass the malleability criterion but personal stigma might, as it is conceivable that a message can convey information that may help people change how they think about their own depression, that is, reduce personal stigma.

McLaren et al. (2023) introduced and tested the seeking mental healthcare model in a prospective study using a sample of 1,368 German adults of whom 983 provided behavioral reports of help-seeking at a 3-month follow-up and/or a 6-month follow-up. Intention and behavior were measured as a composite of expected likelihood of seeking help and actual help-seeking from each of several mental health professionals. Intention was primarily influenced by awareness that symptoms indicate a mental health issue and beliefs about one's capability to seek help. Intention predicted actual help-seeking as assessed 3 to 6 months later. Both awareness and perceived capability can improve as a function of learning processes (Bandura, 1997) and are therefore malleable in principle. In samples of US college students and medical residents, Yzer et al. (2022) and Siegel et al. (2024) found that help-seeking intentions were explained by beliefs about how likely it is that help-seeking results in outcomes such as feeling judged and having someone to talk to (Yzer et al., 2022) and feeling better and shortening how long someone is depressed (Siegel et al., 2024). These outcome expectations are beliefs that people hold and thus malleable in principle, even if it may prove challenging for a message planner to develop a sufficiently persuasive argument.

In conclusion, of the many types of variables that may be associated with help-seeking, only a select few meet the malleability criterion and are thus useful to consider for MCD purposes. Individual level variables, or more specifically, beliefs that people have about various aspects of help-seeking, may be most useful to consider for a message planner's logic model of help-seeking for depression (Hornik & Woolf, 1999).

The Precision Criterion

The precision criterion asks: Is the conceptual definition of the variable clear and specific? A variable can be useful for MCD research only if it is defined clearly and consistently so that the variable is interpreted the same by different researchers and when the variable is sufficiently specific so that it can be easily translated to message content. Ideally, a variable that is selected as a candidate for message content is so clearly defined that if multiple message designers are asked to create a message that translates the variable into content, they produce similar content. If message designers are asked to create a message based on a variable that is not very specific, they may create very different messages that may not resonate with the audience. For example, attitude is defined as an evaluation of a behavior in terms of favorability (Fishbein & Ajzen, 2010). Attitude is often found to be strongly related to help-seeking intentions and behaviors (e.g. Bohon et al., 2016; Shi et al., 2023), but may not be specific enough to offer the message designer clear ideas about content that expresses "favorability." Compare this with outcome expectations, which are defined as the perceived likelihood that engaging in a behavior produces highly specific outcomes (Fishbein & Ajzen, 2010). Siegel et al. (2024) tested outcome expectations such as "help-seeking reduces the duration of depression," which is so specific that it can almost be included verbatim in messaging.

Behavioral Theory as a Basis for Depression Help-Seeking Logic Models

To create a help-seeking logic model, the message planner needs to select variables that are likely to explain help-seeking for depression and that are malleable and defined with precision. In this section we discuss behavioral theory as a good source of such variables. Applied to health domains, behavior change theories "describ[e] rational, emotional, social, and personal predictors of healthy and risk behavior" (Cappella, 2006, p. S265). Research that uses behavior change theory enables comparative analyses across different studies to understand which variables explain help-seeking behavior under which circumstances, strengthens the replicability of findings, and offers opportunities for benefiting from previous research to inform research design, sample selection, and measurement choices.

Theories of behavior change present a set of variables that are proposed to predict behavior. Whereas all behavior change theories acknowledge that non-individual-level variables such as health policies and regulations, neighborhood environment, social networks, or one's media environment contribute to behavior, they differ in the extent to which such variables are the focus of primary behavior change propositions. This is important for MCD considerations, because behavior change theories that emphasize non-individual-level variables do not meet the malleability criterion. Consider community-level theories, such as the community coalition action theory (Butterfoss & Kegler, 2009), and multi-level theories, such as the behavioral ecological model (Hovell et al., 2009; for review, see DiClemente et al., 2009; Sallis et al., 2008). These theories are important for informing multilevel interventions as they can identify non-individual-level intervention targets such as policies and resource accessibility. However, they are not useful for determining message content because a message cannot directly help message recipients change non-individual-level factors.

Many behavior change theories are rooted in social psychology. Whereas there exist a great number of psychological behavior change theories, they are quite similar to each other in that they all emphasize beliefs about advantages and disadvantages of performing the behavior as central to behavior change (Noar & Zimmerman, 2005; Rothman, 2000; for detailed descriptions of widely used psychological theories of behavior change, see Glanz et al., 2015; Westmaas et al., 2011; Yzer & Nagler, 2021). They differ from each other in how they conceptualize those beliefs and the precision and specificity of the conceptualization of these beliefs. For example, applied to seeking help for depression, the health belief model (Janz & Becker, 1984; Rosenstock, 1974) proposes that beliefs about one's susceptibility to depression and the severity of depression, as well as beliefs about benefits of and barriers to seeking help predict help-seeking. Protection motivation theory (Rogers, 1983) proposes that beliefs about one's susceptibility to depression and the severity of depression are evaluated against beliefs about the severity of depression and about the efficacy of seeking help to prevent depression, which shapes intention to seek help.

It is for the message planner to decide which behavioral theory they believe best meets the malleability and precision criteria. They should then test the variables proposed by that theory to predict help-seeking, in order to identify candidates for message content. For illustrative purposes we describe here in more detail the reasoned action approach to predicting and changing behavior (RAA[2]; Fishbein & Ajzen, 2010). We do so because in our assessment the variables that RAA proposes meet the malleability and precision criteria.

Applied to seeking help for depression, RAA proposes that help-seeking ultimately is a function of three types of beliefs that people have about seeking help, that is, behavioral beliefs, normative beliefs, and control beliefs. Behavioral beliefs are conceptually similar to outcome expectations. They are beliefs about how likely it is that seeking help leads to highly specific positive and negative outcomes, such as feeling better or feeling judged. Normative beliefs are expectations of approval or disapproval for seeking help for depression from specific referents, such as one's mother, father, friends, or employer. Control beliefs are expectations of one's ability to successfully seek help under various circumstances, such as if appointments can be made online or if there is a long waitlist for appointments.

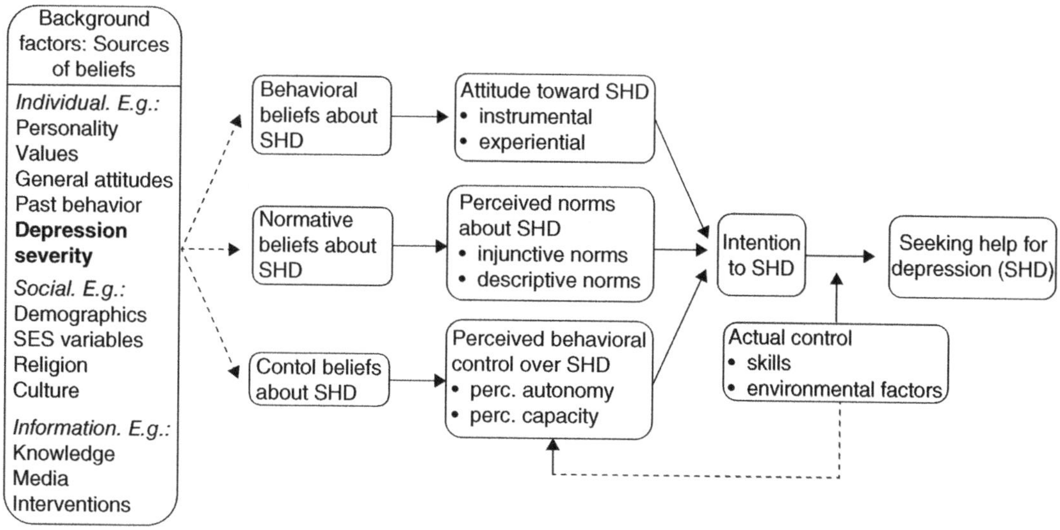

Figure 27.1 *Reasoned action approach applied to seeking help for depression.*
Note. SES, socioeconomic status; SHD, seeking help for depression.

More so than alternative behavior change theories, RAA emphasizes a conceptual separation of highly specific beliefs about seeking help and more general perceptions of performing the behavior (see Figure 27.1). These general perceptions are attitude, perceived norms, and perceived behavioral control, which can be interpreted as cognitive summaries of the full set of highly specific behavioral, normative, and control beliefs. Attitude is one's evaluation of personally seeking help and has an instrumental component—the extent to which someone thinks that their seeking help would have positive or negative attributes (e.g. foolish or wise)—and an experiential component—the extent to which someone thinks that their seeking help would have positive or negative experiences (e.g. pleasant or unpleasant). Perceived norms are the extent to which someone expects normative support for or pressure against seeking help. Perceived norms have an injunctive component—the extent to which someone expects that important referents will approve or disapprove if they would seek help—and a descriptive component—the extent to which someone believes that important referents would seek help themselves if those referents would experience depression. Perceived behavioral control is the extent to which someone expects that they can successfully seek help for depression and has a perceived autonomy component—the extent to which someone believes that the decision to seek help is up to them—and a perceived capacity component—the extent to which someone believes they have the skills to seek help. These six variables are proposed to explain behavioral intention, which is someone's perception of the likelihood that they will seek help if they would experience depression. Intention in turn leads to seeking help as long as the individual possesses the necessary skills and their environment facilitates rather than hinders seeking help for depression.

From an MCD perspective, behavioral beliefs, normative beliefs, and control beliefs are most useful, as beliefs are malleable and in RAA conceptualized with precision. Variables such as attitude, perceived norms, and perceived control are less useful as message content candidates because these are not directly malleable by message recipients and although conceptually well-defined, they do not offer clear ideas for translation to message content. This is consistent with the notion that campaign messages address beliefs (Hornik & Woolf, 1999). If a message planner intends to use RAA to create a help-seeking logic model, they can include all RAA variables and are encouraged to further adapt the model to what they think works best in their population and context. At the very least, however, they should ensure that they include beliefs, as beliefs ultimately are candidates for message content.

Step 4: Identifying Variables as Candidates for Message Content

The final step in the MCD process is to identify which of the variables that were selected for the help-seeking logic model best explain help-seeking outcomes, that is, intentions to seek help or actual help-seeking. To test effects of predictor variables on help-seeking behavior, a longitudinal design is needed. Although this is certainly possible (e.g. see Hornik et al., 2019), longitudinal designs by definition take time, which may be in short supply in campaign contexts. For this reason, help-seeking intentions are a recommended albeit imperfect outcome variable for MCD research, as associations between predictor variables and intention can be assessed in cross-sectional survey data.

A quantitative survey study is designed that includes measures of help-seeking intention as well as measures of all the variables that were specified in the logic model as potential predictors of help-seeking intentions. The survey instrument should also include a depression measure in order to test effects of variations in depression on predictor variables, even in samples that purposively recruited participants with heightened depression (e.g. see Trusty & Swift, 2023).

The analytic strategy involves two major types of analyses. First, examine the mean levels of the predictor variables and intention in order to get a sense of how much room for improvement there is. It is advised to test whether the mean levels of the predictor variables and intention vary as a function of depression. Second, examine the associations of the predictor variables with intention using correlational or regression-based tests. The variables that most strongly correlate with intention and for which there is room to move are then selected as candidates for message content.

An MCD Case Study: The Seeking Help for Depression Beliefs Project

We conclude this chapter with an illustration of how the MCD protocol can deliver a list of variables that can be targeted for message content purposes. For this purpose, we use data from a project that tested beliefs about depression help-seeking, which hereafter we refer to as the seeking help for depression beliefs project (SHD-B; Yzer & Fang, 2023).

Step 1: Definition of Help-Seeking

In the SHD-B project we defined the behavior of interest as "making (*action*) an appointment with a health professional (*context*) to discuss depressive symptoms (*context*) if you were to experience depressive symptoms anytime (*time*) in the next 2 months (*time*)." This definition was included in all questionnaire items.

Step 2: Depression Severity as Audience Stratification Variable

We measured depression severity with the Patient Health Questionnaire-9 (PHQ-9; Kroenke et al., 2001) with the intent to use PHQ-9 scores to test effects of depression severity on beliefs about help-seeking. The PHQ-9 asks how often in the last 7 days people experienced nine depression symptoms (0 = *not at all*, 1 = *several days*, 2 = *more than half the days*, 3 = *nearly every day*). The summed score is interpreted as the level of severity of depressive symptoms; none (a PHQ-9 score of 0–4), mild depression (a score of 5–9), moderate depression (a score of 10–14), moderately severe depression (a score of 15–19), and severe depression (a score of 20–27).

Step 3: Selecting Variables for a Logic Model of Seeking Help for Depression

The SHD-B project used RAA as the basis for a logic model of help-seeking for depression. Figure 27.1 presents all variables in the full RAA model. From these, we selected depression severity as the most important background factor (see step 2), the three belief types (i.e. behavioral, normative, and control beliefs), the six general perception variables (i.e. instrumental and experiential attitude, injunctive and descriptive norms, and perceived autonomy and capacity), and intention to seek help.

Step 4: Identifying Beliefs as Candidates for Message Content

When using RAA as a logic model, two studies are needed to identify the beliefs that should be considered for message content. First, belief elicitation research is recommended to identify the specific beliefs that a population may have about seeking help for depression (Schomerus et al., 2009; Yzer & Gilasevitch, 2019). A belief elicitation study identifies "the set of beliefs that are held with the greatest frequency in the population of interest, that is, the ***modal*** set of salient or readily accessible beliefs" (Fishbein & Ajzen, 2010, p. 102, italics in original). The deliverable of belief elicitation research for MCD is a selection from this modal set of beliefs that will be quantitatively tested in a second study. The second study uses a survey to identify which of the beliefs that were selected from the modal belief set best explain intentions to seek help.

Belief Elicitation Study

We asked 105 US adults open-ended questions about what they thought would be good and bad things that would happen if they would seek help for depression (i.e. behavioral beliefs), people or groups who they thought would approve or not approve seeking help (normative beliefs), and factors that could make it easier or more difficult to seek help (i.e. control beliefs). Of the 105 participants, 19 were not depressed, 27 had mild depression, 23 were moderately depressed, 19 were moderately severely depressed, and 17 were severely depressed.

The 105 participants gave a total of 1,144 responses. Depression severity was associated with mentioning more negative beliefs. The 1,144 responses were categorized into distinct behavioral, normative, and control beliefs based on semantic similarity. This resulted in a modal belief set of 72 behavioral beliefs, 17 normative referents, and 54 control beliefs.

To select beliefs from this modal set for the survey study we rank-ordered all beliefs by how many participants had mentioned them. To select beliefs, one can simply take an arbitrary number of the highest ranking beliefs within each belief type group (e.g. the first 10 beliefs), or select all beliefs within each belief type that are mentioned by a minimum proportion of the sample (e.g. all beliefs that are mentioned by at least 20% of the sample), or, as recommended by Fishbein and Ajzen (2010), within each belief type select the most frequently mentioned beliefs until a desired proportion of the sample's responses have been accounted for. In the SHD-B project, this resulted in 16 behavioral beliefs (e.g. "have someone to talk to," "feel better," "get stronger coping skills," "feel judged by the health professional," "have to pay a great deal of money," and "feel bad about myself"), nine normative referents (e.g. "friends," "mother," "life partner," and "employer"), and 11 control beliefs (e.g. "appointments can be made online," "have telehealth/video appointment options," "feeling too depressed," "financial costs," and "not knowing how to find care").

Survey Study

We asked 564 US adults closed-ended questions about the 16 beliefs that we selected from the belief elicitation study, instrumental and experiential attitude, injunctive and descriptive norms, perceived autonomy and capacity, and intention to seek help. Of the 564 participants, 172 were not depressed, 141 had mild depression, 118 were moderately depressed, 83 were moderately severely depressed, and 50 were severely depressed.

The analytic strategy of the survey data is twofold. First, regression analysis is used to determine the association of the six attitudinal, normative, and control variables with intention. Next, the beliefs that underlie the variables that best explain intention are examined in terms of their correlation with intention. Correlations give a sense of how much gain in help-seeking intentions would be produced if a message effectively improves a belief; for each unit change in a belief, intention would change to the magnitude of the size of the correlation.[3] The beliefs that most strongly correlate with intention and for which there is room to move (that is, mean levels of beliefs are not highly favorable toward seeking help) are then selected as candidates for message content.

In the SHD-B project we stratified the regression results by depression severity categories based on PHQ-9 (i.e. no, mild, moderate, moderately severe, and severe depression). The set of six variables explained substantial proportions of the variance in intention in each of the five depression groups; $0.32 < R^2 < 0.48$. Depression severity affected all predictor variables as well as help-seeking intention in the sense that mean levels of all variables indicated a more negative stance toward help-seeking for participants with heightened depression than for participants with lower depression. Additionally, different variables explained help-seeking intention in groups with different levels of depression severity, which underscores the importance of including depression severity in analyses.

For illustrative purposes, let us assume that we are interested in designing a message for people with moderately severe depression. In this group, intention to seek help was primarily influenced by instrumental attitude ($\beta = 0.40$) and perceived capacity ($\beta = 0.42$). We next examined correlations between the 16 behavioral beliefs (which underlie instrumental attitude) and 11 control beliefs (which underlie perceived capacity) with intention among participants with moderately severe depression. Of these, six behavioral beliefs and one control belief were moderately to strongly correlated with intention. Specifically, the more that participants thought that seeking help would make them feel better ($r = 0.40$), get the help they need ($r = 0.58$), get strong coping skills ($r = 0.35$), help them not feel like a burden to other people ($r = 0.34$), and enjoy life more ($r = 0.40$), the stronger they intended to seek help. The less participants thought they would feel anxious about an appointment, the stronger their intention to seek help ($r = -0.34$). Only one control belief was found to correlate with intention at a meaningful level; the more participants were confident that they could seek help if appointments were easy to get to, the stronger they intended to seek help ($r = 0.28$).

The identification of these seven beliefs as candidates for message content concludes the MCD protocol. From here, message planners would start the creative process of translating these seven beliefs to messages. A first necessary task is to obtain expert advice on the question whether these beliefs can be changed by a message. For example, it may prove very difficult for a message to change beliefs that are based on personal experience, such as having had consistently negative experiences with finding help in the past.

Conclusion

Deciding on the content that a message should convey is a critical step in designing messages that aim to encourage people to seek help for depression. The MCD protocol offers a systematic approach to determining message content. Our case study illustrated the feasibility of analysis methods and effectiveness of data-driven decisions. In the SHD-B project, we found 143 beliefs about seeking help in our belief elicitation study. Whereas this offered great insight in networks of beliefs about help-seeking, for a message planner 143 beliefs is a daunting number to choose from. By following the MCD protocol, we were able to identify seven of these 143 beliefs as promising candidates for message content, which offers message designers an actionable number of themes to work with. This is by far superior to choosing message content by intuition.

The use of the MCD protocol has several advantages. First, when adopted widely, the protocol will aid the standardization of approaches to determining message content, which leads to streamlined future research that can be compared in systematic reviews. Second, a how-to approach and its standardizing features can additionally lead to consistent documentation of methods, which further increases transparency and replicability. Last, the use of MCD increases the effectiveness of messages in encouraging people to adopt the recommended behavior (Albarracin et al., 2006; Hornik et al., 2019; Yang et al., 2023), which offers hope for efforts to relieve the plight of people with depression and other mental illnesses.

Notes

1 We intentionally omitted citations for studies in which people with depression were not analyzed separately. We greatly respect all scholars who seek to advance understanding of how people with depression can be encouraged to seek help. What matters is why analyzing people with depression is critically important and why not doing so can be harmful.

2 RAA is the most recent iteration of theories in the reasoned action tradition. Its predecessors are the theory of reasoned action (Fishbein & Ajzen, 1975), the theory of planned behavior (Ajzen, 1985), and the integrative model of behavioral prediction (Fishbein, 2000).

3 H&W recommend an additional decision metric, that is, the percentage to gain, which considers how many people are available to move (simplified, everyone who does not yet strongly endorse beliefs in favor of the behavior; see Hornik et al., 2019).

References

Ajzen, I. (1985). From intentions to actions: A theory of planned behavior. In J. Kuhl & J. Beckman (Eds.), *Action-control: From cognition to behavior* (pp. 11–39). Springer.

Albarracin, D., Durantini, M. R., & Earl, A. (2006). Empirical and theoretical conclusions of an analysis of outcomes of HIV-prevention interventions. *Current Directions in Psychological Science, 15,* 73–78. https://doi.org/10.1111/j.0963-7214.2006.00410.x

Bandura, A. (1997). *Self-efficacy: The exercise of control.* W. H. Freeman.

Beck, A., & Bredemeier, K. (2016). A unified model of depression: Integrating clinical, cognitive, biological, and evolutionary perspectives. *Clinical Psychological Science, 4*(4), 596–619. https://doi. org/10.1177/2167702616628523

Beck, A. T. (1967). *Depression: Clinical, experimental, and theoretical aspects.* Harper and Row.

Boerema, A. M., Kleiboer, A., Beekman, A. T. F., van Zoonen, K., Dijkshoorn, H., & Cuijpers, P. (2016). Determinants of help-seeking behavior in depression: A cross-sectional study. *BMC Psychiatry, 16,* 1–9. https://doi.org/10.1186/s12888-016-0790-0

Bohon, L. M., Cotter, K. A., Kravitz, R. L., Cello, P. C., Jr., & Fernandez y Garcia, E. (2016). The theory of planned behavior as it predicts intention to seek mental health services for depression among college students. *Journal of American College Health, 64*(8), 593–603. https://doi.org/10.1080/07448481.2016.1207646

Brennan, E., Gibson, L. A., Kybert-Momjian, A., Liu, J., & Hornik, R. C. (2017). Promising themes for antismoking campaigns targeting youth and young adults. *Tobacco Regulatory Science, 3*(1), 29–46. https://doi.org/10.18001/TRS.3.1.4

Butterfoss, F. D., & Kegler, M. C. (2009). The community coalition action theory. In R. J. DiClemente, R. A. Crosby, & M. C. Kegler (Eds.), *Emerging theories in health promotion practice and research* (pp. 237–276). Jossey-Bass.

Cappella, J. N. (2006). Integrating message effects and behavior change theories: Organizing comments and unanswered questions. *Journal of Communication, 56*(S1), S265–S279. https://doi.org/10.1111/j.1460-2466.2006.00293.x

Damghanian, M., & Alijanzadeh, M. (2018). Theory of planned behavior, self-stigma, and perceived barriers explains the behavior of seeking mental health services for people at risk of affective disorders. *Social Health and Behavior, 1*(2), 54–61. https://doi.org/10.4103/SHB.SHB_27_18

DiClemente, R. J., Crosby, R., & Kegler, M. C. (2009). *Emerging theories in health promotion practice and research.* Jossey-Bass.

Fang, S., Wang, X. Q., Yang, B. X., Liu, X. J., Morris, D. L., & Yu, S. H. (2019). Survey of Chinese persons managing depressive symptoms: Help-seeking behaviours and their influencing factors. *Comprehensive Psychiatry, 95,* 152127. https://doi.org/10.1016/j.comppsych.2019.152127

Fishbein, M. (2000). The role of theory in HIV prevention. *AIDS Care, 12,* 273–278. https://doi.org/10.1080/09540120050042918

Fishbein, M., & Ajzen, A. (2010). *Predicting and changing behavior: The reasoned action approach.* Psychology Press.

Fishbein, M., & Ajzen, I. (1975). *Belief, attitude, intention, and behavior: An introduction to theory and research.* Addison-Wesley.

Glanz, K., Rimer, B. K., & Viswanath, K. "V." (2015). *Health behavior: Theory, research, and practice* (5th ed.). Jossey-Bass/Wiley.

Hawkins, R. P., & Dobes, R. W. (1977). Behavioral definitions in applied behavior analysis: Explicit or implicit? In B. C. Etzel, J. M. LeBlanc, & D. M. Baer (Eds.), *New developments in behavioral research: Theory, methods, and application* (pp. 167–188). Erlbaum.

Hornik, R., & Woolf, K. D. (1999). Using cross-sectional surveys to plan message strategies. *Social Marketing Quarterly, 5*(2), 34–41. https://doi.org/10.1080/15245004.1999.9961044

Hornik, R. C., Volinsky, A. C., Mannis, S., Gibson, L. A., Brennan, E., Lee, S. J., & Tan, A. S. L. (2019). Validating the Hornik & Woolf approach to choosing media campaign themes: Do promising beliefs predict behavior change in a longitudinal study? *Communication Methods and Measures, 13*(1), 60–68. https://doi.org/10.1080/19312458.2018.1515902

Hovell, M. F., Wahlgren, D. R., & Adams, M. A. (2009). The logical and empirical basis for the behavioral ecological model. In R. J. DiClemente, R. A. Crosby, & M. C. Kegler (Eds.), *Emerging theories in health promotion practice and research* (pp. 415–450). Jossey-Bass.

Janz, N. K., & Becker, M. H. (1984). The health belief model: A decade later. *Health Education Quarterly, 11*(1), 1–47. https://doi.org/10.1177/109019818401100101

Kroenke, K., Spitzer, R. L., & Williams, J. B. W. (2001). The PHQ-9. Validity of a brief depression severity measure. *Journal of General Internal Medicine, 16*(9), 606–613. https://doi.org/10.1046/j.1525-1497.2001.016009606.x

Lim, G. Y., Tam, W. W., Lu, Y., Ho, C. S., Zhang, M. W., & Ho, R. C. (2018). Prevalence of depression in the community from 30 countries between 1994 and 2014. *Scientific Reports, 8*, 2861. https://doi.org/10.1038/s41598-018-21243-x

McLaren, T., Peter, L., Tomczyk, S., Muehlan, H., Schomerus, G., & Schmidt, S. (2023). The seeking mental health care model: Prediction of help-seeking for depressive symptoms by stigma and mental illness representations. *BMC PublicHealth, 23*, 69. https://doi.org/10.1186/s12889-022-14937-5

Mekonen, T., Chan, G. C. K., Connor, J. P., Hides, L., & Leung, J. (2021). Estimating the global treatment rates for depression: A systematic review and meta-analysis. *Journal of Affective Disorders, 295*, 1234–1242. https://doi.org/10.1016/j.jad.2021.09.038

Michel, C., Schnyder, N., Schmidt, S. J., Groth, N., Schimmelmann, B. G., & Schultze-Lutter, F. (2018). Functioning mediates help-seeking for mental problems in the general population. *European Psychiatry, 54*, 1–9. https://doi.org/10.1016/j.eurpsy.2018.06.009

Nan, X., Iles, I. A., Yang, B., & Ma, Z. (2022). Public health messaging during the COVID-19 pandemic and beyond: Lessons from communication science. *Health Communication, 37*(1), 1–19. https://doi.org/10.1080/10410236.2021.1994910

Noar, S. M., & Zimmerman, R. S. (2005). Health behavior theory and cumulative knowledge regarding health behaviors: Are we moving in the right direction? *Health Education Research, 20*(3), 275–290. https://doi.org/10.1093/her/cyg113

Rath, J. M., Romberg, A. R., Perks, S. N., Edwards, D., Vallone, D. M., & Hair, E. C. (2021). Identifying message themes to prevent e-cigarette use among youth and young adults. *Preventive Medicine, 150*, 106683. https://doi.org/10.1016/j.ypmed.2021.106683

Rogers, R. W. (1983). Cognitive and physiological processes in fear appeals and attitude change: A revised theory of protection motivation. In J. Cacioppo & R. Petty (Eds.), *Social psychophysiology* (pp. 153–176). Guilford.

Rosenstock, I. M. (1974). The health belief model and preventive health behavior. *Health Education Monographs, 2*(4), 354–386. https://doi.org/10.1177/109019817400200405

Rothman, A. J. (2000). Toward a theory-based analysis of behavioral maintenance. *Health Psychology, 19*(S1), 64–69. https://doi.org/10.1037//0278-6133.19

Sallis, J. F., Owen, N., & Fisher, E. B. (2008). Ecological models of health behavior. In K. Glanz, B. K. Rimer, & K. Viswanath (Eds.), *Health behavior and health education: Theory, research, and practice* (4th ed., pp. 465–486). Wiley.

Schomerus, G., Matschinger, H., & Angermeyer, M. C. (2009). Attitudes that determine willingness to seek psychiatric help for depression: A representative population survey applying the theory of planned behavior. *Psychological Medicine, 39*, 1855–1865. https://doi.org/10.1017/S0033291709005832

Shi, W., Donovan, E. E., Quaack, K. R., Mackert, M., Shaffer, A. L., De Luca, D. M., Nolan-Cody, H., & Yang, J. (2023). A reasoned action approach to social connection and mental health: Racial group differences and similarities in attitudes, norms, and intentions. *Health Communication*. Advance online publication. https://doi.org/10.1080/10410236.2023.2259690

Siegel, J. T., Ellis, B., Riazi, G., Brafford, A., Guldner, G., & Wells, J. C. (2024). The paradox of the resident experiencing depression: Higher depression, less favorable help-seeking outcome expectations, and lower help-seeking intentions. *Social Science & Medicine, 344*, 116593. https://doi.org/10.1016/j.socscimed.2024.116593

Siegel, J. T., Lienemann, B. A., & Rosenberg, B. D. (2017). Resistance, reactance, and misinterpretation: Highlighting the challenge of persuading people with depression to seek help. *Social and Personality Psychology Compass, 11*(6), e12322. https://doi.org/10.1111/spc3.12322

Trusty, W. T., & Swift, J. K. (2023). Effort and effort discounting as predictors of seeking psychotherapy among individuals with depression. *Journal of Clinical Psychology, 79*, 2635–2649. https://doi.org/10.1002/jclp.23573

Vos, M. W., Smeets, T., & Everaert, J. (2025). Emotional information-processing bias in psychopathology. In M. C. Yzer & J. T. Siegel (Eds.), *Handbook of mental health mass communication*. Wiley.

Westmaas, J. L., Gil-Rivas, V., & Silver, R. C. (2011). Designing and conducting interventions to enhance physical and mental outcomes. In H. S. Friedman (Ed.), *The Oxford handbook of health psychology* (pp. 73–94). Oxford University Press.

Wisco, B. E. (2009). Depressive cognition: Self-reference and depth of processing. *Clinical Psychology Review, 29*(4), 382–392. https://doi.org/10.1016/j.cpr.2009.03.003

Xiong, J., Lipsitz, O., Nasri, F., Lui, L. M. W., Gill, H., Phan, L., Chen-Li, D., Iacobucci, M., Ho, R., Majeed, A., & McIntyre, R. S. (2021). Impact of COVID-19 pandemic on mental health in the general population: A systematic review. *Journal of Affective Disorders, 277*, 55–64. https://doi.org/10.1016/j.jad.2020.08.001

Yang, S., Shen, L., Gregory, S., Probst, B., Farrar-Edwards, D., & Passmore, S. R. (2023). Applying the Hornik & Woolf approach to identify messaging themes and improve COVID-19 vaccine confidence among federally qualified health centers' workforce in Wisconsin. *Journal of Health Communication, 28*(8), 507–525. https://doi.org/10.1080/10810730.2023.2230929

Yzer, M. & Fang, Y. (2023). *Unpublished data on beliefs about seeking help for depression among two samples of non-depressed and depressed U.S. adults* [Unpublished manuscript]. University of Minnesota.

Yzer, M., & Gilasevitch, J. (2019). Beliefs underlying stress reduction and depression help-seeking among college students: An elicitation study. *Journal of American College Health*, *67*(2), 153–160. https://doi.org/10.1080/07448481.2018.1462828

Yzer, M., Kinzer, H., & Mallone, M. (2022). A reasoned action approach to depression help-seeking messaging for college students: Implications of cognitive biases in depression. *Health Communication*, *37*(14), 1731–1739. https://doi.org/10.1080/10410236.2021.1917744

Yzer, M. C., & Nagler, R. H. (2021). Theories of behavior. In T. Thompson & P. J. Schulz (Eds.), *Health communication theory* (pp. 178–199). Wiley/Blackwell.

Yzer, M., & Siegel, J. T. (in press). Recipient-focused research on depression help-seeking messaging. In G. J. De Bruijn & H. Vandebosch (Eds.), *Handbook of communication science: Vol. 15. Health, media, and communication*. De Gruyter Mouton.

Zorrilla, M. M., Modeste, N., Gleason, P. C., Sealy, D. A., Banta, J. E., & Trieu, S. L. (2019). Depression and help-seeking intention among young adults: The theory of planned behavior. *American Journal of Health Education*, *50*(4), 236–244. https://doi.org/10.1080/19325037.2019.1616014

28

Investigating Help-Seeking Attitudes Among People With Varying Levels of Depressive Symptomatology: An Attitude-Strength Diagnostic Approach

Jason T. Siegel and Cara N. Tan
Claremont Graduate University

Scholars have long acknowledged that an attitude toward an object cannot be fully understood by focusing exclusively on its valence (see Petty & Krosnick's [1995] foundational volume for a discussion). As Krosnick and Smith (1994) described, "Attitudes vary in the degree to which they are crystallized and consequential, and the notion of attitude-strength is meant to capture this variation" (p. 279). Compared to weak attitudes, strong attitudes are more stable, more resistant to change, more influential over information processing and judgments, and more likely to predict behavior (Krosnick & Petty, 1995; Petty et al., 2013). Attitude-strength scholarship has spanned numerous decades and continues to flourish (Feather, 1964; Philipp-Muller et al., 2020).

The current chapter reports on two studies where we conducted ***attitude-strength diagnostics*** of attitudes toward help seeking for depression. We proposed the term attitude-strength diagnostic to refer to an approach where a large variety of attitude-strength antecedents regarding an attitude object are simultaneously assessed. The attitude-strength diagnostic was conducted on attitudes toward help seeking for depression to determine differences in attitude-strength antecedents across levels of depressive symptomatology. The goal was to use the data derived from the diagnostic to explain why attempts to persuade people with depression sometimes struggle and to propose new paths for persuading people with depression to seek help.

Depression

Worldwide, approximately 280 million people experience depression annually (World Health Organization, 2023). The Substance Abuse and Mental Health Services Administration (SAMHSA) estimated that 22,475,000 American adults (8.8%) experienced depression in the past year (SAMHSA, 2023). Depressive symptomatology is associated with higher levels of drug use (e.g., Danek et al., 2023) and increased suicide risk (e.g., Stubbing et al., 2024).

Even though depression is treatable, 38.5% of US adults (8.6 million people) who experienced depression in the past year did not receive professional treatment (SAMHSA, 2023). This is particularly problematic as there is a positive relationship between the length of time depression goes untreated,

The Handbook of Mental Health Communication, First Edition.
Edited by Marco C. Yzer and Jason T. Siegel.

the severity of symptoms, and suicide likelihood (see Ghio et al., 2014 for a review). Moreover, remission from depression without treatment is unlikely (Mekonen et al., 2022).

Increasing help seeking among people with depression can have life-saving implications, and various forms of mental health communication have been tested and implemented to increase the number of people with depression who seek help. Although there have been numerous instances of success (Bossarte et al., 2014; Hammer & Vogel, 2010; Siegel et al., 2015), developing messages that can increase help seeking among people with depression has proved difficult (e.g., Lueck, 2018; see Niederkrotenthaler et al., 2014; Siegel et al., 2017; Yzer & Siegel, 2025, for reviews).

Some attempts to persuade people with depression initially appeared to be successful among the general public but were then revealed to be less effective among people with depression (Goldney & Fisher, 2008). Likewise, Wiglesworth et al. (2021) reported that high-risk participants (i.e., those with heightened depressive symptomatology or a previous suicide attempt) were less likely to recall help-seeking content post-exposure to a suicide message than low-risk participants. Other studies indicate that attempts to increase help seeking can have the opposite effect (Keeler & Siegel, 2016; Lueck, 2018). For example, a message that read, "You are not to blame for the cause of your depression. Depression is treatable if you are willing to seek help," led people with elevated depressive symptomatology—and only people with elevated depressive symptomatology—to report increased perceptions of stigma. Moreover, these perceptions were associated with reduced intentions to seek help (Lienemann et al., 2013; see Klimes-Dougan et al., 2009, for a complementary example).

Siegel et al. (2017) put forth three complementary reasons as to why messages targeting people with depression sometimes struggle. The first has to do with the symptomatology of depression. As described by Beck's (1963, 1987; Beck & Bredemeier, 2016) cognitive theory of depression, people with the disorder process information through a depressogenic schema. The schema results in processing that is steeped in a negative bias (e.g., Beck, 1963, 1964), leading people with depression to have negative views of themselves, the world, and the future (Clark et al., 1999; see Gotlib & Joormann, 2010 and Wisco, 2009, for reviews). The depressogenic schema is also associated with cognitive errors such as arbitrary inference, overgeneralization, and absolutistic dichotomous thinking (Beck, 1987). As Siegel and colleagues described, the same schema that is responsible for the cognitive errors experienced by people with depression also processes the messages that advocate help seeking (also see Yzer & Siegel, 2025, for a review).

Psychological reactance (Brehm, 1966; see Rosenberg & Siegel, 2018 for a review) is a second reason Siegel et al. (2017) put forth, particularly explaining why help-seeking messages that are successful or harmless among those without depression backfire on those with this illness (see Lienemann & Siegel, 2016 for initial theorizing). Psychological reactance is a motivational state aroused by specific threats to, or elimination of, a person's autonomy (Brehm, 1966). As Lienemann and Siegel (2016) described, people experiencing depression likely believe they have the right to seek help or not seek help; therefore, messages advocating help seeking have the potential to cause psychological reactance. Moreover, they proposed that the depressogenic schema and the associated cognitive errors could lead to the perception that a help-seeking message was more controlling and freedom-threatening than it would be otherwise. In support of this possibility, two experimental studies indicated a positive association between depressive symptomatology and psychological reactance to a public service announcement advocating help seeking (see Falco & Rosenberg, 2025, for a further discussion of reactance and depression).

The third reason, and the focus of this chapter, centers on the negative association typically found between levels of depressive symptomatology and help-seeking attitudes (e.g., Huntley & Fisher, 2016; Lienemann & Siegel, 2016; Lueck & Yzer, 2018). From a persuasion perspective, the negative association between depressive symptomatology and help-seeking attitudes is problematic because message receivers with less favorable attitudes generally process messages differently than those with more favorable attitudes (e.g., Crano & Prislin, 2008). As Eaton et al. (2008) described, "Attitudes guide our thoughts, bias our judgments, and influence our interpretations of events" (p. 166). They further noted, "Attitudes also motivate and guide our behaviour, inspiring us to approach objects that we like and avoid objects that we dislike. Thus, attitudes powerfully regulate our interactions with the world around us" (p. 166). Overall, the less favorable a person's attitude, the more they will scrutinize, resist, and counterargue a message advocating on behalf of the attitude object (e.g., help seeking; Knowles & Linn, 2004), rendering a persuasive message less effective and possibly causing iatrogenic effects

(Tormala, 2008; for a review, see Siegel et al., 2017). Fortunately, beyond partially explaining why people with higher levels of depression are more resistant to help-seeking messages than those with lower levels (i.e., less favorable attitudes), attitude scholarship also offers an approach for possibly overcoming this persuasive barrier.

Attitude Strength

Though numerous studies have uncovered a negative association between levels of depressive symptomatology and help-seeking attitudes, attitude valence represents just one aspect of an attitude (Petty & Krosnick, 1995). As noted, attitudes can differ in how much they influence thought and action (Krosnick & Smith, 1994). Strong attitudes, compared to weak ones, are more stable, less easily swayed, and will have greater influence over processing and behavior (Krosnick & Petty, 1995; Petty et al., 2013).

The attitude-strength diagnostic was motivated by scholarship on what has been referred to as attitude-strength attributes, also referred to as attitude-strength antecedents (Luttrell & Sawicki, 2020). As Luttrell and Sawicki described, the extent to which an attitude is durable and impactful can be assessed only through direct observation; however, it is possible to anticipate the strength of an attitude by assessing attitude-strength antecedents. Antecedents commonly used in contemporary research include extremity, elaboration, accessibility, ambivalence, certainty, knowledge, importance, and vested interest (see Table 28.1 for a description of each antecedent). Although there are exceptions, including interactions between antecedents (e.g., Tormala & Rucker, 2007), attitudes are typically expected to be strong when extremity (e.g., Henderson et al., 2008), elaboration (Horcajo & Luttrell, 2016; Petty et al., 1995), accessibility (e.g., Fazio et al., 1982), certainty (e.g., Tormala & Petty, 2002), knowledge (e.g., Farc & Sagarin, 2009), importance (e.g., Brannon et al., 2007), and vested interest (e.g., Crano & Prislin, 1995) are high, and ambivalence (e.g., Clarkson et al., 2008) is low.

Although attitude-strength antecedents are often related, they are empirically and conceptually distinct (Luttrell & Sawicki, 2020; Visser et al., 2006). As Krosnick and Petty (1995) noted, there is "a considerable amount of independence among the individual strength-related dimensions" (p. 16; see Visser et al., 2006, for a discussion). For example, it is possible to attach personal importance to an attitude object, typically predictive of a strong attitude, but only to have limited knowledge, which is generally associated with a weak attitude (Visser et al., 2006). Moreover, causing a change in one attitude-strength antecedent will not necessarily influence other antecedents (Clarkson et al., 2008).

Table 28.1 Attitude-Strength Antecedents Included in the Current Investigation

Antecedent	*Definition*
Accessibility	The speed and ease with which thoughts about an attitude object come to mind (Fazio, 1986; Haddock & Gebauer, 2011).
Ambivalence	The extent to which people hold both positive and negative attitudes toward an attitude object (Kaplan, 1972; Thompson et al., 1995).
Certainty	The degree of confidence people have regarding the accuracy or validity of a particular attitude (see Tormala, 2016; Tormala & Rucker, 2007, for reviews).
Elaboration	The degree to which a person has thought about an attitude object, including its advantages and disadvantages (Barden & Tormala, 2014).
Extremity	The intensity with which the valence of an attitude strays from neutrality (Wegener et al., 1995).
Importance	The amount of significance or concern that an individual attaches to an attitude (Boninger et al., 1995).
Knowledge	The degree to which people perceive themselves experts in regard to an attitude object (Brannon et al., 2007).
Vested Interest	The extent to which the attitude object is perceived as personally important and hedonically relevant (Crano & Prislin, 1995). Vested interest differs from importance in that it is possible to attach a high level of significance to an attitude but not have it be personally important or hedonically relevant (Crano & Prislin, 1995; Eaton et al., 2008).

Help-Seeking Attitudes and Attitude Strength

The possibility that some attitude-strength antecedents might indicate a weak attitude whereas others suggest a strong attitude was at the heart of the attitude-strength diagnostic approach. Our goal was to simultaneously measure numerous attitude-strength antecedents to analyze which antecedents differ based on the level of depressive symptomatology. We wanted to explore how help-seeking attitudes held by people at varying levels of depressive symptomatology differ regarding their help-seeking attitude structure and the antecedents responsible for the attitude's strength. As noted, numerous studies indicate that people with higher levels of depressive symptomatology have less favorable help-seeking attitudes than people with lower levels. Still, the extent to which attitude-strength antecedents differ among those with lower and higher levels of depressive symptomatology has rarely been explored. This approach aligns with the sentiment of Krosnick and Petty (1995), who noted that helpful insight can be obtained by simultaneously considering numerous attitude-strength dimensions (Bassili, 1996; Visser et al., 2006).

We imagined several possible uses of the information derived from the attitude-strength diagnostic. First, we hoped to uncover a deeper understanding of the differences in help-seeking attitudes between those at varying levels of depressive symptomatology. We envisioned that such information could increase knowledge as to why efforts that seem to work among those without depression sometimes fail or backfire on those with the disorder. Beyond explaining why some approaches promoting help seeking sometimes fail or backfire exclusively among people with heightened depressive symptomatology, we hoped that the findings could serve as a roadmap for future persuasive efforts. We expected the attitude-strength diagnostic to reveal the aspects of help-seeking attitudes most vulnerable to persuasion and let us know how to influence help-seeking attitudes. For example, if people with depression have positive help-seeking attitudes that are less certain than those without depression, increasing certainty about the positive aspects of help seeking among people with depression could make their help-seeking attitudes more similar to people without depression.

The Current Studies

The current chapter reports the results of two attitude-strength diagnostics of help-seeking attitudes, focusing on correlations between attitude-strength antecedents and levels of depressive symptomatology. Study 1 examined the relationships between levels of depressive symptomatology, attitudes toward help seeking from the participants' most likely help-seeking source (e.g., romantic partner, mental health professional, website), and a range of attitude-strength antecedents associated with global (nonvalenced) help-seeking attitudes, positive help-seeking attitudes, and negative help-seeking attitudes: extremity, elaboration, accessibility, felt ambivalence (i.e., ambivalence measured directly), potential ambivalence (i.e., ambivalence measured indirectly), certainty, knowledge, importance, and vested interest. Study 2 was an exact replication of Study 1 to ensure the data were reliable. These studies were not preregistered, as they were largely exploratory. Files for all studies, materials, data, codebooks, and analysis syntax can be found at https://osf.io/xqmnp/. We report all exclusions for all studies, and all measured variables are included in the uploaded data sets.

Study 1: Method

Participants

According to an a priori power analysis (G*Power v. 3.1.9.7) for a two-tailed test of a correlation (point biserial model), a sample of 343 participants would allow for the detection of a small-moderate effect size ($\rho = 0.15$; $1\text{-}\beta = 0.80$; $\alpha = 0.05$). Data were collected through Amazon's Mechanical Turk (MTurk) from 414 adults currently living within the United States. Participants were screened for successful completion of attention checks. Their responses were removed if they were presently seeking help for depression or if they had a duplicate IP address (see Table 28.2). More participants were screened out than anticipated, resulting in a final sample of 300 (see Table 28.6 for demographics).

Table 28.2 Screening Criteria and Final Sample Sizes for Studies 1 and 2

	Study 1	*Study 2*
Initial sample	414	415
Did not complete the survey	[a]	1
Did not pass attention checks	51	49
Currently seeking help	44	49
Duplicate IP address	17	15
Final sample	300	302

[a] Not used as exclusion criteria in this study.

Table 28.3 Sample Items and Sources for Measures

	Source	*Sample item*
Extremity	Bassili & Krosnick, 2000[a]	N/A
Elaboration (G)	Tormala et al., 2006[a]	In the past 2 weeks, how much effort have you put into thinking about seeking help for depression from (chosen source)?
Elaboration (P/N)		In the past 2 weeks, how much effort have you put into thinking about **the positive/negative aspects of** seeking help for depression from (chosen source)?
Accessibility (G)	Haddock & Gebauer, 2011	How slowly or quickly do thoughts about seeking help from (chosen source) come to mind?
Accessibility (P/N)		How slowly or quickly do **positive/negative** thoughts about seeking help from (chosen source) come to mind?
Felt Ambivalence	Bassili, 1996[a]	When you think about seeking help for depression from (chosen source) you are ***not at all indecisive/extremely indecisive.***
Potential Ambivalence	Armitage & Conner, 2000	How **positive/negative** do you feel about seeking help for depression from (chosen source)?
Certainty (G)	Clarkson et al., 2008[a]	How certain are you of your impressions about seeking help for depression from (chosen source)?
Certainty (P/N)		How certain are you of your impressions about **the positive/ negative aspects of** seeking help for depression from (chosen source)?
Knowledge (G)	Farc & Sagarin, 2009[a]	How knowledgeable are you about what will happen if you seek help for depression from (chosen source)?
Knowledge (P/N)		How knowledgeable are you about **the positive/negative aspects of** what will happen if you seek help for depression from (chosen source)?
Importance (G)	Krosnick et al., 1993[a]	How important is seeking help for depression from (chosen source) to you personally?
Importance (P/N)		How important **are the positive/negative aspects of** seeking help for depression from (chosen source) to you personally?
Vested Interest (G)	Boninger et al., 1995[a]	When it comes to seeking help for depression from (chosen source), how much do you have at stake?
Vested Interest (P/N)		When it comes to **the positive/negative aspects of** seeking help for depression from (chosen source), how much do you have at stake?

Note. G, Global; N, Negative; P, Positive.
[a] Multiple sources were used to develop the questions for this scale; this was a primary influence.

Materials and Procedure

After providing consent, participants were administered measures of depressive symptomatology, global attitudes toward help seeking and attitude-strength antecedents (e.g., certainty about help-seeking attitudes), attitude-strength antecedents regarding positive attitudes (e.g., certainty about positive attitudes) and negative attitudes (e.g., certainty about negative attitudes), depression history, and demographics. They were then debriefed and compensated $1.75 for their time. See Table 28.3 for sample items and Table 28.4 for the number of items, method of computation, and Cronbach's alphas.

Table 28.4 Number of Items, Computation Method, and Internal Consistencies From Studies 1–2

	Number of items	*Study 1* α	*Study 2* α
BDI-II[1]	21	0.94	0.95
Attitude	6	0.94	0.94
Extremity[2]	[a]	[a]	[a]
Elaboration	3	0.94	0.95
Positive	3	0.97	0.97
Negative	3	0.95	0.96
Accessibility	2	0.88	0.90
Positive	2	0.95	0.96
Negative	2	0.96	0.95
Felt Ambivalence	3	0.95	0.96
Potential Ambivalence[3]	2	[a]	[a]
Certainty	3	0.94	0.94
Positive	3	0.97	0.96
Negative	3	0.96	0.95
Knowledge	3	0.90	0.90
Positive	3	0.94	0.95
Negative	3	0.94	0.95
Importance	4	0.96	0.96
Positive	4	0.96	0.97
Negative	4	0.96	0.96
Vested interest	3	0.80	0.84
Positive	3	0.81	0.89
Negative	3	0.92	0.93

Note. An average of the items was used for all scales, with response sets ranging from 1 to 7, with the exceptions of: [1] BDI-II, which was summed, with possible scores of 0–63; [2]Extremity, which was computed using the formula |Attitude – 4|, with possible scores ranging from 0 to 3; [3]Potential ambivalence, which was computed using the Griffin equation (Thompson et al., 1995), with possible scores ranging from 0 to 9.
[a] Not applicable.

Beck Depression Inventory-II

Participants were given the Beck Depression Inventory-II (BDI-II; Beck et al., 1996) to assess depressive symptomatology. This measure contains 21 items with a 4-point scale (0–3) comprising statements with increasing severity. For example, one item assessed sadness, with statements ranging from 0 = ***I do not feel sad*** to 3 = ***I am so sad or unhappy that I can't stand it.*** Participants selected the statement that best described their feelings during the past two weeks. Scores were summed, resulting in a possible range from 0 to 63, with higher scores indicating higher depressive symptomatology.

Help-Seeking Source

Participants were then asked to indicate who they would most likely seek help from if they were experiencing depression (see Table 28.5). This information was used to personalize the help-seeking attitude and attitude-strength antecedent measures (discussed later) so that questions were about help seeking from their specified source. We collapsed all data across the different most-likely help-seeking sources.

Attitudes Toward Help Seeking for Depression

In line with common approaches for attitude measurement, attitudes toward help seeking were measured using a 7-point semantic differential scale. Participants were asked, "How would you describe your thoughts and feelings about seeking help for depression from (chosen source)?" Anchor pairs included ***negative/positive, bad/good, unfavorable/favorable, harmful/beneficial, foolish/wise,*** and ***undesirable/desirable*** (e.g., Farc & Sagarin, 2009; Tormala & Petty, 2002).

Table 28.5 Study 1 and 2 Chosen Help-Seeking Source

	Study 1		*Study 2*	
	n	*Percentage (%)*	*n*	*Percentage (%)*
Romantic partner	93	31.0	71	23.6
Close friend	41	13.7	33	11.0
Parent	24	8.0	27	9.0
Family member (nonparent)	11	3.7	11	3.7
Mental health professional	73	24.3	88	29.2
Support group	7	2.3	3	1.0
Helpline	1	0.3	5	1.7
Depression website	22	7.3	29	9.6
Doctor/general practitioner	28	9.3	34	11.3

Table 28.6 Demographics for Studies 1 and 2

	Study 1	*Study 2*
Age (*M*)	36.53	38.84
Age (*SD*)	10.83	12.34
Sex		
Male	51.3%	48.3%
Female	48.3%	51.3%
Non-binary	0.3%	0.0%
Other	0.0%	0.3%
Declined to respond	0.0%	0.0%
Race or ethnicity		
White	74.0%	77.5%
Black	9.0%	6.6%
Hispanic	5.3%	6.0%
Asian or Pacific Islander	8.0%	6.3%
Native American	1.3%	0.0%
Multiethnic	2.0%	3.6%
Other	0.0%	0.0%
Declined to respond	0.3%	0.0%

Attitude-Strength Antecedents

Several antecedents of global attitude strength were assessed in the following order: elaboration, accessibility, felt ambivalence, potential ambivalence, knowledge, certainty, importance, and vested interest. We also computed extremity based on responses to the attitude measure. In addition to the global measures, elaboration, accessibility, knowledge, certainty, importance, and vested interest were split to separately assess the positive and negative aspects of help seeking for depression. The order of positive and negative attitude-strength antecedents was randomly assigned, with 49.8% of participants receiving positive and 50.2% receiving negative questions first. For all scales, higher scores indicate higher levels of the attitude-strength antecedent. See Table 28.3 for sample items and Table 28.4 for the number of items, method of computation, and Cronbach's alphas for both data collections.

Depression History

To determine if participants were in the population of interest (i.e., those who were experiencing heightened depressive symptomatology, and considered themselves to be depressed, but were not currently seeking help for their symptoms), they were first asked if they considered themselves to be presently depressed; if so, they were then asked if they were currently seeking help. Those who indicated that they did not consider themselves to be depressed or that they were presently seeking help were screened out of the survey.

Demographics

Participants were asked for their sex, age, ethnicity, and level of education. They were then debriefed and thanked for their time.

Study 1: Results

A correlation table reports whether attitude-strength elements were related to depressive symptomatology (see Table 28.7). Spearman's ρ was used rather than Pearson's r because BDI-II scores did not approximate a normal distribution ($M = 9.42$, $SD = 10.32$, Skew = 1.52, $SE_{skew} = 0.14$, Kurtosis = 2.13, $SE_{kurtosis} = 0.28$).

As indicated in Table 28.7, the diagnostic indicated a negative association between levels of depressive symptomatology and attitudes toward seeking help from participants' most likely help-seeking source. People with higher levels of depressive symptomatology also reported help-seeking attitudes (global) from their most likely help-seeking source that were less extreme, elaborated on to a greater extent, less accessible, more ambivalent (felt and potential), and less certain. People with higher levels of depressive symptomatology also perceived themselves as less knowledgeable regarding help seeking. Regarding positive attitudes, people with higher levels of depressive symptomatology held positive help-seeking attitudes that were elaborated to a greater extent, less accessible, less certain, and perceived to be based on less knowledge. People with higher levels of depressive symptomatology also reported having negative help-seeking attitudes that were elaborated on to a greater extent, more accessible, perceived as more important, and held with greater vested interest. There were not significant associations between levels of depressive symptomatology and importance (global), certainty (negative), knowledge (negative), importance (positive), or vested interest (positive).

Table 28.7 Study 1 and 2 Correlations With BDI-II Scores

	Study 1 (N = 300)		*Study 2 (N = 301)*	
	ρ	*95% CI*	ρ	*95% CI*
Attitude	−.24***	[−0.347, −0.131]	−.29***	[−0.393, −0.182]
Extremity	−.22***	[−0.325, −0.107]	−.27***	[−0.369, −0.155]
Elaboration	.44***	[0.337, 0.529]	.43***	[0.332, 0.524]
Positive	.25***	[0.140, 0.356]	.29***	[0.178, 0.389]
Negative	.35***	[0.242, 0.447]	.46***	[0.360, 0.548]
Accessibility	−.21***	[−0.314, −0.095]	−.10†	[−0.213, 0.011]
Positive	−.30***	[−0.406, −0.195]	−.27***	[−0.373, −0.160]
Negative	.33***	[0.218, 0.426]	.34***	[0.237, 0.443]
Felt Ambivalence	.38***	[0.279, 0.480]	.36***	[0.251, 0.455]
Potential Ambivalence	.24***	[0.129, 0.345]	.26***	[0.144, 0.359]
Certainty	−.26***	[−0.367, −0.152]	−.29***	[−0.395, −0.184]
Positive	−.22***	[−0.324, −0.105]	−.29***	[−0.389, −0.178]
Negative	−.05	[−0.157, 0.069]	−.03	[−0.142, 0.084]
Knowledge	−.22***	[−0.328, −0.110]	−.10†	[−0.215, 0.009]
Positive	−.19***	[−0.298, −0.077]	−.11†	[−0.218, 0.006]
Negative	.04	[−0.071, 0.156]	.15*	[0.032, 0.254]
Importance	−.05	[−0.164, 0.062]	−.13*	[−0.237, −0.014]
Positive	−.08	[−0.193, 0.033]	−.04	[−0.153, 0.072]
Negative	.17**	[0.056, 0.278]	.21***	[0.100, 0.319]
Vested interest	.04	[−0.075, 0.152]	−.03	[−0.138, 0.088]
Positive	−.01	[−0.126, 0.100]	.01	[−0.107, 0.119]
Negative	.13*	[0.012, 0.236]	.22***	[0.103, 0.321]

Note. ***$p < .001$, **$p < .01$, *$p < .05$, †$p < .10$.

In addition to these analyses, we conducted bivariate correlations between BDI-II scores and the single items used to compute potential ambivalence, as these items exclusively inquired about how positive/negative respondents felt about seeking help for depression from their chosen source. There was a significant negative correlation between BDI-II scores and positive attitude toward help seeking for depression ($\rho = -.26$, $N = 300$, $p < .001$, 95% CI [−0.360, −0.145]) and a significant positive correlation between BDI-II scores and negative attitude toward help seeking for depression ($\rho = .28$, $N = 300$, $p < .001$, 95% CI [0.173, 0.386]).

Finally, as there were positive correlations between BDI-II scores and the elaboration of positive and negative attitudes, we decided to explore whether these correlations were significantly different. Using a *z*-test (Lenhard & Lenhard, 2014), we found that the correlations between BDI-II scores and positive elaboration ($\rho = .25$) and negative elaboration ($\rho = .35$) were significantly different, $z = -2.01$, $p = .044$, two-tailed.

Study 2: Method

Participants

Study 2 was an exact replication conducted to assess the reliability of Study 1 results. Using the same power analysis and screening rationale as Study 1, we recruited 415 adults living within the United States through MTurk (see Table 28.2 for removal rationale). This resulted in a final sample of 301 participants (see Table 28.6 for demographics). Although we had fewer participants than planned, given we had a similar number of participants as Study 1, where correlations as low as $\rho = 0.126$ were statistically significant, we decided to proceed with analyses.

Materials and Procedure

The same materials and procedures used in Study 1 were used in Study 2. See Table 28.3 for sample items and Table 28.4 for the number of items, method of computation, and Cronbach's alphas.

Study 2: Results

Table 28.7 reports the correlations between attitude-strength antecedents and depressive symptomatology. Spearman's ρ was used rather than Pearson's *r* because BDI-II scores did not approximate a normal distribution ($M = 9.30$, $SD = 8.89$, Skew = 1.18, $SE_{skew} = 0.14$, Kurtosis = 1.22, $SE_{kurtosis} = 0.28$).

Replicating the results of Study 1, there was a negative association between levels of depressive symptomatology and global attitudes toward seeking help from the most likely help-seeking source. Also, like Study 1, people with higher levels of depressive symptomatology reported help-seeking attitudes (global) from their most likely source that were less extreme, elaborated on to a greater extent, more ambivalent (felt and potential), and less certain. Two of the significant correlations from Study 1 (i.e., negative correlation between levels of depressive symptomatology and accessibility, as well as knowledge) were marginally significant in Study 2. Regarding positive help-seeking attitudes, akin to Study 1, people with higher levels of depressive symptomatology reported positive help-seeking attitudes that were elaborated on to a greater extent, less accessible, and less certain. Unlike Study 1, where there was a significant negative correlation between levels of depressive symptomatology and knowledge about positive help-seeking attitudes, this association was marginally significant in Study 2. Regarding negative help-seeking attitudes, and replicating Study 1 results, people with higher levels of depressive symptomatology reported negative help-seeking attitudes that were elaborated on to a greater extent, more accessible, more important, and held with a higher vested interest. There was also a significant positive correlation between levels of depressive symptomatology and the knowledge on which negative help-seeking attitudes were based, which was not present in Study 1. Mirroring

Study 1, there was not a significant association between levels of depressive symptomatology and vested interest (global), certainty (negative), importance (positive), or vested interest (positive).

As in the previous study, we also conducted bivariate correlations between BDI-II and the single items used to compute potential ambivalence. There was a significant negative correlation between BDI-II scores and positive attitude toward help seeking for depression ($\rho = -.24$, $N = 301$, $p < .001$, 95% CI [−0.342, −0.126]) and a significant positive correlation between BDI-II scores and negative attitude toward help seeking for depression ($\rho = .36$, $N = 301$, $p < .001$, 95% CI [0.252, 0.456]).

Finally, similar to Study 1, a z-test (Lenhard & Lenhard, 2014) indicated that the correlations between BDI-II scores and positive elaboration ($\rho = .29$) and negative elaboration ($\rho = .46$) were significantly different, $z = -4.05$, $p < .001$, two-tailed.

General Discussion

Motivated by the challenges sometimes faced when attempting to persuade people with depression to seek help, we conducted attitude-strength diagnostics on attitudes toward help seeking for depression. This involved exploring relationships between levels of depressive symptomatology and various help-seeking attitude-strength antecedents. The results of these studies offer insight into why prior campaign efforts were sometimes less effective on those with higher levels of depressive symptomatology and provide a potential path for increasing the persuasive strength of future messaging attempts.

Help-Seeking Attitudes and Level of Depressive Symptomatology

Both studies indicated a negative relationship between depressive symptomatology and attitudes toward seeking help from participants' most likely help-seeking source. The attitude-strength diagnostic also revealed that higher levels of depressive symptomatology were associated with higher levels of negative help-seeking attitudes and lower levels of positive help-seeking attitudes. Given people with depression have more negative thoughts than people without depression (Beck, 1987), this is not surprising. This finding is in line with Clark et al.'s (1999) observation that "increases in depressive symptomatology will be associated with a corresponding increase in negative cognitions at each level of depression severity" (p. 168). To be sure, people with depressive symptomatology do not have purely negative help-seeking attitudes; instead, they have help-seeking attitudes that are less positive than those without depression. As less favorable attitudes are generally associated with a greater tendency to counterargue information advocating the position, thus impairing the persuasive strength of the message (Knowles & Lynn, 2004), these data provide initial insight into why some help-seeking approaches were less successful for people with heightened depressive symptomatology.

Global Help-Seeking Attitude-Strength Antecedents

Given that many efforts have failed to change help-seeking attitudes among people with depression, we expected most attitude-strength antecedents at a global level (e.g., certainty of help-seeking attitudes without reference to valence) would be indicative of stronger help-seeking attitudes among those with higher levels of depressive symptomatology (e.g., more extreme, greater elaboration, accessibility, certainty, knowledge, importance, vested interest, and less ambivalent). We were wrong. The only finding in line with this expectation was that people with higher levels of depressive symptomatology reported more elaboration, which is typically associated with stronger attitudes (Petty et al., 1995). All other attitude-strength antecedents regarding global help-seeking attitudes either indicated weaker attitudes, or showed no significant relationship with depressive symptomatology (see Table 28.7). People with higher levels of depressive symptomatology reported global help-seeking attitudes that were less extreme, less accessible, more ambivalent, less certain, and based on less knowledge. Rather than offering insight into why prior persuasive attempts have sometimes backfired among those with elevated depressive symptomatology (Lienemann et al., 2013), the data indicated that persuasive help-seeking attempts should be more successful among those with higher levels of symptomatology. Fortunately, in line with Cacioppo et al.'s (1997) theorizing regarding the benefits of treating positive and negative attitudes as bivariate rather than bipolar, we also measured attitude-strength antecedents of negative and positive help-seeking attitudes.

Help-Seeking Attitude-Strength Antecedents (Positive and Negative)

The current data consistently indicated that people with higher levels of depressive symptomatology elaborated on their positive and negative help-seeking attitudes to a greater extent than those with lower levels. Moreover, there was a stronger correlation between depressive symptomatology and the elaboration of negative help-seeking attitudes than positive ones. Helping explain the struggle to persuade people with depression to seek help, one result of elaboration is that it increases resistance to persuasion—the more people think about an issue, the more they believe that "considerable thought accompanied opinion formation" (p. 119, Petty et al., 1995). This makes it so that highly elaborated attitudes are more resistant to persuasive attempts than attitudes that are not (see Petty et al., 1995, for a review).

The positive correlation between depressive symptomatology and accessibility of negative help-seeking attitudes—and reduced accessibility of positive attitudes—is also consistent with prior scholarship. People with higher levels of depressive symptomatology have negative thoughts that are more accessible (Riskind & Rholes, 1984). The reduced accessibility of positive help-seeking attitudes is in line with studies indicating that people experiencing depression experience a deactivation of positive schemas (Beck & Bredemeier, 2016), including the minimization of positive materials (Clark et al., 1999). As described by persuasion scholars, when attitudes are accessible, they orient attention (Roskos-Ewoldsen & Fazio, 1992) and influence information processing (Fazio & Williams, 1986). As people will generally evaluate information in a manner that is agreeable to their accessible attitudes, it follows that messages advocating help seeking will be evaluated less favorably by people with higher levels of depressive symptomatology due to their negative attitudes being more accessible and their positive attitudes less accessible.

There was not a significant association between levels of depressive symptomatology and certainty of negative help-seeking attitudes in either study. However, both studies indicated a negative association between levels of depressive symptomatology and certainty of positive help-seeking attitudes. The lower levels of positive help-seeking attitude certainty offer further insight into the challenges faced when trying to persuade people experiencing depression to seek help. When attitudes are less certain (i.e., the degree of confidence that people have regarding the accuracy or validity of a particular attitude; see Tormala, 2016; Tormala & Rucker, 2007, 2018, for reviews), they are viewed as less accurate and will act as weaker guides for message processing and future judgments.

People with higher levels of depressive symptomatology also had negative help-seeking attitudes that were perceived as more important. However, there was not a significant correlation between levels of depressive symptomatology and the importance of positive help-seeking attitudes. The increased importance of negative attitudes further explains the challenge of persuading people with depression to seek help. Howe and Krosnick (2017) described attitude importance as one of the most investigated aspects of attitude strength. They noted that if an attitude object is highly important, people become motivated to protect it. More important attitudes are more stable and resistant to change (Krosnick & Smith, 1994; Visser et al., 2017), even when counterattitudinal information is presented.

A positive association was found between levels of depressive symptomatology and vested interest in negative help-seeking attitudes; however, there was no association with vested interest in positive help-seeking attitudes. The finding that higher levels of depressive symptomatology were associated with a greater vested interest in negative help-seeking attitudes is somewhat in line with Hevey et al.'s (2017) finding that people with depression have higher punishment sensitivity. The higher punishment sensitivity could lead people with higher levels of depressive symptomatology to perceive the negative outcomes as having more personal and important consequences. These associations are also in line with data indicating that people with depression have greater expectations of adverse outcomes of help seeking (Yzer et al., 2022). As people with higher levels of depressive symptomatology are more vested in their negative attitudes than those with lower levels of depressive symptomatology, it follows that the behavior of people with higher levels of depressive symptomatology will be more challenging to influence.

Altogether, the attitude-strength diagnostic provided insight into the challenge of increasing help seeking among people experiencing depression that goes beyond the previously reported negative association between help-seeking attitudes and depressive symptomatology (e.g., Siegel et al., 2015). Beyond having help-seeking attitudes that are more negative, nearly every attitude-strength antecedent regarding negative help-seeking attitudes was indicative of people with higher levels of depressive symptomatology having negative attitudes that are stronger than those with lower levels. Moreover, although people with higher levels of depressive symptomatology elaborate on their positive attitudes to a greater extent than those with lower levels, numerous other attitude-strength antecedents are indicative of weaker positive help-seeking attitudes. Among people with higher levels of depressive symptomatology, their positive attitudes are less accessible, held with less certainty, and somewhat perceived to be based on less knowledge. These data indicate that persuasive attempts to increase help seeking should be expected to be met with stronger negative and weaker positive help-seeking attitudes, thus making attitude change more difficult. Simply, these findings explain why attempts to persuade people with depression to seek help will likely be met with strong resistance, and any success should be considered an accomplishment. Fortunately, the same data we used to explain the reasons for prior struggles to persuade people with depression to seek help can also be used to devise approaches for increasing help seeking among people with elevated depressive symptomatology.

Identifying Targets for Persuasive Influence

Although attitude-strength antecedents are typically used to predict attitude strength rather than guide persuasive approaches, we believe it is feasible to do so. As noted, people with higher levels of depressive symptomatology elaborate on positive attitudes to a greater extent than those with lower levels, but these positive attitudes are less accessible, held with less certainty, and somewhat perceived to be based on less knowledge. This combination provides an image of people with higher levels of depressive symptomatology striving to think positive thoughts about help seeking (i.e., higher levels of elaboration of positive help-seeking attitudes) but not being able to do so (i.e., less accessible positive help-seeking attitudes), and lacking confidence in those thoughts when they arise (i.e., less certainty of positive help-seeking attitudes and positive help-seeking attitudes that are based in somewhat less knowledge).

As such, mental health communication might find success by strategically increasing the accessibility and certainty of positive help-seeking attitudes. Increasing perceived knowledge associated with help-seeking attitudes could also be useful. The higher levels of elaboration of positive attitudes that were found among people with higher levels of depressive symptomatology can serve to increase the likelihood that people experiencing depression will internalize these more accessible and more certain positive help-seeking attitudes. This could lead to positive help-seeking attitudes that are stronger and more favorable, causing positive help-seeking attitudes of those with higher levels of depressive symptomatology to be more like those with lower levels.

The attitude-strength diagnostic focused on negative help-seeking attitudes also provides a potential, albeit less promising, persuasive pathway. Among people with higher levels of depressive symptomatology, negative help-seeking attitudes are elaborated on to a greater extent, more accessible, perceived to be more important, held with a greater vested interest, and possibly perceived to be based on more accurate knowledge. Therefore, messages that can strategically reduce the importance of, vested interest in, and perceived expertise of negative help-seeking attitudes could be helpful. This could possibly be accomplished by letting people with depression know their feared adverse outcomes are unlikely. However, it might be challenging to do so without increasing negative attitude accessibility and elaboration. Once negative material becomes top of mind among people experiencing depression, there is difficulty in disengaging from the material (see Gotlib & Joormann, 2010, for a review). This could counteract any possible gains or cause a backfire effect. As such, we are less confident in this approach, and pilot testing is critical.

Limitations

One limitation involves our measurement of accessibility via self-report. Although other studies have taken this approach (Pfau et al., 2003) or combined a self-report measure with response latencies (Haddock & Gebauer, 2011), most studies use response latency as an indicator of accessibility (e.g., Fazio, 1995). Future studies could overcome this limitation by measuring response latency and assessing whether the same pattern of results emerges. Also, the data in the current studies only allow for assessing the associations between variables rather than determining causal links. Future studies could overcome this limitation by conducting longitudinal research to evaluate if there is a causal relationship between higher levels of depressive symptomatology and help-seeking attitudes or if a third variable is responsible for these associations.

Future Directions

As described, one goal of the current set of studies was to uncover approaches for persuading people with heightened levels of depressive symptomatology to seek help. Crafting messages or tasks that increase the accessibility and certainty of positive attitudes represents a highly promising approach. A critical future direction is assessing whether the diagnostic's guidance can lead to the development of successful persuasive messages. Another possibility, albeit less promising, is to convince people with depression that their negative help-seeking attitudes are less important and have fewer personal consequences. Regardless of which approach is taken, extensive pilot testing is necessary, as backfire effects could occur. Moreover, given the differences in help-seeking attitudes and attitude-strength antecedents based on levels of depressive symptomatology, it would be critical to conduct such pilot testing on people with heightened levels of depressive symptomatology. Doing otherwise could lead to misleading results (see Siegel et al., 2017, and Yzer & Siegel, 2025, for a discussion).

Future studies will ideally further assess the patterns that are not so easily explained. For example, people with higher levels of depressive symptomatology have positive help-seeking attitudes that are less certain. Still, there was no significant association between levels of depressive symptomatology and positive help-seeking attitude importance or vested interest. Negative help-seeking attitudes were seen as more important and were held with greater vested interest among people with higher levels of depressive symptomatology. However, there was not a significant association between levels of depressive symptomatology and the certainty of negative attitudes. This pattern of results would not be obvious without the attitude-strength diagnostic, and the exploration of these associations could be fruitful. Similarly, the use of the attitude-strength diagnostic in other contexts could be beneficial.

Conclusion

Current results indicated that people with higher levels of depressive symptomatology, compared to those with lower levels, have negative attitudes that are more accessible, perceived as more important, held with a greater vested interest, and possibly perceived to be based on more accurate information. People with higher levels of depressive symptomatology also had positive attitudes that were less accessible, less certain, and likely perceived to be based on less accurate information. Moreover, although there was increased elaboration of positive help-seeking attitudes among those with higher levels of depressive symptomatology, the association between depressive symptomatology and elaboration of negative attitudes was significantly stronger. As these associations are nearly all predictive of greater resistance to persuasive messages, these results highlight and explain the challenge of persuading people with depression. These results also offer a possible path for persuading people with depression to seek out the help they need (i.e., increasing positive attitude certainty, accessibility, and possibly knowledge). These findings will ideally lead to a greater appreciation of the challenge of persuading people with depression to seek help and offer guidance for future help-seeking interventions.

References

Armitage, C. J., & Conner, M. (2000). Attitudinal ambivalence: A test of three key hypotheses. *Personality and Social Psychology Bulletin*, *26*(11), 1421–1432. https://doi.org/10.1177/0146167200263009

Barden, J., & Tormala, Z. L. (2014). Elaboration and attitude-strength: The new meta-cognitive perspective. *Social and Personality Psychology Compass*, *8*(1), 17–29. https://doi.org/10.1111/spc3.12078

Bassili, J. N. (1996). Meta-judgmental versus operative indexes of psychological antecedents: The case of measures of attitude-strength. *Journal of Personality and Social Psychology*, *71*(4), 637–653. https://psycnet.apa.org/doi/10.1037/0022-3514.71.4.637

Bassili, J. N., & Krosnick, J. A. (2000). Do strength-related attitude properties determine susceptibility to response effects? New evidence from response latency, attitude extremity, and aggregate indices. *Political Psychology*, *21*(1), 107–132. https://doi.org/10.1111/0162-895X.00179

Beck, A. T. (1963). Thinking and depression I. Idiosyncratic content and cognitive distortions. *Archives of General Psychiatry*, *9*, 324–333.

Beck, A. T. (1964). Thinking and depression II. Theory and therapy. *Archives of General Psychiatry*, *10*, 561–571.

Beck, A. T. (1987). Cognitive models of depression. *Journal of Cognitive Psychotherapy*, *1*(1), 5–37.

Beck, A. T., & Bredemeier, K. (2016). A unified model of depression: Integrating clinical, cognitive, biological, and evolutionary perspectives. *Clinical Psychological Science*, *4*(4), 596–619. https://doi.org/10.1177/2167702616628523

Beck, A. T., Steer, R. A., & Brown, G. K. (1996). *Manual for the Beck Depression Inventory-II*. Psychological Corporation.

Boninger, D. S., Krosnick, J. A., & Berent, M. K. (1995). Origins of attitude importance: Self-interest, social identification, and value relevance. *Journal of Personality and Social Psychology*, *68*(1), 61–80. https://doi.org/10.1037//0022-3514.68.1.61

Bossarte, R. M., Karras, E., Naiji, L., Xin, T., Stephens, B., Draper, J., & Kemp, J. E. (2014). Associations between the Department of Veterans Affairs' suicide prevention campaign and calls to related crisis lines. *Public Health Reports*, *129*, 516–525. https://doi.org/10.1177/003335491412900610

Brannon, L. A., Tagler, M. J., & Eagly, A. H. (2007). The moderating role of attitude-strength in selective exposure to information. *Journal of Experimental Social Psychology*, *43*(4), 611–617. https://doi.org/10.1016/j.jesp.2006.05.001

Brehm, J. W. (1966). *A theory of psychological reactance*. Academic Press.

Cacioppo, J. T., Gardner, W. L., & Bemtson, G. G. (1997). Beyond bipolar conceptualizations and measures: The case of attitudes and evaluative space. *Personality and Social Psychology Review*, *1*, 3–25. https://doi.org/10.1207/s15327957pspr0101_2

Clark, D. A., Beck, A. T., & with Alford, B. A. (1999). *Scientific foundations of cognitive theory and therapy of depression*. Wiley.

Clarkson, J. J., Tormala, Z. L., & Rucker, D. D. (2008). A new look at the consequences of attitude certainty: The amplification hypothesis. *Journal of Personality and Social Psychology*, *95*(4), 810–825. https://doi.org/10.1037/a0013192

Crano, W. D., & Prislin, R. (1995). Components of vested interest and attitude-behavior consistency. *Basic and Applied Social Psychology*, *17*(1–2), 1–21. https://doi.org/10.1080/01973533.1995.9646129

Crano, W. D., & Prislin, R. (2008). *Attitudes and attitude change*. Psychology Press.

Danek, R., Blackburn, J., Greene, M., Mazurenko, O., & Menachemi, N. (2023). Unmet mental health need and subsequent substance use in individuals with a history of depression: Are there differences between metro and nonmetro areas? *American Journal on Addictions*, *32*(4), 360–366. https://doi.org/10.1111/ajad.13393

Eaton, A. A., Majka, E. A., & Visser, P. S. (2008). Emerging perspectives on the structure and function of attitude-strength. *European Review of Social Psychology*, *19*, 165–201. https://doi.org/10.1080/10463280802383791

Falco, C. M., & Rosenberg, B. D. (2025). Minimizing reactance to increase help-seeking for depression. In M. C. Yzer & J. T. Siegel (Eds.), *Handbook of mental health communication*. Wiley.

Farc, M. M., & Sagarin, B. J. (2009). Using attitude strength to predict registration and voting behavior in the 2004 US presidential elections. *Basic and Applied Social Psychology*, *31*(2), 160–173. https://doi.org/10.1080/01973530902880498

Fazio, R. (1995). Attitudes as object-evaluation associations: Determinants, consequences, and correlates of attitude accessibility. In R. Petty & J. Krosnick (Eds.), *Attitude strength: Antecedents and consequences* (pp. 247–282). Lawrence Erlbaum.

Fazio, R. H. (1986). How do attitudes guide behavior? In R. M. Sorrentino & E. T. Higgins (Eds.), *Handbook of motivation and cognition: Foundations of social behavior* (pp. 204–243). Guilford Press.

Fazio, R. H., Chen, J., McDonel, E. C., & Sherman, S. J. (1982). Attitude accessibility, attitude-behavior consistency, and the strength of the object-evaluation association. *Journal of Experimental Social Psychology*, *18*(4), 339–357. https://doi.org/10.1016/0022-1031(82)90058-0

Fazio, R. H., & Williams, C. J. (1986). Attitude accessibility as a moderator of the attitude–perception and attitude–behavior relations: An investigation of the 1984 presidential election. *Journal of Personality and Social Psychology, 51*(3), 505–514. https://doi.org/10.1037//0022-3514.51.3.505

Feather, N. T. (1964). Acceptance and rejection of arguments in relation to attitude strength, critical ability, and intolerance of inconsistency. *Journal of Abnormal and Social Psychology, 69*(2), 127–136. https://doi.org/10.1037/h0046290

Ghio, L., Gotelli, S., Marcenaro, M., Amore, M., & Natta, W. (2014). Duration of untreated illness and outcomes in unipolar depression: A systematic review and meta-analysis. *Journal of Affective Disorders, 152–154*, 45–51. https://doi.org/10.1016/j.jad.2013.10.002

Goldney, R. D., & Fisher, L. J. (2008). Have broad-based community and professional education programs influenced mental health literacy and treatment seeking of those with major depression and suicidal ideation? *Suicide & Life-Threatening Behavior, 38*(2), 129–142. https://doi.org/10.1521/suli.2008.38.2.12

Gotlib, I. H., & Joormann, J. (2010). Cognition and depression: Current status and future directions. *Annual Review of Clinical Psychology, 6*, 285–312. https://doi.org/10.1146/annurev.clinpsy.121208.131305

Haddock, G., & Gebauer, J. E. (2011). Defensive self-esteem impacts attention, attitude-strength, and self-affirmation processes. *Journal of Experimental Social Psychology, 47*(6), 1276–1284. https://doi.org/10.1016/j.jesp.2011.05.020

Hammer, J. H., & Vogel, D. L. (2010). Men's help seeking for depression: The efficacy of a male-sensitive brochure about counseling. *Counseling Psychologist, 38*(2), 296–313. https://doi.org/10.1177/0011000009351937

Henderson, M. D., de Liver, Y., & Gollwitzer, P. M. (2008). The effects of an implemental mind-set on attitude strength. *Journal of Personality and Social Psychology, 94*(3), 396–411. https://doi.org/10.1037/0022-3514.94.3.396

Hevey, D., Thomas, K., Laureano-Schelten, S., Looney, K., & Booth, R. (2017). Clinical depression and punishment sensitivity on the BART. *Frontiers in Psychology, 8*, 670. https://doi.org/10.3389/fpsyg.2017.00670

Horcajo, J., & Luttrell, A. (2016). The effects of elaboration on the strength of doping-related attitudes: Resistance to change and behavioral intentions. *Journal of Sport & Exercise Psychology, 38*(3), 236–246. https://doi.org/10.1123/jsep.2015-0316

Howe, L. C., & Krosnick, J. A. (2017). Attitude-strength. *Annual Review of Psychology, 68*, 327–351. https://doi.org/10.1146/annurev-psych-122414-033600

Huntley, C. D., & Fisher, P. L. (2016). Examining the role of positive and negative metacognitive beliefs in depression. *Scandinavian Journal of Psychology, 57*(5), 446–452. https://doi.org/10.1111/sjop.12306

Kaplan, K. J. (1972). On the ambivalence-indifference problem in attitude theory and measurement: A suggested modification of the semantic differential technique. *Psychological Bulletin, 77*(5), 361–372. https://doi.org/10.1037/h0032590

Keeler, A., & Siegel, J. T. (2016). Depression, help seeking, and perceived family functioning among Hispanics and non-Hispanics whites. *Journal of Affective Disorders, 202*, 236–246. https://doi.org/10.1016/j.jad.2016.05.017

Klimes-Dougan, B., Yuan, C., Lee, S., & Houri, A. K. (2009). Suicide prevention with adolescents: Considering potential benefits and untoward effects of public service announcements. *Crisis: The Journal of Crisis Intervention and Suicide Prevention, 30*(3), 128–135. https://doi.org/10.1027/0227-5910.30.3.128

Knowles, E. S., & Linn, J. A. (2004). *Resistance and persuasion*. Lawrence Erlbaum Associates, Inc.

Krosnick, J. A., Boninger, D. S., Chuang, Y. C., Berent, M. K., & Carnot, C. G. (1993). Attitude strength: One construct or many related constructs? *Journal of Personality and Social Psychology, 65*, 1132–1151. https://doi.org/10.1037/0022-3514.65.6.1132

Krosnick, J. A., & Petty, R. E. (1995). Attitude-strength: An overview. In R. E. Petty & J. A. Krosnick (Eds.), *Attitude-strength: Antecedents and consequences* (pp. 1–24). Lawrence Erlbaum Associates, Inc.

Krosnick, J. A., & Smith, W. A. (1994). Attitude-strength. In V. S. Ramachandran (Ed.), *Encyclopedia of human behavior* (Vol. 1, pp. 279–289). Academic Press.

Lenhard, W., & Lenhard, A. (2014). Testing the significance of correlations. *Psychometrica*. http://dx.doi.org/10.13140/RG.2.1.2954.1367

Lienemann, B. A., & Siegel, J. T. (2016). State psychological reactance to depression public service announcements among people with varying levels of depressive symptomatology. *Health Communication, 31*(1), 102–116. https://doi.org/10.1080/10410236.2014.940668

Lienemann, B. A., Siegel, J. T., & Crano, W. D. (2013). Persuading people with depression to seek help: Respect the boomerang. *Health Communication, 28*(7), 718–728. https://doi.org/10.1080/10410236.2012.712091

Lueck, J., & Yzer, M. (2018). Explaining intentions to seek help for depressive symptoms in the context of responsibility message framing. *Health Communication, 33*(8), 946–953. https://doi.org/10.1080/10410236.2017.1322857

Lueck, J. A. (2018). Respecting the "stages" of depression: Considering depression severity and readiness to seek help. *Patient Education and Counseling, 101*(7), 1276–1282. https://doi.org/10.1016/j.pec.2018.02.007

Luttrell, A., & Sawicki, V. (2020). Attitude-strength: Distinguishing predictors versus defining features. *Social and Personality Psychology Compass, 14*(8). https://doi.org/10.1111/spc3.12555

Mekonen, T., Ford, S., Chan, G. C. K., Hides, L., Connor, J. P., & Leung, J. (2022). What is the short-term remission rate for people with untreated depression? A systematic review and meta-analysis. *Journal of Affective Disorders, 296*, 17–25. https://doi.org/10.1016/j.jad.2021.09.046

Niederkrotenthaler, T., Reidenberg, D. J., Till, B., & Gould, M. S. (2014). Increasing help-seeking and referrals for individuals at risk for suicide by decreasing stigma: The role of mass media. *American Journal of Preventive Medicine, 47*(3 Suppl. 2), S235–S243. https://doi.org/10.1016/j.amepre.2014.06.010

Petty, R. E., Haugtvedt, C. P., & Smith, S. M. (1995). Elaboration as a determinant of attitude strength: Creating attitudes that are persistent, resistant, and predictive of behavior. In R. E. Petty & J. A. Krosnick (Eds.), *Attitude-strength: Antecedents and consequences* (pp. 93–130). Lawrence Erlbaum Associates, Inc.

Petty, R. E., & Krosnick, J. A. (1995). *Attitude-strength: Antecedents and consequences.* Lawrence Erlbaum Associates, Inc.

Petty, R. E., Wheeler, S. C., & Tormala, Z. L. (2013). Persuasion and attitude change. In H. Tennen, J. Suls, & I. B. Weiner (Eds.), *Handbook of psychology: Vol. 5. Personality and social psychology* (2nd ed., pp. 369–389). John Wiley & Sons.

Pfau, M., Roskos-Ewoldsen, D., Wood, M., Yin, S., Cho, J., Lu, K.-H., & Shen, L. (2003). Attitude accessibility as an alternative explanation for how inoculation confers resistance. *Communication Monographs, 70*(1), 39–51. https://doi.org/10.1080/715114663

Philipp-Muller, A. Z., Wallace, L. E., & Wegener, D. T. (2020). Where does moral conviction fit?: A factor analytic approach examining antecedents to attitude-strength. *Journal of Experimental Social Psychology, 86.* https://doi.org/10.1016/j.jesp.2019.103900

Riskind, J. H., & Rholes, W. S. (1984). Cognitive accessibility and the capacity of cognitions to predict future depression: A theoretical note. *Cognitive Therapy and Research, 8*(1), 1–12. https://doi.org/10.1007/BF01315092

Rosenberg, B. D., & Siegel, J. T. (2018). A 50-year review of psychological reactance theory: Do not read this article. *Motivation Science, 4*, 281–300. http://dx.doi.org/10.1037/mot0000091

Roskos-Ewoldsen, D. R., & Fazio, R. H. (1992). On the orienting value of attitudes: Attitude accessibility as a determinant of an object's attraction of visual attention. *Journal of Personality and Social Psychology, 63*(2), 198–211. https://doi.org/10.1037/0022-3514.63.2.198

Siegel, J. T., Lienemann, B. A., & Rosenberg, B. D. (2017). Resistance, reactance, and misinterpretation: Highlighting the challenge of persuading people with depression to seek help. *Social and Personality Psychology Compass, 11*(6), e12322. https://doi.org/10.1111/spc3.12322

Siegel, J. T., Lienemann, B. A., & Tan, C. N. (2015). Influencing help-seeking among people with elevated depressive symptomatology: Mistargeting as a persuasive technique. *Clinical Psychological Science, 3*(2), 242–255. https://doi.org/10.1177/2167702614542846

Siegel, J. T., & Yzer, M. C. (2025). Maximizing mental health communication: The IIFF model of help-seeking for depression. In M. C. Yzer & J. T. Siegel (Eds.), *Handbook of mental health communication.* Wiley.

Stubbing, J., Tolin, D. F., Sain, K. S., Everhardt, K., Rudd, M. D., & Diefenbach, G. J. (2024). Borderline personality traits do not moderate the relationship between depression, beliefs, and suicidal thoughts and behaviors. *Archives of Suicide Research, 29*, 1–15. https://doi.org/10.1080/13811118.2024.2345168

Substance Abuse and Mental Health Services Administration. (2023). *Key substance use and mental health indicators in the United States: Results from the 2022 National Survey on Drug Use and Health* (HHS Publication No. PEP23-07-01-006, NSDUH Series H-58). Center for Behavioral Health Statistics and Quality, Substance Abuse and Mental Health Services Administration.

Thompson, M. M., Zanna, M. P., & Griffin, D. W. (1995). Let's not be indifferent about (attitudinal) ambivalence. In R. E. Petty & J. A. Krosnick (Eds.), *Attitude-strength: Antecedents and consequences* (pp. 361–386). Lawrence Erlbaum Associates, Inc.

Tormala, Z. L. (2008). A new framework for resistance to persuasion: The resistance appraisals hypothesis. In W. D. Crano & R. Prislin (Eds.), *Attitudes and attitude change* (pp. 213–234). Psychology Press.

Tormala, Z. L. (2016). The role of certainty (and uncertainty) in attitudes and persuasion. *Current Opinion in Psychology, 10*, 6–11. https://doi.org/10.1016/j.copsyc.2015.10.017

Tormala, Z. L., Briñol, P., & Petty, R. E. (2006). When credibility attacks: The reverse impact of source credibility on persuasion. *Journal of Experimental Social Psychology, 42*(6), 684–691. https://doi.org/10.1016/j.jesp.2005.10.005

Tormala, Z. L., & Petty, R. E. (2002). What doesn't kill me makes me stronger: The effects of resisting persuasion on attitude certainty. *Journal of Personality and Social Psychology, 83*(6), 1298–1313. https://doi.org/10.1037//0022-3514.83.6.1298

Tormala, Z. L., & Rucker, D. D. (2007). Attitude certainty: A review of past findings and emerging perspectives. *Social and Personality Psychology Compass, 1*(1), 469–492. https://doi.org/10.1111/j.1751-9004.2007.00025.x

Tormala, Z. L., & Rucker, D. D. (2018). Attitude certainty: Antecedents, consequences, and new directions. *Consumer Psychology Review, 1*(1), 72–89. https://doi.org/10.1002/arcp.1004

Visser, P. S., Bizer, G. Y., & Krosnick, J. A. (2006). Exploring the latent structure of strength-related attitude antecedents. *Advances in Experimental Social Psychology, 38*, 1–67. https://doi.org/10.1016/S0065-2601(06)38001-X

Visser, P. S., Krosnick, J. A., & Norris, C. J. (2017). Attitude importance and attitude-relevant knowledge: Motivator and enabler. In J. A. Krosnick, I.-C. A. Chiang, & T. H. Stark (Eds.), *Political psychology: New explorations* (pp. 203–245). Routledge/Taylor & Francis Group.

Wegener, D. T., Downing, J., Krosnick, J. A., & Petty, R. E. (1995). Measures and manipulations of strength-related properties of attitudes: Current practice and future directions. In R. E. Petty & J. A. Krosnick (Eds.), *Attitude-strength: Antecedents and consequences* (pp. 455–487). Lawrence Erlbaum Associates, Inc.

Wiglesworth, A., Abate, J. P., & Klimes-Dougan, B. (2021). Suicide prevention public service announcements: Recall biases associated with increased risk for suicide. *Crisis: The Journal of Crisis Intervention and Suicide Prevention, 42*(6), 448–454. https://doi.org/10.1027/0227-5910/a000744

Wisco, B. E. (2009). Depressive cognition: Self-reference and depth of processing. *Clinical Psychology Review, 29*(4), 382–392. https://doi.org/10.1016/j.cpr.2009.03.003

World Health Organization. (2023). *Depressive disorder (depression)* https://www.who.int/news-room/fact-sheets/detail/depression

Yzer, M., Kinzer, H., & Mallone, M. (2022). A reasoned action approach to depression help-seeking messaging for college students: Implications of cognitive biases in depression. *Health Communication, 37*(14), 1731–1739. https://doi.org/10.1080/10410236.2021.1917744

Yzer, M. C., & Siegel, J. T. (2025). Cognitive biases in depression: Implications for help-seeking messaging. In G. J. de Bruijn & H. Vandebosch (Eds.), *Health, media, and communication* (pp. 391–410). De Gruyter Mouton. https://doi.org/10.1515/9783110775426-021

Part VII

Lessons Learned

29

My Third Child: The Journal *Health Communication* and Some Lessons for Mental Health Communication

Teresa L. Thompson
University of Dayton and University of Kansas-Edwards

I have three children: Alyse is 36, Tony is 32, and the journal *Health Communication* is 35. I started accepting submissions for *Health Communication* (*HC*) when I was pregnant with Alyse. The first issue of the journal came out shortly after Alyse turned one. I once told Eileen Berlin Ray that if I was ever lucky enough to have a second baby, I would probably need to stop editing the journal. But, apparently, by the time Tony was born I had learned enough about editing a journal to keep going even though I had two human children. I have long thought of *HC* as my third child, as it grew as my children did. I hope, therefore, that I can be forgiven for my emphasis on scholarship that has been published in this journal as I present a few thoughts on mental health communication.

I have been studying and teaching about health communication for a long time. My early scholarship focused on communication and disability issues, which merged into the new area of study that we call health communication in the early 1980s. I first began receiving submissions for the journal for which I served as the founding and long-term editor, *Health Communication*, in Fall 1987. As I write this essay, I am in my last year as editor-in-chief of the journal. I have coedited three editions of the *Routledge Handbook of Health Communication*, the three-volume, 600-entry *Sage Encyclopedia of Health Communication*, and a volume on health communication theory as well as writing or editing several other books and many articles. During that time, I have heard a lot of discussion of the need to study the communicative dimensions of mental health. Over those many years, however, very little was done about actually studying mental health. I am sure that it was 20 or 30 years ago that I first heard such an inquiry suggested, again by Eileen Berlin Ray. And now we finally have a book that begins to provide this focus for us!

I am especially pleased to be participating in this volume because I was the person who first suggested to the publisher that there was a need for a book on this topic. Wiley/Blackwell had published the book that I mentioned earlier on health communication theory and I was zooming with Nicole Allen from Wiley when she asked for my ideas about other books that were needed in the field of health communication. I suggested this topic and that she contact Marco Yzer about it. Marco and I had been communicating about scholarship on this topic for many years and I knew of his expertise and interest in mental health communication. We both knew of Jason Siegel's work in the area, as well, and Jason quickly became involved. Thus, I feel that I am in some ways the grandmother of this book. As being a grandmother (I am called Mimi by my four wonderful grandbabies) is my favorite role EVER in life, thinking of myself as the grandmother of this book brings great joy to me. You can see that I am on a roll with family metaphors . . . !

The Handbook of Mental Health Communication, First Edition.
Edited by Marco C. Yzer and Jason T. Siegel.

In this essay, however, I would like to share with you some of the lessons that I have learned about health communication scholarship as well as mention various topics related to mental health communication that the journal *Health Communication* has covered in the 36 years I have been editing it. I will also make note of some directions that I would like to see research move toward in the future. I apologize in advance that this review will not be inclusive of all the important work that has been conducted; there is too much good work for me to adequately cover it here. I encourage you to read the various flagship health communication journals to broaden your horizons on this scholarship.

The Early Years

The field of communication and the corresponding subfield of health communication encompass study on a variety of contexts, including interpersonal, organizational, mass-mediated, rhetorical, performance, instructional, intercultural, political, and applied communication. Mental health issues are related to all of these, but the emphasis of the present volume is appropriately on that aspect of health communication that has been the subject of more scholarship than the other areas: mass-mediated communication. As a side note, I should mention that the early years of the study of mental health and communication did include a more interpersonal focus, in that some of it was grounded in the perspective that came out of the work of Gregory Bateson and those who studied with him. This is exemplified by the ground-breaking volume *The Pragmatics of Human Communication* (Watzlawick et al., 1967). The principles of communication defined within that volume were foundational for how we as a field have come to look at the constitutive nature of communicative processes (although the term "constitutive" was not used in that book) and have direct and important application to our understanding of communication and mental health. The perspective, however, with its discussion of the relational dimension of communication, led us to look at how relationships are created by communication.

This Batesonian perspective primarily drew the attention of interpersonal scholars and very early health communication scholars. This influence is made evident when we note that the early discussions among those who founded the Health Communication Division of the International Communication Association in the late 1970s evidenced that they were torn between labeling it "health communication," "medical communication," and "therapeutic communication." The potential name "therapeutic communication" brings with it an understanding of communicative processes as they relate to not only therapy but also families/relationships and mental health. An examination of the *Pragmatics* book also makes this clear. The volume is based upon a systemic, cybernetic conceptualization and is where the oft-cited axiom, "One cannot not communicate" comes from Watzlawick et al. (1967, p. 48). The tradition of the inclusion of mental health issues in the study of interpersonal communication is, thus, also a long one, but has not been the focus of as much scholarship in recent years as has mass-mediated mental health communication.

Before we turn to the various contexts in which mental health communication has been studied, I should mention one of the important concepts that has been addressed in the health communication scholarship. This is the need for a context-specific focus on "mental health literacy" (Jorm, 2015). The notion of health literacy is an important one in the field and narrowing this focus to an emphasis on mental health "has had policy impacts and led to the development of interventions" and assessments that, Jorm (2015, p. 1166) asserts, likely would not have otherwise occurred.

Other Contexts of Mental Health Communication

Although it is unlikely that many would argue that mental health issues are uniquely relevant to mass-mediated channels of communication, it is probably indisputable that mass communication plays an important role in the lives of those living in most areas of the globe. Future volumes and scholars will focus their attention on those other contexts of communication that are also fundamental to our understanding of the role of health communication and mental health. Let me mention at this point, however, some scholarship that has looked at other contexts of communication, just to spark the attention of the reader. Some of these studies are not context specific, whereas others are focused upon a particular channel or context. Again, the studies I will mention are, I hope, representative rather than inclusive of the scholarship on mental health communication.

A recent important piece on the theoretical grounding of interpersonal health communication-related mental health interventions (Caban et al., 2022) reported that very few of the interventions were grounded in theory. This is an important limitation that must be rectified in future work and has been overcome in some mental health communication scholarship. Exemplary theoretical approaches are evident in W. Shi et al.'s (2023) application of the reasoned action approach to social connection and mental health and J. Shi and Kim's (2019) use of the risk perception attitude framework and the theory of planned behavior to predict mental health promotion behaviors in young adults, for instance. Several other studies that are discussed here are also framed in theory. Another study taking a broader focus on seeking help for mental health concerns, although the target population was military service members, is work by Clark-Hitt et al. (2011) on message creation. This work is applicable to all channels and contexts of communication, but the presentation of the results is organized around source, message, channel, and receiver factors. Similarly, Segrin et al. (2021) looked at neighborhood disadvantage and mental health, bringing a parallel mediation model to examine social support and negative emotionality.

Focusing more specifically on families, a particularly important context for mental health scholarship, we have seen work examining adolescents' disclosure of mental health concerns to parents (Rasmussen et al., 2022), on the dilemmas families face in talking with returning military service members about seeking professional help for mental health issues (Wilson et al., 2014), and that on memorable messages about mental health (Greenwell, 2019) as well as parental memorable messages about depression (Flood-Grady et al., 2021). Flood-Grady and Koenig (2018) have also studied the narratives about mental health told in families. In other interpersonal contexts, memorable messages as they relate to resilience and mental health (Kuang et al., 2023), narratives of mental health among migrant domestic workers (Kaur-Gill & Dutta, 2021), coping for partners of those with mental health conditions (Acevedo Callejas & Thompson, 2017), and client–clinician shared decision making about psychotropic mediations (Mikesell et al., 2016) have been studied. Also related to the therapeutic context is work on patient-centered communication in equine-assisted mental health (Nieforth & Craig, 2021) and breaking down barriers in pediatric mental health consultation, with a particular focus on patients' use of "I don't know" (Hesson & Pichler, 2017).

Taking an intercultural focus is work on Chinese international students and help-seeking for mental health (Ma et al., 2022), undocumented students' willingness to talk to a mental health professional (Kam et al., 2022), the role of communication perceptions in the mental health of older adults in Thailand and the United States (Keaton et al., 2016), as well as the willingness of Muslim immigrant women in Canada to talk about mental health issues (Ahmed & Mao, 2023). In the political communication context, we know that US presidential candidates communicate about mental health by "swapping insults, neglecting policy" (Parrott & Allen, 2023). Moving on to the organizational communication context, we see work by Wu and Chen (2024) on leadership health support on employee mental health during crises.

As is apparent in many of the chapters in this volume, mental health stigma is a frequent focus of research. It has been examined in veterans with PTSD (Roscoe, 2021), in the children of incarcerated parents (Kumar, 2023), in families in which a parent is an alcoholic (Haverfield & Theiss, 2015), as it influences responses to favor requests (Imai & Dailey, 2015), in terms of how interactivity of a medium influences mental health stigma (Kim & Stout, 2010), in pro-anorexia websites (Chang & Bazarova, 2016; Yeshua-Katz & Martin, 2013), as well as in studies examining suicide stigma in online social interaction (An & Lee, 2019) and as influenced by attributions of cause (Lee & An, 2015). Related to and strongly influenced by stigma is disclosure about mental health within friendships (Chernichky-Karcher et al., 2022) and to family and friends (Wilson et al., 2021).

Suicide, an important mental health issue, is one of the topics that has been most frequently studied in the mental health communication scholarship. Coverage of suicide by the press has frequently been discussed in the health communication literature, as it influences copy-cat suicides. This topic is thoroughly covered by Niederkrotenthaler et al. (2025).

Mass-Mediated Contexts

In addition to the topics covered within this volume, the journal *Health Communication* has published articles on several aspects of mass communication as they relate to mental health. Some of these focus on traditional/legacy media (see, for instance, Wang's 2020 study of depression as a primary versus an incidental topic in important US media outlets and her 2017 comparison of depression coverage in US versus Spanish outlets), but more examine electronic or other social media or the arts. Research has looked at how mental health information is optimally presented on social media (Quintero Johnson et al., 2016); peer support for mental health concerns in advocacy groups' social media messages (Smith-Frigerio, 2020); at how mental illness is discussed on social media in China (Wang & Liu, 2015); the perceived helpfulness of mental illness information in Australia (Graham et al., 2017); how mental health is defined by what was formerly called Twitter, focusing on frames, emotions, and stigma (Pavlova & Berkers, 2020); the "gobbledygook" published in parent-focused online information about kids' mental health (Wozney et al., 2017); mothers' self-discrepancy and postpartum mental health as related to exposure to online parenting content (Sun et al., 2022), how Black, Indigenous, and People of Color young adults perceive and engage with the media (To et al., 2023); and sharing on social network sites following Carrie Fisher's death (Hoffner, 2019). In addition to Carrie Fisher, scholarship has looked at the mental health-related outcomes of Robin Williams' death, examining parasocial relations and media exposure (Hoffner & Cohen, 2017) and reactions to Kid Cudi's disclosure of depression (Francis, 2019). Some of the work looks at mental health as it relates to enjoyment of Facebook use (Kaufmann et al., 2016), video streamers' mental health disclosures as they affect viewers' risk perceptions (Lee et al., 2020), and mental health organizations' use of visuals on Instagram (Jia et al., 2023). Note the interesting emphasis in several of these studies on parents', especially mothers', mental health.

Another notable emphasis on mental health communication research is apparent in scholarship on news that covers mass shootings (Zhang, 2020). Such research has focused on perceived media bias and intention to engage in discursive activities for mental health (Zhang, 2020) and framing mass shootings as a public health crisis (DeFoster & Swalve, 2017). Olufowote and Matusitz (2016) examined how the clergy framed the Sandy Hook shootings in the United States. Work has also looked at several aspects of mental illness interventions, including computerized mental health programs (Kuosmanen et al., 2017)

Yet other research has examined the representations of mental health in various modes of art, as exemplified by the work of Kresovich (2020). This research looked at pop songs referencing anxiety, depression, and suicidal ideation as the songs influence mental health empathy, stigma, and behavioral intentions.

Some Possible Directions

One of the developments I would like to see in future research on mental health communication is a change from just encouraging message receivers to "seek help" to instead urge people to seek specific kinds of help. Incorporation of such a view would be more helpful than current campaigns/messages typically emphasize. The implication of many messages is that searching for help means seeking counseling but such advice is rather broad. What kind of counseling could be sought? As we focus on the various avenues through which counseling may be extended more specificity may be appropriate. We have numerous online counseling options available, which are likely to be more appealing to some individuals and less appealing to others. Targeting and tailoring of messages is appropriate as these messages are constructed. The many approaches that are now commonly used in campaigns research would be useful for mental health-seeking research. The "Promising Strategies" section of the present volume provides relevant suggestions for this work.

Relatedly, message research needs to emphasize the possible success or impact of various approaches. Many individuals know that they need help with their mental health concerns but must be convinced that counseling will actually provide that help. What theoretical frameworks that focus on persuasion/behavior change can be used to convince individuals that counseling ***can*** help them? Similarly, what message strategies might convince people of the value of social support in coping with mental health issues?

As noted earlier, the field of health communication has many roots in the study of therapeutic interaction. We have yet to adequately embrace and build upon those early directions in scholarship to focus upon what actually goes on during therapeutic interaction, however. These are communicative interactions, but we as communication scholars have contributed little to an understanding of such processes and could do much more. Conversation Analytic work would be promising in the examination of these processes.

Theoretical Directions

There are many theoretical approaches related to persuasion, mass communication, and interpersonal communication that would be appropriate to apply to our understanding of mental health communication. The theories that are commonly used by health communication scholars are summarized in Thompson and Schulz's (2021) *Health Communication Theory*. Some of the theories that I will mention were primarily developed by one or one group of scholars, so I will identify them by the name of that scholar or scholars. Others encompass multiple conceptualizations, so I will not limit my mention of them to a particular scholar but will provide a relevant citation for interested readers.

Particularly relevant theories include such interpersonal perspectives as Giles's (2016) communication accommodation theory, Petronio's (Petronio & Sargent, 2011) communication privacy management theory, and Waldron's (Waldron & Kelley, 2015) theory of negotiated morality. Theories such as the double ABCX model of family stress and coping (McCubbin & Patterson, 1983), Olson's (1993) circumplex model of marital and family systems, LePoire's (1995) inconsistent nurturing as control perspective, and Floyd's (2001) affection exchange theory pertain particularly to family communication contexts. Also focusing on an interpersonal level are such theories as those on Charon's (2006) view on narrative medicine, argumentation theory (Labrie & Schulz, 2014), Millar and Rogers' (1987) relational communication model, Baxter's (1990) focus on dialectical tensions, Smith's (2007) stigma theory, and Meisenbach's (2010) stigma management communication theory.

Moving to a focus on information-processing and cognitive theories, we have available to us such perspectives as the multiple motive heuristic systematic model, attribution theory, the health belief model, Rimal and Real's (2003) risk perception attitude framework, Griffin et al.'s (1999) risk information seeking and processing model, and Kahlor's (2010) planned risk information seeking model. As we are focusing in part on attitude and behavior change, various theories of affective impact are also relevant. These include Brehm and Brehm's (1981) psychological reactance theory, Festinger's (1957) dissonance theory, and fear-based theories such as Rogers' (1975) protection motivation theory and Witte's (1992) extended parallel process model. The theories of affective impact also represent action tendency emotions, such as anger and hope. More general theories of emotional influence are also available, including Nabi's (1999) cognitive-functional model as well as her emotions as frames (Nabi, 2003) and emotional flow models (Nabi, 2015).

As we attempt to influence behavior, we may apply such perspectives as Bandura's social cognitive theory, Fishbein and Ajzen's (2010) reasoned action theory and theory of planned behavior (1975), and Prochaska and DiClemente's (1983) transtheoretical model of behavior change. Applicable to message effects are such theories as McCombs and Shaw's (1972) work on agenda setting, Gerbner et al.'s (2002) cultivation theory, the narrative engagement framework (Miller-Day & Hecht, 2013), framing theory (O'Keefe & Jensen, 2007), inoculation theory (McGuire, 1964), uses and gratifications theory (Katz et al., 1974), and media complementarity theory (Dutta-Bergman, 2004). Broader social psychological theoretical frameworks include Rogers' (2003) diffusion of innovation conceptualization, Sherif and Hovland's (1961) social judgment theory, Ryan and Deci's (2000) self-determination theory, and Festinger's (1954) social comparison theory.

A fundamental process affecting all health communication is uncertainty. Various theories on this concept that could be applied to our understanding of mental health communication include the harm reduction framework, Brashers' (2001) uncertainty management theory, Afifi's (2015) theory of motivated information management, and Babrow's (1992) problematic integration theory. Cultural theories that are useful for our understanding of health communication are represented by various ecological perspectives (Street, 2003) as well as work on culture as critique (Lupton, 1994). Most notable in the study of health communication is Dutta's (2007) culture-centered approach.

In light of the broad application of digital media technology to our understanding of mental health communication, it is important to mention several theoretical cues and action routes. Notable among the cue routes is Sundar's (2008a) MAIN (modality-agency-interactivity-navigability) model as well as the concept of social contagion developed by Christakis and Fowler (2013). This area of study also benefits from application of Yee et al.'s (2009) Proteus effect. The action route can be best understood by such theories as the agency model (Sundar, 2008b); the selective exposure self- and affect-management model (Knobloch-Westerwick, 2015); the motivational technology model (Sundar et al., 2012); gamification (Peng et al., 2012), which builds on self-determination theory; Sundar's (2007) interactivity effects model; and the notion of captology (Fogg, 2003).

Conclusion

The study of mental health communication has come far in the 10–15 years in which scholars have been studying it, but there is much work that is still needed. It is hoped that a considerable amount of this work can be based on the theoretical perspectives that have been mentioned in the final portion of this chapter. Reliance on theory rather than a focus on problem increases the generalizability and application of work. Although we normally think of generalizability as being based on sampling and ecological validity, scholarship that is grounded in theory can be applied to other contexts to which the theoretical framework is also relevant. Such an approach will greatly increase the value of our work and the contributions we can make to an understanding of mental health communication.

I started editing *HC* when I had my first child. Mental health communication (MHC) is starting to burgeon as my grandchildren, Connor, Coco, Miles, and Evie, are starting to grow. Perhaps I am MHC's grandparent. Without *HC*, there would not be MHC. MHC is the child of my children.

As I retire from my *HC* editorship, MHC is indeed like having a grandchild. I get to have all the fun but none of the responsibility. I hope that I have earned the privilege of sitting back and watching MHC grow without any day-to-day headaches. In other words, I can watch MHC blossom while relaxing, knowing that others are responsible for changing the diapers.

References

Acevedo Callejas, M. L., & Thompson, C. M. (2017). Stress, frequency of challenges, and coping for partners of individuals with mental health conditions. *Health Communication*, *32*(7), 880–889. https://doi.org/10.1080/10410236.2016.1196408

Afifi, W. A. (2015). Theory of motivated information management. In C. R. Berger & M. E. Roloff (Eds.), *International encyclopedia of interpersonal communication* (pp. 1756–1765). Wiley Blackwell.

Ahmed, R., & Mao, Y. (2023). An intersectional approach to understanding beliefs and attitudes toward mental health issues among Muslim immigrant women in Canada. *Health Communication*, 1–12. https://doi.org/10.1080/10410236.2023.2252644

An, S., & Lee, H. (2019). Suicide stigma in online social interactions: Impacts of social capital and suicide literacy. *Health Communication*, *34*(11), 1340–1349. https://doi.org/10.1080/10410236.2018.1486691

Babrow, A. S. (1992). Communication and problematic integration: Understanding diverging probability and value, ambiguity, ambivalence, and impossibility. *Communication Theory*, *2*(2), 95–130. https://doi.org/10.1111/j.1468-2885.1992.tb00031.x

Baxter, L. A. (1990). Dialectical contradictions in relationship development. *Journal of Social and Personal Relationships*, *7*(1), 69–88. https://doi.org/10.1177/0265407590071004

Brashers, D. E. (2001). Communication and uncertainty management. *Journal of Communication*, *51*(3), 477–497. https://doi.org/10.1111/j.1460-2466.2001.tb02892.x

Brehm, S. S., & Brehm, J. W. (1981). *Psychological reactance: A theory of freedom and control*. Academic Press.

Caban, S., Makos, S., & Thompson, C. M. (2022). The role of interpersonal communication in mental health literacy interventions for young people: A theoretical review. *Health Communication*, *38*(13), 2818–2832. https://doi.org/10.1080/10410236.2022.2121473

Chang, P. F., & Bazarova, N. N. (2016). Managing stigma: Disclosure-response communication patterns in aro-anorexic websites. *Health Communication*, *31*(2), 217–229. https://doi.org/10.1080/10410236.2014.946218

Charon, R. (2006). *Narrative medicine: Honoring the stories of illness*. Oxford University Press.

Chernichky-Karcher, S., Venetis, M. K., & Getting, P. E. (2022). Revealing mental health information in friendships: The role of disclosure strategy and perceived recipient response on disclosure outcomes. *Health Communication*, *37*(7), 909–918. https://doi.org/10.1080/10410236.2021.1876325

Christakis, N. A., & Fowler, J. H. (2013). Social contagion theory: Examining dynamic social networks and human behavior. *Statistics in Medicine*, *32*(4), 556–577. https://doi.org/10.1002/sim.5408

Clark-Hitt, R., Smith, S. W., & Broderick, J. S. (2011). Help a buddy take a knee: Creating persuasive messages for military service members to encourage others to seek mental health help. *Health Communication*, *27*(5), 429–438. https://doi.org/10.1080/10410236.2011.606525

DeFoster, R., & Swalve, N. (2017). Guns, culture or mental health? Framing mass shootings as a public health crisis. *Health Communication*, *33*(10), 1211–1222. https://doi.org/10.1080/10410236.2017.1350907

Dutta, M. J. (2007). Communicating about culture and health: Theorizing culture-centered and cultural sensitivity approaches. *Communication Theory*, *17*(3), 304–328. https://doi.org/10.1111/j.1468-2885.2007.00297.x

Dutta-Bergman, M. J. (2004). Interpersonal communication after 9/11 via telephone and internet: A theory of channel complementarity. *New Media & Society*, *6*(5), 659–673. https://doi.org/10.1177/146144804047086

Festinger, L. (1954). A theory of social comparison processes. *Human Relations*, *7*, 117–140. https://doi.org/10.1177/001872675400700202

Festinger, L. (1957). *A theory of cognitive dissonance*. Stanford University Press.

Fishbein, M., & Ajzen, I. (1975). *Belief, attitude, intention, and behavior: An introduction to theory and research*. Addison-Wesley.

Fishbein, M., & Ajzen, I. (2010). *Predicting and changing behavior: The reasoned action approach*. Psychology Press.

Flood-Grady, E., & Koenig Kellas, J. (2018). Sense-making, socialization, and stigma: Exploring narratives told in families about mental illness. *Health Communication*, *34*(6), 607–617. https://doi.org/10.1080/10410236.2018.1431016

Flood-Grady, E., Starcher, S. C., & Bergquist, G. L. (2021). Parental memorable messages about depression: Implications for perceived support, stigma, relational satisfaction, and treatment-seeking among young adults with depression. *Health Communication*, *38*(1), 11–20. https://doi.org/10.1080/10410236.2021.1926108

Floyd, K. (2001). Human affection exchange: I. Reproductive probability as a predictor of men's affection with their sons. *Journal of Men's Studies*, *10*(1), 39–50. https://doi.org/10.3149/jms.1001.39

Fogg, B. J. (2003). *Persuasive technology: Using computers to change what we think and do*. Morgan Kaufmann.

Francis, D. B. (2019). "Twitter is really therapeutic at times": Examination of Black men's Twitter conversations following hip-hop artist kid Cudi's depression disclosure. *Health Communication*, *36*(4), 448–456. https://doi.org/10.1080/10410236.2019.1700436

Gerbner, G., Gross, L., Morgan, M., Signorielli, N., & Shanahan, J. (2002). Growing up with television: Cultivation processes. In J. Bryant & D. Zillmann (Eds.), *Media effects: Advances in theory and research* (2nd ed., pp. 43–67). Lawrence Erlbaum.

Giles, H. (2016). *Communication accommodation theory: Negotiating personal relationships and social identities across contexts*. Cambridge University Press.

Graham, A. L., Brooker, J., Hasking, P., Clarke, D., & Meadows, G. (2017). Receipt and perceived helpfulness of mental illness information: Findings from the Australian National Survey of Mental Health Wellbeing. *Health Communication*, *34*(1), 39–45. https://doi.org/10.1080/10410236.2017.1384355

Greenwell, M. R. (2019). Memorable messages from family members about mental health: Young adult perceptions of relational closeness, message satisfaction, and clinical help-seeking attitudes. *Health Communication*, *34*(6), 652–660. https://doi.org/10.1080/10410236.2018.1431021

Griffin, R. J., Dunwoody, S., & Neuwirth, K. (1999). Proposed model of the relationship of risk information seeking and processing to the development of preventive behaviors. *Environmental Research*, *80*(2 Pt 2), S230–S245. https://doi.org/10.1006/enrs.1998.3940

Haverfield, M. C., & Theiss, J. A. (2015). Parent's alcoholism severity and family topic avoidance about alcohol as predictors of perceived stigma among adult children of alcoholics: Implications for emotional and psychological resilience. *Health Communication*, *31*(5), 606–616. https://doi.org/10.1080/10410236.2014.981665

Hesson, A. M., & Pichler, H. (2017). Breaking down barriers in pediatric mental health consultations: Understanding patients' use of I DON'T KNOW. *Health Communication*, *33*(7), 867–876. https://doi.org/10.1080/10410236.2017.1321160

Hoffner, C. A. (2019). Sharing on social network sites following Carrie Fisher's death: Responses to her mental health advocacy. *Health Communication*, *35*(12), 1475–1486. https://doi.org/10.1080/10410236.2019.1652383

Hoffner, C. A., & Cohen, E. L. (2017). Mental health-related outcomes of Robin Williams' death: The role of parasocial relations and media exposure in stigma, help-seeking, and outreach. *Health Communication*, *33*(12), 1573–1582. https://doi.org/10.1080/10410236.2017.1384348

Imai, T., & Dailey, R. (2015). Influences of mental illness stigma on perceptions of and responses to requests for favors. *Health Communication*, *31*(7), 863–872. https://doi.org/10.1080/10410236.2015.1012630

Jia, M., Ju, R., & Zhu, J. (2023). Understanding mental health organizations' Instagram through visuals: A content analysis. *Health Communication*, *39*(4), 767–777. https://doi.org/10.1080/10410236.2023.2185350

Jorm, A. F. (2015). Why we need the concept of "Mental health literacy.". *Health Communication*, *30*(12), 1166–1168. https://doi.org/10.1080/10410236.2015.1037423

Kahlor, L. (2010). PRISM: A planned risk information seeking model. *Health Communication*, *25*(4), 345–356. http://dx.doi.org/10.1080/10410231003775172

Kam, J., Mendez Murillo, R., Cornejo, M., & Mendoza, N. (2022). The importance of norms and efficacy in predicting undocumented college students' intentions to talk to an on-campus mental health professional. *Health Communication*, *37*(2), 230–241. https://doi.org/10.1080/10410236.2020.1834208

Katz, E., Blumler, J. G., & Gurevitch, M. (1974). Utilization of mass communication by the individual. In J. G. Blumbler & E. Katz (Eds.), *The uses of mass communications: Current perspectives on gratifications research* (pp. 19–34). Sage.

Kaufmann, R., Buckner, M. M., & Ledbetter, A. M. (2016). Having fun on Facebook?: Mothers' enjoyment as a moderator of mental health and Facebook use. *Health Communication*, *32*(8), 1014–1023. https://doi.org/10.1080/10410236.2016.1196513

Kaur-Gill, S., & Dutta, M. J. (2021). Structure as depressant: Theorizing narratives of mental health among migrant domestic workers. *Health Communication*, *36*(12), 1464–1475. https://doi.org/10.1080/10410236.2020.1767448

Keaton, S. A., McCann, R. M., & Giles, H. (2016). The role of communication perceptions in the mental health of older adults: Views from Thailand and the United States. *Health Communication*, *32*(1), 92–102. https://doi.org/10.1080/10410236.2015.1099507

Kim, H., & Stout, P. A. (2010). The effects of interactivity on information processing and attitude change: Implications for mental health stigma. *Health Communication*, *25*(2), 142–154. https://doi.org/10.1080/10410230903544936

Knobloch-Westerwick, S. (2015). The selective exposure self- and affect-management (SESAM) model: Applications in the realms of race, politics, and health. *Communication Research*, *42*(7), 959–985. https://doi.org/10.1177/0093650214539173

Kresovich, A. (2020). The influence of pop songs referencing anxiety, depression, and suicidal ideation on college students' mental health empathy, stigma, and behavioral intentions. *Health Communication*, *37*(5), 617–627. https://doi.org/10.1080/10410236.2020.1859724

Kuang, K., Tian, Z., Wilson, S. R., & Buzzanell, P. M. (2023). Memorable messages as anticipatory resilience: Examining associations among memorable messages, communication resilience processes, and mental health. *Health Communication*, *38*(6), 1136–1145. https://doi.org/10.1080/10410236.2021.1993585

Kumar, R. (2023). Agency and identity negotiations of "good DNA" by children with incarcerated parents amidst stigmatizing mental health structures: A culture-centered analysis. *Health Communication*, *39*(6), 1140–1148. https://doi.org/10.1080/10410236.2023.2207239

Kuosmanen, T., Fleming, T. M., & Barry, M. M. (2017). Using computerized mental health programs in alternative education: Understanding the requirements of students and staff. *Health Communication*, *33*(6), 753–761. https://doi.org/10.1080/10410236.2017.1309620

Labrie, N., & Schulz, P. (2014). Does argumentation matter? A systematic literature review on the role of argumentation in doctor-patient communication. *Health Communication*, *29*(10), 996–1008. https://doi.org/10.1080/10410236.2013.829018

Lee, H., & An, S. (2015). Social stigma toward suicide: Effects of group categorization and attributions in Korean health news. *Health Communication*, *31*(4), 468–477. https://doi.org/10.1080/10410236.2014.966894

Lee, Y. H., Yuan, C. W., & Wohn, D. Y. (2020). How video streamers' mental health disclosures affect viewers' risk perceptions. *Health Communication*, *36*(14), 1931–1941. http://dx.doi.org/10.1080/10410236.2020.1808405

LePoire, B. (1995). Inconsistent nurturing as control theory: Implications for communication-based research and treatment programs. *Journal of Applied Communication Research*, *23*(1), 60–74. https://doi.org/10.1080/00909889509365414

Lupton, D. (1994). Toward the development of critical health communication praxis. *Health Communication*, *6*(1), 55–67. https://doi.org/10.1207/s15327027hc0601_4

Ma, S., Zhu, Y., & Bresnahan, M. (2022). Chinese international students' face concerns, self-stigma, linguistic factors, and help-seeking intentions for mental health. *Health Communication*, *37*(13), 1631–1639. https://doi.org/10.1080/10410236.2021.1910167

McCombs, M. E., & Shaw, D. L. (1972). The agenda-setting function of mass media. *Public Opinion Quarterly*, *36*(2), 176–187. http://www.jstor.org/stable/2747787

McCubbin, H. I., & Patterson, J. (1983). The family stress process: The double ABCX model of adjustment and adaptation. In H. McCubbin, M. Sussman, & J. Patterson (Eds.), *Social stress and the family: Advances and developments in the family stress theory and research* (pp. 7–37). Haworth Press.

McGuire, W. J. (1964). Inducing resistance to persuasion: Some contemporary approaches. In L. Berkowitz (Ed.), *Advances in experimental social psychology* (Vol. 1, pp. 191–220). Academic Press.

Meisenbach, R. J. (2010). Stigma management communication: A theory and agenda for applied research on how individuals manage moments of stigmatized identity. *Journal of Applied Communication Research, 38*(3), 268–292. https://doi.org/10.1080/00909882.2010.490841

Mikesell, L., Bromley, E., Young, A. S., Vona, P., & Zima, B. (2016). Integrating client and clinician perspectives on psychotropic medication decisions: Developing a communication-centered epistemic model of shared decision making for mental health contexts. *Health Communication, 31*(6), 707–717. https://doi.org/10.1080/10410236.2014.993296

Millar, F. E., & Rogers, L. E. (1987). Relational dimensions of interpersonal dynamics. In M. E. Roloff & G. R. Miller (Eds.), *Interpersonal processes: New directions in communication research* (pp. 117–139). Sage.

Miller-Day, M., & Hecht, M. L. (2013). Narrative means to preventative ends: A narrative engagement framework for designing prevention interventions. *Health Communication, 28*(7), 657–670. https://doi.org/10.1080/10410236.2012.762861

Nabi, R. (1999). A cognitive-functional model for the effects of discrete negative emotions on information processing, attitude change, and recall. *Communication Theory, 9*(3), 292–320. https://doi.org/10.1111/j.1468-2885.1999.tb00172.x

Nabi, R. L. (2003). Exploring the framing effects of emotion: Do discrete emotions differentially influence information accessibility, information seeking, and policy preference? *Communication Research, 30*(2), 224–247. https://doi.org/10.1177/0093650202250881

Nabi, R. L. (2015). Emotional flow in persuasive health messages. *Health Communication, 30*(2), 114–124. https://doi.org/10.1080/10410236.2014.974129

Niederkrotenthaler, T., Kirchner, S., Till, B., Nicholas, A., Ftanou, M., & Pirkis, J. (2025). Suicide prevention media campaigns: An application of the *Papageno effect*. In M. C. Yzer & J. T. Siegel (Eds.), *Handbook of mental health communication*. Wiley.

Nieforth, L. O., & Craig, E. A. (2021). Patient-centered communication (PCC) in equine assisted mental health. *Health Communication, 36*(13), 1656–1665. https://doi.org/10.1080/10410236.2020.1785376

O'Keefe, D. J., & Jensen, J. D. (2007). The relative persuasiveness of gain-framed and loss-framed messages for encouraging disease prevention behaviors: A meta-analytic review. *Journal of Health Communication, 12*(7), 623–644. https://doi.org/10.1080/10810730701615198

Olson, D. H. (1993). Circumplex model of marital and family systems: Assessing family functioning. In F. Walsh (Ed.), *Normative family processes* (pp. 104–137). Guilford.

Olufowote, J. O., & Matusitz, J. (2016). "How dark a world it is . . . where mental health is poorly treated": Mental illness frames in sermons given after the Sandy Hook shootings. *Health Communication, 31*(12), 1539–1547. https://doi.org/10.1080/10410236.2015.1089458

Parrott, S., & Allen, H. C. (2023). Swapping insults, neglecting policy: How U.S. presidential candidates communicate about mental health. *Health Communication, 38*(5), 866–874. https://doi.org/10.1080/10410236.2921.1989252

Pavlova, A., & Berkers, P. (2020). "Mental health" as defined by Twitter: Frames, emotions, stigma. *Health Communication, 37*(5), 637–647. https://doi.org/10.1080/10410236.2020.1862396

Peng, W., Lin, J.-H., Pfeiffer, K. A., & Winn, B. (2012). Need satisfaction supportive game features as motivational determinants: An experimental study of a self-determination theory guided exergame. *Media Psychology, 15*(2), 175–196. https://doi.org/10.1080/15213269.2012.673850

Petronio, S., & Sargent, J. (2011). Disclosure predicaments arising during the course of patient care: Nurses' privacy management. *Health Communication, 26*(3), 255–266. https://doi.org/10.1080/10410236.2010.549812

Prochaska, J. O., & DiClemente, C. C. (1983). Stages and processes of self-change of smoking: Toward an integration model of change. *Journal of Counseling and Clinical Psychology, 51*(3), 390–395. https://doi.org/10.1037//0022-006x.51.3.390

Quintero Johnson, J. M., Yilmaz, G., & Najarian, K. (2016). Optimizing the presentation of mental health information in social media: The effects of health testimonials and platform on source perceptions, message processing, and health outcomes. *Health Communication, 32*(9), 1121–1132. https://doi.org/10.1080/10410236.2016.1214218

Rasmussen, E. E., Shannon, K. L., & Pitchford, B. (2022). Adolescents' disclosure of mental illness to parents: Preferences and barriers. *Health Communication, 37*(3), 346–355. https://doi.org/10.1080/10410236.2020.1839201

Rimal, R. N., & Real, K. (2003). Perceived risk and efficacy beliefs as motivators of change: Use of the risk perception attitude (RPA) framework to understand health behaviors. *Human Communication Research, 29*(3), 370–399. https://doi.org/10.1093/hcr/29.3.370

Rogers, E. M. (2003). *Diffusion of innovations* (5th ed.). Free Press.

Rogers, R. W. (1975). A protection motivation theory of fear appeals and attitude change 1. *Journal of Psychology, 91*(1), 93–114. https://doi.org/10.1080/00223980.1975.9915803

Roscoe, R. A. (2021). The battle against mental health stigma: Examining how veterans with PTSD communicatively manage stigma. *Health Communication, 36*(11), 1378–1387. https://doi.org/10.1080/10410236.2020.1754587

Ryan, R. M., & Deci, E. L. (2000). Self-determination theory and the facilitation of intrinsic motivation, social development, and well-being. *American Psychologist, 55*(1), 68–78. https://doi.org/10.1037/0003-066X.55.1.68

Segrin, C., Jiao, J., & Cooper, R. A. (2021). Neighborhood disadvantage and mental health: Test of a parallel mediation model through social support and negative emotionality. *Health Communication, 37*(13), 1581–1589. https://doi.org/10.1080/10410236.2021.1903733

Sherif, M., & Hovland, C. I. (1961). *Social judgment: Assimilation and contrast effects in communication and attitude change.* Yale University Press.

Shi, J., & Kim, H. K. (2019). Integrating risk perception attitude framework and the theory of planned behavior to predict mental health promotion behaviors among young adults. *Health Communication, 35*(5), 597–606. https://doi.org/10.1080/10410236.2019.1573298

Shi, W., Donovan, E. E., Quaack, K. R., Mackert, M., Shaffer, A. L., De Luca, D. M., Nolan-Cody, H., & Yang, J. (2023). A reasoned action approach to social connection and mental health: Racial group differences and similarities in attitudes, norms, and intentions. *Health Communication, 1–14.* https://doi.org/10.1080/10410236.2023.2259690

Smith, R. A. (2007). Language of the lost: An explication of stigma communication. *Communication Theory, 17*(4), 462–485. https://doi.org/10.1111/j.1468-2885.2007.00307.x

Smith-Frigerio, S. (2020). "You are not alone": Linking peer support to information and resources for mental health concerns in advocacy groups' social media messaging. *Health Communication, 36*(14), 1980–1989. https://doi.org/10.1080/10410236.2020.1808415

Street, R. L. (2003). Communication medical encounters. An ecological perspective. In T. L. Thompson, A. M. Dorsey, K. I. Miller, & R. Parrott (Eds.), *Handbook of health communication* (pp. 63–89). Erlbaum.

Sun, Y., Chia, S. C., & Shi, Y. (2022). How exposure to online parenting content relates to mothers' self-discrepancy and postpartum mental health. *Health Communication, 38*(12), 2782–2794. https://doi.org/10.1080/10410236.2022.2114769

Sundar, S. (2007). Social psychology of interactivity in human-website interaction. In A. Johnson, K. McKenna, T. Postmes, & U.-D. Reips (Eds.), *The Oxford handbook of internet psychology* (pp. 89–104). Oxford University Press.

Sundar, S. (2008a). The MAIN model: A heuristic approach to understanding technology effects on credibility. In M. J. Metzger & A. J. Flanagin (Eds.), *Digital media, youth, and credibility* (pp. 73–100). MIT Press. https://doi.org/10.1162/dmal.9780262562324.073

Sundar, S. (2008b). Self as source: Agency and customization in interactive media. In E. Konijn, S. Uta, M. Tanis, & S. Barnes (Eds.), *Mediated interpersonal communication* (pp. 58–74). Routledge.

Sundar, S. S., Bellur, S., & Jia, H. (2012). Motivational technologies: A theoretical framework for designing preventive health applications. In M. Bang & E. L. Ragnemalm (Eds.), *Proceedings of the 7th international conference on persuasive technology* (pp. 112–122). Springer.

Thompson, T. L., & Schulz, P. J. (2021). *Health communication theory.* Wiley/Blackwell.

To, S. B., Gray, J., Jain, P., Porter, J. H., & Comello, M. L. G. (2023). Advocating, unlearning, tearing it all down? How BIPOC young adults with mental health concerns perceive and engage with the media. *Health Communication, 1–13.* https://doi.org/10.1080/10410236.2023.2290882

Waldron, V., & Kelley, D. (2015). *Moral talk across the lifespan: Creating good relationships.* Peter Lang.

Wang, W. (2017). Stigma and counter-stigma frames, cues, and exemplification: Comparing news coverage of depression in the English- and Spanish-language media in the U.S. *Health Communication, 34*(2), 172–179. https://doi.org/10.1080/10410236.2017.1399505

Wang, W. (2020). Exemplification and stigmatization of the depressed: Depression as the main topic versus an incidental topic in national US news coverage. *Health Communication, 35*(8), 1033–1041. https://doi.org/10.1080/10410236.2019.1606874

Wang, W., & Liu, Y. (2015). Discussing mental illness in Chinese social media: The impact of influential sources on stigmatization and support among their followers. *Health Communication, 31*(3), 355–363. http://dx.doi.org/10.1080/10410236.2014.957376

Watzlawick, P., Beavin, J., & Jackson, D. (1967). *The pragmatics of human communication.* W. W. Norton.

Wilson, S. R., Gettings, P. E., Hall, E. D., & Pastor, R. G. (2014). Dilemmas families face in talking with returning U.S. military service members about seeking professional help for mental health issues. *Health Communication, 30*(8), 772–783. https://doi.org/10.1080/10410236.2014.899659

Wilson, S. R., Hintz, E. A., MacDermid Wadsworth, S. M., Topp, D. B., Southwell, K. H., & Spoont, M. (2021). Female U.S. military veterans' (non)disclosure of mental health issues with family and friends: Privacy rules and boundary management. *Health Communication, 36*(4), 412–423. https://doi.org/10.1080/10410236.2019.1693128

Witte, K. (1992). Putting the fear back into fear appeals: The extended parallel process model. *Communication Monographs, 59*(4), 329–349. https://doi.org/10.1080/03637759209376276

Wozney, L., Radomski, A. D., & Newton, A. S. (2017). The gobbledygook in online parent-focused information about child and adolescent mental health. *Health Communication*, *33*(6), 710–715. https://doi.org/10.1080/10410236.2017.1306475

Wu, Q. L., & Chen, F. (2024). A dual-process model of promoting employee mental health in crises: Impacts of leadership health support and organizational leaders' crisis communication in COVID-19. *Health Communication*, *39*(9), 1705–1713. https://doi.org/10.1080/10410236.2023.2231283

Yee, N., Bailenson, J. N., & Ducheneaut, N. (2009). The Proteus effect. *Communication Research*, *36*(2), 285–312. https://doi.org/10.1177/0093650208330254

Yeshua-Katz, D., & Martins, N. (2013). Communicating stigma: The pro-ana paradox. *Health Communication*, *28*(5), 499–508. https://doi.org/10.1080/10410236.2012.699889

Zhang, X. (2020). Perceived media bias and intention to engage in discursive activities for mental health: Testing corrective action hypothesis in the context of mass shooting news. *Health Communication*, *36*(14), 1921–1930. https://doi.org/10.1080/10410236.2020.1808404

30

The Efficacy of Multi-Behavior Interventions: From Physical Health to Mental Health

Wenhao Dai[1] and Dolores Albarracín[2]

[1] Lawrence University
[2] University of Pennsylvania

The increasing prevalence of mental health illness is a growing health concern both nationally and internationally. According to the National Institute of Mental Health (NIMH), about one in five adults experience some forms of mental illness each year (NIMH, 2021). Specifically, depression has been found to affect approximately 8 percent of the US adult population (Hasin et al., 2018), and anxiety disorders affect around 31 percent of US adults at some point during their lifetime (Kessler et al., 2005). Other disorders, such as alcohol and substance use, contribute to about 4 percent of total mortality (Rehm et al., 2009) and have been linked to other health issues, such as reduced memory capacity and higher rates of motorcycle accidents (Filbey et al., 2015). As a result, designing efficacious intervention programs to improve mental health is a priority for health researchers and practitioners.

Although mental health illnesses do not directly stem from problematic behaviors, they are often still closely associated with clusters of risky behaviors that can either heighten one's risk of certain mental illness (Firth et al., 2020) or pose risks to one's overall well-being (Kim et al., 2020; Okello et al., 2013). Consequently, in addition to prescribing psychiatric medications to alleviate symptoms, most mental health practitioners have also adopted cognitive-behavioral approaches to modify risky behaviors and promote healthy behaviors through either communicative methods (e.g., motivational interviews; Ewing et al., 2021; Satre et al., 2016) or messaging technology (e.g., via smartphones; Aharonovich et al., 2017; Himelhoch et al., 2017). Furthermore, recognizing the interrelations among human behaviors (Di Benedetto et al., 2020; Mahon et al., 2022), many intervention programs attempt to target more than one behavior at a time, through what is known as ***multiple-behavior intervention programs*** (Wilson et al., 2015) or ***integrated interventions*** (Prochaska et al., 2008). Despite the success of such programs at modifying behaviors (Botvin, 2000; Salas-Salvadó et al., 2019; Tucker et al., 2017) and improving physical health outcomes (Dai et al., 2020; Sunderrajan et al., 2021; Zhang et al., 2024), the study of their efficacy in improving mental health outcomes is not yet clear (Bourke et al., 2022; Gómez-Gómez et al., 2020; Wong et al., 2021).

This chapter begins by reviewing our own research demonstrating the general success of multi-behavioral interventions in improving behavioral and physical health in a variety of domains (e.g., lifestyle, HIV behaviors, alcohol, and substance use) as well as their domain-specific performance and underlying mechanisms. We then describe the limited research on multi-behavior programs for mental health conditions, which, as mentioned, has yielded mixed evidence regarding efficacy. Following that, we identify four major challenges for multi-behavior interventions to efficaciously improve mental health outcomes, namely, (a) integrating multiple independent behavioral domains, (b) addressing the multifaceted nature of mental health, (c) tailoring the impaired cognitive capacity of individuals with a mental health diagnosis, and (d) delivering personalized interventions. We also raise important questions for future research along the way.

The Handbook of Mental Health Communication, First Edition.
Edited by Marco C. Yzer and Jason T. Siegel.

Efficacy of Multi-Behavior Interventions in Improving Behavioral and Physical Health

Human behaviors are often interrelated, forming clusters of behaviors that often heighten risk for both physical and mental health (Borrell-Carrió et al., 2004; Di Benedetto et al., 2020; Mahon et al., 2022; Wattanapisit et al., 2022). For example, alcohol use and drug use are often highly correlated, leading to a higher chance of substance use disorder (Agosti et al., 2002; Regier et al., 1990). Compared with people who do not drink alcohol, people who drink alcohol are 35 times more likely to also use cocaine, 17 times more likely to use sedatives, and 13 times more likely to use opioids (Agosti et al., 2002; Helzer & Pryzbeck, 1988; Stinson et al., 2005). Similarly, smoking behaviors and alcohol use have also been commonly associated (Drobes, 2002; Hughes, 1993) among both adolescents (Torabi et al., 1993) and college students (Reed et al., 2007). Unsafe sexual behaviors and substance use have also been shown to affect each other and both co-contribute to higher HIV transmission rates (Kalichman et al., 2007; Robinson et al., 2016). Lastly, lifestyle factors, such as sleep duration and quality, choice of diet, and self-care behaviors, have all been shown to co-contribute to protecting mental health (Di Benedetto et al., 2020; Wang et al., 2017).

Recognizing the existence of clusters of behavioral risks, innovative intervention programs often target multiple behaviors that co-contribute to the same health problem by including messages that make multiple behavioral recommendations to recipients. Such multi-behavioral interventions have been shown successful in modifying a variety of behaviors and improving physical health outcomes (Botvin, 2000; Salas-Salvadó et al., 2019; Tucker et al., 2017). For example, interventions that simultaneously address diet and physical exercise have been shown to decrease cardiovascular risk (Salas-Salvadó et al., 2019). Other integrated interventions have also been successful in simultaneously decreasing both substance use and risky sexual practices (Mouttapa et al., 2009; Tucker et al., 2017).

We have also conducted a series of meta-analyses to test the efficacy of multi-behavior intervention across different health domains, namely, lifestyle, HIV, and substance use. These meta-analyses synthesized randomized controlled trials (RCTs) with more than one recommendation, such as both quitting smoking and increasing physical activity, reducing consumption of both marijuana and cocaine, or both performing regular test for HIV and initiating PrEP (pre-exposure prophylaxis, a medicine to prevent HIV). We counted the number of recommendations presented to participants in the trials and obtained a *d* reflecting improvements in each behavioral and/or clinical outcomes (e.g., changes in diet and amount of weight loss; self-reported smoking and nicotine in blood). The results from these meta-analyses (Dai et al., 2020; Sunderrajan et al., 2021; Wilson et al., 2015; Zhang et al., 2024) are summarized in Table 30.1, which presents either the amount of change observed across conditions (i.e., multi-behavior vs. single-behavior interventions) or the regression term depicting the linear effect of number of recommendations on behavioral and/or clinical changes. As shown, for the two meta-analyses that compared efficacy of multi-behavior interventions with that of single-behavior interventions (Sunderrajan et al., 2021; Wilson et al., 2015), interventions that contained multi-behavioral recommendations (versus single-behavioral recommendation) elicited larger behavioral and clinical changes in both the lifestyle and HIV prevention and care domains.

When examining the linear and quadratic effects of number of recommendations on behavioral change, Wilson et al. (2015) found significant linear and quadratic effects, such that the lifestyle intervention programs brought most behavioral change in smoking, diet, and physical activity when they presented two or three recommendations compared with when they introduced less than two, with more than four recommendations producing a small decrease in efficacy. Furthermore, both Sunderrajan et al. (2021) and Dai et al. (2020) found a strong linear effect of the number of recommendations on behavioral/clinical change in domains of HIV and substance use, such that more recommendations elicit greater changes in sexual and substance use behaviors.

These linear and quadratic patterns resonate with the findings from our own laboratory experiments (McDonald et al., 2017) suggesting that more recommendations tend to be more beneficial in cases where the recommended behaviors can interchangeably contribute to the health outcome but less

Table 30.1 Summary of Meta-analyses on the Efficacy of Multi-Behavior Intervention Programs on Improving Behavioral and Physical Health

Reference and domain	*Type of intervention*	*Statistics*	*k*
	Multi-behavior vs. single-behavior interventions		
Wilson et al. (2015), smoking, physical activity, and diet	Multi-behavior conditions	$d = 0.17$[a] 95% CI [0.16, 0.118]	216
	Single-behavior conditions	$d = 0.07$[a] 95% CI [0.02, 0.13]	15
Sunderrajan et al. (2021), HIV	Multi-behavior conditions	$d = 0.44$[a] 95% CI [0.27, 0.60]	205
	Single-behavior conditions	$d = 0.21$ 95% CI [0.00, 0.43]	38
	Linear and quadratic effect of number of recommendations		
Wilson et al. (2015), smoking, physical activity, and diet	Quadratic effect of number of recommendations	$B = -0.016$[b]	267
Sunderrajan et al. (2021), HIV	Linear effect of number of recommendations	$B = 0.07$[a], $SE = 0.01$	243
Dai et al. (2020), substance use	Linear effect of number of recommendations (all outcomes)	$B = 0.073$[a], $SE = 0.016$	233
	Linear effect of number of recommendations (alcohol use outcomes)	$B = 0.046$[b], $SE = 0.017$	118
	Linear effect of number of recommendations (drug use outcomes)	$B = 0.085$[c], $SE = 0.025$	91
Zhang et al. (2024), all domains	Linear effect of number of recommendations	$B = 0.03$[a], $SE = 0.01$	216

d = weighted-mean Cohen's *d*; CI = confidence interval; *B* = unstandardized coefficients; SE = standard error; *k* = number of effect sizes.
[a] $p < 0.001$.
[b] $p < 0.05$.
[c] $p < 0.01$.

beneficial when all recommended behaviors jointly contribute to the outcome. For example, sexual practices (e.g., HIV testing, prevention, and treatment) and use of multiple substances (e.g., alcohol use, cannabis use, cocaine use) tend to be more interrelated and interchangeable. Consequently, a larger number of recommendations may facilitate changes in at least a subset of recommended behaviors, and that may be sufficient to bring health benefits. If people follow the recommendations to perform regular HIV testing and engage in HIV prevention, they may not become infected with HIV and thus may not need to follow the recommendations for HIV treatment. Similarly, use of one substance tends to be related to use of other substances (Drobes, 2002; Hughes, 1993), so reducing the use of any substance may automatically reduce consumption of other substances as well. However, behaviors in different lifestyle domains (e.g., smoking, diet, and physical exercises) tend to work more jointly to bring real health benefits. Therefore, a moderate number of recommendations may be optimal to ensure that the recipients will perform the complete set of recommended behaviors to maximize the benefits.

In addition to the domain-specific meta-analyses presented in Table 30.1, we have investigated the extent to which the execution of each type of recommendation can facilitate performing other recommended behaviors. This was the main question in a recent meta-analysis of 803 independent samples from 364 research reports examining the association between the number of behavioral recommendations in multi-behavior interventions and behavioral change across eight health domains: diet, smoking, exercise, HIV prevention, HIV testing, HIV treatment, alcohol use, and substance use (Zhang et al., 2024). As shown at the bottom of Table 30.1, the number of behavioral recommendations produced a positive, linear effect on behavioral change, suggesting that presenting more behavioral recommendations is generally more beneficial than less recommendations within the range of domains this meta-analysis covered.

In this comprehensive meta-analysis (Zhang et al., 2024), we also studied the possibility that behavioral cueing might facilitate the impact of multiple recommendations after these recommendations are introduced. According to the idea of classical conditioning (Pavlov, 1927) and behavioral priming (Bargh et al., 1996; Dijksterhuis et al., 2000), an environmental stimulus can provide automatic cues for behavior and in turn leads to habitual behaviors, defined as occurring with a high level of automaticity are tied to consistent environmental cues (Verplanken & Orbell, 2003; Wood & Neal, 2007). For example, many individuals report going to the bathroom to brush their teeth automatically once they start their bedtime routine (McCloskey & Johnson, 2019). In the case of behavioral cueing, we hypothesized that one behavioral recommendation may activate others through similar automatic processes. For example, if one is asked to stop consuming both alcohol and cocaine, performing the two behaviors together a few times after the recommendations may increase the probability of one behavior being activated when the other is. Such a mechanism would potentiate the greater behavioral changes produced by multi-behavioral interventions.

In this meta-analysis (Zhang et al., 2024), we conducted analyses to determine if behavioral cueing explained the positive effects of presenting more behavioral recommendations during the interventions. Specifically, we determined if changes in smoking were associated with changes in diet and exercise, for example. We found that changes in HIV behaviors (e.g., using condoms and regular testing), as well as changes in alcohol and drug use, were associated with changes in other behaviors, whereas changes in smoking and physical exercise were not. These findings provide good explanations for the different patterns found in the previous meta-analyses such that more recommendations are beneficial for HIV and substance use behaviors but not necessarily for lifestyle behaviors. Presumably, HIV, alcohol use, and drug use behaviors often co-occur in ways that ensure co-habituation of these behaviors and potentiation of changes when one behavior changes, but lifestyle behaviors (e.g., smoking and exercise) tend to operate on their own and do not provide the same opportunities for co-habituation.

In sum, our meta-analyses have confirmed that multi-behavioral interventions are generally successful in improving behavioral and physical health across domains, but the effect of number of behavioral recommendations may still vary across domains. For behaviors that more often co-occur, multiple behavioral recommendations appear to elicit more automatic mechanisms that supplement the effects of single-behavioral recommendations on behavioral and clinical outcomes. Specifically, if one behavior is executed following a recommendation, other behaviors are also executed due to behavioral cueing. These behaviors then become mutually reinforcing and on average increase the impact of each intervention recommendations. However, for behaviors that occur separately, these automatic processes may not be activated, and thus a moderate number of recommendations may be optimal to maximize behavioral and clinical change.

Efficacy of Multi-Behavioral Interventions in Improving Mental Health

Like physical health, many mental health conditions are associated with clusters of risky behaviors (Firth et al., 2020; Kim et al., 2020; Okello et al., 2013), and addressing these behaviors has been shown to effectively reduce mental health symptoms (Firth et al., 2019, 2020; Schuch et al., 2016). For example, one meta-analysis (Firth et al., 2019) showed that dietary improvement can significantly reduce depression symptoms ($g = 0.28$, 95% confidence interval [CI] [0.10, 0.45]). Similarly, another meta-analysis (Schuch et al., 2016) showed that physical exercise can be an effective treatment for depression ($d = 1.11$, 95% CI [0.79, 1.43]). Despite the success of these single-behavior interventions, the efficacy of multi-behavior interventions in treating mental health issues has been far less studied and thus remains an open question. To the best of our knowledge, only three small-scale meta-analyses have considered specifically depression and anxiety, finding mixed evidence about the efficacy of multi-behavior interventions in improving mental health (Bourke et al., 2022; Gómez-Gómez et al., 2020; Wong et al., 2021). However, Zhang et al. (2024) considered the impact of multi-behavior interventions on psychological well-being in the domains of lifestyle, HIV, and substance use. The results from these four meta-analyses are presented in Table 30.2.

Table 30.2 Summary of Meta-analyses on the Efficacy of Multi-Behavior Intervention Programs on Improving Mental Health

Reference and domain	*Type of intervention/outcome/effect*	*Statistics*	*k*
	Multi-behavior vs. single-behavior interventions		
Gómez-Gómez et al. (2020), depression	Multirisk lifestyle interventions in reducing depression (compared with control)	$d = -0.18$[a] 95% CI [−0.31, −0.06]	20
	Multirisk lifestyle interventions in reducing depression (compared with control and including only RCTs of low risk of bias)	$d = -0.09$ 95% CI [−0.21, 0.03]	9
Wong et al. (2021), depression	Multicomponent LM intervention in reducing depression (compared with CAU)	$d = -0.20$[a] 95% CI [−0.29, −0.10]	33
	Multicomponent LM intervention in reducing depression (compared with WL/NI)	$d = -0.22$[b] 95% CI [−0.36, −0.08]	15
	Multicomponent LM intervention in reducing depression (compared with AC)	$d = 0.11$ 95% CI [−0.04, 0.26]	2
Bourke et al. (2022), depression and anxiety	Interventions targeting multiple modifiable health behaviors on reducing depression (for selective population and compared with control)	$d = -0.28$[b] 95% CI [−0.52, −0.05]	9
	Interventions targeting multiple modifiable health behaviors on reducing depression (for universal population and compared with control)	$d = 0.08$ 95% CI [−0.03, 0.18]	4
	Interventions targeting multiple modifiable health behaviors on reducing anxiety (compared with control)	$d = -0.55$ 95% CI [−1.36, 0.26]	6
Zhang et al. (2024), psychological well-being	Linear effect of number of behavioral recommendations in multi-behavior interventions on psychological well-being	$B = 0.12$[b], $SE = 0.05$	91

d = weighted-mean Cohen's *d*; CI = confidence interval; *k* = number of effect sizes; LM = lifestyle-medicine; CAU = care as usual; WL = waitlisted; NI = no interventions; AC = attention control.

[a] $p < 0.01$.

[b] $p < 0.0$.

A first meta-analysis (Gómez-Gómez et al., 2020) assessed the effectiveness of multiple-risk lifestyle interventions (i.e., promoting a healthy diet, physical activity, and/or smoking cessation) to reduce depression symptoms among adults. It synthesized results from 20 eligible RCTs and found a small but significant effect of multiple-risk lifestyle interventions on reducing depression symptoms ($d = -0.18$, 95% CI [−0.31, −0.06], $p = 0.005$, $I^2 = 72\%$). However, this effect, which was heterogeneous, disappeared when only studies with a low risk of bias were included. Thus, the authors concluded that the overall evidence for efficacy of multiple-risk lifestyle interventions in reducing depression symptoms was weak and further evidence is required.

The second meta-analysis (Wong et al., 2021) similarly assessed whether multicomponent lifestyle interventions (i.e., physical activity, nutritional advice, sleep management, and/or stress management) were effective in reducing depression symptoms compared with different control groups. This synthesis included 50 studies and found that the efficacy of multicomponent lifestyle interventions largely depended on the control group being used. Specifically, the researchers found a significant effect of integrated interventions on reducing depression symptoms when compared with usual-care control conditions ($d = -0.20$, $p < 0.01$) or waitlist/no intervention control conditions ($d = -0.22$, $p < 0.05$) but not attention control conditions ($d = 0.11$, $p > 0.05$). Furthermore, the intervention effects appeared to last for only a short period of time (i.e., 1–3 – month follow-up) but disappeared in the medium or longer term. Lastly, the moderator analyses showed that the effects of multi-behavior interventions depended on the exact number of lifestyle factors involved. Specifically, targeting two ($d = -0.17$, $p < 0.05$) or three ($d = -0.27$, $p < 0.05$) lifestyle factors were shown to be most effective in reducing depression symptoms, while targeting four lifestyle factors ($d = 0.01$, $p < 0.05$) seemed to bring no benefits.

The last specific meta-analysis (Bourke et al., 2022) assessed the effect of interventions that target multiple modifiable health behaviors (i.e., physical activity/sedentary behaviors, nutrition/diet, sleep, substance use) on reducing symptoms of depression and anxiety in young populations. It synthesized 14 trials for depression and 6 trials for anxiety but found nonsignificant effects of multi-behavior programs in reducing either depression or anxiety. However, when breaking down the trials by intervention types, interventions targeting multiple modifiable health behaviors delivered to groups of young people with an elevated risk of depression did reduce symptoms of depression more than control groups ($d = -0.28$, $p < 0.05$), suggesting the potential of such interventions in vulnerable populations.

All in all, these three specific meta-analyses showed some evidence of the efficacy of multi-behavior interventions in treating mental health illness (e.g., depression), but the overall evidence was weak. In addition, the size of the effect appears to be contingent on a variety of factors, including the time interval, the type of control conditions, the number of domains targeted, and the target population. However, Zhang et al. (2024) considered psychological well-being, which they measured as decreases in stress, anxiety, and depression, both to ascertain the impact of multiple behaviors on well-being and to determine if changes in well-being mediated the linear effects of multiple behavior interventions on behavioral and clinical change. The rationale was that low psychological well-being (e.g., anxiety, stress, or depression) increases risky behaviors such as binge eating, alcohol use, substance use, and risky sex (e.g., Appelhans et al., 2012; Thoits, 2010) and unhealthy behaviors, such as smoking, comprising a risk factor for psychological disorders (Firth et al., 2020). Accordingly, a higher number of health–behavior recommendations may increase psychological well-being, in part because behavioral activation lifts depression, possibly through dopaminergic mechanisms (Salamone et al., 2016) that may come into play when people engage in the multiple behaviors an intervention recommends.

To examine effects on psychological well-being, we (Zhang et al., 2024) obtained effect sizes for:

- Depression and mania, reverse-scored through our effect size calculation:
  - Calgary Depression Scale (Addington et al., 1993)
  - Center for Epidemiological Studies-Depression (Radloff, 1977)
  - Patient Health Questionnaire-9 (Kroenke et al., 2001)
  - Clinical Global Impressions Scale-Bipolar Version-Overall and Mania + Depression subscales (Spearing et al., 1997)
  - Montgomery–Åsberg Depression Rating Scale (Montgomery & Asberg, 1979)
  - Edinburgh Postnatal Depression Scale (Cox et al., 1987)
  - Hamilton Depression Rating Scale (Hamilton, 1960)
  - Beck Depression Inventory (Beck et al., 1961)
  - Mental health subscale of the Addiction Severity Index (McLellan et al., 1992)
- Psychological quality of life:
  - Medical Outcomes Study 36-item short-form health survey (McHorney et al., 1993)
  - Health Promoting Lifestyle scale (Walker & Hill-Polerecky, 1996)
  - EuroQol Visual Analogue Scale (EuroQol Group, 1990)
  - Acceptance and Action Questionnaire–II (Bond et al., 2011)
  - Self-reported mindfulness (self-reported trauma)
- Anxiety and stress, reverse-scored through our effect size calculation:
  - Symptom Checklist-90 (Derogatis et al., 1973)
  - Anxiety subscale of the Depression Anxiety Stress Scale-21 (Henry & Crawford, 2005)
  - Self-report items
- Social quality of life:
  - Social Functioning item from the Medical Outcomes Study 36-item short-form health survey (Ware & Sherbourne, 1992)
  - Community engagement, social support, and social function items (self-reported victimization)

- Positive mood:
  - Positive and Negative Affect Schedule (Watson et al., 1988)
  - Profile of Mood States (McNair et al., 1971)
- Coping:
  - High self-reported positive reinterpretation; low self-reported behavioral disengagement

These effects were averaged and then analyzed as a function of the number of recommendations included in an intervention.

The analyses conducted by Zhang et al. (2024) showed that the number of behavioral recommendations contained in interventions predicted improvement in psychological well-being, which in turn predicted behavioral–clinical improvement. The results indicated that the addition of each behavioral recommendation led to a $d = 0.05$ behavioral and clinical improvement, thus showing benefits in mental health outcomes themselves but also broader impacts on physical health.

Challenges and Future Directions for Multi-Behavior Messages and Other Interventions to Improve Mental Health Outcomes

Although multi-behavior interventions through communicative methods or messaging technology have been promising for modifying risky behaviors and improving physical health outcomes, their application to improving mental health has certain limitations. For one example, most current work has focused on depression (with some on anxiety disorders), but not much work has been done to examine the effect of multi-behavior message interventions on treating other psychological conditions (e.g., bipolar disorder, posttraumatic stress disorder, suicidal ideation). Due to the limitations, the full potential of different types of multi-behavior messages and other interventions for treating different mental illness is not completely clear at this time. Thus, in the final sections of this chapter, we describe four ongoing research challenges concerning the use of multi-behavior interventions to improve mental health outcomes.

Integrating Multiple Independent Behavioral Domains

Unlike the domains of sexual health or substance use, which often involve a set of interrelated behaviors, many mental health conditions are associated with a wide range of relatively independent behavioral domains, such as physical exercise, diet and nutrition, smoking, and sleep (Firth et al., 2020). As suggested by our own meta-analyses (Dai et al., 2020; Sunderrajan et al., 2021; Wilson et al., 2015; Zhang et al., 2024), more behavioral recommendations are often more effective when the targeted behaviors are interchangeable (e.g., use of multiple substances, HIV prevention and treatment) but not necessarily so when the behaviors need to jointly contribute to a health outcome (e.g., when targeting physical exercise and smoking). The reason is that execution of one behavioral recommendation may act as a behavioral cue and facilitate execution of other recommendations as well when these behaviors are co-habituated before (Zhang et al., 2024), but such automatic effect may not happen for behaviors that do not often co-occur, such as exercise and smoking. Consequently, when a lifestyle–medicine intervention program tries to integrate behavioral recommendations from multiple independent domains to improve mental health, these recommendations may not facilitate each other but instead interfere with each other. In such cases, targeting a moderate number of domains (i.e., two or three) may be ideal (Wong et al., 2021). If more recommendations were to be given, finding ways to combine multiple recommendations into a central theme or training co-habituation among independent behaviors may be important for maximizing the benefits. For example, training patients to go for a jog every time they crave cigarettes may establish the conditioning between stopping smoking and starting physical exercise, thus facilitating both behaviors in the future.

Addressing the Multifaceted Nature of Mental Health

Psychological symptoms are often complex and multifaceted, involving not just behavioral, but also a range of biological, psychological, and social factors (Fried, 2022; Remes et al., 2021). Consequently, addressing multiple behaviors at risk may modify these behavioral outcomes but is not sufficient to bring direct benefits to the mental health outcomes if they are not targeting the other underlying factors at the same time. Therefore, successful mental health interventions need to integrate not only behavioral recommendations from different domains but also various efforts including improving medication availability and therapy, strengthening social support, and reducing social stigma. For example, Przybylko et al. (2021) suggested that integrating lifestyle–medicine recommendations (i.e., physical activity and improving diet) with practices from positive psychology (e.g., practice skills in expressing gratitude and embracing positive affects) could be an effective way to improve well-being during and beyond the COVID-19 pandemic. Similarly, a meta-analysis (Asarnow et al., 2015) on integrated medical–behavioral interventions showed that integrating behavioral health care into the regular medical primary care was more successful in improving child and adolescents' behavioral and mental health compared with the regular care by itself. Thus, future message interventions should continue to seek innovative ways to integrate behavioral recommendations with medical care and social support to maximize their effects.

Tailoring the Impaired Cognitive Capacity of Mental Health Patients

Simultaneously changing multiple behaviors is often cognitively demanding and relies on the cognitive capacity to process, memorize, and execute multiple behaviors, thus posing a limit on how many recommendations one person can follow at a time (McDonald et al., 2017; Shiffrin & Nosofsky, 1994; Zhang et al., 2024). This limit may be even lower for patients with psychological conditions because many such conditions have been shown to impair patients' cognitive capacity. For example, a meta-analysis (Bora & Pantelis, 2015) showed that patients with a first-episode bipolar disorder have cognitive impairment in all cognitive domains, including memory, attention, verbal fluency, and reasoning. Another meta-analysis (Rock et al., 2014) found similar cognitive impairment in executive function, memory, and attention among patients diagnosed with depression. Considering different levels of cognitive impairment, future research should determine the optimal number of behavioral recommendations to include in messages and interventions for patients with each mental illness. Additionally, finding innovative ways to combine multiple recommendations into a higher-order single recommendation and training co-habituation among different recommendations may be especially important for patients with impaired cognitive capacity.

Delivering Personalized Messages

Mental health needs vary from patient to patient, thus requiring personalized mental health intervention programs (Zilcha-Mano et al., 2022). In line with this notion, Bourke et al.'s (2022) meta-analysis suggested that multi-behavior interventions were most effective in reducing depression symptoms when they specifically targeted groups of young people with elevated risk of depression as opposed to the general population. Thus, to fully realize multi-behavior interventions' potential in improving mental health outcomes, individualized interventions that target personalized behaviors through tailored messages may be necessary to address the unique needs and circumstances of each population. Specifically, the intervention approaches should seek to achieve a diversity of aims, measure a diversity of health outcomes, depend on a variety of information to determine the tailoring, and rely on a variety of research designs to evaluate the quality of the approaches (Zilcha-Mano et al., 2022).

Concluding Remarks

Considering the correlation between different psychological conditions with a range of unhealthy behaviors (Firth et al., 2020), as well as a high rate of comorbidity among different conditions (e.g., Spinhoven et al., 2014; Swendsen & Merikangas, 2000), multi-behavior messages and interventions hold promise in addressing the behavioral, physical, and mental health needs of important populations. However, research on such applications will require further evidence to fully ascertain the feasibility and efficacy of such messages and interventions for improving mental health outcomes. In particular, integrating behaviors from independent domains through co-habituation, integrating behavioral treatment with medical care and social support, tailoring recommendations to patients with impaired cognitive capacity, and providing individualized mental health services may be critical to better serve the need for people with mental illness.

References

Addington, D., Addington, J., & Maticka-Tyndale, E. (1993). Assessing depression in schizophrenia: The Calgary depression scale. *British Journal of Psychiatry*, *163*(S22), 39–44. http://dx.doi.org/10.1192/s0007125000292581

Agosti, V., Nunes, E., & Levin, F. (2002). Rates of psychiatric comorbidity among U.S. residents with lifetime cannabis dependence. *American Journal of Drug and Alcohol Abuse*, *28*(4), 643–652. http://dx.doi.org/10.1081/ADA-120015873

Aharonovich, E., Stohl, M., Cannizzaro, D., & Hasin, D. (2017). HealthCall delivered via smartphone to reduce co-occurring drug and alcohol use in HIV-infected adults: A randomized pilot trial. *Journal of Substance Abuse Treatment*, *83*, 15–26. http://dx.doi.org/10.1016/j.jsat.2017.09.013

Appelhans, B. M., Whited, M. C., Schneider, K. L., Ma, Y., Oleski, J. L., Merriam, P. A., Waring, M. E., Olendzki, B. C., Mann, D. M., Ockene, I. S., & Pagoto, S. L. (2012). Depression severity, diet quality, and physical activity in women with obesity and depression. *Journal of the Academy of Nutrition and Dietetics*, *112*(5), 693–698. http://dx.doi.org/10.1016/j.jand.2012.02.006

Asarnow, J. R., Rozenman, M., Wiblin, J., & Zeltzer, L. (2015). Integrated medical-behavioral care compared with usual primary care for child and adolescent behavioral health: A meta-analysis. *JAMA Pediatrics*, *169*(10), 929–937. http://dx.doi.org/10.1001/jamapediatrics.2015.1141

Bargh, J. A., Chen, M., & Burrows, L. (1996). Automaticity of social behavior: Direct effects of trait construct and stereotype activation on action. *Journal of Personality and Social Psychology*, *71*(2), 230–244. http://dx.doi.org/10.1037/0022-3514.71.2.230

Beck, A. T., Ward, C. H., Mendelson, M., Mock, J., & Erbaugh, J. (1961). An inventory for measuring depression. *Archives of General Psychiatry*, *4*(6), 561–571. http://dx.doi.org/10.1001/archpsyc.1961.01710120031004

Bond, F. W., Hayes, S. C., Baer, R. A., Carpenter, K. M., Guenole, N., Orcutt, H. K., Waltz, T., & Zettle, R. D. (2011). Preliminary psychometric properties of the acceptance and action questionnaire-II: A revised measure of psychological inflexibility and experiential avoidance. *Behavior Therapy*, *42*(4), 676–688. http://dx.doi.org/10.1016/j.beth.2011.03.007

Bora, E., & Pantelis, C. (2015). Meta-analysis of cognitive impairment in first-episode bipolar disorder: Comparison with first-episode schizophrenia and healthy controls. *Schizophrenia Bulletin*, *41*(5), 1095–1104. http://dx.doi.org/10.1093/schbul/sbu198

Borrell-Carrió, F., Suchman, A. L., & Epstein, R. M. (2004). The biopsychosocial model 25 years later: Principles, practice, and scientific inquiry. *Annals of Family Medicine*, *2*(6), 576–582. http://dx.doi.org/10.1370/afm.245

Botvin, G. J. (2000). Preventing drug abuse in schools. *Addictive Behaviors*, *25*(6), 887–897. http://dx.doi.org/10.1016/s0306-4603(00)00119-2

Bourke, M., Patten, R. K., Dash, S., Pascoe, M., Craike, M., Firth, J., Bailey, A., Jacka, F., & Parker, A. G. (2022). The effect of interventions that target multiple modifiable health behaviors on symptoms of anxiety and depression in young people: A meta-analysis of randomized controlled trials. *Journal of Adolescent Health*, *70*(2), 208–219. http://dx.doi.org/10.1016/j.jadohealth.2021.08.005

Cox, J. L., Holden, J. M., & Sagovsky, R. (1987). Detection of postnatal depression: Development of the 10-item Edinburgh postnatal depression scale. *British Journal of Psychiatry*, *150*(6), 782–786. http://dx.doi.org/10.1192/bjp.150.6.782

Dai, W., Palmer, R., Sunderrajan, A., Durantini, M., Sánchez, F., Glasman, L. R., … Albarracín, D. (2020). More behavioral recommendations produce more change: A meta-analysis of efficacy of multibehavior recommendations to reduce nonmedical substance use. *Psychology of Addictive Behaviors*, *34*(7), 709. http://dx.doi.org/10.1037/adb0000586

Derogatis, L. R., Lipman, R. S., & Covi, L. (1973). SCL-90: An outpatient psychiatric rating scale–preliminary report. *Psychopharmacology Bulletin*, *9*(1), 13–28.

Di Benedetto, M., Towt, C. J., & Jackson, M. L. (2020). A cluster analysis of sleep quality, self-care behaviors, and mental health risk in Australian university students. *Behavioral Sleep Medicine*, *18*(3), 309–320. http://dx.doi.org/10.1080/15402002.2019.1580194

Dijksterhuis, A., Aarts, H., Bargh, J. A., & Van Knippenberg, A. (2000). On the relation between associative strength and automatic behavior. *Journal of Experimental Social Psychology*, *36*(5), 531–544. http://dx.doi.org/10.1006/jesp.2000.1427

Drobes, D. J. (2002). Cue reactivity in alcohol and tobacco dependence. *Alcoholism: Clinical and Experimental Research, 26*(12), 1928–1929. http://dx.doi.org/10.1111/j.1530-0277.2002.tb02506.x

EuroQol Group. (1990). EuroQol—A new facility for the measurement of health-related quality of life. *Health Policy, 16*(3), 199–208. https://doi.org/10.1016/0168-8510(90)90421-9

Ewing, S. F., Bryan, A. D., Dash, G. F., Lovejoy, T. I., Borsari, B., & Schmiege, S. J. (2021). Randomized controlled trial of motivational interviewing for alcohol and cannabis use within a predominantly Hispanic adolescent sample. *Experimental and Clinical Psychopharmacology, 30*(3), 287–299. http://dx.doi.org/10.1037/pha0000445

Filbey, F. M., McQueeny, T., DeWitt, S. J., & Mishra, V. (2015). Preliminary findings demonstrating latent effects of early adolescent marijuana use onset on cortical architecture. *Developmental Cognitive Neuroscience, 16*, 16–22. http://dx.doi.org/10.1016/j.dcn.2015.10.001

Firth, J., Marx, W., Dash, S., Carney, R., Teasdale, S. B., Solmi, M., Stubbs, B., Schuch, F. B., Carvalho, A. F., Jacka, F., & Sarris, J. (2019). The effects of dietary improvement on symptoms of depression and anxiety: A meta-analysis of randomized controlled trials. *Psychosomatic Medicine, 81*(3), 265–280. http://dx.doi.org/10.1097/PSY.0000000000000673

Firth, J., Solmi, M., Wootton, R. E., Vancampfort, D., Schuch, F. B., Hoare, E., Gilbody, S., Torous, J., Teasdale, S. B., Jackson, S. E., Smith, L., Eaton, M., Jacka, F. N., Veronese, N., Marx, W., Ashdown-Franks, G., Siskind, D., Sarris, J., Rosenbaum, S., … Stubbs, B. (2020). A meta-review of "lifestyle psychiatry": The role of exercise, smoking, diet and sleep in the prevention and treatment of mental disorders. *World Psychiatry, 19*(3), 360–380. http://dx.doi.org/10.1002/wps.20773

Fried, E. I. (2022). Studying mental health problems as systems, not syndromes. *Current Directions in Psychological Science, 31*(6), 500–508. http://dx.doi.org/10.1177/09637214221114089

Gómez-Gómez, I., Bellón, J., Resurrección, D. M., Cuijpers, P., Moreno-Peral, P., Rigabert, A., Maderuelo-Fernández, J. Á., & Motrico, E. (2020). Effectiveness of universal multiple-risk lifestyle interventions in reducing depressive symptoms: Systematic review and meta-analysis. *Preventive Medicine, 134*, 106067. http://dx.doi.org/10.1016/j.ypmed.2020.106067

Hamilton, M. (1960). A rating scale for depression. *Journal of Neurology, Neurosurgery, and Psychiatry, 23*(1), 56–62. http://dx.doi.org/10.1136/jnnp.23.1.56

Hasin, D. S., Sarvet, A. L., Meyers, J. L., Saha, T. D., Ruan, W. J., Stohl, M., & Grant, B. F. (2018). Epidemiology of adult DSM-5 major depressive disorder and its specifiers in the United States. *JAMA Psychiatry, 75*(4), 336–346. http://dx.doi.org/10.1001/jamapsychiatry.2017.4602

Helzer, J. E., & Pryzbeck, T. R. (1988). The co-occurrence of alcoholism with other psychiatric disorders in the general population and its impact on treatment. *Journal of Studies on Alcohol, 49*(3), 219–224. https://doi.org/10.15288/jsa.1988.49.219

Henry, J. D., & Crawford, J. R. (2005). The short-form version of the depression anxiety stress scales (DASS-21): Construct validity and normative data in a large non-clinical sample. *British Journal of Clinical Psychology, 44*(2), 227–239. http://dx.doi.org/10.1348/014466505X29657

Himelhoch, S., Kreyenbuhl, J., Palmer-Bacon, J., Chu, M., Brown, C., & Potts, W. (2017). Pilot feasibility study of Heart2HAART: A smartphone application to assist with adherence among substance users living with HIV. *AIDS Care, 29*(7), 898–904. http://dx.doi.org/10.1080/09540121.2016.1259454

Hughes, J. R. (1993). Treatment of smoking cessation in smokers with past alcohol/drug problems. *Journal of Substance Abuse Treatment, 10*(2), 181–187. http://dx.doi.org/10.1016/0740-5472(93)90043-2

Kalichman, S. C., Simbayi, L. C., Kaufman, M., Cain, D., & Jooste, S. (2007). Alcohol use and sexual risks for HIV/AIDS in sub-Saharan Africa: Systematic review of empirical findings. *Prevention Science, 8*, 141–151. http://dx.doi.org/10.1007/s11121-006-0061-2

Kessler, R. C., Wai, T. C., Demler, O., & Walters, E. E. (2005). Prevalence, severity, and comorbidity of 12-month DSM-IV disorders in the National Comorbidity Survey Replication. *Archives of General Psychiatry, 62*(6), 617–627. http://dx.doi.org/10.1001/archpsyc.62.6.617

Kim, E. M., Kim, H., & Park, E. (2020). How are depression and suicidal ideation associated with multiple health risk behaviours among adolescents? A secondary data analysis using the 2016 Korea Youth Risk Behavior Web-based survey. *Journal of Psychiatric and Mental Health Nursing, 27*(5), 595–606. http://dx.doi.org/10.1111/jpm.12610

Kroenke, K., Spitzer, R. L., & Williams, J. B. W. (2001). The PHQ-9: Validity of a brief depression severity measure. *Journal of General Internal Medicine, 16*(9), 606–613. http://dx.doi.org/10.1046/j.1525-1497.2001.016009606.x

Mahon, C., Howard, E., O'Reilly, A., Dooley, B., & Fitzgerald, A. (2022). A cluster analysis of health behaviours and their relationship to mental health difficulties, life satisfaction and functioning in adolescents. *Preventive Medicine, 164*, 107332. http://dx.doi.org/10.1016/j.ypmed.2022.107332

McCloskey, K., & Johnson, B. T. (2019). Habits, quick and easy: Perceived complexity moderates the associations of contextual stability and rewards with behavioral automaticity. *Frontiers in Psychology, 10*, 460055. http://dx.doi.org/10.3389/fpsyg.2019.01556

McDonald, J., McDonald, P., Hughes, C., & Albarracín, D. (2017). Recalling and intending to enact health recommendations: Optimal number of prescribed behaviors in multibehavior messages. *Clinical Psychological Science, 5*(5), 858–865. http://dx.doi.org/10.1177/2167702617704453

McHorney, C. A., Ware, J. E., & Raczek, A. E. (1993). The MOS 36-item short-form health survey (Sf-36): II. Psychometric and clinical tests of validity in measuring physical and mental health constructs. *Medical Care, 31*(3), 247–263. http://dx.doi.org/10.1097/00005650-199303000-00006

McLellan, A. T., Kushner, H., Metzger, D., Peters, R., Smith, I., Grissom, G., Pettinati, H., & Argeriou, M. (1992). The fifth edition of the addiction severity index. *Journal of Substance Abuse Treatment, 9*(3), 199–213. https://doi.org/10.1016/0740-5472(92)90062-S

McNair, D. M., Loor, M., & Droppleman, L. F. (1971). *EITS manual for the profile of mood states.* Educational and Industrial Testing Service.

Montgomery, S. A., & Asberg, M. (1979). A new depression scale designed to be sensitive to change. *British Journal of Psychiatry, 134*(4), 382–389. http://dx.doi.org/10.1192/bjp.134.4.382

Mouttapa, M., Watson, D., McCuller, W., Reiber, C., & Tsai, W. (2009). Substance use and HIV prevention for youth in correctional facilities. *Journal of Correctional Education, 60*(4), 289–315. https://www.jstor.org/stable/44944667

National Institute of Mental Health. (2021). *Mental illness.* https://www.nimh.nih.gov/health/statistics/mental-illness

Okello, J., Nakimuli-Mpungu, E., Musisi, S., Broekaert, E., & Derluyn, I. (2013). War-related trauma exposure and multiple risk behaviors among school-going adolescents in northern Uganda: The mediating role of depression symptoms. *Journal of Affective Disorders, 151*(2), 715–721. http://dx.doi.org/10.1016/j.jad.2013.07.030

Pavlov, I. P. (1927). *Conditioned reflexes: An investigation of the physiological activity of the cerebral cortex.* Oxford University Press.

Prochaska, J. J., Spring, B., & Nigg, C. R. (2008). Multiple health behavior change research: An introduction and overview. *Preventive Medicine, 46*(3), 181–188. http://dx.doi.org/10.1016/j.ypmed.2008.02.001

Przybylko, G., Morton, D. P., & Renfrew, M. E. (2021). Addressing the COVID-19 mental health crisis: A perspective on using interdisciplinary universal interventions. *Frontiers in Psychology, 12*, 644337. http://dx.doi.org/10.3389/fpsyg.2021.644337

Radloff, L. S. (1977). The CES-D scale: A self-report depression scale for research in the general population. *Applied Psychological Measurement, 1*(3), 385–401. http://dx.doi.org/10.1177/014662167700100306

Reed, M. B., Wang, R., Shillington, A. M., Clapp, J. D., & Lange, J. E. (2007). The relationship between alcohol use and cigarette smoking in a sample of undergraduate college students. *Addictive Behaviors, 32*(3), 449–464. http://dx.doi.org/10.1016/j.addbeh.2006.05.016

Regier, D. A., Farmer, M. E., Rae, D. S., Locke, B. Z., Keith, S. J., Judd, L. L., & Goodwin, F. K. (1990). Comorbidity of mental disorders with alcohol and other drug abuse: Results from the epidemiologic catchment area (ECA) study. *JAMA: The Journal of the American Medical Association, 264*(19), 2511–2518. http://dx.doi.org/10.1001/jama.1990.03450190043026

Rehm, J., Mathers, C., Popova, S., Thavorncharoensap, M., Teerawattananon, Y., & Patra, J. (2009). Global burden of disease and injury and economic cost attributable to alcohol use and alcohol-use disorders. *The Lancet, 373*(9682), 2223–2233. http://dx.doi.org/10.1016/S0140-6736(09)60746-7

Remes, O., Francisco, J., & Templeton, P. (2021). Biological, psychological, and social determinants of depression: A review of recent literature. *Brain Sciences, 11*(12), 1633. http://dx.doi.org/10.3390/brainsci11121633

Robinson, A. C., Knowlton, A. R., Gielen, A. C., & Gallo, J. J. (2016). Substance use, mental illness, and familial conflict non-negotiation among HIV-positive African-Americans: Latent class regression and a new syndemic framework. *Journal of Behavioral Medicine, 39*, 1–12. http://dx.doi.org/10.1007/s10865-015-9670-1

Rock, P. L., Roiser, J. P., Riedel, W. J., & Blackwell, A. D. (2014). Cognitive impairment in depression: A systematic review and meta-analysis. *Psychological Medicine, 44*(10), 2029–2040. http://dx.doi.org/10.1017/S0033291713002535

Salamone, J. D., Pardo, M., Yohn, S. E., López-Cruz, L., SanMiguel, N., & Correa, M. (2016). Mesolimbic dopamine and the regulation of motivated behavior. In E. Simpson & P. Balsam (Eds.), *Behavioral neuroscience of motivation* (pp. 231–257). Springer. http://dx.doi.org/10.1007/7854_2015_383

Salas-Salvadó, J., Díaz-López, A., Ruiz-Canela, M., Basora, J., Fitó, M., Corella, D., Serra-Majem, L., Wärnberg, J., Romaguera, D., Estruch, R., Vidal, J., Alfredo Martínez, J., Arós, F., Vázquez, C., Ros, E., Vioque, J., López-Miranda, J., Bueno-Cavanillas, A., Tur, J. A., … Martínez-González, M. (2019). Effect of a lifestyle intervention program with energy-restricted Mediterranean diet and exercise on weight loss and cardiovascular risk factors: One-year results of the PREDIMED-plus trial. *Diabetes Care, 42*(5), 777–788. http://dx.doi.org/10.2337/dc18-0836

Satre, D. D., Leibowitz, A., Sterling, S. A., Lu, Y., Travis, A., & Weisner, C. (2016). A randomized clinical trial of motivational interviewing to reduce alcohol and drug use among patients with depression. *Journal of Consulting and Clinical Psychology, 84*(7), 571–579. http://dx.doi.org/10.1037/ccp0000096

Schuch, F. B., Vancampfort, D., Richards, J., Rosenbaum, S., Ward, P. B., & Stubbs, B. (2016). Exercise as a treatment for depression: A meta-analysis adjusting for publication bias. *Journal of Psychiatric Research, 77*, 42–51. http://dx.doi.org/10.1016/j.jpsychires.2016.02.023

Shiffrin, R. M., & Nosofsky, R. M. (1994). Seven plus or minus two: A commentary on capacity limitations. *Psychological Review, 101*(2), 357–361. http://dx.doi.org/10.1037/0033-295X.101.2.357

Spearing, M. K., Post, R. M., Leverich, G. S., Brandt, D., & Nolen, W. (1997). Modification of the clinical global impressions (CGI) scale for use in bipolar illness (BP): The CGI-BP. *Psychiatry Research, 73*(3), 159–171. http://dx.doi.org/10.1016/S0165-1781(97)00123-6

Spinhoven, P., Penninx, B. W., van Hemert, A. M., de Rooij, M., & Elzinga, B. M. (2014). Comorbidity of PTSD in anxiety and depressive disorders: Prevalence and shared risk factors. *Child Abuse and Neglect*, *38*(8), 1320–1330. http://dx.doi.org/10.1016/j.chiabu.2014.01.017

Stinson, F. S., Grant, B. F., Dawson, D. A., Ruan, W. J., Huang, B., & Saha, T. (2005). Comorbidity between DSM-IV alcohol and specific drug use disorders in the United States: Results from the National Epidemiologic Survey on Alcohol and Related Conditions. *Drug and Alcohol Dependence*, *80*(1), 105–116. http://dx.doi.org/10.1016/j.drugalcdep.2005.03.009

Sunderrajan, A., White, B., Durantini, M., Sanchez, F., Glasman, L., & Albarracín, D. (2021). Complex solutions for a complex problem: A meta-analysis of the efficacy of multiple-behavior interventions on change in outcomes related to HIV. *Health Psychology*, *40*(9), 642–653. http://dx.doi.org/10.1037/hea0001088

Swendsen, J. D., & Merikangas, K. R. (2000). The comorbidity of depression and substance use disorders. *Clinical Psychology Review*, *20*(2), 173–189. http://dx.doi.org/10.1016/S0272-7358(99)00026-4

Thoits, P. A. (2010). Stress and health: Major findings and policy implications. *Journal of Health and Social Behavior*, *51*(1_suppl), S41–S53. http://dx.doi.org/10.1177/0022146510383499

Torabi, M. R., Bailey, W. J., & Majd-Jabbari, M. (1993). Cigarette smoking as a predictor of alcohol and other drug use by children and adolescents: Evidence of the "gateway drug effect". *Journal of School Health*, *63*(7), 302–306. http://dx.doi.org/10.1111/j.1746-1561.1993.tb06150.x

Tucker, J. S., D'Amico, E. J., Ewing, B. A., Miles, J. N. V., & Pedersen, E. R. (2017). A group-based motivational interviewing brief intervention to reduce substance use and sexual risk behavior among homeless young adults. *Journal of Substance Abuse Treatment*, *76*, 20–27. http://dx.doi.org/10.1016/j.jsat.2017.02.008

Verplanken, B., & Orbell, S. (2003). Reflections on past behavior: A self-report index of habit strength. *Journal of Applied Social Psychology*, *33*(6), 1313–1330. http://dx.doi.org/10.1111/j.1559-1816.2003.tb01951.x

Walker, S.N., & Hill-Polerecky, D.M. (1996). *Psychometric evaluation of the Health-Promoting Lifestyle Profile II* [Unpublished manuscript].

Wang, S., Wu, Y., Ungvari, G. S., Ng, C. H., Forester, B. P., Gatchel, J. R., Chiu, H. F. K., Kou, C., Fu, Y., Qi, Y., Yu, Y., Li, B., & Xiang, Y. T. (2017). Sleep duration and its association with demographics, lifestyle factors, poor mental health and chronic diseases in older Chinese adults. *Psychiatry Research*, *257*, 212–218. http://dx.doi.org/10.1016/j.psychres.2017.07.036

Ware, J. E., & Sherbourne, C. D. (1992). The MOS 36-item short-form health survey (Sf-36): I. Conceptual framework and item selection. *Medical Care*, *30*(6), 473–483. http://dx.doi.org/10.1097/00005650-199206000-00002

Watson, D., Clark, L. A., & Tellegen, A. (1988). Development and validation of brief measures of positive and negative affect: The PANAS scales. *Journal of Personality and Social Psychology*, *54*(6), 1063–1070. http://dx.doi.org/10.1037/0022-3514.54.6.1063

Wattanapisit, A., Abdul Rahman, H., Car, J., Abdul-Mumin, K. H., de la Cruz, M. H. T. O., Chia, M., Rosenberg, M., Ho, M., Ho, R., Chaiyasong, S., Mahmudiono, T., Rodjarkpai, Y., Dinov, I. D., Ottom, M., & Amornsriwatanakul, A. (2022). The clusters of health-risk behaviours and mental wellbeing and their sociodemographic correlates: A study of 15,366 ASEAN university students. *BMC Public Health*, *22*(1), 1840. http://dx.doi.org/10.1186/s12889-022-14233-2

Wilson, K., Senay, I., Durantini, M., Sánchez, F., Hennessy, M., Spring, B., & Albarracín, D. (2015). When it comes to lifestyle recommendations, more is sometimes less: A meta-analysis of theoretical assumptions underlying the effectiveness of interventions promoting multiple behavior domain change. *Psychological Bulletin*, *141*(2), 474–509. http://dx.doi.org/10.1037/a0038295

Wong, V. W. H., Ho, F. Y. Y., Shi, N. K., Sarris, J., Chung, K. F., & Yeung, W. F. (2021). Lifestyle medicine for depression: A meta-analysis of randomized controlled trials. *Journal of Affective Disorders*, *284*, 203–216. http://dx.doi.org/10.1016/j.jad.2021.02.012

Wood, W., & Neal, D. T. (2007). A new look at habits and the habit-goal interface. *Psychological Review*, *114*(4), 843–863. http://dx.doi.org/10.1037/0033-295X.114.4.843

Zhang, A., Liu, S., White, B., Liu, X., Durantini, M., Chan, S., Dai, W. Y. Z., Leung, M., Ye, Q. D. O., Palmese, L., & Albarracín, D. (2024). Multiple-behavior interventions to promote health: A meta-analysis of general and behavior-specific processes of change. *Psychological Bulletin*. Advance online publication. https://doi.org/10.1037/bul0000427

Zilcha-Mano, S., Constantino, M. J., & Eubanks, C. F. (2022). Evidence-based tailoring of treatment to patients, providers, and processes: Introduction to the special issue. *Journal of Consulting and Clinical Psychology*, *90*(1), 1–4. http://dx.doi.org/10.1037/ccp0000694

31

Lessons from Digital Health Research

Jenna Reno[1], Kevin Wombacher[2], and Brian Southwell[1]
[1] RTI International
[2] University of Illinois–Chicago

The proliferation of digital media in recent decades has shaped possibilities for people to encounter, seek, promote, and share information related to health. Efforts to understand how best to navigate this new digital landscape across the spectrum of health behaviors have generated lessons that are applicable to practitioners interested in improving mental health. Understanding some common pitfalls that exist in the realm of digital health promotion can help practitioners avoid these same mistakes and can provide guidance on how best to structure attempts to influence conversations about mental health. Past observations of digital health projects also suggest insights regarding health outcome measurement and the potential effectiveness of digital campaigns.

Opportunities to Encourage Health Behavior via Digital Media

Digital Media Campaigns and Interventions

Media campaigns and interventions in support of population health and well-being have drawn on digital media tools in various ways in recent years. Public health campaigns have a robust history of utilizing mass media to educate the public and encourage positive health behaviors, yet one challenge such efforts have faced has been the limitations of content reach and timing for relevant audiences. A television advertisement can reach many people but can be costly to create and will reach only specific audiences. The evolution of digital media as widely available and somewhat inexpensive tools has created numerous opportunities for reaching a diverse range of audiences quickly with messages that can be updated over time and responsive to audience input.

In 2013, for example, the Centers for Disease Control and Prevention (CDC) added a suite of digital media—online video ads, display ads, mobile ads, and paid search linked to the campaign website—to its national anti-smoking campaign (Centers for Disease Control and Prevention, 2012). Markets with higher saturation with digital advertising than television advertising demonstrated higher levels of overall ad awareness than those where television ads were more highly placed than digital (Davis et al., 2016). A report evaluating the *Tips* campaign between 2012 and 2018 showed that it was responsible for 16.4 million quit attempts and 1,005,419 sustained quits (Murphy-Hoefer et al., 2020).

Social media—platforms in which individual users can post their content and connect directly and interact with other users—also have shown promise as platforms for health campaigns. The use of social media for awareness initiatives has demonstrated effectiveness as practitioners have used social media to increase reach, knowledge, and engagement in various health initiatives. Ghahramani et al. (2022)

The Handbook of Mental Health Communication, First Edition.
Edited by Marco C. Yzer and Jason T. Siegel.

concluded in their review that social media–based interventions can have small but significantly beneficial effects on changing health behavior.

We know that the online information environment can encourage patient engagement with specific health information. For example, the Minnesota Heart Health Program launched a media campaign called *Ask About Aspirin* to encourage patients to talk with health care professionals about the use of aspirin for cardiovascular disease prevention in 2012 (Zauche & Berra, 2012). In 2015, the campaign began the online promotion of a web-based assessment tool that patients could use to consider their risk. That online promotion prompted patient behavior. Time-series evidence using data from September 2014 to September 2017 suggested population use of the online tool to be a function of the amount of paid search promotion sponsored by the campaign over and above factors such as simple topical search trends (Southwell et al., 2018). In other words, digital media campaigns can encourage health information-seeking among patients.

Social media activities also have been shown to increase awareness and raise money for health research. The ALS [amyotrophic lateral sclerosis] Ice Bucket Challenge may be one of the most memorable examples. In this social media challenge, users were encouraged to record a video of themselves dumping a bucket of ice-cold water over their heads and then challenging other users to do the same. The goal of this challenge was to raise awareness of the disease and money for research. Pressgrove et al. (2018) posit that part of what made this challenge successful was that it allowed users to gain social currency while engaging with it, that it stirred a positive emotional response, and that it was done in a way that was public and easy to share. Understanding what factors allowed the ALS Ice Bucket Challenge to be successful can help guide future health behavior change campaigns.

Multiple campaigns also have found success in building general awareness of health issues via social media (Patel et al., 2020). The hashtag #WorldCancerDay as well as social media efforts related to National Breast Cancer Awareness Month have found success in generating engagement on social media as well as increasing relevant web searches about cancer. In 2020, the #GetMePPE movement on Twitter along with the website GetUsPPE.org were able to coordinate personal protective equipment (PPE) donation and distribution via public engagement and advocacy on social media (He et al., 2020).

The success of digital media health campaigns provides multiple examples and principles that can be translated to the mental health field. Effective campaigns use multiple digital channels targeting channels popular among core audiences. Integrating social media allows for capitalizing upon features that promote engagement among users as well as between users and health communicators. Users are motivated by campaigns that provide social currency via advocacy and activism or "slacktivism" efforts (McCafferty, 2011). By employing proven digital media strategies, mental health communicators can create campaigns and interventions that produce positive mental health outcomes.

Mobile Applications and Wearables

Mobile applications (apps) and wearables also have demonstrated potential for improving health outcomes. Apps have been used to track and improve nutrition, to increase physical activity, and to improve sleep. A 2019 review assessed long-term and short-term outcomes from the use of apps for managing type 2 diabetes (Wu et al., 2019). Their meta-analysis of 11 studies showed a significant reduction in the mean HbA1c levels (a primary clinical outcome for diabetes control) among participants who presumably used apps for lifestyle modification.

Some health-focused applications now include elements of so-called gamification, which potentially make apps more engaging to users by using game design elements (Berglund et al., 2022). Montagni et al. (2020) examined the use of gamified digital tools for vaccine promotion and found evidence for positive effects on intended outcomes (e.g., behavior, cognition, use, and acceptability) across seven studies.

Carlier et al. (2023) have drawn on available literature to suggest considerations for designing effective health interventions using gamification. Their framework focuses on the roles and responsibilities of project partners in the design process to enhance the reusability, formalization, and transferability of their expertise to simplify the design process. By following best practices for design, research, and app development, teams can optimize the results of digital health interventions and avoid the limitations of designing content without sufficient audience input.

The field of mental health has provided a rich landscape for the adoption of mobile applications (many of which incorporate gamification elements) as well as wearables that can be used for monitoring vitals (e.g., heart rate, breathing) and behaviors associated with improved mental health (e.g., movement, exercise). However, while many mental health apps have seen commercial success, they have failed to generate consistent evidence of improved clinical outcomes (Goldberg et al., 2022). Opportunities exist for mental health communicators and researchers to meet this gap by contributing to the development of apps and the integration of wearables by integrating best practices for digital health interventions.

Online Support Groups and Health Communities

Many people use forms of digital and social media as a forum for finding health information from other people similar to themselves. Rupert et al. (2016) examined where, when, and why users seek peer-generated health information and found that they often stumble upon health information unintentionally by engaging social networks online. They often find value in this information as it presents alternative perspectives—and often use it to supplement other health information–seeking efforts or to generate questions to discuss with their health care providers. At other times, people will look for health information online because it allows them to ask health questions anonymously. Wombacher et al. (2018) found that college students used a popular social media app to ask questions or seek advice about a wide range of health topics—including many risky health behaviors.

Social media and online platforms also have facilitated the creation of spaces for users to connect over common health conditions and diseases. Online health communities serve as places where people can find health information as well as seek social support. Many social media platforms such as Facebook, X (formerly Twitter), and Reddit provide forums that focus on specific health care topics. Online support groups in which people who share common medical diagnoses can bond over their common experiences can be particularly valuable for users (Southwell & Rupert, 2016). Rueger et al. (2021) analyzed 12 years of interaction data from a question and answer (Q&A) online health community. They found that information delivered from similar others was valued more than information from those without similar interests. Information that was delivered by those who were quick to access new information or who had diverse areas of lay expertise is also valued more highly. A study by Wang et al. (2017) found that providing informational support, seeking emotional support, and companionship predicted the longevity of participation in online health communities.

These studies reveal opportunities for mental health communicators to take advantage of the socially supportive contexts and norms found on many social media platforms for promoting mental health. For example, social media accounts or online groups could be structured to engage and connect youth with similar others to provide the type of emotional and information support found in one study of transgender youth (Selkie et al., 2020). Digital communication channels may also be able to replace or supplement traditional forms of in-person communication such as using video calling platforms to facilitate therapy sessions or support groups like Alcoholics Anonymous (AA), thus increasing accessibility.

Challenges Posed by Digital Media

Social Media Connections Can Be Harmful

While social media offers an opportunity to connect with others across the globe, these connections are not always beneficial. Just as social media communities can encourage users to engage in healthy behaviors and adopt a healthy lifestyle, they can also promote and support the enactment of harmful behaviors.

Wombacher et al. (2017) explored how powerful viral trends can be used to promote binge drinking in their study of the social media phenomenon NekNominate, in which users would binge drink and then challenge other users to try drinking more than them. This example illustrates how some of the same mechanisms that can be used to support prosocial behavior, like the ALS Ice Bucket Challenge to raise awareness and money for ALS, can be used to promote harmful behaviors.

The internet and social media have also opened up new avenues for people seeking social support, and while this is often a good thing, it is not universally good. Social support provides not just information but also emotional and even tangible support for its users. Many of the social support networks that form online are meant to help users as they struggle with health issues like addiction, obesity, or mental illness. However, some social support communities provide support for harmful behaviors like substance abuse or disordered eating. Wombacher et al. (2020) examined how Reddit was used to provide social support for people using and abusing substances. They were able to seek out information and support on a number of topics including how much to take, how to assess the quality of substances, how to deal with relational turbulence that was caused by substance use, and how to avoid negative repercussions like arrest or robbery.

The ability to easily disseminate messages on a large scale has also made it easier than ever for misinformation to spread. Although misinformation has been available since long before the advent of digital media, our current environment facilitates a quicker pace of information spread than ever before. During the COVID-19 pandemic, research showed a relationship between exposure to misinformation and reduced compliance with social distancing and other protective measures (Bridgman et al., 2020) with misinformation being shared more widely across social media platforms rather than through traditional media channels. If social media users see other members of their network whom they trust sharing misinformation, they may be more likely to accept that misinformation as being accurate (Southwell, 2017).

Another factor to consider when assessing the use of social media and other digital media for health promotion campaigns is that access to reliable internet and online health information is not equal across populations. Research has shown that there is a digital divide with more vulnerable populations often having less access to online health information (Kelley et al., 2016). If your message is being disseminated only digitally, you may be inadvertently contributing to disparities in access to health information.

Social media can be a powerful tool for positive change, but it is important to recognize that not every social media user has prosocial motives. The existence of bad actors and people who intentionally engage in antisocial behavior online is an important challenge that should be considered whenever deciding how to best leverage social media. Just as every user is not a good fit for your message, not every platform will be a good fit. Being intentional about identifying what your goals are and then identifying platforms that have matching affordances is important. For instance, if your goal is to spread awareness, you would look for a platform that allows users to easily share your message to magnify its reach.

Different Media Offer Different Affordances

Social media platforms vary greatly in the different affordances that they offer to users, and these affordances often help to shape how users interact with one another on these platforms. Some of these affordances make it easier for prosocial connections to be forged, while others can make it easier for users to engage in bullying or the promotion of harmful behaviors.

For example, platforms differ in the level of anonymity that is offered to users. Some, like Facebook, encourage people to use their real name, while other platforms offer partial or complete anonymity. Anonymity is not an inherently bad affordance and can be beneficial, especially for those who want to discuss stigmatized topics. However, research has also shown that when users have a high level of anonymity, they may choose to use it to promote risky health behaviors (Wombacher et al., 2018) or to engage in bullying of other users. When considering platforms, consider what level of anonymity is offered to users on that platform and how that could either help or hinder your ability to achieve your goals.

Some platforms offer affordances that allow users to vote or react to a user's post in a way that functions as a normative mechanism. Users can leverage these mechanisms to communicate whether they agree or disagree with a message. In some platforms, users can like a post to indicate a measure of support for a message. In other platforms (like Reddit), users have the option to vote up or down on a message or reply to indicate that they agree or disagree with it.

Another affordance to consider is the extent to which a platform is geographically limited, or the ability of the platform to deliver specific content to users within a geographic area. Some platforms are ubiquitous and allow users from anywhere in the world; if your campaign has a specific geographic focus, however, you will want to select a platform that allows you to selectively target users from that area. For instance, Reddit generally does not have a geographic limitation; however, you may be able to access specific communities (i.e., subreddits,) that do have a geographic focus. Some platforms may offer the ability to target advertisements or messages to users that meet specific geographic criteria.

One of the most important affordances to understand when considering using social media for health promotion is the ability for users to share or amplify a message. The ability for a user to share the post with their community and other users is important when trying to reach a broad audience. Messages that can be easily shared or rebroadcast can spread more easily than messages that are static. Many platforms have different mechanisms that accomplish this, although they may have different terminology associated with the ability to rebroadcast a message to a user's network.

Picking a social media platform with affordances in line with your messaging goals is vital to the success of any social media promotion effort. Failing to align your messaging strategy with a platform that has the correct affordances will reduce the likelihood that your message spreads and has the intended impact on your audience or even reaches your intended audience at all. It is important to understand that which affordances are best is contextual, as what may work best for one type of audience or campaign may be a very poor choice for another. You may also want to consider using more than one platform and having multiple messaging strategies that match the different affordances each platform offers.

Measuring Health Outcomes: Opportunities and Challenges to Health Research

Digital media—including social media—allow for access to a multitude of digital analytics for tracking everything from weblink clicks to online conversations to biometric data (from wearables). Often these analytics are built into the platform and automatically track user activity. This presents a plethora of opportunities for measuring user behaviors and recording diverse outcome metrics. For example, Reno and Dempsey (2021) used Facebook advertisements to test the effectiveness of messages promoting an online human papillomavirus (HPV) educational tool by comparing advertisement metrics. By varying the geotargeting of ad placement, they were able to conduct an experimental design where exposure to different messages was controlled across user segments.

Other challenges relate to the diversity of metrics that often lack the specificity required to be truly meaningful. Many studies of digital and social media have focused on engagement metrics—link clicks, comments, sharing content, and other online content interactions—as measures of effectiveness. Engagement metrics can often serve as measures of reach and awareness replacing traditional media measures like gross rating points, yet we are still learning about the degree to which engagement can reliably predict behavior change (Eppes et al., 2023; Simeon et al., 2020; Yang, 2017). Online interactions do not necessarily translate to offline effects. The interpretation of digital metrics is also not always straightforward. For example, many platforms provide the number of impressions—the times an ad has been shown to a user—however, in environments where users actively scroll past ads, there is no way of knowing whether their brains actively registered seeing the ad. Social media platforms allow users to like a post—but what does a like mean? Does the user actually like the content, or are they trying to indicate some other meaning? Moreover, different platforms use different symbols (i.e., a thumbs-up, a heart) to indicate a like. Just as patterns and styles of use vary between different social media platforms, the meaning of a like likely varies as well. How should we compare the meaning of likes on Facebook to likes on the platform X (formerly Twitter)? These are questions with which mental health researchers will have to wrestle in considering the use of digital media platforms that allow endorsement.

Although social media platforms provide digital analytics to track content performance, most utilize complex proprietary algorithms for displaying content to users. These algorithms differ between platforms and are updated over time. The relative effectiveness of content when measured by reach or engagement metrics is necessarily impacted and potentially skewed by the algorithms. Without being able to fully account for how algorithms impact content, comparisons between posts across platforms are inherently confounded. To successfully apply principles of scientific methodologies to the study of digital media, it is necessary for researchers to address issues of reliability and validity among digital metrics.

Additionally, as the use of electronic health records has become almost universal, there are opportunities to link online user behavior to clinical health outcomes. Previous research has explored the roles social media use has on outcomes such as sexual and mental health (Keles et al., 2020). Record linkage methods could allow researchers to take this work a step further linking an individual's online activity with their health records. However, this type of record linkage across platforms is harder to accomplish than it is to conceptualize. Many institutions are reluctant to share data for the purposes of research—or lack personnel with the skills to pull data in a readily linkable format. Issues of data privacy often prevent the unauthorized sharing of personal data. Additionally, a lack of universal use of unique identifiers (such as social security numbers) presents challenges to matching records correctly across datasets. That is, how do you know that John Smith in one dataset is the same John Smith in another dataset? Advances in record linkage processes and technologies are helping to address some of these issues but still have a long way to go before the potential of record linkage across multiple contexts and platforms is realized.

Surveillance Using Digital Media

As social media use has expanded, so have the ways public health practitioners have engaged in disease surveillance and behavioral research (Aiello et al., 2020; Ellis et al., 2021; Radin et al., 2022). While this surveillance can be useful, it is not without ethical considerations, including concerns about how social media surveillance can be seen as an invasion of privacy. Users may not feel comfortable having private or governmental organizations collecting information about their health that is deeply personal or, in some cases, potentially stigmatizing. Some users may not even be aware that their posts may be collected or surveilled, which represents a threat to informed consent. In some situations, there may not be appropriate oversight and accountability for groups that engage in large-scale social media surveillance (Mello & Wang, 2020). Once data are collected, they could be sold for marketing purposes or accidentally made public through a data breach.

The practice of deidentifying individual patient health records and then selling them on a secondary health data market also raises concerns (Mandl & Perakslis, 2021). Data purchased on the secondary market can pose problems for research when researchers do not have access to the original data or an understanding of data collection methods. Patients also may not be comfortable knowing that their health data were packaged and sold as a product.

A 2014 study using manipulated Facebook feeds to research emotional contagion illustrates another set of concerns about the use of social media data for research (Kramer et al., 2014). Much criticism of the study has focused on the potential violation of the rights of research participants due to the lack of informed consent (Selinger & Hartzog, 2016). Although many digital media users unwittingly agree to share their data by quickly marking their consent to terms of use agreements required to use the platform, institutional review boards at organizations where many mental health researchers work will hold researchers to higher ethical standards than are sometimes required by social media platforms.

While digital media provide a wealth of opportunities for collecting and linking novel types of data, it is essential for mental health communication researchers to understand the limitations of their application as well as the ethical implications surrounding collecting or accessing data from users where true informed consent is missing or implausible. Digital media have become increasingly popular for mental health promotion and delivering mental health interventions. However, challenges exist when employing digital analytics to evaluate the potential impact on clinical outcomes (Kostkova, 2015). Future research should focus on developing best practices and methodologies for evaluating digital mental health interventions.

Questions for Future Inquiry

Considerations for Intervention Design on Digital Platforms

A common practice among commercial digital media entities is to tailor advertisements based on a user's web browsing history or other digital footprints, which affords opportunities and challenges. Some users have accepted that after looking at a website to potentially buy new shoes, they will later see those shoes advertised to them on another website or on their favorite social media platform. Media professionals can use this same kind of data to personalize health information (Bol et al., 2020). Previous research has found that using tailored messaging based on previously collected data can generate small but positive effects on health behavior and related constructs (Lustria et al., 2013), yet message tailoring effects are highly reliant on the rigor of the message design process—including the application of theory and which elements are tailored (Harrington & Noar, 2012). Tailoring based on digital media data may be challenging.

In one example, a study by Reno et al. (2023) found that tailored messaging was equally effective to untailored messages for promoting HPV vaccination intent. They concluded that the tailored messages failed to produce greater effects in part due to how messages were tailored to participants—demonstrating the need to control for message order as well as content. Nguyen et al. (2020) found that allowing users to have control over the customization of content presentation (as opposed to being entirely computer programmed) increased the effectiveness of the intervention. Pope et al. (2018) proposed using a Comprehensive Messaging Strategy for Sustained Behavior Change (CMSSBC) to tailor messages to individuals' stage of change and framing messages to emphasize self-determined motives and intrinsic goals. Although digital media applications can provide a trove of data for tailoring messages, we need continued research to determine how to optimize the integration of data into the design and delivery of messages that stimulate sustained behavior change.

Optimizing Engagement: Encouraging Positive Interactions While Limiting the Negative

Another challenge that can arise in using digital media for health promotion lies in the tendency of many projects to focus on engagement, which often is operationalized in terms of clicks or interaction between users (Barger et al., 2016; Welch et al., 2016). Not all forms of engagement are necessarily positive for population health, however. Many platforms allow users to leave open text comments on content wherein the content creator has little to no ability to control the types of comments received. For example, a comments section could quickly become overrun with negative forms of engagement that undermine the effects and effectiveness behind the initial post's content. During the COVID-19 pandemic, information shared via social media by public health organizations often was met with comments promoting anti-public health sentiments and misinformation (Arbane et al., 2023; Gunasekeran et al., 2022; Oyebode et al., 2021).

The negative impact of health misinformation shared in digital spaces is a leading concern among health practitioners. Social media platforms offer both some opportunities to mitigate the spread of misinformation and a potentially deceptive invitation for campaign staff to assume social media posts alone could adequately counteract all misinformation about mental health. On one hand, direct correction of misinformation at the point of exposure seems to hold promise for mitigation strategies based on social media (Bode & Vraga, 2015). At the same time, trust in information sources is a vital aspect of the influence of those sources (Southwell et al., 2021), and the development of trust over time may require ongoing effort over time, effort which could involve digital communication, but which nonetheless likely requires long-term investment on the part of intervention staff. Social media is unlikely to offer an easy remedy for misinformation mitigation unless campaign staff have established relationships with audiences.

How best to respond to negative comments on social media is unclear; we can find a range of commentary and suggestions but still need more empirical evidence. While some observers have identified strategies for responding to misleading comments, others advise ignoring or downplaying comments to prevent them from gaining further attention (Barger et al., 2016; Rim & Song, 2016). We need further research to understand how to best engage users via platforms that support conversations and allow for comments to be added with limited to no moderation.

Research Recruitment on Social Media

Social media presents new opportunities for research recruitment. Using social media advertising allows recruitment ads to be targeted to certain demographics as well as users interested in topics of interest (e.g., vaping, exercise, eating healthy, cancer). Since much digital advertising is not specifically built for research participant recruitment, however, we need more research to inform exactly how to use these tools to solicit research study enrollment or participation in health interventions as opposed to selling products.

In one example, McInnis et al. (2022) looked at the use of social media platforms Facebook, Instagram, and Pinterest for the recruitment of study participants. They recruited expectant and new mothers to sign up for an online newborn screening research study and compared the effectiveness of each platform based on the number of link clicks and subsequent participant enrollments each ad generated along with the relative cost for each. They found that in order to optimize recruitment and limit costs they needed to use different strategies for each of the platforms.

In another example, Reno and Dempsey (2021) looked at the use of Facebook advertising to promote an educational website on HPV vaccination. They assessed differences in the effectiveness of different message types by looking at link click-throughs and website engagement metrics. Although ads were successful at inviting click-throughs, the bounce rate (number of users who left the website immediately) also was high, with only a handful of users staying on the site for more than a few seconds, underlining challenges for converting social media users into engaged users of other platforms. We need more research on how to use different social media platforms for recruiting participants for research.

Conclusion

Our current information environment offers many opportunities for supporting health. Digital media tools can help to improve intervention reach, allow user interaction, and afford flexibility in content timing. At the same time, digital media tools are not a panacea for health behavior change when applied without theoretical justification or message design insights. Moreover, digital media also pose challenges for mental health professionals as a source of stress, distraction, and misinformation.

Mental health professionals can consider digital media environments and tools as both causes for concern and potential assets. Digital media offer affordances and opportunities to reach and engage with audiences through novel and often unprecedented means. Digital media can be used to provide mental health services via virtual appointments or digital health interventions reaching people who may live in more rural areas or who face transportation barriers. It is critical for mental health practitioners and researchers who seek to employ digital media to understand the benefits, challenges, and limitations of these platforms to optimize their potential to promote mental health.

References

Aiello, A. E., Renson, A., & Zivich, P. (2020). Social media-and internet-based disease surveillance for public health. *Annual Review of Public Health, 41*(1), 101–118. https://doi.org/10.1146/annurev-publhealth-040119-094402

Arbane, M., Benlamri, R., Brik, Y., & Alahmar, A. D. (2023). Social media-based COVID-19 sentiment classification model using bi-LSTM. *Expert Systems with Applications, 212*, 118710. https://doi.org/10.1016/j.eswa.2022.118710

Barger, V., Peltier, J. W., & Schultz, D. E. (2016). Social media and consumer engagement: A review and research agenda. *Journal of Research in Interactive Marketing, 10*(4), 268–287. https://doi.org/10.1108/JRIM-06-2016-0065

Berglund, A., Jaarsma, T., Berglund, E., Strömberg, A., & Klompstra, L. (2022). Understanding and assessing gamification in digital healthcare interventions for patients with cardiovascular disease. *European Journal of Cardiovascular Nursing, 21*(6), 630–638. https://doi.org/10.1093/eurjcn/zvac048

Bode, L., & Vraga, E. K. (2015). In related news, that was wrong: The correction of misinformation through related stories functionality in social media. *Journal of Communication, 65*(4), 619–638. https://doi.org/10.1111/jcom.12166

Bol, N., Smit, E. S., & Lustria, M. L. A. (2020). Tailored health communication: Opportunities and challenges in the digital era. *DIGITAL HEALTH, 6*, 2055207620958913. https://doi.org/10.1177/2055207620958913

Bridgman, A., Merkley, E., Loewen, P. J., Owen, T., Ruths, D., Teichmann, L., & Zhilin, O. (2020). The causes and consequences of COVID-19 misperceptions: Understanding the role of news and social media. *The Harvard Kennedy School Misinformation Review*. https://doi.org/10.37016/mr-2020-028

Carlier, S., Naessens, V., Backere, F. D., & Turck, F. D. (2023). A software engineering framework for reusable design of personalized serious games for health: Development study. *JMIR Serious Games, 11*(1), e40054. https://doi.org/10.2196/40054

Centers for Disease Control and Prevention. (2012). *Tips from former smokers campaign*. https://www.cdc.gov/tobacco/campaign/tips/index.html

Davis, K. C., Shafer, P. R., Rodes, R., Kim, A., Hansen, H., Patel, D., Coln, C., & Beistle, D. (2016). Does digital video advertising increase population-level reach of multimedia campaigns? Evidence from the 2013 tips from former smokers campaign. *Journal of Medical Internet Research, 18*(9), e5683. https://doi.org/10.2196/jmir.5683

Ellis, R. B., Wright, J., Miller, L. S., Jake-Schoffman, D., Hekler, E. B., Goldstein, C. M., Arigo, D., & Nebeker, C. (2021). Lessons learned: Beta-testing the digital health checklist for researchers prompts a call to action by behavioral scientists. *Journal of Medical Internet Research, 23*(12), e25414. https://doi.org/10.2196/25414

Eppes, E. V., Augustyn, M., Gross, S. M., Vernon, P., Caulfield, L. E., & Paige, D. M. (2023). Engagement with and acceptability of digital media platforms for use in improving health behaviors among vulnerable families: Systematic review. *Journal of Medical Internet Research, 25*(1), e40934. https://doi.org/10.2196/40934

Ghahramani, A., de Courten, M., & Prokofieva, M. (2022). The potential of social media in health promotion beyond creating awareness: An integrative review. *BMC Public Health, 22*(1), 2402. https://doi.org/10.1186/s12889-022-14885-0

Goldberg, S. B., Lam, S. U., Simonsson, O., Torous, J., & Sun, S. (2022). Mobile phone-based interventions for mental health: A systematic meta-review of 14 meta-analyses of randomized controlled trials. *PLOS Digital Health, 1*(1), e0000002. https://doi.org/10.1371/journal.pdig.0000002

Gunasekeran, D. V., Chew, A., Chandrasekar, E. K., Rajendram, P., Kandarpa, V., Rajendram, M., Chia, A., Smith, H., & Leong, C. K. (2022). The impact and applications of social media platforms for public health responses before and during the COVID-19 pandemic: Systematic literature review. *Journal of Medical Internet Research, 24*(4), e33680. https://doi.org/10.2196/33680

Harrington, N. G., & Noar, S. M. (2012). Reporting standards for studies of tailored interventions. *Health Education Research, 27*(2), 331–342. https://doi.org/10.1093/her/cyr108

He, S., Ojo, A., Beckman, A. L., Gondi, S., Ranney, M., Betz, M., Faust, J. S., Choo, E., Kass, D., & Raja, A. S. (2020). The story of #GetMePPE and http://GetUsPPE.org to mobilize health care response to COVID-19: Rapidly deploying digital tools for better health care. *Journal of Medical Internet Research, 22*(7), e20469. https://doi.org/10.2196/20469

Keles, B., McCrae, N., & Grealish, A. (2020). A systematic review: The influence of social media on depression, anxiety and psychological distress in adolescents. *International Journal of Adolescence and Youth, 25*(1), 79–93. https://doi.org/10.1080/02673843.2019.1590851

Kelley, M. S., Su, D., & Britigan, D. H. (2016). Disparities in health information access: Results of a county-wide survey and implications for health communication. *Health Communication, 31*(5), 575–582. https://doi.org/10.1080/10410236.2014.979976

Kostkova, P. (2015). Grand challenges in digital health. *Frontiers in Public Health, 3*, 147199. https://doi.org/10.3389/fpubh.2015.00134

Kramer, A. D. I., Guillory, J. E., & Hancock, J. T. (2014). Experimental evidence of massive-scale emotional contagion through social networks. *Proceedings of the National Academy of Sciences, 111*(24), 8788–8790. https://doi.org/10.1073/pnas.1320040111

Lustria, M. L. A., Noar, S. M., Cortese, J., Van Stee, S. K., Glueckauf, R. L., & Lee, J. (2013). A meta-analysis of web-delivered tailored health behavior change interventions. *Journal of Health Communication, 18*(9), 1039–1069. https://doi.org/10.1080/10810730.2013.768727

Mandl, K. D., & Perakslis, E. D. (2021). HIPAA and the leak of "deidentified" EHR data. *The New England Journal of Medicine, 384*, 2171–2173. https://doi.org/10.1056/NEJMp2102616

McCafferty, D. (2011). Activism vs slacktivism. *Communications of the ACM, 54*(12), 17–19. https://doi.org/10.1145/2043174.2043182

McInnis, S., Sobolewski, J., Dass, M., Gehtland, L. M., & Bailey, D. B. (2022). Using Facebook, Instagram, and Pinterest advertising campaigns to increase enrollment in newborn screening research. *Frontiers in Communication, 7*, 1052355. https://doi.org/10.3389/fcomm.2022.1052355

Mello, M. M., & Wang, C. J. (2020). Ethics and governance for digital disease surveillance. *Science, 368*(6494), 951–954. https://doi.org/10.1126/science.abb9045

Montagni, I., Mabchour, I., & Tzourio, C. (2020). Digital gamification to enhance vaccine knowledge and uptake: Scoping review. *JMIR Serious Games, 8*(2), e16983. https://doi.org/10.2196/16983

Murphy-Hoefer, R., Davis, K. C., King, B. A., Beistle, D., Rodes, R., & Graffunder, C. (2020). Association between the tips from former smokers campaign and smoking cessation among adults, United States, 2012–2018. *Preventing Chronic Disease, 17*, E97. https://doi.org/10.5888/pcd17.200052

Nguyen, M. H., Bol, N., & Lustria, M. L. A. (2020). Perceived active control over online health information: Underlying mechanisms of mode tailoring effects on website attitude and information recall. *Journal of Health Communication, 25*(4), 271–282. https://doi.org/10.1080/10810730.2020.1743797

Oyebode, O., Ndulue, C., Adib, A., Mulchandani, D., Suruliraj, B., Orji, F. A., Chambers, C. T., Meier, S., & Orji, R. (2021). Health, psychosocial, and social issues emanating from the COVID-19 pandemic based on social media comments: Text mining and thematic analysis approach. *JMIR Medical Informatics, 9*(4), e22734. https://doi.org/10.2196/22734

Patel, M. S., Halpern, J. A., Desai, A. S., Keeter, M. K., Bennett, N. E., & Brannigan, R. E. (2020). Success of prostate and testicular cancer awareness campaigns compared to breast cancer awareness month according to internet search volumes: A Google trends analysis. *Urology, 139*, 64–70. https://doi.org/10.1016/j.urology.2019.11.062

Pope, J. P., Pelletier, L., & Guertin, C. (2018). Starting off on the best foot: A review of message framing and message tailoring, and recommendations for the comprehensive messaging strategy for sustained behavior change. *Health Communication, 33*(9), 1068–1077. https://doi.org/10.1080/10410236.2017.1331305

Pressgrove, G., McKeever, B. W., & Jang, S. M. (2018). What is contagious? Exploring why content goes viral on Twitter: A case study of the ALS ice bucket challenge. *International Journal of Nonprofit and Voluntary Sector Marketing, 23*(1), e1586. https://doi.org/10.1002/nvsm.1586

Radin, J. M., Quer, G., Pandit, J. A., Gadaleta, M., Baca-Motes, K., Ramos, E., Coughlin, E., Quartuccio, K., Kheterpal, V., Wolansky, L. M., Steinhubl, S. R., & Topol, E. J. (2022). Sensor-based surveillance for digitising real-time COVID-19 tracking in the USA (DETECT): A multivariable, population-based, modelling study. *The Lancet Digital Health, 4*(11), e777–e786. https://doi.org/10.1016/S2589-7500(22)00156-X

Reno, J. E., & Dempsey, A. F. (2021). Testing messages on Facebook to promote use of an HPV educational web-intervention. *Frontiers in Digital Health, 3*, 648555. https://doi.org/10.3389/fdgth.2021.648555

Reno, J. E., Sevick, C., Maertens, J., & Dempsey, A. F. (2023). Is tailored messaging more effective? An analysis of a digital health intervention to promote HPV vaccination intent among Latinx. *Journal of Behavioral Medicine, 46*(1), 335–345. https://doi.org/10.1007/s10865-022-00340-3

Rim, H., & Song, D. (2016). "How negative becomes less negative": Understanding the effects of comment valence and response sidedness in social media. *Journal of Communication, 66*(3), 475–495. https://doi.org/10.1111/jcom.12205

Rueger, J., Dolfsma, W., & Aalbers, R. (2021). Perception of peer advice in online health communities: Access to lay expertise. *Social Science & Medicine, 277*, 113117. https://doi.org/10.1016/j.socscimed.2020.113117

Rupert, D. J., Gard Read, J., Amoozegar, J. B., Moultrie, R. R., Taylor, O. M., O'Donoghue, A. C., & Sullivan, H. W. (2016). Peer-generated health information: The role of online communities in patient and caregiver health decisions. *Journal of Health Communication, 21*(11), 1187–1197. https://doi.org/10.1080/10810730.2016.1237592

Selinger, E., & Hartzog, W. (2016). Facebook's emotional contagion study and the ethical problem of co-opted identity in mediated environments where users lack control. *Research Ethics, 12*(1), 35–43. https://doi.org/10.1177/1747016115579531

Selkie, E., Adkins, V., Masters, E., Bajpai, A., & Shumer, D. (2020). Transgender adolescents' uses of social media for social support. *Journal of Adolescent Health, 66*(3), 275–280. https://doi.org/10.1016/j.jadohealth.2019.08.011

Simeon, R., Dewidar, O., Trawin, J., Duench, S., Manson, H., Pardo, J. P., Petkovic, J., Roberts, J. H., Tugwell, P., Yoganathan, M., Presseau, J., & Welch, V. (2020). Behavior change techniques included in reports of social media interventions for promoting health behaviors in adults: Content analysis within a systematic review. *Journal of Medical Internet Research, 22*(6), e16002. https://doi.org/10.2196/16002

Southwell, B. (2017). Promoting popular understanding of science and health through social networks. In K. H. Jamieson, D. Scheufele, & D. Kahan (Eds.), *The Oxford handbook on the science of science communication* (pp. 345–359). Oxford University Press.

Southwell, B., Corin, D., Eck, M., Hessenius, A., Li, L., Magnuson, A., Parkman, J., Sauer, R., Turner, C., & Stansbury, S. (2021). Dimensions of trust and information seeking on natural disasters, hazards, and extreme weather in North Carolina (USA) (EMS2021-25). *EMS2021*. Copernicus Meetings. 10.5194/ems2021-25

Southwell, B. G., Eder, M., Finnegan, J., Hirsch, A. T., Luepker, R. V., Duval, S., Russell, C., & O'Byrne, S. (2018). The utility of online promotion to encourage patient awareness of aspirin use to prevent heart attack and stroke. *Journal of Epidemiology and Community Health, 72*, 1059–1063. https://doi.org/10.1136/jech-2018-210676

Southwell, B. G., & Rupert, D. J. (2016). Future challenges and opportunities in online prescription drug promotion research. *International Journal of Health Policy and Management, 5*(3), 211–213. https://doi.org/10.15171/ijhpm.2016.05

Wang, X., Zhao, K., & Street, N. (2017). Analyzing and predicting user participations in online health communities: A social support perspective. *Journal of Medical Internet Research, 19*(4), e130.

Welch, V., Petkovic, J., Pardo, J. P., Rader, T., & Tugwell, P. (2016). Interactive social media interventions to promote health equity: An overview of reviews. *Health Promotion and Chronic Disease Prevention in Canada: Research, Policy and Practice, 36*(4), 63–75. https://doi.org/10.24095/hpcdp.36.4.01

Wombacher, K., Reno, J. E., & Veil, S. R. (2017). NekNominate: Social norms, social media, and binge drinking. *Health Communication, 32*(5), 596–602. https://doi.org/10.1080/10410236.2016.1146567

Wombacher, K., Reno, J. E., Williams, G. A., & Johnson, L. (2018). Does Yik Yak promote risky health behavior on college campuses? *Health Communication, 33*(4), 372–378. https://doi.org/10.1080/10410236.2016.1266577

Wombacher, K., Sheff, S. E., & Itrich, N. (2020). Social support for active substance users: A content analysis of r/drugs. *Health Communication, 35*(6), 756–765. https://doi.org/10.1080/10410236.2019.1587691

Wu, X., Guo, X., & Zhang, Z. (2019). The efficacy of mobile phone apps for lifestyle modification in diabetes: Systematic review and meta-analysis. *JMIR mHealth and uHealth, 7*(1), e12297. https://doi.org/10.2196/12297

Yang, Q. (2017). Are social networking sites making health behavior change interventions more effective? A meta-analytic review. *Journal of Health Communication, 22*(3), 223–233. https://doi.org/10.1080/10810730.2016.1271065

Zauche, D., Berra, K. (2012). *ASK ABOUT ASPIRIN A Case Study on the Minnesota Heart Health Program's Aspirin-Based Cardiovascular Disease Prevention Initiative.* https://askaboutaspirin.umn.edu/wp-content/uploads/2016/12/Minnesota-case-study-FINAL-PDF-3-14-16.pdf

32

Persuasive Prevention Strategies in Health Communication

William D. Crano
Claremont Graduate University

The potential of the behavioral sciences to contribute to the public good has only recently been recognized by much of the health establishment. This is reasonable, if overdue, as available evidence supporting the effectiveness of science-based behavioral interventions in medicine is long-standing and undeniable. Research published in the *Journal of the National Cancer Institute* indicated "behaviors such as poor diet, alcohol consumption, tobacco use, sedentary behavior, and excessive ultraviolet exposure account for nearly one-half of all cancer morbidity and mortality" (Klein et al., 2022, p. 179). Imagine halving cancer rates by 50%, thereby negating the need for the painful and sometimes deadly effects of current chemotherapy and radiation treatments often used. In the United States alone, these observations are of monumental importance. It is crucial to understand that the behaviors noted by Klein and associates are voluntary. The Centers for Disease Control and Prevention (2022) estimated that tobacco use, a voluntary behavior (at least in the early phases of nicotine addiction), accounted "for more than 480,000 deaths every year, or about 1 in 5 deaths." Cornelius et al. (2023) estimated 46 million US adults used some form of combustible tobacco product in 2021, then nearly 18.7% of the population. Although the sober facts might be used to influence these trends, it is patently obvious that more than mere information is needed to make a significant dent in combustible tobacco's toll. The rising cost of cigarettes deters some youth from initiation, but the trending rise of vaping in the country more than offsets the loss among adolescents. Vaping has reversed the otherwise optimistic trend of declining cigarette use among a highly vulnerable segment of the population, 8th–12th-grade school students (Miech et al., 2023). The National Institutes of Health provide copious and useful information about the ways voluntary behaviors may prove dangerous to health and ways to avoid their grim outcomes, but thus far the battle over nicotine addiction is yet to be won. Now that tobacco has lost its mistaken reputation as a sign of adolescent rebellion, thanks in part to Florida's dearly departed "truth campaign" (1998–2003) and the like, the advent of electronic nicotine delivery systems (aka e-cigarettes or vapes) has thrown a lifeline to the immoral adults profiting from Big Tobacco's apparent attempt to poison young people for no reason other than profit. Filthy lucre has never been so filthy.

National Institute on Drug Abuse

The National Institute on Drug Abuse (NIDA, http://www.nida.nih.gov) makes available a wealth of evidence-based information about many dangerous and addictive psychoactive substances, legal and not, how they work, and why they should be avoided. It offers special advice for parents and current, contemplating, and former substance use–dependent individuals about how they might avoid

The Handbook of Mental Health Communication, First Edition.
Edited by Marco C. Yzer and Jason T. Siegel.

future use, and a director's page that deals with many evolving issues of importance in prevention. Like the National Cancer Institute, NIDA also offers information about ways to avoid the dangers of risky substance use and the many organizations that offer help for those dependent on psychoactive substances if other available information proves insufficient or is ignored. Even so, the annual Monitoring the Future study reports continuing and unacceptably high levels of risky substance use among America's youth, with 41% of high school students in 2022 reporting lifetime use of "any illicit drug" (Miech et al., 2023, p. 82). These data are discouraging considering the millions spent over the years on demand reduction and the even more expensive efforts to defeat drug importation and trafficking. Even more discouraging are current ill-advised and medically unsupportable actions of many of our state legislators to decriminalize use of marijuana among adults in their states. These actions betray a severe lack of understanding and knowledge or concern about the deflection of illicit or even legal (for adults) drugs into the adolescent population. Had they bothered to read a superb monograph by some of our best scientists, they would know that prolonged use of marijuana can stop brain development in its tracks (see National Academies of Sciences & Medicine, 2017). For those who have attained the age of majority plus 5 years (on average), recreational use may not prove overly dangerous. However, legalizing marijuana in light of its rapid deflection into a population whose brains have yet to develop fully seems criminally negligent. Marijuana-based substances whose delta-9-tetrahydrocannabino (THC) content has been enhanced to an incredible 90% are easily available. The National Academies' monograph was based on the unadulterated varieties available in legal dispensaries. The modified versions (dabs, wax) of considerably higher THC levels seem likely to have more damaging long-term effects. The widespread rationalization defense, "It's natural," is frequently used to argue for the use of cannabis over prescription pharmaceuticals, but there is not much of the unadulterated natural cannabis to be found in street products that often are favored because of their higher potency and lower cost than in the varieties dispensed in legal dispensaries. The illogical and annoying "It's natural" argument begs the question of the many natural substances that are not health promotive, as Socrates learned.

National Heart, Lung, and Blood Institute

The National Heart, Lung, and Blood Institute promotes prevention and treatment of cardiovascular issues and related lung and blood matters. As part of its mission, the institute is concerned with the hidden dangers of high blood pressure and the steps needed to avoid dangers without major adjustments to one's lifestyle. These may involve minimizing salt in one's diet, maintaining a healthy body mass index, and engaging in moderate exercise. As numerous studies have shown, however, medical compliance with moderate regimens appears difficult to maintain even when failure to do so could prove fatal. For example, McDermott et al. (1997) found noncompliance with medical advice had a negative impact on heart disease patients. In related research, Bennett et al. (2005) showed that up to 76% of heart patients indicated that curbing salt use was a barrier to compliance—78% found compliance disruptive to their normal sleep cycle.

This is not to diminish either reason for noncompliance, but it is inescapable that these self-reported barriers to compliance do not bode well for good health. Using an e-health self-management intervention, even the clear danger of HIV infection progressing to full-blown AIDS was not enough to convince individuals to comply with antiretroviral therapy (ART; Schnall et al., 2023). A study of longitudinal adherence to an ART intervention conducted in California showed an encouraging overall adherence rate of 85% over 210 weeks (Tchakoute et al., 2022), but large sociodemographic differences (e.g. age and race) indicated a clear need for more tailored interventions to reach all those afflicted. One size does not fit all.

National Institute of Mental Health

Along with many state and nongovernmental organizations (NGOs), the National Institute of Mental Health has consistently warned of the dangers of depression and where help can be found to assist the many thousands who suffer the debilitating effects of this condition. Most of these organizations offer helpful information that is online and free to anyone wishing to use it. Yet depression remains one of the most debilitating diseases humankind faces. The World Health Organization (2019, 2022) reported more than 280 million people were living with depression across the globe. Clearly, much needs to be accomplished, but some recent research has shown that depressed individuals can be persuaded to seek help through mass-mediated intervention approaches, which clearly are needed given the vast scope of the problem (e.g. Siegel et al., 2017; Siegel & Thomson, 2017; Straszewski & Siegel, 2021). As found in considerable research on persuasive prevention, tailored interventions appear most effective (e.g. Lienemann & Siegel, 2018; Noar, 2006), but using the appropriate method of presenting health-relevant preventive communications to attain the greatest effect is critical.

The list could be extended almost indefinitely, but the moral of this story is the same. For many in the field, the information necessary to address health-relevant concerns across a wide variety of afflictions is there for the taking, and well-meaning dedicated people across a range of governmental institutes and NGOs are willing to assist. However, the key to creating conditions that impel individuals to take advantage of the help on offer is another issue. Given our relatively long-term lack of success, it might be time to reexamine some of the working assumptions that have been a consistent feature of health communications over the years. Had these assumptions been investigated more thoughtfully and rigorously evaluated, it is conceivable that progress would have been advanced.

Some Reasonable Assumptions in Need of Reconsideration

Information ≠ Action

A common element of almost all the health promotion organizations' communications cited here, and most others not cited, is the promise that health can be improved or attained if the information on offer is absorbed and the appropriate behaviors subsequently adopted. Information—or better, knowledge—is the implied key to good health. It facilitates the ways people might change or modify their behaviors to avoid unnecessary health risks. For those who ignored, were unaware, or somehow did not absorb the advice provided, additional approaches may be mounted to inform the uninformed or convert the defiant or resistant. The safety net provided by prosocial government institutes and NGOs is well conceived and often semi-effective, but it clearly is insufficient considering ample evidence, which relates unhealthy behaviors to subsequent morbidity and mortality indices. Information clearly is necessary. The point seems obvious. One might not avoid the dangers of fentanyl overdose if the dangers of the substance are not known and not addressed in the relevant health promotion communications. Why would an individual who uses illicit injection substances avoid use of fentanyl if the danger inherent in its use is not known? But here's the rub: Even if provided, information alone often is not sufficient to induce behavior change. For example, most smokers are well aware of the dangers of smoking; yet many find it nearly impossible to quit. The World Health Organization (2024) estimated 39 million people worldwide are living with HIV, which probably often was not contracted via routes other than sexual transmission or misuse of injection tools. These numbers and the long history of the HIV/AIDS pandemic indicate that the effects of logic, knowledge, and apparent self-interest on behavior often are limited.

These simple facts reveal that dissemination of valid and useful information—a central goal of many health-promoting communications—although obviously necessary, is obviously insufficient. The insufficiency is the result of an incorrect assumption that information alone is enough to ensure proper action. Usually, it is not. Preventing risky behavior requires more than knowledge; it involves some way of motivating receivers to act on it consistently and persistently. Understanding that proffered actions are clearly in the receiver's self-interest appears needed to ensure their compliance with good advice. Knowing something and doing something consistent with what is known are different, and this is where health communications dealing with avoidance of unhealthy behaviors often fail. The issue involves not merely informing; rather, the information must be actionable and incite action. Further, the incitement to action must trump other behaviors that might motivate alternate behaviors diametrically opposed to those suggested.

In our view, the incitement involves the application of established principles of persuasion, paired with a rationale that takes advantage of the imparted information. The combination seems obvious, but in practice the integration often is not seen. The assumption of prosocial health communication is that people value good health, often above other concerns; if this assumption is incorrect, then logically, such preventive communications are a waste of effort. Thus, attending to the assumptions underlying our health-promoting messages is indicated. If information is necessary but not sufficient to affect behavior, then a pure information model is unlikely to have the effects that would seem the logical goal of our prevention activities. The assumption needs to be altered.

Prevention ≠ Cure

There is an important and obvious distinction between prevention and treatment, but in some settings the distinction becomes muddled. The two processes, although complementary, are distinct in their aims and processes. Communication-based prevention approaches are not likely to succeed in changing committed, ongoing risky behaviors. A persuasive communication intervention designed to prevent a behavior that is a part of an individual's behavioral repertoire will not usually succeed. In the current context, prevention is focused on mitigating the initiation of risky behaviors. However, once they are engaged and become part of the ongoing behavior pattern of the individual, prevention ceases to be relevant. Obviously, curative clinical intervention involves persuasion, but the persuasion model of prevention is wholly different from clinical treatment.

A second distinction between prevention and treatment concerns the relative support for the necessary activities of prevention and treatment. By almost any metric, it is patently obvious that the bulk of available public funding is provided to treat problems after they have developed rather than to prevent the problems from developing in the first place.[1] There is an undeniable logic to the lopsided support provided treatment over prevention in the United States. After all, a person presenting with symptoms of acute coronary distress is better served by appropriate medical interventions than by lectures about the dangers of smoking while morbidly obese. When the house is burning, we require water, not a treatise on the nature of fire. However, the vast discontinuity between support for treatment over funding may condemn our efforts to a continuous cycle of disease, for without prevention we may be doomed to fix the same problems (along with new ones that occur) with no end to the dismal cycle. Simple logic would seem to lead to an infusion of funding for preventive activities to a substantially greater extent than has been evident for many years. Prior and recent cost–benefit analyses indicate the enormous returns on investments in prevention, which considerably eclipse similar analyses bearing on the relative benefit-to-cost of treatment outcomes. The National Center for Drug Abuse Statistics showed the average investment in US Federal Drug Control spending on prevention averaged $1.71 billion per year over the years 2014–2020. In 2008, spending was $1.8 billion. During the period 2014–2020 Federal Drug Control spending on treatment averaged $12.26 billion per year. In 2008, spending was $6.7 billion. Differences in spending growth between prevention and treatment support require no hyperbole (see https://www.Drugabusestatistics.org). Pointing out this disparity should not be taken as an argument to cut treatment funding in favor of prevention. This issue cannot be viewed as a zero-sum game. Treatment is fundamental, but if current practices were restructured such that a more even distribution were to occur, both fields might be better served. The disproportionate funding of treatment over prevention must be addressed, and with the onslaught of fentanyl and other synthetic drugs, sooner is better than later, as later may be too late.

Why Has Prevention Been Shortchanged?

Possibly the reason prevention, writ large, has been underfunded relative to treatment is that evidence demonstrating preventive successes is not readily forthcoming. Why throw money at an approach that has only irregularly produced the anticipated findings or, worse yet, that sometimes has produced outcomes opposite those expected, the dreaded iatrogenic effect? Such backfires are rare, but they are noticed when they occur, especially when their costs are high (Hornik et al., 2008). Even when iatrogenesis is not evident, simple failures to produce successful outcomes of costly social interventions often have dampened enthusiasm for pouring more support into approaches that have failed to deliver expected results.

Such reactions, however, often are misguided. For example, not long ago in the face of some costly failures of media-based prevention activities, the European Monitoring Center for Drugs and Drug Addiction (EMCDDA) found that nearly 30% of its members had scrubbed or seriously cut back on the funding of such preventive activities. The reason for this drastic action noted by EMCDDA seemed obvious to some: Media-based drug prevention efforts were not successful in moderating substance use, as shown by the continued intransigence of usage rates; hence, stop spending valuable prevention euros on the media. The logic of this conclusion, however, demands further consideration. It seems analogous to throwing a beautiful dinner plate into the trash because the dinner was not to one's liking. The media are mere servants of the message. McLuhan was not correct; the medium is not the message (McLuhan, 1964). The message is the message, and if the message is not persuasive, there's little chance that it will attain the desired persuasive results no matter its medium of dissemination—which in EMCDDA's case was an attenuation of media-based substance use prevention in some of its member states. Admittedly, the media are far from a panacea, but no one ever claimed they were. However, there should be no doubt that they can be and have proved to be a powerful ally in the service of prevention; this is true only if the messages the media are made to convey are persuasive and not merely informative. Without the added ingredient of persuasion, information rarely translates into action, even when the stakes may be life or death. To succeed, the information that is conveyed must be acted on. The mere fact that one knows something is no guarantee that the knowledge will be transformed into behavior or even attitude change. This holds even in contexts in which the communication is of existential moment. If the message does not involve one's vested interest, its effects on behavior will be trivial. It is good to remember: information $\neq$ persuasion.

Persuasive Prevention

It is a major premise of this chapter that persuasive prevention communications can be exceptionally valuable resources in health communication. This is not arguable for many in behavioral science, but it is clearly not common knowledge among many decision-makers whose behavior belies this position. We have argued the provision of information alone is almost never sufficient to motivate action. Something more must be added, and we have shown that ingredient is persuasion (Crano et al., 2013, 2015; Crano & Alvaro, 2013; Crano, Alvaro, & Siegel, 2019; Crano & Burgoon, 2002; Crano & Ruybal, 2020; Siegel et al., 2015, 2017, 2019).[2] We have tried information. Now it is time to wed information with persuasion, an approach we might term *persuasive prevention*. To show the utility of this approach and the dangers of its circumvention, consider a recent massive failure of media-based prevention, presented in high definition on almost every television screen in America: the campaign to stop the fatal effects of COVID-19 on an initially unaware public and the role preventive persuasion might have played.

Some Background

One of the most established findings in communication and persuasion was produced by Carl Hovland and associates (1953), who were interested in the features of a communication source that influenced its power to persuade. In their research, conducted more than 80 years ago, they found that two factors worked hand in hand to establish source credibility, a crucial feature because credible sources can affect attitude change. They termed these features *expertise*, the perceived capacity of a message source to provide valid information, and *trustworthiness*, the perception that the source was not providing information for its own benefit (and often, to the detriment of the message receiver). The source credibility effect has been demonstrated innumerable times. It is practically an article of faith in communication science and social psychology.

Now consider the common prevention model evident at the height of the COVID-19 pandemic. In addition to the massive effort to create a vaccine that could shield the populace from the potentially fatal infection, the government mounted an all-hands-on-deck social communication attack to inform the populace and influence their behavior (e.g. close bars, theaters, and schools; be inoculated, wear masks). An unanticipatedly large proportion of the population resisted all these preventive actions. In their effort to persuade the unpersuaded, the Donald Trump administration trotted out some noteworthy scientific talent, including Dr. Anthony Fauci, a hero to many dating from his efforts during the HIV/AIDS panic of the 1970s. Fauci, along with then-president Trump, was onstage seemingly daily, urging people to be inoculated and to behave in ways that would help them avoid COVID infection, which was killing citizens in alarming numbers. Those who were in Fauci's corner probably were inoculated as soon as the vaccine became available, but many were not in his corner and continually refused to follow his advice. Why? If Hovland were around, he would have told the government that Fauci was the very last person to deliver the prevention message to so-called COVID resisters, as he was probably the least credible spokesperson imaginable to that audience. They may have distrusted Fauci because of Trump's own disdain for Fauci, conveyed in terms of the president's creative alternative approaches to confront the virus (e.g. ingesting bleach or large animal tranquilizers) and his tacit lack of agreement with the good doctor's advice. Too many resisted, and some of them paid for their intransigence with their lives.

Why did those in charge continue to match a message source with those least likely to find the source credible? Why did they continue after the apparent ineffectiveness of their efforts? Their actions were wasteful, almost certain to fail, and most good behavioral scientists anticipated this outcome. Indeed, some even might have recommended alternative courses of action. But the failed approach persisted, and the question remains. A possible answer is that those in charge did not know a simple and often replicated result that had been a part of the persuasion literature from the 1950s. That might be a plausible hypothesis were it not for some who tried desperately to make this point to any authority (including those scientists on the anti-COVID team) who would listen, to no avail. The campaign failed, or at least was not as successful as it might have been. Brief consideration of the mortality statistics renders this statement unarguable. But it is not the media that failed. In this case it was the messenger, who through no fault of his own was doomed to fail from the start. This is not a criticism of Fauci, a hero of contemporary medical science, but of the intransigent political experts whose certain knowledge of what to do was based on little more than conjecture. Hubris kills.

What Might Have Been

Assume the powers that be had listened to advice from qualified behavioral scientists. The first thing they might have done is determine the source of their audience's reluctance. Then, they might have found a messenger (communication source) who was universally or near universally trusted and viewed as highly knowledgeable, or credible in Hovland et al.'s (1953) terminology. Certainly, such people exist, but they were rarely, if ever drafted in service of the cause. Our point is not to blame the administration for a poor choice of spokespersons but rather to show how with relatively little effort they might have saved hundreds of thousands of people who otherwise might be alive today. This should weigh heavily on the experts who rejected clear, evidence-based calls to revise their failed approach.

Some simple persuasive strategies that might have been tried, assuming a proper message source (or sources) had been identified, would be to identify influential individuals in their communities—remember, in persuasion, one size does not fit all. Today, such influential individuals have been termed *opinion leaders*, whose views have a powerful influence on their opinion followers. Opinion leaders have a powerful influence on the outcome of media-based campaigns because they have strong effects on their followers' interpretations and evaluations of mass-mediated communications (Crano et al., 2017; Lazarsfeld et al., 1944). Identifying such opinion leaders would not have proven unduly difficult, and this change alone likely would have had a powerful impact on inoculation rates among resistant group members.

Choosing the proper message source clearly is crucial in the persuasion process, but equally important is the source's message and the management of a persuasion campaign. How could a source of proinoculation communications persuade a reluctant (but not hostile) audience to consider changing their attitudes toward COVID inoculation? The answer takes many forms, but placing the proper source at the table's head is a great first step. Without this, there isn't a second step. Assuming the best, a properly chosen source would need to create a series of persuasive communications, as a single message in a persuasion campaign is not likely to succeed (Crano et al., 2015). This would facilitate persuasion, but what would these speakers say and how would their messages be structured for maximal impact?

The EQUIP Model of Communication Development

The structure of successful media-based prevention communications appears to follow a regular pattern. We have distilled this knowledge in a simple acronym that summarizes the steps the communicator must take, and their order of precedence when developing effective persuasive communications. These steps are summarized in the acronym EQUIP (Crano, Alvaro, & Siegel, 2019a), which is shorthand for engage, question, undermine, inform, and persuade. The model is based on an evidence base built on results of hundreds of persuasion studies conducted over the years.

Engage

The process requires the communicator to ***engage*** the audience throughout the presentation of the persuasive message. Most communication professionals will not find this particularly challenging. Visual effects, quick cuts in a video, unexpected colors or print sizes on posters or billboards, and so forth all attract attention. Following engagement, message content presented in the following sections of the persuasive message must carry the burden of maintaining engagement. In a 30- to 60-second video clip, this requirement should not prove overly onerous.

Question

Immediately following, or as part of the engagement process itself, the next requirement of the communication is to raise a ***question***. The question should not threaten or contest the expected answer but rather signal communication receivers that not everyone believes as they do. Simply raising the question begins to weaken the assumed consensus that acts as a bolster of the individual's belief. Assuming everyone else agrees with our belief can provide a powerful underpinning of the belief. Raising a question about belief consensus begins to raise doubts about the assumed widespread agreement of the belief and renders it more susceptible to subsequent persuasive argumentation.

Undermine

A simple question to a person reluctant to receive a Covid inoculation might be, "Do you think the Moderna (or Pfizer) vaccine is ineffective (risky, dangerous)?" Having asked the question, the next step of the EQUIP model is to ***undermine*** the answer that is given. Sometimes this might be accomplished by providing an incontestable expert on the issue under consideration, who provides strong evidence that is difficult to counterargue; or we could cite facts from news sources or other publications the audience member finds nearly irrefutable because to do so would unbalance other strongly held beliefs.

Inform

This EQUIP phase is designed to provide the ammunition necessary to rebut the answer received in the question phase (e.g. "Actually, some of our best medical schools have shown the vaccine is highly effective," "exceptionally safe," or "has been developed based on one of the largest social health campaigns in the history of the world"). This part of the message, in conjunction with the earlier phases, is designed to add to the uncertainty of the targeted individual. The stark rebuttal of the undermining is followed by, or combined in the EQUIP model's inform stage, where evidence is brought to bear on the validity of the undermining retort. Strong messages combined with highly credible sources are needed in this context, as these factors both bear on the likelihood of message acceptance (see Hovland et al., 1953; Petty & Krosnick, 1995).

Persuade

The final phase of the EQUIP model's attitude change procedure involves acceptance of persuasive communication. The persuade phase brings all the various EQUIP features together. It is designed to link positive outcomes with message acceptance. Indicating why the proffered information should be accepted. It can take many forms. For example, it might show why compliance with persuasive communication supports the targets' vested interest (Donaldson et al., 2016, 2020; Siegel et al., 2019), or it could be merely that one's association with a positively regarded message source is reinforcing. A strong message also can help resolve nagging doubts. In addition, the cognitive equilibrium resulting from the resolution of attitude ambivalence also can prove reinforcing, and the induced change is likely to be maintained (Crano, Donaldson, et al., 2019b). The particular form of reinforcement for message acceptance that is offered will depend on the issues and audience and will prove a decisive factor in the success of the messages advanced in the campaign.

The persuade phase requires the interventionist to take advantage of the many factors identified in the literature over the years as effective adjuncts to the persuasion process. Some of these adjuncts are distraction (Petty et al., 1976), misdirection (Crano et al., 2007; Siegel et al., 2015), innuendo (Wegner et al., 1981), vested interest (Adame, 2020; Siegel et al., 2019) and a host of other subtle tactics that induce attention and attitude change.

Lasswell's two-step flow of communication, rarely tested experimentally, can prove a powerful adjunct to the behavior change process (e.g., Crano et al., 2017). Strong and relevant message sources, targeted or tailored messages relevant to the targeted individual, and many other features established over the past half-century in the persuasion literature are relevant and can be employed without undue effort. Of course, the propriety of persuasive health communication interventions must be honored, its truth must be unassailable, and the ethical treatment of all must be absolute.

If all the phases of the EQUIP model are followed rigorously and in order, the process is most likely to produce persuasive preventive communications. Of course, many other factors will influence persuasive success. Targeting the appropriate audience or tailoring the communication to critical features of the audience has been shown to accelerate persuasive message acceptance (Lustria et al., 2013; Noar, 2006; Willoughby & Noar, 2022). Normative interventions, which may be brought to bear in the information phase of the EQUIP model, also may have positive implications for persuasive success (Blanton & Burkley, 2008; Neighbors et al., 2019). Using a misdirected communication approach also reduces reactance or resistance to a persuasive message (Crano et al., 2007; Siegel et al., 2015). The literature is replete with research on tactics of persuasion that operate powerfully in the appropriate contexts. These must be considered when creating persuasive communications. Once these contexts are identified, the EQUIP model provides guidelines for developing persuasive communications that maximize the chances for success. It is hoped that this advice will be considered when the next major health threat occurs. Meanwhile, it is reasonable to get ahead of the needed work by refining our message development strategies and understanding features of the contexts in which our research and applications will be employed. Together, these factors may add considerable strength to health-relevant interventions.

In Short

The persuasion process is at once simple and complex. It is simple because at heart persuasion involves convincing another to believe or act in a way that, without force or coercion, they initially opposed. Without the implied element of conflict, the context does not initiate persuasion. Threats, coercion, and brute force are not elements of persuasion, which is focused on others' acceptance of a source's communication. However, this does not suggest that persuasion for ignoble purposes cannot succeed.

Accordingly, it might prove wise for those who wish to use persuasion to promote mental health to consider the advice offered herein.

The fundamental goal of the persuasion process is to achieve others' acceptance of a position that another had not considered initially, or that was different from or strongly at odds with their initial views. A central feature of persuasion is its focus on overcoming apathy or resistance to the proffered position. Obvious tactics to *avoid* include fear-arousing or disgusting appeals; exaggerated, unbelievable, or overblown messages; humorous appeals that focus more on being funny than on persuading; and using language that commands rather than suggests, as the former indicates a lack of respect for the audience. What should be done? Remember the first necessity is to overcome resistance. Target or tailor the message to the proclivities, interests, and susceptibilities of the audience. Use the EQUIP model to develop communications that resonate with the audience's interests and needs. You will appreciate how these suggestions may be most usefully enacted by learning as much as possible about the people you are hoping to influence on the road to better health.

Concluding Comments

The use of persuasive communications in health promotion contexts has been shown to have a powerful preventive impact on many risky behaviors, including adolescent vaping (e.g. Ma et al., 2023), smoking prevention in cancer patients (Yingst et al., 2023), obesity prevention (Parsons et al., 2023), and many other health areas. Media-based persuasive persuasion can help ameliorate a veritable host of health conditions that are susceptible to behavioral interventions. The evidence base exists to aid creators of interventions planned for local, regional, national, or international venues to encourage mounting strong interventions across a range of health-relevant conditions. To base campaigns on what seems to be common sense is usually an excuse to avoid doing the work necessary for success. Dereliction of duty may be another way of putting it. Perhaps we should change our approach. The use of evidence and science will help.

Notes

1 Miller & Hendrie (2008), estimated an $18 return on every prevention dollar spent, whereas the President's Office of National Drug Policy (2012) estimated that approximately $4 were returned for every treatment dollar spent. More recent estimates are largely of the same order of magnitude.

2 In persuasion, redundance often proves necessary. One-shot exposures rarely suffice.

References

Adame, B. J. (2020). Connecting attitudes and motivating behavior: Vested interest theory. In H. D. O'Hair & M. J. O'Hair (Eds.), *The handbook of applied communication research* (Vol. 1, pp. 47–62). John Wiley & Sons.

Bennett, S. J., Lane, K. A., Welch, J., Perkins, S. M., Brater, D. C., & Murray, M. D. (2005). Medication and dietary compliance beliefs in heart failure. *Western Journal of Nursing Research, 27*(8), 977–993. https://doi.org/10.1177/0193945905280253

Blanton, H., & Burkley, M. (2008). Deviance regulation theory: Applications to adolescent social influence. In M. J. Prinstein & K. A. Dodge (Eds.), *Understanding peer influence in children and adolescents* (pp. 94–121). Guilford Press.

Centers for Disease Control and Prevention. (2022). *Health effects of cigarette smoking*. https://www.cdc.gov/tobacco/data_statistics/fact_sheets/health_effects/effects_cig_smoking

Cornelius, M. E., Loretan, C. G., Mamal, A., Lynn, B. C., Mayer, M., Alcantara, I. C., & Neff, L. (2023). Tobacco product use among adults—United States, 2021. *Morbidity and Mortality Weekly Report, 72*(18), 475–483.

Crano, W. D., & Alvaro, E. M. (2013). Social factors that affect the processing and subsequent effect of persuasive communications. In J. P. Forgas, O. Vincze, & J. Laszlo (Eds.), *Social cognition and communication* (pp. 297–312). Psychology Press.

Crano, W. D., Alvaro, E. M., & Siegel, J. T. (2015). The media campaign as a focal prevention strategy: A guide to design, implementation, and evaluation. In L. M. Scheier (Ed.), *Handbook of adolescent drug use prevention: Research, intervention strategies, and practice* (pp. 397–414). American Psychological Association. https://doi.org/10.1037/14550-023

Crano, W. D., Alvaro, E. M., & Siegel, J. T. (2019a). Creating persuasive substance-use prevention communications: The EQUIP model. In Z. Sloboda, H. Petras, E. Robertson, & R. W. Hingson (Eds.), *Prevention of substance use* (pp. 303–318). Springer Nature Switzerland.

Crano, W. D., Alvaro, E. M., Tan, C. N., & Siegel, J. T. (2017). Social mediation of persuasive media in adolescent substance prevention. *Psychology of Addictive Behaviors, 31*(4), 479–487. https://doi.org/10.1037/adb0000265

Crano, W. D., & Burgoon, M. (2002). *Mass media and drug prevention: Classic and contemporary theories and research.* Lawrence Erlbaum Associates Publishers.

Crano, W. D., Donaldson, C. D., Siegel, J. T., Alvaro, E. M., & O'Brien, E. K. (2019b). Selective invalidation of ambivalent pro-marijuana attitude components. *Addictive Behaviors, 97*, 77–83. https://doi.org/10.1016/j.addbeh.2019.05.020

Crano, W. D., & Ruybal, A. L. (2020). Social psychological contributions to the mitigation of adolescent depression. In J. P. Forgas, W. D. Crano, & K. Fiedler (Eds.), *Applications of social psychology: How social psychology can contribute to the solution of real-world problems* (pp. 207–230). Routledge/Taylor & Francis Group. https://doi.org/10.4324/9780367816407-11

Crano, W. D., Siegel, J. T., & Alvaro, E. M. (2013). The siren's call: Mass media and drug prevention. In J. P. Dillard & L. Shen (Eds.), *The SAGE handbook of persuasion: Developments in theory and practice* (2nd ed., pp. 296–313). Sage.

Crano, W. D., Siegel, J. T., Alvaro, E. M., & Patel, N. M. (2007). Overcoming adolescents' resistance to anti-inhalant appeals. *Psychology of Addictive Behaviors, 21*, 516–524. https://doi.org/10.1037/0893-164x.21.4.516

Donaldson, C. D., Siegel, J. T., & Crano, W. D. (2016). Nonmedical use of prescription stimulants in college students: Attitudes, intentions, and vested interest. *Addictive Behaviors, 53*, 101–107. https://doi.org/10.1016/j.addbeh.2015.10.007

Donaldson, C. D., Siegel, J. T., & Crano, W. D. (2020). Preventing college student nonmedical prescription stimulant use: Development of vested interest theory-based persuasive messages. *Addictive Behaviors, 108*. https://doi.org/10.1016/j.addbeh.2020.106440

Hornik, R. C., Jacobsohn, L., Orwin, R., Piese, A., & Kalton, G. (2008). Effects of the National Youth Anti-Drug Media Campaign on youths. *American Journal of Public Health, 98*, 2229–2236. https://doi.org/10.2105/ajph.2007.125849

Hovland, C. I., Janis, I. L., & Kelley, H. H. (1953). *Communication and persuasion. Psychological studies of opinion change.* Yale University Press.

Klein, W. M. P., O'Connell, M. E., Bloch, M. H., Czajkowski, S. M., Green, P. A., Han, P. K. J., Moser, R. P., Nebeling, L. C., & Vanderpool, R. C. (2022). Behavioral research in cancer prevention and control: Emerging challenges and opportunities. *Journal of the National Cancer Institute, 114*(2), 179–186. https://doi.org/10.1093/jnci/djab139

Lazarsfeld, P. F., Berelson, B., & Gaudet, H. (1944). *The people's choice.* Duell, Sloan and Pearce.

Lienemann, B. A., & Siegel, J. T. (2018). Increasing help-seeking outcomes among people with elevated depressive symptomatology with public service announcements: An examination of function matching and message sidedness. *Journal of Health Communication, 23*, 28–39. https://doi.org/10.1080/10810730.2017.1396630

Lustria, M. L. A., Noar, S. M., Cortese, J., Van Stee, S. K., Glueckauf, R. L., & Lee, J. (2013). A meta-analysis of web-delivered tailored health behavior change interventions. *Journal of Health Communication, 18*(9), 1039–1069. https://doi.org/10.1080/10810730.2013.768727

Ma, H., Kieu, T. K.-T., Ribisl, K. M., & Noar, S. M. (2023). Do vaping prevention messages impact adolescents and young adults? A meta-analysis of experimental studies. *Health Communication, 38*(8), 1709–1722. https://doi.org/10.1080/10410236.2023.2185578

McDermott, M. M., Schmitt, B., & Wallner, E. (1997). Impact of medication nonadherence on coronary heart disease outcomes. A critical review. *Archives of Internal Medicine, 157*(17), 1921–1929. https://doi.org/10.1001/archinte.1997.00440380023002

McLuhan, M. (1964). *Understanding media: The extensions of man.* Routledge.

Miech, R. A., Johnston, L. D., Patrick, M. E., O'Malley, P. M., Bachman, J. G., & Schulenberg, J. E. (2023). *Monitoring the future national survey results on drug use, 1975–2022: Secondary school students.* Institute for Social Research, The University of Michigan. https://monitoringthefuture.org/wp-content/uploads/2022/12/mtf2022.pdf

Miller, T., & Hendrie, D. (2008). *Substance abuse prevention dollars and cents: A cost-benefit analysis. DHHS Pub. No. (SMA) 07-4298.* Center for Substance Abuse Prevention, Substance Abuse and Mental Health Services Administration.

National Academies of Sciences & Medicine. (2017). *The health effects of cannabis and cannabinoids: The current state of evidence and recommendations for research.* National Academies Press. https://doi.org/10.17226/24625

Neighbors, C., DiBello, A. M., Young, C. M., Steers, M.-L. N., Rinker, D. V., Rodriguez, L. M., Ryamond Knee, C., Blanton, H., & Lewis, M. A. (2019). Personalized normative feedback for heavy drinking: An application of deviance regulation theory. *Behaviour Research and Therapy, 115*, 73–82. https://doi.org/10.1016/j.brat.2018.11.004

Noar, S. M. (2006). A 10-year retrospective of research in health mass media campaigns: Where do we go from here? *Journal of Health Communication, 11*, 21–42. https://doi.org/10.1080/10810730500461059

Office of National Drug Control Policy. (2012). *Cost benefits of investing early in substance abuse treatment. Fact sheet.* Executive Office of the President. https://obamawhitehouse.archives.gov/sites/default/files/ondcp/Fact_Sheets/investing_in_treatment_5-23-12.pdf

Parsons, K., Payne, S., Codling, S., & Murphy, M. (2023). A reflection on the co-design approach to the development of the Medway Can campaign; a whole systems approach to obesity prevention using COM-B. *Health Marketing Quarterly, 41*(1), 33–49. https://doi.org/10.1080/07359683.2023.2235501

Petty, R. E., & Krosnick, J. A. (1995). *Attitude strength: Antecedents and consequences.* Lawrence Erlbaum Associates, Inc.

Petty, R. E., Wells, G. L., & Brock, T. C. (1976). Distraction can enhance or reduce yielding to propaganda: Thought disruption versus effort justification. *Journal of Personality and Social Psychology, 34*(5), 874–884. https://doi.org/10.1037/0022-3514.34.5.874

Schnall, R., Sanabria, G., Jia, H., Cho, H., Bushover, B., Reynolds, N. R., Gradilla, M., Mohr, D. C., Ganzhorn, S., & Olender, S. (2023). Efficacy of an mHealth self-management intervention for persons living with HIV: The WiseApp randomized clinical trial. *Journal of the American Medical Informatics Association, 30*(3), 418–426. https://doi.org/10.1093/jamia/ocac233

Siegel, J. T., Donaldson, C. D., & Crano, W. D. (2019). Application of vested interest theory to prevention of non-medical prescription stimulant and marijuana use: Unforeseen benefits of attitude-behavior inconsistency. *Drug and Alcohol Dependence, 194*, 210–215. https://doi.org/10.1016/j.drugalcdep.2018.10.007

Siegel, J. T., Leinemann, B. A., & Tan, C. (2015). Influencing help-seeking among people with elevated depressive symptomatology: Mistargeting as a persuasive technique. *Clinical Psychological Science, 3*(2), 242–255. https://doi.org/10.1177/2167702614542846

Siegel, J. T., Lienemann, B. A., & Rosenberg, B. D. (2017). Resistance, reactance, and misinterpretation: Highlighting the challenge of persuading people with depression to seek help. *Social and Personality Psychology Compass, 11*, e12322. https://doi.org/10.1111/spc3.12322

Siegel, J. T., & Thomson, A. T. (2017). Positive emotion infusions of elevation and gratitude: Increasing help-seeking among people with elevated levels of depressive symptomatology. *Journal of Positive Psychology, 12*, 509–524. https://doi.org/10.1080/17439760.2016.1221125

Straszewski, T., & Siegel, J. T. (2021). From writing tasks to a public service announcement: Experimentally assessing savoring as a means of increasing help-seeking for depression. *Social Science & Medicine, 287.* https://doi.org/10.1016/j.socscimed.2021.114362

Tchakoute, C., Rhee, S. Y., Hare, C. B., Shafer, R. W., & Sainani, K. (2022). Adherence to contemporary antiretroviral treatment regimens and impact on immunological and virologic outcomes in a US healthcare system. *PLoS One, 17*(2), e0263742. https://doi.org/10.1371/journal.pone.0263742

Wegner, D. M., Wenzlaff, R., Kerker, R. M., & Beattie, A. E. (1981). Incrimination through innuendo: Can media questions become public answers? *Journal of Personality and Social Psychology, 40*(5), 822–832. https://doi.org/10.1037/0022-3514.40.5.822

Willoughby, J. F., & Noar, S. M. (2022). Fifteen years after a 10-year retrospective: The state of health mass mediated campaigns. *Journal of Health Communication, 27*(6), 362–374. https://doi.org/10.1080/10810730.2022.2110627

World Health Organization. (2019). *Mental health.* https://www.who.int/health-topics/mental-health#tab=tab_1

World Health Organization. (2022, June 8). *Mental disorders.* https://www.who.int/news-room/fact-sheets/detail/mental-disorders

World Health Organization. (2024). *HIV.* https://www.who.int/data/gho/data/themes/hiv-aids

Yingst, J. M., Carrillo, M., Chan, K. H., Choi, K., Dao, J., Kulkarni, P., Bordner, C., Goyal, N., Foulds, J., & Bascom, R. (2023). Effectiveness of smoking cessation interventions among persons with cancer: A systematic review. *Psycho-Oncology, 32*(8), 1147–1162. https://doi.org/10.1002/pon.6171

33

Maximizing Mental Health Communication: The IIFF Model of Help Seeking for Depression

Jason T. Siegel[1] and Marco C. Yzer[2]

[1] Claremont Graduate University
[2] University of Minnesota

This chapter proposes the IIFF model of help seeking for depression. Derived from the IIFF model of organ donor registration (Siegel et al., 2010a), the model includes four cognitive and behavioral supports: information, immediate help-seeking mechanism, favorable activation, and focused engagement. When these elements are present simultaneously, they can maximize the likelihood that group-based and mass communication efforts will be successful in increasing help seeking. A complementary objective of the model is to maximize the quality and quantity of support people experiencing depression will receive when help seeking occurs. Many model components have previously been used to facilitate the help-seeking process or increase social support for people with depression (e.g., mental health literacy; Jorm, 2025); however, they have rarely been brought together as a unified approach.

Depression

Nearly 300 million people suffer from depression worldwide (World Health Organization, 2023). This pervasive ailment is associated with myriad adverse outcomes, including an increased risk of suicide (e.g., Riera-Serra et al., 2023). Depression can be understood as an information-processing disorder. As Beck's (1963, 1964, 1987) cognitive theory of depression describes, people with the disorder process information through a depressogenic schema. The schema results in processing that is steeped in a negative bias (e.g., Beck, 1964), leading people experiencing depression to have negative views of themselves, the world, and the future (Clark et al., 1999; for a review, see Wisco, 2009). People experiencing depression have consistent and involuntary thoughts of failure and loss that dominate information processing (Clark et al., 1999; Gotlib & Joormann, 2010). The depressogenic schema is also associated with cognitive errors such as arbitrary inference, overgeneralization, and absolutistic dichotomous thinking (Beck, 1987).

Although effective treatment exists (Canbeyli, 2022), increasing help seeking among people experiencing depression is fraught with challenges. As described throughout this *Handbook of Mental Health Communication*[1] (Yzer & Siegel, 2025a), increasing help seeking among people experiencing depression requires a mix of science, creativity, and precision. Unlike other contexts, where increased ailment severity is associated with increased help-seeking inclinations (e.g., substance

The Handbook of Mental Health Communication, First Edition.
Edited by Marco C. Yzer and Jason T. Siegel.

abuse; Corliss et al., 2006), people with higher levels of depressive symptomatology typically report less favorable help-seeking attitudes and intentions than those with lower levels (e.g., Huntley & Fisher, 2016; Siegel et al., 2024).

Consistent with the negative association between levels of depressive symptomatology and help-seeking attitudes, although some attempts to persuade people experiencing depression to seek help have been successful (Hammer & Vogel, 2010), others have struggled to find success (e.g., Costin et al., 2009), and backfiring effects have occurred (Christensen et al., 2006; Lueck, 2018). Some backfiring effects of attempts to increase help seeking have occurred exclusively among people with heightened levels of depressive symptomatology (Klimes-Dougan & Lee, 2010; Lienemann et al., 2013). Such results are not necessarily surprising, as help-seeking messages are processed by the same depressogenic schema that is responsible for the adverse outcomes associated with the disorder. As described by Siegel et al. (2017), campaign messages targeting people experiencing depression are up against a combination of resistance, reactance, and misinterpretation (for information about reactance and messages about help seeking, see Lienemann & Siegel, 2016, and Falco & Rosenberg, 2025).

The IIFF Model of Help Seeking for Depression

The IIFF model proposes that the simultaneous presence of four cognitive and behavioral supports can maximize the likelihood that intervention efforts to increase help seeking will be successful: (a) information, (b) immediate help-seeking mechanism, (c) focused engagement, and (d) favorable activation. The expectation is that the simultaneous presence of all four elements, when properly implemented, will provide crucial information while circumventing or minimizing the influence of the depressogenic schema, thus maximizing the likelihood that people experiencing depression will seek help when presented with the opportunity. A complementary function of the model is to increase the support received when people experiencing depression let their loved ones know about their struggles.

The Origin of the IIFF Model

The IIFF model of help seeking for depression was derived from its counterpart, the IIFF model of organ donor registration (Siegel et al., 2010a). The IIFF model of organ donor registration was developed to maximize the likelihood that people who already had positive attitudes about organ donor registration would register as donors. The challenge in the organ donor registration context was translating positive attitudes into action when most people were not highly vested in organ donor registration, and their attitudes and beliefs about the topic were rarely top of mind (also see Alvaro et al., 2011; Siegel, Alvaro, Crano, et al., 2010b; Siegel, Alvaro, Tan, et al., 2016a; Siegel, Tan, Rosenberg, et al., 2016b). The challenge in the depression help-seeking domain is quite different, but the four components of the IIFF model are equally valuable. The immediate help-seeking mechanism was the first component of the IIFF model of organ donation that was translated into the depression domain (Siegel & Thomson, 2017), but the realization that all components were useful soon followed (Siegel, 2021). The IIFF model of help seeking for depression was initially proposed for group-based interventions. However, we believe the IIFF model can help guide mental health mass communication (e.g., public service announcements [PSAs]). We now present each of the model's components. Although it is named the IIFF model of help seeking for depression, we will present the components in the order they would likely be experienced by those receiving the group-based intervention to mental health mass communication: (a) focused engagement, (b) favorable activation, (c) information, and (d) immediate help-seeking mechanism.

Focused Engagement

Focused engagement refers to ensuring that people actively engage with and process the material. If the intervention targets are not exposed to or ignore the material, all efforts will be for naught. Maximizing engagement will increase the likelihood that the information will be processed through the central route, increasing the likelihood of attitude change (Petty & Cacioppo, 1986; for a discussion, see Quick et al., 2025). Steps for maximizing engagement must also be considered because people experiencing depression have impaired cognitive effort motivation (Ang et al., 2023) and cognitive deficits (Ahern, 2025). As the relationship between depression and processing capabilities is complex (Hammar et al., 2003; Yost & Weary, 1996), materials must be tested on individuals who are experiencing depression to ensure success and avoid causing harm. Among all the model components, focused engagement is the one that will vary most depending on whether the context is a group setting or mental health mass communication.

Group Setting

The recommendation to conduct sessions in a group setting was highly motivated by the focused engagement aspect of the model. A workplace requiring employees to attend an information session on helping co-workers with depression, a guidance counselor visiting a classroom, or a webinar session on mental wellness are all contexts where focused engagement is likely to be achieved. Changing the modes of instruction throughout the session (e.g., lecture, videos, and activities) can maximize participant engagement. Where appropriate, monitoring learning (e.g., quizzes throughout the session) can also maximize engagement.

Mass Communication

Numerous campaigns have failed due to a lack of exposure (for a review, see Wakefield et al., 2010). Moreover, the IIFF model of help seeking for depression does not just require exposure; the information must also be engaged with (a concept labeled *encoded exposure*; Southwell et al., 2002). This could be challenging in many contexts, but it is possible. The communication literature is replete with information about message features that can help draw attention to, and maximize engagement with, messages. These include emotional shifts (Peinado & Nabi, 2024), message sensation value (Palmgreen et al., 1991; Yang et al., 2023), expectation violations (Siegel & Burgoon, 2002), high levels of readability (Pancer et al., 2019), and narratives (Green & Brock, 2000), to name a few. Because all these options have been tested as means for increasing attention and engagement outside the mental health domain, they must be pilot tested on people experiencing depression prior to implementation. As often noted, approaches that are useful among the general population could be useless or harmful when applied to people experiencing depression (Siegel et al., 2019; Yzer & Siegel, 2025b).

Favorable Activation

Two elements are involved regarding favorable activation: (a) inducing positive emotions and (b) avoiding negative activation. The depressogenic schema, including the tendency for people experiencing depression to be unable to disengage from negatively valenced material, has been well described (e.g., Vos et al., 2025; Ying et al., 2025). The tendency for messages to sometimes backfire among people experiencing depression has also been illustrated on numerous occasions (for reviews, see Siegel et al., 2017; Yzer & Siegel, 2025c). It is, therefore, imperative to put people experiencing depression in a mindset that maximizes the success of persuasive attempts and avoid negative materials that would be challenging for people experiencing depression to disengage from. Although the specific ways positive emotions will be induced might vary based on whether the intervention is in a group setting or a mental health mass communication, both elements should be present regardless of the context.

Inducing Positive Emotions

As noted earlier, the initial catalyst for applying the IIFF model of organ donor registration to the help-seeking domain occurred when Siegel and Thomson (2017) encountered Beck's (2002) theorizing about how a temporary reduction of dysphoria is possible. Beck's theorizing led Siegel and Thomson to consider how this temporary reduction of dysphoria could be created. Based on Siegel and Thomson's research on positive emotions in general (Graham et al., 2019) and elevation (i.e., the emotion experienced when exposed to moral beauty; Haidt, 2000) in particular (Siegel et al., 2014; Thomson et al., 2014; see Thomson & Siegel, 2017, and Liu & Siegel, 2023 for reviews), they proposed ***positive emotion infusions*** (PEIs) as a means for creating a temporary change in perceptions among people with depression (see Straszewski & Siegel, 2025, for a review).

Guided by research indicating that positive emotions can increase the likelihood of positive evaluations (Gorn et al., 1993), cognitive flexibility (Isen, 1990), future-oriented thinking (Pyone & Isen, 2011), social connectedness (Isen, 1990), and approach behaviors (Cacioppo et al., 1997), while undoing negative emotions (Fredrickson, 2001), Siegel and Thomson (2017) reasoned that if they could infuse people with positive emotions, they might be able to temporarily change how people experiencing depression perceive help seeking. They acknowledged that this window of change would be brief but also posited that if an immediate means of help seeking could be simultaneously provided, the result could be help-seeking behavior that would not occur otherwise.

Since the initial proposal of the PEI approach, several experimental studies have indicated that it is possible to temporarily infuse people experiencing depression with positive emotions (for a review, see Straszewski & Siegel, 2025). Siegel and Thomson (2017) infused people experiencing depression with elevation and gratitude in their initial studies. Straszewski and Siegel (2018) found success by asking people experiencing depression to savor a positive experience. They also found success when asking participants experiencing depression to savor a calm memory or an exciting one (Straszewski & Siegel, 2020). Roy and Siegel (2025) led people experiencing depression to make affective forecasting errors, thereby increasing positive affect. Hussain and Alhabash (2022) found an increase in positive emotions when they exposed college students to a depression PSA that included a nostalgia appeal compared to one that did not. The totality of these studies indicates that it is possible to infuse people experiencing depression with a temporary burst of positive emotions.

Although it is possible to infuse people experiencing depression with positive emotions, doing so is not a guarantee that help-seeking intentions will be influenced. For example, Siegel and Thomson (2017) found a direct effect of their story-based elevation induction but less success with a story-based gratitude induction; moreover, the elevation recall induction was less successful than the story-based one. Straszewski and Siegel (2018) found both a direct effect of savoring on help-seeking intentions and an indirect effect through positive affect. However, follow-up studies (Straszewski & Siegel, 2020) indicated that although savoring an exciting memory was associated with increased help seeking, savoring a calm memory was not. Further, whereas Straszewski and Siegel (2021) succeeded in directly increasing help-seeking intentions among people experiencing depression who reported paying attention during the study through a relational savoring writing task, the same approach failed when implemented through a depression PSA. Although Roy and Siegel (2025) increased positive affect, their affective forecasting approach did not directly affect help-seeking intentions. Likewise, Hussain and Alhabash (2022) successfully induced positive emotions but did not affect help-seeking intentions.

These studies highlight the feasibility of infusing people experiencing depression with positive emotions; however, they also indicate that not every successful positive emotion induction will increase help-seeking intentions. We still recommend PEIs as part of interventions to increase help seeking, as success is possible. Thus far, writing tasks focused on elevation, especially in response to a story, and writing tasks focused on savoring exciting positive experiences seem to have had the most uniform success at infusing positive emotions and increasing help-seeking intentions (e.g., Siegel & Thomson, 2017; Straszewski & Siegel, 2018, 2020). However, there is reason to believe that mental health mass communication messages can be created for people with depressive symptomatology that induce positive emotions and will also increase help seeking. For example, a video-based advertisement could tell an elevating story that infuses feelings of elevation and then switch to information about helping people experiencing depression. It might also be possible to do so without relating the two videos. For example, one 30-second message could evoke feelings of elevation, and then the very next message, seemingly unrelated to the first, could focus on the other elements of the IIFF model (Siegel & Straszewski, 2019).

Avoiding Negative Activation

We recommend that information be focused on the positive (e.g., benefits of help seeking) rather than counterarguing the negative. For example, we do not recommend bringing up stigma and then counterarguing it, or noting help-seeking barriers and then describing how they can be overcome (see Zhu et al., 2025, for a review on stigma and communication). As Ahern (2025) explained, people experiencing depression have an inclination toward the processing of negative content. Moreover, people experiencing depression struggle with disengagement from negative stimuli (Gotlib & Joormann, 2010). Therefore, if a message or meeting describes help-seeking barriers, once the barriers are recalled, a person with depression could begin to ruminate on such barriers (Gotlib & Joormann, 2010) despite information about how the obstacles can be overcome. As described by Vos et al. (2025), people experiencing depression have difficulty updating negative interpretations.

A set of studies supports the importance of avoiding negative activation. Tan and Siegel (2025) created two writing tasks designed to either strengthen positive attitudes or weaken negative ones. They randomly assigned participants to imagine they were talking to a loved one and either list two reasons why someone would want to seek help for depression (group 1) or write two reasons why someone would *not* want to do so (group 2). Participants were then asked to imagine talking to a loved one who was experiencing depression and write down what they might say to convince them that either the positive outcomes will occur (group 1) or why the adverse outcomes will not (group 2). Across three studies, the positive outcome writing task increased help-seeking attitudes. The positive outcome writing task also increased help-seeking intentions in the two studies that help-seeking intentions were included as an outcome variable. The negative outcome writing task was only tested in one study. It failed to increase help-seeking attitudes and caused participants to perceive themselves as having a greater stake in the adverse outcomes associated with help seeking.

Tan and Siegel (2025) theorized that once participants with depression thought of two reasons that people might not want to seek help for depression, the participants might have struggled to stop thinking about those barriers, even if they wrote about why those outcomes would not happen (e.g., Gotlib & Joormann, 2010). The hyperfocus on the outcomes was likely automatic and not possible to shut off (Beck, 1987). This occurred even though the writing task was put forth to minimize self-relevance (i.e., participants were to imagine talking to a loved one who was experiencing depression and write down what they might say to convince the loved one that negative outcomes would not occur).

Along these lines, we do not recommend directly talking about stigma. Stigma can be combated through text such as, "Tell your loved one with depression that depression can be temporary." However, if stigma is explicitly noted, it could confirm fears that are held by people experiencing depression (e.g., "They mentioned that we should not worry about stigma; that means there is a stigma"). We do not believe focusing on the negative will be problematic for the loved ones of people experiencing depression. However, as messages will be seen, and group-based meetings (e.g., classroom sessions) will be attended by people with and without depressive symptomatology, it is best to stay focused on the positive.

Information

The information component has three aspects: (a) how to present the information, (b) what information should be presented, and (c) who should present the information (i.e., the message source).

How to Present the Information: Overheard Communication

A central challenge in the provision of information is that people with depressive symptomatology have more accessible negative help-seeking attitudes and less accessible positive help-seeking attitudes (Siegel & Tan, 2025). Accordingly, people experiencing depression respond to information differently than those without depression (Siegel et al., 2017). Interventions must be strategically implemented with the depressogenic schema in mind. Fortunately, decades of scholarship on the processing patterns of people experiencing depression (for a review, see Wisco, 2009) and persuasive techniques (for a review, see Dillard & Shen, 2013) offer a roadmap. Whether an intervention is in the form of a mass media message or a group meeting, it should be framed as information for teaching people how to assist someone with depression. Messages should ask, "Do you know someone experiencing depression?" instead of, "Are you experiencing depression?" We now provide the rationale for this suggestion.

As Bargh and Tota (1988) described, "There is evidence that the negative thought of the depressed person is confined to the self and does not extend to thinking about other people" (p. 926). Similarly, Vos et al.'s (2025) review notes how self-relevant information could trigger cognitive bias, a view also supported by Clark et al. (1999). If a message or a group-based intervention directly targets people experiencing depression, the negative cognitive bias will likely be made more extreme. Fortunately, Walster and Festinger (1962) offered a different way: the overheard communication technique. Walster and Festinger stated, "It is widely believed that a communication, if inadvertently overheard, is more likely to be effective in changing the opinion of the listener than if it had been deliberately addressed to him" (1962, p. 395). Although not focused on people experiencing depression, they demonstrated that communication perceived to be overheard was more persuasive than when the receiver knew it was intended for them.

The combination of theorizing about the depressogenic schema and Walster and Festinger's (1962) overheard communication technique motivated Siegel et al. (2015) to conduct two studies that experimentally pitted direct messages (e.g., "Are you feeling distressed? . . . You might be depressed") against overheard messages (e.g., "Do you know someone who is feeling distressed? . . . They might be depressed"). The first experiment compared a direct print advertisement to an overheard one. The overheard message resulted in more favorable help-seeking intentions from most sources among participants with the highest levels of depressive symptomatology. The second study used video messages and added a no-message control condition. Participants who received the overheard message (e.g., "It is not their fault they are depressed") reported more favorable help-seeking outcome expectations (HSOEs), attitudes, and intentions than both the direct and control conditions. However, those who received the direct message (e.g., "It is not your fault you are depressed") reported HSOEs, attitudes, and intentions that were not statistically significantly different from participants who received no message. A follow-up study further supported the utility of the approach (Siegel & Marshburn, 2025). Note that a message that is overheard for people experiencing depression will be a direct message for the loved ones of those with the disorder. Siegel and Marshburn's (2025) data indicated that whether a message directly targets loved ones of those with depression or does so in an indirect manner, it is equally effective.

Additional Considerations

There are additional techniques that could complement the overheard communication approach. These include using gender-sensitive language (Hammer & Vogel, 2010), attitude-function matching (Lienemann & Siegel, 2018), and self-distancing (Hollar & Siegel, 2020). An explanation of each of these approaches is beyond the scope of this chapter. Still, these approaches have been found to increase help seeking among people with elevated depressive symptomatology.

What Information Should Be Presented

The information goal associated with the IIFF model of help seeking for depression is to provide knowledge that will lead people experiencing depression to seek help at the end of the intervention, and to give information to those without depression so that they can offer assistance and support to those with depression. Much of the information we recommend providing aligns with Jorm's (2025) description of mental health literacy. The list of information options we will present is not all-encompassing, and there are likely specific facets of information that the particular context will determine (for a review, see Yzer & Zhu, 2025), but we hope to provide a foundation from which to build. Concerning intervention format/modality, a one-hour meeting will allow more information to be presented with greater detail than a 60-second PSA. Besides that limitation, the overall approach should not differ based on whether presented in a group context or mass media format.

Recognizing Depressive Symptomatology

We recommend providing information that will allow people to recognize depressive symptomatology. People are unlikely to seek help for depression if they do not recognize themselves as depressed. Further, people cannot suggest their loved ones seek help if they are unable to recognize depressive symptomatology. The ability to recognize symptoms of mental health disorders is part of Jorm's definition of mental health literacy (see Jorm, 2025, for a review). In support of the importance of being able to recognize one's own depressive symptomatology, Straszewski and Siegel (2020) reported that the effect size of their positive emotion infusion on help-seeking intentions more than doubled when they limited their sample to people who perceived themselves as experiencing depressive symptomatology (also see Straszewski & Siegel, 2025). Fortunately, education along these lines is feasible. Although not focused on people with depression, Hernandez and Organista (2013) used Entertainment–Education to increase people's knowledge of the symptoms of depression and their ability to recognize depression in themselves and others.

Help-Seeking Outcome Expectations

Information provided as part of an IIFF-guided intervention, whether a group-based intervention or mental health mass communication, should include information about the benefits of seeking help. As Jorm (2025) described, mental health literacy includes knowledge about evidence-based options for treatment, which implies that people experiencing depression believe that seeking help will lead to desirable outcomes. Illustrative of the challenge of persuading people experiencing depression to seek help, there is a negative association between levels of depressive symptomatology and HSOEs (Lueck & Yzer, 2018; Siegel et al., 2015; Yzer et al., 2022). Moreover, Siegel et al. (2024) found that HSOEs mediated the negative association between depressive symptomatology and help-seeking intentions among medical residents.

Demonstrating the value of increasing HSOEs, Jorm et al. (2003) conducted a randomized controlled trial indicating that there are benefits to informing people experiencing depression about the effectiveness of various treatments. Although not all outcomes were statistically significant, there were several significant effects (e.g., trying self-help treatment, the number of interventions rated as effective) indicating the promise of interventions that tout the effectiveness of treatments. Moreover, experimental studies have indicated that HSOEs are malleable (Lienemann & Siegel, 2018; Siegel et al., 2015; Siegel & Marshburn, 2025). A complementary benefit is that informing potential supporters that the disorder is treatable can maximize the amount of support that people experiencing depression will receive (for a review, see Muschetto & Siegel, 2025a,b).

Attributions

Information provided as part of an IIFF-guided intervention will ideally convey to participants that people experiencing depression are putting forth effort to overcome their disorder, that no one deserves to be depressed, that people experiencing depression are not responsible for their ailment, and that depression can be temporary (for a review, see Muschetto & Siegel, 2025a,b). Attribution-based efforts have more commonly been used to increase the support that people with depression will receive, so we begin there.

Guided by Weiner's (1980) attribution-emotion-action model, numerous studies have explored how making attributions more favorable or salient can lead to desirable outcomes (e.g., Yao & Siegel, 2021, 2024). Experimental studies have revealed that adding a couple of sentences to PSAs that highlight the temporary nature of depression (Muschetto & Siegel, 2020), the effort being put forth by the person with depression (Ruybal & Siegel, 2021), or how no one deserves to be depressed (Muschetto & Siegel, 2025a,b) can increase favorable emotions toward people with depression, make social support seem more valuable, and indirectly increase willingness to provide social support. This approach has avoided the backfiring effects that some anti-stigma campaigns have faced (for a review, see Twiss et al., 2025).

Turning to the impact of the attribution approach on people with depression, the main content of the overheard communication studies discussed earlier (Siegel et al., 2015) leaned on attribution theory for the central content. The messages included information about responsibility (e.g., "They are not weak. They did nothing wrong") and stability (e.g., "They have an illness—an illness that can be overcome! They will not be depressed forever"; see Siegel & Marshburn, 2025, for additional support). As described earlier, these messages increased help-seeking attitudes and intentions among those with heightened depressive symptomatology. Therefore, we recommend including overheard content along these lines. Although Siegel et al. (2015) did not test if this influence occurred through the reduction of self-stigma of seeking help (see Vogel et al., 2025, for a review), it is possible some of the effects of the attribution approach occurred through this mechanism.

Attribution-based approaches targeting people with depression must be delivered in an overheard manner. When attribution messages are presented to people experiencing depression in a direct fashion (e.g., "Depression is not your fault"), the messages are minimally effective (i.e., they moved HSOEs but not attitudes nor intentions; Siegel & Marshburn, 2025), ineffective (Siegel et al., 2015), or cause a backfire effect (Lienemann et al., 2013) among people experiencing depression. Ultimately, by adding content such as, "Please let your loved ones with depression know that depression can be temporary, people experiencing depression are trying to overcome their ailment, and no one deserves to be depressed," people experiencing depression should be more inclined to seek help and should be more likely to receive support when they do.

Context-Specific Information About Obtaining Future Assistance

The central goal of the IIFF-guided intervention is to have people with depression seek help at the end of the intervention when the immediate mechanism is provided. However, there will also be audience members who are not currently depressed but can benefit from insight into how to support others or themselves if they experience depression in the future. For example, if the message targets a specific college population, it would be beneficial to include information about where help can be obtained on campus. If the intervention targets lawyers at a particular firm, adding information about the firm's resources would be helpful.

Additional Information Targets

In addition to the critical categories of content just described (i.e., symptoms, HSOEs, attributions, obtaining future assistance), other information targets should be considered.

Social Norms. Though over 60% of people who experienced depression in the United States received professional help in the prior year (Substance Abuse and Mental Health Services Administration, 2023), people with depressive symptomatology assume this rate is about 30% (Falco & Siegel, 2025). This is important, as there is a positive association between descriptive norms and help-seeking intentions (Lueck, 2018; Lueck & Yzer, 2018; Yzer et al., 2022). Falco and Siegel (2025) experimentally tested messages that used the overheard approach and either did or did not include information about static or trending norms. Both messages changed perceived norms, but neither directly affected help-seeking outcome expectations, attitudes, or intentions. Relative to the message without information about norms, both norm messages indirectly affected intentions through changes in perceived norms. Due to the limited strength of these effects, we do not recommend a campaign focused solely on norms at this time, but they could be part of a broader campaign.

Perceived Effort. Trusty and Swift (2023) reported a positive association between levels of depressive symptomatology and the perceived effort associated with seeking professional help. A follow-up assessment conducted three months later indicated that higher levels of perceived effort had a negative association with having initiated psychotherapy. Although it is unknown whether perceptions of effort can be readily influenced, or if doing so will affect help seeking, Trusty and Swift's research offers a promising new direction.

Depression as a Functional Signal. Schroder et al. (2023) have conducted interesting work framing depression as a functional signal (e.g., "depression also serves a really important function. Depression is a signal that something in our lives needs more attention. Depression is telling us that something is not working for us, and our needs are not being met"; p. 5). Although this approach has been compared only to the biogenetic approach (i.e., an approach that explains depression as having biological, chemical, or genetic origins) and has yet to be compared to a true control, it shows promise.

Gain and Loss Framing. Gain and loss framing could also prove helpful, but the results have not been consistent thus far. Gain and loss messages have often been operationalized as how seeking help is useful (i.e., gain frame) and how not seeking help can worsen symptoms (i.e., loss frame; Shi & Dai, 2022). Some studies showed benefits in loss framing (Lueck, 2018; Shi & Dai, 2022; Suka et al., 2019), whereas some indicated gain frames to be superior (Mavandadi et al., 2018), and others revealed mixed results depending on the level of depressive symptomatology, including backfiring effects (Lueck, 2018). Ideally, future studies can untangle these results and determine the best approach.

Who Should Present the Information

When providing information, another consideration is who will be the most credible source (e.g., Hovland et al., 1953; for reviews, see Quick et al., 2025; RW et al., 2025). Scholars have long noted that the message's source can significantly affect the extent to which the information is believed and internalized (Pornpitakpan, 2004). Dimensions such as expertise and trustworthiness (Hovland et al., 1953; O'Keefe, 2015) have long been considered hallmarks of source credibility. Caring/goodwill has also been touted as an important factor of source credibility (McCroskey & Teven, 1999). Additional features have also been investigated (e.g., the benefit of speaker–recipient similarity; Chen et al., 2024). Although there is limited research specific to the sources that people with depressive symptomatology perceive as most credible regarding help-seeking information, it is crucial to ensure that information sources are perceived as credible by people experiencing depression before implementation.

Immediate Help-Seeking Mechanism

The immediate help-seeking mechanism is the cornerstone of the IIFF model of help seeking for depression. Without the immediate help-seeking mechanism, the likelihood that people with depression will seek help as a result of the intervention will be vastly reduced. As noted, the immediate help-seeking mechanism catalyzed thought on taking the IIFF model of organ donation (Siegel, Alvaro, & Hohman, 2010a) and applying it to the depression help-seeking domain. This occurred when Siegel and Thomson (2017), who were investigating ways to increase help seeking for people experiencing depression, came across Beck's (2002) theorizing on temporarily reducing dysphoria experienced by people experiencing depression: "Even though situations may be favorable and indeed may temporarily reduce dysphoria and introduce some satisfaction, the overall set of futility persists" (Beck, 2002, p. 36). Siegel and Thomson were also working on an article involving the IIFF donor registration model at the time (Siegel, Tan, Rosenberg, et al., 2016b), and they began thinking about how the model's immediate donor registration mechanism could be translated into the depression domain (i.e., an immediate help-seeking mechanism) to increase help seeking among people with depression. With Beck's theorizing in mind, they realized that if an immediate help-seeking mechanism could be provided to people experiencing depression at the very time dysphoria is temporarily reduced and perceptions of help seeking are more favorable, the temporary nature of the changes would not be problematic.

Critical to the implementation of the IIFF model of help seeking for depression is the awareness that the intervention is not meant to permanently change help-seeking perceptions among people with depression. As Beck (2002) described, dysphoria can be temporarily reduced, and this temporary reduction is the target of the IIFF model of help seeking for depression. The model seeks to create a temporary window where perceptions of help seeking become more favorable. It is specifically designed to motivate a specific action at a particular time. As noted, the direct benefit of the intervention will be vastly minimized if the immediate opportunity is not provided at the time of delivery.

Because the influence of the intervention on people experiencing depression is expected to be fleeting, it is critical to include an immediate mechanism such that the person with depression can immediately reach out for help at the time that the other components of the IIFF model are present. This might involve immediately scheduling an appointment or having the person with depression email someone who will reach out to them in the very near future. The idea is that the person with depression will be able to make "first contact" with someone who can directly provide help or facilitate assistance and ensure that help seeking continues. Whether the IIFF model of help seeking for depression is implemented in a mass media format or a group setting, the immediate help-seeking mechanism should be provided.

Implementing an immediate help-seeking mechanism could be challenging, so we fear that, of the four IIFF components, the immediate help-seeking mechanism is most likely to be scrapped. This would be a terrible mistake. As Beck (2002) described, "Even though situations may be favorable and indeed may temporarily reduce dysphoria and introduce some satisfaction, the overall set of futility persists" (p. 36). This was supported by Horner et al. (2014), who successfully induced positive affect in participants with and without major depressive disorder. However, the positive affect declined far quicker among participants experiencing depression. Likewise, when describing positive emotion infusions, Siegel and Thomson (2017) noted that the intervention is only expected to open a brief window where help-seeking perceptions are changed.

If the IIFF model of help seeking for depression is part of a video message, there could be a QR code to be scanned at the end of the message, taking the person to a website where help can be immediately received or, if not possible, an immediate appointment can be made. An immediate link could be provided if the message is part of a social media effort. Suppose the IIFF model is part of a group intervention (e.g., classroom-based presentation). In that case, participants could be asked to evaluate the session, and the mechanism could be the first thing provided during the evaluation.

The mechanism should be set up to ensure that help is readily accessible without requiring additional effort from the person seeking help, and it should be promoted as such. Help seeking should be conveyed as being as effortless as possible (Trusty & Swift, 2023), which could reduce concerns about whether the person feels capable of seeking help. This might be particularly relevant given the cognitive deficits associated with depression (e.g., concentrating and memory difficulties; for a review, see Ahern, 2025), as it is common for people with depression to perceive problems as "complex, severe, and difficult to solve" (Andrews & Thomson, 2009, p. 620).

Implementing the IIFF Model of Help Seeking for Depression

The IIFF model of help seeking for depression can guide efforts to increase help seeking, whether implemented in a group context or as a mental health mass communication. The critical question is whether all four elements of the IIFF model can be simultaneously implemented. There are advantages and disadvantages of each format (i.e., group context and mass communication). A group setting has advantages in that it can do more to guarantee that the focused engagement requirement of the model is met, and a help-seeking mechanism can be provided as part of an evaluation form. However, this approach will only be able to reach a limited number of people at a time compared to a mass media campaign. Mental health mass communication also has the benefit of repeated exposure, which is favorably impactful among people experiencing depression (Suka et al., 2020). However, not all mass communication approaches make it easy for all four elements of the model to be simultaneously present. For example, including immediate help-seeking mechanisms is critical; to do so in a radio message might not be highly feasible. Imagine someone with depression listening to a radio-based PSA while driving. Even if the PSA convinces the person to seek help, the message's persuasive punch would likely be less influential when the person arrives at their destination. However, an immediate help-seeking mechanism could be provided as part of a message that appears on Instagram, TikTok, or another social media outlet.

Regardless of the context, the IIFF model of help seeking for depression should be implemented only where those who reach out can get help. If people reach out but help is not received, it could make matters worse for those with the disorder. Although a discussion of the range of providers is out of the scope of this chapter, advancements in various forms of telehealth might allow help to be received by a broader range of people (see Jabeen et al., 2025, and Lau et al., 2025, for reviews). However, privacy concerns must also be considered (see Dellinger, 2025, for a review). We now illustrate how implementation can occur in group-based settings or through mental health mass communication.

Group-Based Settings

We can imagine a group-based implementation that is advertised as a session for learning how to help loved ones, colleagues, or classmates who are experiencing depression. The session could begin with a PEI framed as a means of getting everyone relaxed and ready for the information that would be provided. Next, the content of the message, framed as information for helping others with depression, could be provided through a combination of lectures, videos, and possibly interactive games. Participants could then be asked to do a writing task such as the one used by Tan and Siegel (2025), in which people were asked to write about why someone else would want to seek help and why those positive outcomes would occur. Another PEI could be given, followed by the immediate help-seeking mechanism.

In group-based settings, there can be differences in the challenge of implementing different components based on the specific context in which it is implemented. For example, it might be easier to have all four components simultaneously present as part of a school-based intervention (for a review of school-based interventions, see Johnston et al., 2025), but it could be more difficult in a rural area where community members are spread out and internet access is limited (see Barksdale et al., 2025, for a discussion about mental health equity). Ideally, the need to ensure that a mechanism for seeking help is provided would not exacerbate inequities, but rather motivate interventionists to find ways to ensure that help is received by people who are often ignored or disadvantaged (see Marciano et al., 2025, for a review). Also, specific content might differ based on the audience. The information provided to a group of medical residents might not need to include the symptoms of depression. However, it would have to address other challenges, such as the reluctance to take on the role of the patient (for a review, see Menezes & Guldner, 2025).

Mental Health Mass Communication

Mental health mass communication could be a one-way message or, if delivered through social media, it could be interactive to maximize engagement. The message could infuse positive emotion either before the message or as part of it. Steps could be taken to ensure the message draws attention and maintains it. The message, which should be written in an overheard manner, could, at a minimum, describe how to recognize depression, frame depression to maximize positive attributions (e.g., "Depression can be temporary"), note the benefits of help seeking, describe means of seeking help and the feasibility of doing so, and then offer an immediate help-seeking mechanism. The mechanism could be framed as a means of getting help and obtaining additional information about techniques for helping loved ones. Mental health mass communication messages must consider how the immediate help-seeking mechanism will be able to facilitate help seeking across the range of geographies in which the message might be viewed. This will be more challenging in some communities than others; however, mental health equity must be considered (for a review, see Barksdale et al., 2025).

Evaluating the IIFF Model of Help-Seeking for Depression

It will be critical to evaluate efforts both prior to implementation and after. Given that efforts to increase help seeking among people experiencing depression have backfired (e.g., Keeler & Siegel, 2016), and anti-stigma messages that target the general public have sometimes been found to backfire among people experiencing depression (Siegel et al., 2019), all intervention components must be tested on people experiencing depression prior to implementation (Siegel et al., 2017; Yzer & Siegel, 2025b,c). Given that anti-stigma messages have also backfired on the public (Twiss et al., 2025), intervention components must also be tested on the general population. Perceived message effectiveness measures are a valuable outcome for evaluating the intervention in pilot research (Noar et al., 2025). Although there are many approaches to testing messages, online peer communities represent an underexplored option (see Griffith & Simmons, 2025, for a review).

Once implemented, the most critical measure of success is the number of people who use the immediate help-seeking mechanism or seek information to help others. This might be the only feasible measure for mental health mass communication efforts. A group-based setting can have a more robust evaluation that, in addition to the immediate help-seeking mechanism, it can also possibly include measures to assess gains in knowledge, help-seeking attitudes and outcome expectations, changes in attributions and emotional responses to people experiencing depression, and anything else that could be of interest that will not overburden the attendees. Measures of stigma can be helpful, as an intervention guided by the IIFF model of help seeking for depression can influence self-stigma and public stigma (for reviews on measuring these constructs, see Fox et al., 2025, and Vogel et al., 2025). Measuring mental health literacy, as described by Jorm (2025), can also be helpful as an intervention guided by the IIFF model of help seeking for depression should increase mental health literacy among those experiencing depression and those who support people with the disorder.

Future Directions

The most imperative future direction is to empirically test the IIFF model of help seeking for depression. Although many of the model's components have been empirically assessed, the totality of the model has not been tested in the depression domain. The process to do so has begun, and an IIFF-based intervention is currently being developed for military members.

Another future direction is to apply the model to other areas of mental health (for an argument for expanding research on all mental illnesses, see Yzer & Siegel, 2025c). The general approach and its components are not specific to depression. The IIFF model might help motivate help seeking for issues such as substance abuse (Charuvastra et al., 2002) and gaming disorder (see Woodman & Weber, 2025, for a review), but specific aspects of the approach will likely need to be altered, albeit to varying degrees.

Conclusion

The IIFF model of help seeking for depression is a guide for maximizing the utility of mass communication interventions and communication in group settings such as classrooms. Four components must be simultaneously present to maximize success: (a) immediate help-seeking mechanism, (b) information, (c) focused engagement, and (d) favorable activation. The central audience is the person experiencing depression, and the main goal is to have that person reach out for assistance and make first contact before the message or intervention is over. The secondary audience is the people who will support those experiencing depression whose assist should increase by the end of the intervention or messaging.

Creating messages and finding settings where all four components of the IIFF model of help seeking for depression are present could be challenging. However, we believe that, when components of the model are implemented successfully, the likelihood that people experiencing depression will reach out for assistance and receive support when they do so will substantially increase. We also see the IIFF model of help seeking for depression as a work in progress that can benefit from classic and contemporary scholarship that has yet to be applied in this domain. The importance of persuading people with mental illness to seek help warrants approaches that span academic disciplines and combine theories not typically put together. Increasing help seeking among people with mental illnesses and increasing the support they receive is difficult—but it can have life saving implications.

Note

1 The current chapter is the final one of the *Handbook of Mental Health Communication*. We intentionally referenced most of these chapters in the current one to highlight the complementary nature of the content.

References

Ahern, E. (2025). Cognitive deficits in major depression: Characteristics, role, and relevance. In M. C. Yzer & J. T. Siegel (Eds.), *Handbook of mental health communication*. Wiley.

Alvaro, E. A., Siegel, J. T., & Jones, S. P. (2011). Increasing organ donor registration rates by providing an immediate and complete registration opportunity: An experimental assessment of the IIFF model. *Psychology, Health and Medicine*, *16*(6), 686–694. https://doi.org/10.1080/13548506.2011.564353

Andrews, P. W., & Thomson, J. A., Jr. (2009). The bright side of being blue: Depression as an adaptation for analyzing complex problems. *Psychological Review*, *116*(3), 620–654. https://doi.org/10.1037%2Fa0016242

Ang, Y.-S., Gelda, S. E., & Pizzagalli, D. A. (2023). Cognitive effort-based decision-making in major depressive disorder. *Psychological Medicine*, *53*(9), 4228–4235. https://doi.org/10.1017/S0033291722000964

Bargh, J. A., & Tota, M. E. (1988). Context-dependent automatic processing in depression: Accessibility of negative constructs with regard to self but not others. *Journal of Personality and Social Psychology*, *54*(6), 925–939. https://doi.org/10.1037/0022-3514.54.6.925

Barksdale, C. L., Lawhorn, C., Alvidrez, J., & Schwartz, K. (2025). Considerations for optimizing mental health communication to advance mental health equity. In M. C. Yzer & J. T. Siegel (Eds.), *Handbook of mental health communication*. Wiley.

Beck, A. T. (1963). Thinking and depression: I. Idiosyncratic content and cognitive distortions. *Archives of General Psychiatry*, *9*(4), 324–333. https://doi.org/10.1001/archpsyc.1963.01720160014002

Beck, A. T. (1964). Thinking and depression: II. Theory and therapy. *Archives of General Psychiatry*, *10*(6), 561–571. https://doi.org/10.1001/archpsyc.1964.01720240015003

Beck, A. T. (1987). Cognitive models of depression. *Journal of Cognitive Psychotherapy*, *1*, 5–37.

Beck, A. T. (2002). Cognitive models of depression. In L. Robert & E. T. Dowd (Eds.), *Clinical advances in cognitive psychotherapy: Theory and application* (pp. 29–61). Springer Publishing Company.

Cacioppo, J. T., Gardner, W. L., & Berntson, G. G. (1997). Beyond bipolar conceptualizations and measures: The case of attitudes and evaluative space. *Personality and Social Psychology Review*, *1*(1), 3–25. https://doi.org/10.1207/s15327957pspr0101_2

Canbeyli, R. (2022). Sensory stimulation via the visual, auditory, olfactory and gustatory systems can modulate mood and depression. *European Journal of Neuroscience*, *55*(1), 244–263. https://doi.org/10.1111/ejn.15507

Charuvastra, A., Anderson, B. J., Friedmann, P. D., & Stein, M. D. (2002). Perceived addiction treatment needs among alcohol using injection drug users. *Journal of Addictive Diseases*, *21*(4), 93–107. https://doi.org/10.1300/j069v21n04_09

Chen, M., Dong, Y., & Wang, J. (2024). A meta-analysis examining the role of character-recipient similarity in narrative persuasion. *Communication Research*, *51*(1), 56–82. https://doi.org/10.1177/00936502231204834

Christensen, H., Leach, L. S., Barney, L., Mackinnon, A. J., & Griffiths, K. M. (2006). The effect of web based depression interventions on self reported help seeking: Randomised controlled trial [ISRCTN77824516]. *BMC Psychiatry*, *6*(13). https://doi.org/10.1186/1471-244X-6-13

Clark, D. A., Beck, A. T., & Alford, B. A. (1999). *Scientific foundations of cognitive theory and therapy of depression*. John Wiley & Sons, Inc.

Corliss, H. L., Grella, C. E., Mays, V. M., & Cochran, S. D. (2006). Drug use, drug severity, and help-seeking behaviors of lesbian and bisexual women. *Journal of Women's Health (2002)*, *15*(5), 556–568. https://doi.org/10.1089/jwh.2006.15.556

Costin, D. L., Mackinnon, A. J., Griffiths, K. M., Batterham, P. J., Bennett, A. J., Bennett, K., & Christensen, H. (2009). Health e-cards as a means of encouraging help seeking for depression among young adults: Randomized controlled trial. *Journal of Medical Internet Research*, *11*(4). e42. https://doi.org/10.2196/jmir.1294

Dellinger, J. (2025). Mental health apps and privacy: Misunderstandings and messaging. In M. C. Yzer & J. T. Siegel (Eds.), *Handbook of mental health communication*. Wiley.

Dillard, J. P., & Shen, L. (2013). *The SAGE handbook of persuasion: Developments in theory and practice* (2nd ed.). SAGE. https://doi.org/10.4135/9781452218410

Falco, C. M., & Rosenberg, B. D. (2025). Minimizing reactance to increase help-seeking for depression. In M. C. Yzer & J. T. Siegel (Eds.), *Handbook of mental health communication*. Wiley.

Falco, C. M., & Siegel, J. T. (2024). *Increasing help-seeking for depression: An empirical assessment of a static and trending norms approach* [Manuscript in preparation]. Department of Behavioral and Organizational Sciences, Claremont Graduate University.

Fox, A. B., Qiu, X., Mousavi, M. E., & Earnshaw, V. A. (2025). Advancing the measurement of mental illness stigma: Considerations of time, structural stigma, and intersectionality. In M. C. Yzer & J. T. Siegel (Eds.), *Handbook of mental health communication*. Wiley.

Fredrickson, B. L. (2001). The role of positive emotions in positive psychology: The broaden-and-build theory of positive emotions. *American Psychologist, 56*(3), 218–226. https://doi.org/10.1037/0003-066X.56.3.218

Gorn, G. J., Goldberg, M. E., & Basu, K. (1993). Mood, awareness, and product evaluation. *Journal of Consumer Psychology, 2*(3), 237–256. https://doi.org/10.1016/S1057-7408(08)80016-2

Gotlib, I. H., & Joormann, J. (2010). Cognition and depression: Current status and future directions. *Annual Review of Clinical Psychology, 6*, 285–312. https://doi.org/10.1146/annurev.clinpsy.121208.131305

Graham, L. E., Thomson, A. L., Nakamura, J., Brandt, I. A., & Siegel, J. T. (2019). Finding a family: A categorization of enjoyable emotions. *Journal of Positive Psychology, 19*(2), 206–229. https://doi.org/10.1080/17439760.2017.1402074

Green, M. C., & Brock, T. C. (2000). The role of transportation in the persuasiveness of public narratives. *Journal of Personality and Social Psychology, 79*(5), 701–721. https://doi.org/10.1037/0022-3514.79.5.701

Griffith, F. J., & Simmons, S. C. (2025). Affinity and advocacy: Online communities for people experiencing mental illness. In M. C. Yzer & J. T. Siegel (Eds.), *Handbook of mental health communication*. Wiley.

Haidt, J. (2000). The positive emotion of elevation. *Prevention & Treatment, 3*(1), Article 3c. https://doi.org/10.1037/1522-3736.3.1.33c

Hammar, A., Lund, A., & Hugdahl, K. (2003). Selective impairment in effortful information processing in major depression. *Journal of the International Neuropsychological Society, 9*(6), 954–959. https://doi.org/10.1017/S1355617703960152

Hammer, J. H., & Vogel, D. L. (2010). Men's help seeking for depression: The efficacy of a male-sensitive brochure about counseling. *Counseling Psychologist, 38*(2), 296–313. https://doi.org/10.1177/0011000009351937

Hernandez, M. Y., & Organista, K. C. (2013). Entertainment–education? A fotonovela? A new strategy to improve depression literacy and help-seeking behaviors in at-risk immigrant Latinas. *American Journal of Community Psychology, 52*, 224–235. https://doi.org/10.1007/s10464-013-9587-1

Hollar, S. M., & Siegel, J. T. (2020). Self-distancing as a path to help-seeking for people with depression. *Social Science & Medicine, 245*, Article 112700. https://doi.org/10.1016/j.socscimed.2019.112700

Horner, M. S., Siegle, G. J., Schwartz, R. M., Price, R. B., Haggerty, A. E., Collier, A., & Friedman, E. S. (2014). C'mon get happy: Reduced magnitude and duration of response during a positive-affect induction in depression. *Depression and Anxiety, 31*(11), 952–960. https://doi.org/10.1002/da.22244

Hovland, C. I., Janis, I. L., & Kelley, H. H. (1953). *Communication and persuasion*. Yale University Press.

Huntley, C. D., & Fisher, P. L. (2016). Examining the role of positive and negative metacognitive beliefs in depression. *Scandinavian Journal of Psychology, 57*(5), 446–452. https://doi.org/10.1111/sjop.12306

Hussain, S. A., & Alhabash, S. (2022). Effect of nostalgia as a motivational force for depressed students to seek professional psychological help. *Journal of American College Health, 70*(2), 484–492. https://doi.org/10.1080/07448481.2020.1754838

Isen, A. M. (1990). The influence of positive and negative affect on cognitive organization: Some implications for development. In N. Stein, B. Leventhal, & T. Trabasso (Eds.), *Psychological and biological approaches to emotion* (pp. 75–94). Lawrence Erlbaum Associates.

Jabeen, F., de Brujin, G., & Bosse, T. (2025). Chatbots for mental health: A network-oriented modeling perspective. In M. C. Yzer & J. T. Siegel (Eds.), *Handbook of mental health communication*. Wiley.

Johnston, A., Supriya, M., Banawa, R., Anagnost, J., & Eisenberg, D. (2025). Reducing mental health stigma through school-based interventions: Assessing the evidence and translating it into practice. In M. C. Yzer & J. T. Siegel (Eds.), *Handbook of mental health communication*. Wiley.

Jorm, A. F. (2025). Refining the concept of mental health literacy: Criteria for determining what the public needs to know. In M. C. Yzer & J. T. Siegel (Eds.), *Handbook of mental health communication*. Wiley.

Jorm, A. F., Griffiths, K. M., Christensen, H., Korten, A. E., Parslow, R. A., & Rogers, B. (2003). Providing information about the effectiveness of treatment options to depressed people in the community: A randomized controlled trial of effects on mental health literacy, help-seeking and symptoms. *Psychological Medicine, 33*(6), 1071–1079. https://doi.org/10.1017/S0033291703008079

Keeler, A. R., & Siegel, J. T. (2016). Depression, help-seeking perceptions, and perceived family functioning among Spanish-dominant Hispanics and non-Hispanic whites. *Journal of Affective Disorders, 202*, 236–246. https://doi.org/10.1016/j.jad.2016.05.017

Klimes-Dougan, B., & Lee, C. Y. (2010). Suicide prevention public service announcements: Perceptions of young adults. *Crisis, 31*(5), 247–254. https://doi.org/10.1027/0227-5910/a000032

Lau, N., Kola, L., Zhao, X., Asafo, S., Attah, D., & Ben-Zeev, D. (2025). mHealth for mental health: Expanding the reach of care. In M. C. Yzer & J. T. Siegel (Eds.), *Handbook of mental health communication*. Wiley.

Lienemann, B. A., & Siegel, J. T. (2016). Reactance to depression public service announcements among people with depression. *Health Communication, 31*(1), 102–116. https://doi.org/10.1080/10410236.2014.940668

Lienemann, B. A., & Siegel, J. T. (2018). Increasing help-seeking outcomes among people with elevated depressive symptomatology with public service announcements: An examination of function matching and message sidedness. *Journal of Health Communication, 23*(1), 28–39. https://doi.org/10.1080/10810730.2017.1396630

Lienemann, B. A., Siegel, J. T., & Crano, W. D. (2013). Persuading people with depression to seek help: Respect the boomerang. *Health Communication*, *28*(7), 718–728. https://doi.org/10.1080/10410236.2012.712091
Liu, X., & Siegel, J. T. (2023). Elevation and heroism. In S. T. Allison, J. K. Beggan, & G. R. Goethals (Eds.), *Encyclopedia of heroism studies* (pp. 1–7). Springer.
Lueck, J., & Yzer, M. C. (2018). Explaining intentions to seek help for depressive symptoms in the context of responsibility message framing. *Health Communication*, *33*(8), 946–953. https://doi.org/10.1080/10410236.2017.1322857
Lueck, J. A. (2018). Examining determinants of seeking help for depression: Implications for effective health promotion messages. *Journal of Communication in Healthcare*, *11*(1), 19–29. https://doi.org/10.1080/17538068.2017/1417957
Marciano, L., Kikut-Stein, A., & Viswanath, K. (2025). Communication, equity, and mental well-being: The road ahead. In M. C. Yzer & J. T. Siegel (Eds.), *Handbook of mental health communication*. Wiley.
Mavandadi, S., Wright, E., Klaus, J., & Oslin, D. (2018). Message framing and engagement in specialty mental health care. *Psychiatric Services*, *69*(3), 308–314. https://doi.org/10.1176/appi.ps.201700251
McCroskey, J. C., & Teven, J. J. (1999). Goodwill: A reexamination of the construct and its measurement. *Communication Monographs*, *66*(1), 90–103. https://doi.org/10.1080/03637759909376464
Menezes, S., & Guldner, G. (2025). Well-being among physicians in training: Barriers to treatment and efforts to increase help-seeking for depression. In M. C. Yzer & J. T. Siegel (Eds.), *Handbook of mental health communication*. Wiley.
Muschetto, T., & Siegel, J. T. (2020). Use of attribution vignettes and public service announcements to influence perceived stability of depression: The impact on affect, outcome expectancy, and helping judgments. *Stigma and Health*, *5*(1), 69–78. https://doi.org/10.1037/sah0000174
Muschetto, T., & Siegel, J. T. (2025). *Reactions to others with depression: An investigation of responsibility and deservingness judgments* [Manuscript under review]. Claremont Graduate University.
Muschetto, T., & Siegel, J. T. (2025). Application of Weiner's attribution-emotion-action model to increase support for people with depression. In M. C. Yzer & J. T. Siegel (Eds.), *Handbook of mental health communication*. Wiley.
Noar, S. M., Ma, H., & Rohde, J. A. (2025). Pretesting and selecting messages using perceived message effectiveness (PME) ratings. In M. C. Yzer & J. T. Siegel (Eds.), *Handbook of mental health communication*. Wiley.
O'Keefe, D. J. (2015). *Persuasion: Theory and research* (3rd ed.). Sage.
Palmgreen, P., Donohew, L., Lorch, E. P., Rogus, M., Helm, D., & Grant, N. (1991). Sensation seeking, message sensation value, and drug use as mediators of PSA effectiveness. *Health Communication*, *3*(4), 217–227. https://doi.org/10.1207/s15327027hc0304_4
Pancer, E., Poole, M., Chandler, V., & Noseworthy, T. J. (2019). How readability shapes social media engagement. *Journal of Consumer Psychology*, *29*(2), 262–270. https://doi.org/10.1002/jcpy.1073
Peinado, S., & Nabi, R. L. (2024). Emotional shifts in health messages as a strategy for generating talk and behavior change. *Health Communication*. Advance online publication. https://doi.org/10.1080/10410236.2024.2305552
Petty, R. E., & Cacioppo, J. T. (1986). The elaboration likelihood model of persuasion. *Advances in Experimental Social Psychology*, *19*, 123–205. https://doi.org/10.1016/S0065-2601(08)60214-2
Pornpitakpan, C. (2004). The persuasiveness of source credibility: A critical review of five decades' evidence. *Journal of Applied Social Psychology*, *34*(2), 243–281. https://doi.org/10.1111/j.1559-1816.2004.tb02547.x
Pyone, J. S., & Isen, A. M. (2011). Positive affect, intertemporal choice, and levels of thinking: Increasing consumers' willingness to wait. *Journal of Marketing Research*, *48*(3), 532–543. https://doi.org/10.1509/jmkr.48.3.532
Quick, B., Caban, S., Chung, M., & Yan, J. (2025). Introducing health communication science to mental health researchers: An examination of information seeking, processing, and dissemination frameworks. In M. C. Yzer & J. T. Siegel (Eds.), *Handbook of mental health communication*. Wiley.
Riera-Serra, P., Navarra-Ventura, G., Castro, A., Gili, M., Salazar-Cedillo, A., Ricci-Cabello, I., Roldán-Espínola, L., Coronado-Simsic, V., García-Toro, M., Gómez-Juanes, R., & Roca, M. (2023). Clinical predictors of suicidal ideation, suicide attempts and suicide death in depressive disorder: A systematic review and meta-analysis. *European Archives of Psychiatry and Clinical Neuroscience*, Advance online publication. https://doi.org/10.1007/s00406-023-01716-5
Roy, S., & Siegel, J. T. (2025). *A new form of positive emotion infusion: Using affective forecasting errors for good among individuals experiencing depression* [Manuscript under review].
Ruybal, A., & Siegel, J. T. (2021). Increasing social support for women with postpartum depression through attribution theory guided vignettes and video messages: The understudied role of effort. *Journal of Experimental Social Psychology*, *97*. https://doi.org/10.1016/j.jesp.2021.104197
RW, R., Xingman, W., Kim, R. S., & Nan, X. (2025). A typology of health communication variables relevant for mental health. In M. C. Yzer & J. T. Siegel (Eds.), *Handbook of mental health communication*. Wiley.
Schroder, H. S., Devendorf, A., & Zikmund-Fisher, B. J. (2023). Framing depression as a functional signal, not a disease: Rationale and initial randomized controlled trial. *Social Science & Medicine*, *328*, Article 115995.
Shi, J., & Dai, Y. (2022). Promoting favorable attitudes toward seeking counseling among people with depressive symptomatology: A masspersonal communication approach. *Health Communication*, *37*(2), 242–254. https://doi.org/10.1080/10410236.2020.1834209
Siegel, J. T. (2021, June 1). Reducing stigma and increasing help-seeking for your people struggling with depression [Webinar]. *Claremont Graduate University Public Sector Leadership Webinar Series*. https://www.youtube.com/watch?v=i-bUjZLdzTo

Siegel, J. T., Alvaro, E. A., Crano, W. D., Gonzalez, A., Tang, J., & Jones, S. P. (2010b). Passive-positive organ donor registration behavior: A mixed method assessment of the IIFF model. *Psychology, Health and Medicine, 15*(2), 198–209. https://doi.org/10.1080/13548501003623922

Siegel, J. T., Alvaro, E. A., & Hohman, Z. (2010a). A dawning recognition of factors for increasing donor registration: The IIFF model. In J. T. Siegel & E. A. Alvaro (Eds.), *Understanding organ donation: Applied behavioral science approaches* (pp. 313–330). Blackwell-Wiley.

Siegel, J. T., Alvaro, E. M., Tan, C. N., Navarro, M. A., Garner, L. R., & Jones, S. P. (2016a). The potential (f)utility of a passive organ donor registration opportunity: A conceptual replication. *Progress in Transplantation, 26*(2), 103–108. https://doi.org/10.1177/1526924816641814

Siegel, J. T., & Burgoon, J. K. (2002). Expectancy theory approaches to prevention: Violating adolescent expectations to increase the effectiveness of public service announcements. In W. D. Crano & M. Burgoon (Eds.), *Mass media and drug prevention: Classic and contemporary theories and research* (pp. 163–186). Lawrence Erlbaum Associates, Inc.

Siegel, J. T., Ellis, B., Riazi, G., Brafford, A., Guldner, G., & Wells, J. C. (2024). The paradox of the resident experiencing depression: Higher depression, less favorable help-seeking outcome expectations, and lower help-seeking intentions. *Social Science & Medicine, 344*, Article 116593. https://doi.org/10.1016/j.socscimed.2024.116593

Siegel, J. T., Flores-Mendal, E., Martinez, D., & Berger, D. E. (2019). Can mental health anti-stigma messages have untoward effects on some people with depression? An exploratory study. *Journal of Health Communication, 24*(11), 821–828. https://doi.org/10.1080/10810730.2019.1672838

Siegel, J. T., Lienemann, B. A., & Rosenberg, B. D. (2017). Resistance, reactance, and misinterpretation: Highlighting the challenge of persuading people with depression to seek help. *Social and Personality Psychology Compass, 11*(6), Article e12322. https://doi.org/10.1111/spc3.12322

Siegel, J. T., Lienemann, B. A., & Tan, C. (2015). The overheard communication technique: Influencing people with depression to seek help. *Clinical Psychological Science, 3*(2), 242–255. https://doi.org/10.1177/2167702614542846

Siegel, J. T. & Marshburn, A. (2025). *Increasing help-seeking and social support for people with depression: A dual dependent variable approach* [Manuscript submitted for publication]. Department of Behavioral and Organizational Sciences, Claremont Graduate University.

Siegel, J. T. & Straszewski, T. (2019, May). *The influence of elevation on help-seeking intentions and PSA effectiveness* [Panel presentation]. Association for Psychological Science 2019 Annual Conference, Washington, DC.

Siegel, J. T., & Tan, C. N. (2025). Investigating help-seeking attitudes among people with varying levels of depressive symptomatology: An attitude-strength diagnostic approach. In M. C. Yzer & J. T. Siegel (Eds.), *Handbook of mental health communication*. Wiley.

Siegel, J. T., Tan, C. N., Rosenberg, B. D., Navarro, M. A., Thomson, A. L., Lyrintzis, E. A., Alvaro, E. M., & Jones, N. D. (2016b). Anger, frustration, boredom and the Department of Motor Vehicles: Can negative emotions impede organ donor registration? *Social Science & Medicine, 153*, 174–181. https://doi.org/10.1016/j.socscimed.2016.02.013

Siegel, J. T., & Thomson, A. L. (2017). Positive emotion infusions of elevation and gratitude: Increasing help-seeking intentions among people with heightened levels of depressive symptomatology. *Journal of Positive Psychology, 12*(6), 509–524. https://doi.org/10.1080/17439760.2016.1221125

Siegel, J. T., Thomson, A. L., & Navarro, M. A. (2014). Experimentally distinguishing elevation from gratitude: Oh, the morality. *Journal of Positive Psychology, 9*(5), 414–427. https://doi.org/10.1080/17439760.2014.910825

Southwell, B. G., Barmada, C. H., Hornik, R. C., & Maklan, D. M. (2002). Can we measure encoded exposure? Validation evidence from a national campaign. *Journal of Health Communication, 7*(5), 445–453. https://doi.org/10.1080/10810730290001800

Straszewski, T., & Siegel, J. T. (2018). Positive emotion infusions: Can savoring increase help-seeking intentions among people with depression? *Applied Psychology: Health and Well-Being, 10*(1), 171–190. https://doi.org/10.1111/aphw.12122

Straszewski, T., & Siegel, J. T. (2020). Differential effects of high- and low-arousal positive emotions on help-seeking for depression. *Applied Psychology. Health and Well-Being, 12*(3), 887–906. https://doi.org/10.1111/aphw.12214

Straszewski, T., & Siegel, J. T. (2021). From writing tasks to a public service announcement: Experimentally assessing savoring as a means of increasing help-seeking for depression. *Social Science and Medicine, 287*(3), 114362. https://doi.org/10.1016/j.socscimed.2021.114362

Straszewski, T., & Siegel, J. T. (2025). Positive emotion infusions as a means of increasing help-seeking among people experiencing depression: Savoring, elevation, and gratitude. In M. C. Yzer & J. T. Siegel (Eds.), *Handbook of mental health communication*. Wiley.

Substance Abuse and Mental Health Service Administration. (2023). *Key substance use and mental health indicators in the United States: Results from the 2022 national survey on drug use and health*. Center for Behavioral Health Statistics and Quality, Substance Abuse and Mental Health Services Administration. https://www.samhsa.gov/data/sites/default/files/reports/rpt42731/2022-nsduh-nnr.pdf

Suka, M., Yamauchi, T., & Yanagisawa, H. (2019). Responses to persuasive messages encouraging professional help seeking for depression: Comparison between individuals with and without psychological distress. *Environmental Health and Preventive Medicine, 24*, Article 29. https://doi.org/10.1186/s12199-019-0786-8

Suka, M., Yamauchi, T., & Yanagisawa, H. (2020). Persuasive messages can be more effective when repeated: A comparative survey assessing a message to seek help for depression among Japanese adults. *Patient Education and Counseling*, *103*(4), 811–818. https://doi.org/10.1016/j.pec.2019.11.008

Tan, C. N., & Siegel, J. T. (2025). *Strengthening positive, and weakening negative, help-seeking attitudes among people with depressive symptomatology: Applying results from an attitude-strength diagnostic* [Manuscript in preparation]. Department of Behavioral and Organizational Sciences, Claremont Graduate University.

Thomson, A. L., Nakamura, J., Siegel, J. T., & Csikszentmihalyi, M. (2014). Elevation and mentoring: An experimental assessment of causal relations. *Journal of Positive Psychology*, *9*(5), 402–413. https://doi.org/10.1080/17439760.2014.910824

Thomson, A. L., & Siegel, J. T. (2017). Elevation: A review of scholarship on a moral and other-praising emotion. *Journal of Positive Psychology*, *12*(6), 628–638. https://doi.org/10.1080/17439760.2016.1269184

Trusty, W. T., & Swift, J. K. (2023). Effort and effort discounting as predictors of seeking psychotherapy among individuals with depression. *Journal of Clinical Psychology*, *79*(11), 2635–2649. https://doi.org/10.1002/jclp.23573

Twiss, M., Turchmanovych, N., & Corrigan, P. (2025). The benefits and unintended consequences of anti-stigma campaigns. In M. C. Yzer & J. T. Siegel (Eds.), *Handbook of mental health communication*. Wiley.

Vogel, D. L., Heath, P. J., Brenner, R. E., Lannin, D. G., & Zhao, N. (2025). The conceptualization, measurement, and reduction of self-stigma of seeking help. In M. C. Yzer & J. T. Siegel (Eds.), *Handbook of mental health communication*. Wiley.

Vos, L. M. W., Smeets, T., & Everaert, J. (2025). Emotional information-processing biases in psychopathology. In M. C. Yzer & J. T. Siegel (Eds.), *Handbook of mental health communication*. Wiley.

Wakefield, M. A., Loken, B., & Hornik, R. (2010). Use of mass media campaigns to change health behavior. *Lancet*, *376*(9748), 1261–1271. https://doi.org/10.1016/S0140-6736(10)60809-4

Walster, E., & Festinger, L. (1962). The effectiveness of "overheard" persuasive communications. *Journal of Abnormal and Social Psychology*, *65*(6), 395–402. https://doi.org/10.1037/h0041172

Weiner, B. (1980). A cognitive (attribution)–emotion–action model of motivated behavior: An analysis of judgments of help-giving. *Journal of Personality and Social Psychology*, *39*(2), 186–200. https://doi.org/10.1037/0022-3514.39.2.186

Wisco, B. E. (2009). Depressive cognition: Self-reference and depth of processing. *Clinical Psychology Review*, *29*(4), 382–392. https://doi.org/10.1016/j.cpr.2009.03.003

Woodman, K., & Weber, R. (2025). Cracking the code of gaming disorder: Effective communication for parents, children, and policy makers. In M. C. Yzer & J. T. Siegel (Eds.), *Handbook of mental health communication*. Wiley.

World Health Organization. (2023, March 31). *Depressive disorder (depression)*. https://www.who.int/news-room/fact-sheets/detail/depression

Yang, B., Li, Y., Terán, L., Choi, E., & Choi, Y. (2023). COVID-19 vaccines #ForYou: Analyzing COVID-19 vaccine videos on TikTok during the early phase of the vaccine rollout in the U.S. *Health Communication*, *39*(8), 1594–1605. https://doi.org/10.1080/10410236.2023.2227431

Yao, E., & Siegel, J. T. (2021). Examining the role of interpersonal relationship on attribution, emotion, and depression support provision: Experimental evidence from the People's Republic of China. *Motivation Science*, *7*(1), 46–55. https://doi.org/10.1037/mot0000180

Yao, E., & Siegel, J. T. (2024). Weiner's attribution-emotion-action model: Uncovering the mediating role of self-blame and the moderating effect of the Helper's responsibility for the help Recipient's behavior. *Personality and Social Psychology Bulletin*. Advance online publication https://doi.org/10.1177/0146167224123813

Ying, F., Murphy, G. C. M., & Dozois, D. J. A. (2025). The impact of self- and partner-schemas on information processing and treatment-seeking in depression. In M. C. Yzer & J. T. Siegel (Eds.), *Handbook of mental health communication*. Wiley.

Yost, J. H., & Weary, G. (1996). Depression and the correspondent inference bias: Evidence for more effortful cognitive processing. *Personality and Social Psychology Bulletin*, *22*(2), 192–200. https://doi.org/10.1177/0146167296222008

Yzer, M. C., Kinzer, H., & Malone, M. (2022). A reasoned action approach to depression help-seeking messaging for college students: Implications of cognitive biases in 52 depression. *Health Communication*, *37*(14), 1731–1739. https://doi.org/10.1080/10410236.2021.1917744

Yzer, M. C., & Siegel, J. T. (2025a). *Handbook of mental health communication*. Wiley.

Yzer, M. C., & Siegel, J. T. (2025b). Cognitive biases in depression: Implications for help-seeking messaging. In G. J. de Bruijn & H. Vandebosch (Eds.), *Handbook Health, media, and communication* (pp. 391–410). De Gruyter Mouton. https://doi.org/10.1515/9783110775426-021

Yzer, M. C., & Siegel, J. T. (2025c). Mental health communication: Using messages to relieve the plight of people with mental illness. In M. C. Yzer & J. T. Siegel (Eds.), *Handbook of mental health communication*. Wiley.

Yzer, M. C., & Zhu, X. (2025). A research protocol for determining depression help-seeking message content. In M. C. Yzer & J. T. Siegel (Eds.), *Handbook of mental health communication*. Wiley.

Zhu, X., Smith, R. A., & Osoro, R. A. (2025). Stigmatizing communication and mental health. In M. C. Yzer & J. T. Siegel (Eds.), *Handbook of mental health communication*. Wiley.

Index

The Handbook of Mental Health Communication, First Edition.
Edited by Marco C. Yzer and Jason T. Siegel.

Printed and bound by CPI Group (UK) Ltd, Croydon, CR0 4YY
17/09/2026
14964250-0004